HUMAN NUTRITION

A health perspective

SECOND EDITION

Mary E. Barasi

BA, BSc, MSc, R. Nutr.
Principal Lecturer in Nutrition,
University of Wales Institute, Cardiff, UK

Illustrations by Megan Morris

Hodder Arnold

A MEMBER OF THE HODDER HEADLINE GROUP

LONDON

First published in Great Britain in 2003 by
Hodder Arnold, a member of the Hodder Headline Group,
338 Euston Road, London NW1 3BH

http://www.hoddereducation.com

Distributed in the United States of America by
Oxford University Press Inc.,
198 Madison Avenue, New York, NY10016
Oxford is a registered trademark of Oxford University Press

Whilst the advice and information in this book are believed to be true and
accurate at the date of going to press, neither the author nor the publisher
can accept any legal responsibility or liability for any errors or omissions
that may be made. In particular (but without limiting the generality of the
preceding disclaimer) every effort has been made to check drug dosages;
however, it is still possible that errors have been missed. Furthermore,
dosage schedules are constantly being revised and new side-effects
recognized. For these reasons the reader is strongly urged to consult the
drug companies' printed instructions before administering any of the drugs
recommended in this book.

British Library Cataloguing in Publication Data
A catalogue record for this book is available from the British Library

Library of Congress Cataloging-in-Publication Data
A catalog record for this book is available from the Library of Congress

ISBN-10: 0 340 81025 4
ISBN-13: 978 0 340 81025 5

5 6 7 8 9 10

Commissioning Editor: Georgina Bentliff
Development Editor: Heather Smith
Project Editor: Wendy Rooke
Production Controller: Lindsay Smith
Cover Design: Amina Dudhia

Hodder Headline's policy is to use papers that are natural, renewable and
recyclable products and made from wood grown in sustainable forests.
The logging and manufacturing processes are expected to conform to the
environmental regulations of the country of origin.

Typeset in RotisSerif 9.5/12 by Charon Tec Ltd (A Macmillan Company), Chennai, India
Printed and bound in Spain.

What do you think about this book? Or any other Hodder Arnold title?
Please send your comments to www.hoddereducation.com

CONTENTS

The need for a second edition of this book stems from the continuing rapid changes occurring in our understanding of nutrition. A number of these developments can be identified here. Advances have taken place in the way that information is collected and reviewed and the concept of an evidence base informing practice has become established. Research findings from many studies can be subjected to reviews, using an approach that should be both systematic and clear in its methodology. In this way, it is increasingly possible to provide some answers to important questions, on the basis of a body of research evidence that has been thoroughly analysed and combined with data from similar studies to produce quantitative outcomes. This approach of systematic review strengthens the conclusions that are made, and provides a sound basis for policy or practice to be developed. The Cochrane Database contains information relating to clinical systematic reviews and is a prime example of the application of this methodology. In the future, all practice should be evidence based, and patients and consumers should expect this.

A technological advance that has sometimes worked counter to the concept of an evidence base has been the widespread use of the Internet, with the proliferation of web-based resources. These can provide almost instant access to good quality information through online databases and access to scientific publications and reputable web sites, often with extensive links to related information. However, there is also the opportunity for much unscientific and uncontrolled information to be presented, and this may be confusing, inaccurate, misleading and potentially dangerous. For users of such information, there is a real need to have some basic nutrition knowledge to enable them to discern truth from fiction.

One of the most exciting developments at the beginning of the new millennium has been the human genome project, with mapping of human DNA. This reflects the enormous advances that have occurred in molecular biology in recent years. These are already having their impact in nutrition, with research outcomes identifying genetic variants that explain some of the recognized differences in the way individuals respond to nutrients or exhibit increased susceptibility to nutritional disorders. There is a great deal to be discovered in this field. At some point in the future, we will understand much more about the way that genes and nutrients interact.

The moves towards healthy eating in the last two decades of the twentieth century led to recognition that food and nutrition can have positive health benefits. From this has developed a concept of optimal nutrition, wherein food or nutrients can be actively used to promote health, in ways that are additional to their nutritional role. This has generated new developments within the food industry to produce functional or smart foods that aim to address these demands. At present, there is a lack of sound evidence about the mechanisms of action or the benefits in humans for some of these components. Consequently, the amounts required to be consumed for optimal benefit are also unknown, and more research in this area is needed.

The importance of nutrition as part of public health is now recognized at Government level. The Food Standards Agency (FSA) has been established since 2001 to take the lead in the UK. The Nutrition Strategy Framework* identifies a number of objectives to improve both knowledge and practical aspects of nutrition throughout society. In order to achieve these, practical guidance on nutritional issues will be needed at various levels in society and will require informed educators. Traditionally, health professionals have been responsible for health-related issues, including nutrition. Those with the greatest responsibility are dietitians and nutritionists, yet doctors and nurses may be the people who are most readily accessible to the general population. It has been recognized that all health professionals need nutritional knowledge at some

---

*Food Standards Agency 2000: *Your food – farm to fork.* London: FSA.

level. This, in turn, needs to be disseminated to others working within communities who can help to further disseminate the messages about dietary improvements.

This new edition of the book retains the structure of the first edition, but has been substantially updated and extended. A new chapter has been added to include optimal nutrition and smart or functional foods.

The book takes a practical approach, involving the reader in thinking about their own nutrition, in order to understand better why people eat as they do, and the difficulties that others may have in changing their food intake. There are activities and study questions within each chapter that are intended to stimulate further thought and practise problem-solving. References for further reading are provided at the end of each chapter for those who wish to pursue further study.

Sections in the book include an introduction to the study of nutrition and the foundations of healthy eating. This is followed by a section on the macronutrients and micronutrients, and includes a consideration of energy balance and

a new section on the need for fluids. The final section of the book considers more applied aspects of nutrition during the normal stages of the life cycle, in situations that challenge nutritional status as well as the relationship between nutrition and major diseases. Optimal nutrition, and nutrition policy and health promotion are considered in this section.

The author is grateful to all those who have helped in the development of the book, including colleagues and students who offer endless challenges with interesting and stimulating questions. I would also like to thank Megan Morris for her imaginative contribution in the illustrations throughout the text. The production of the book has been efficiently managed by Georgina Bentliff and Heather Smith from the publishers.

Thank you also to my family for their support throughout the work on this edition.

Mary Barasi
Cardiff
2003

LIST OF TABLES

LIST OF FIGURES

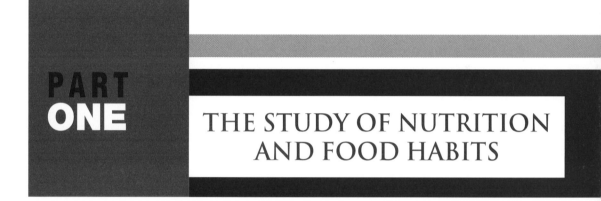

PART ONE

THE STUDY OF NUTRITION AND FOOD HABITS

The aims of this chapter are to:

❏ define nutrition as a discipline for study and reflect on its importance;
❏ look at ways in which dietary information is collected;
❏ encourage the reader to think about their own food intake, their own and others' perceptions of nutrition;
❏ consider why nutrition is important and how it is included in nutrition policies.

On completing the study of this chapter, you should be able to:

❏ think about nutrition and food in relation to yourself;
❏ understand what is meant by nutrition, and why it is an important science, involving many different disciplines;
❏ explain and discuss the various ways in which nutrition is studied, together with their advantages and disadvantages;
❏ understand and evaluate the information about nutrition that is disseminated in the scientific as well as the non-specialist literature;
❏ explain how nutritional status can be assessed;
❏ understand the basis on which nutrition policy may be made at government level.

DEFINITIONS OF NUTRITION

Everybody has their own experience of food and eating, so it is likely that people will have different ideas about what is meant by nutrition. Some may see eating as a means of meeting our basic physiological needs and warding off hunger, and others as a pleasurable experience in its own right and something to anticipate and plan. These represent the two extremes implied by the sayings 'eat to live' and 'live to eat'.

In reality, eating is far more complicated than this, involving aspects of our psychological make-up and current state of mind, our genetic blueprint, the social environment of which we are a part, our economic situation and external factors relating to the availability of the food. These will be explored in more detail in Chapter 2. Eating also does more than just keep us alive. When insufficient food or specific nutrients are supplied, some physiological adaptation may

occur to minimize the consequences. Eventually, however, a deficiency state will arise.

At the beginning of the twentieth century, most of the science of nutrition was directed at discovering the essential nutrients, studying the effects of insufficient intakes and determining the quantities needed to prevent deficiency states. Since then it has gradually been recognized that good nutrition is not simply a matter of providing enough of all the nutrients. We now realize that diets in the affluent Western countries, although apparently containing all the necessary nutrients, are probably contributing to many of the diseases afflicting these populations. Much research has been focused on finding which nutrients are linked to which diseases, in an effort to promote a change in the dietary intake and hence an improvement in health. Since the 1970s a great deal of advice has been aimed at encouraging people to eat a healthier balance of foods, thereby reducing disease. The emphasis in the twenty-first century has started to move towards promoting positive health through diet, know as optimum nutrition. However, nutritionists recognize that altering people's food intake is complicated because diets are influenced by many factors other than the need to eat and the desire for well-being.

It can be seen that arriving at a definition of nutrition is far from straightforward. Two rather different definitions have been suggested, describing nutrition as:

> 'the study of foods and nutrients vital to health and how the body uses these to promote and support growth, maintenance and reproduction of cells' or

> 'the study of the relationship between people and their food'.

The first definition deals only with the nutrients, what happens to them within the human body and what the results are if insufficient amounts are provided. However, people do not eat nutrients, they eat food. This definition ignores all the external factors that play a role in our approach to food and that are crucial in any study of what people are eating. These factors are different for each individual, depending on cultural background and the circumstances of a person's life.

The second definition takes a much broader perspective, from the supply of food and all the influences thereon, to the individual's food selection and, finally, to the physiological and biochemical effects of the nutrients in the human body, and the consequences for health and survival. It also recognizes that nutritionists do not only study the effects of nutrients on biochemical and physiological functioning, they have an additional responsibility to translate their knowledge for those who produce, process and market the foods. Furthermore, nutritionists must be involved in the formulation of policy that determines the access by consumers to food. Finally, consumers need the help of nutritionists to enable them to make the best of the food available. Only by broadening our definition of the subject across the full range of human relationships with food can nutrition have its justified place in human well-being.

WHY IS NUTRITION IMPORTANT?

To answer this question, it is perhaps useful to consider the various levels at which nutrition can be studied. Table 1.1 illustrates some examples of the application of nutritional science in other fields of study. In each case, nutrition plays a specific role, and the emphasis required may differ from its application in all other roles. Thus, nutrition is a science with many different applications and meanings to different specialists. Nevertheless, each of these specialists, working in their own particular field of expertise, needs to have knowledge of nutrition in order to apply the findings of their work to the nutritional context.

There has been an upsurge of general interest in nutrition in the last 20–30 years; this has not just been among the scientific community, but also among the general population. Why has this happened?

First, it is notable that dietary intakes have been and are changing rapidly. In the Western world, we have an ever-increasing selection of foods available to us. People can now eat every day the foods our ancestors had only on special occasions. New foods are appearing that have been conceived and developed by food

Activity 1.1

Why are you studying nutrition?

At what level will you be applying your nutritional knowledge?

At what level might the following be using nutrition:

nurse	pharmacist
dietitian	journalist
obstetrician	parent?
home economist	

Try to think of some other examples of people working with nutrition, at each of the different levels in Table 1.1.

TABLE 1.1 Different levels of studying nutrition

Level of study	Examples of application
Macro/population studies	Government statistics (for formulation of policy, e.g. about agriculture, or health)
	Epidemiology (to study relationship between diet and disease)
	Food producers (to respond to changes in consumer demand and to lead demand)
Individual/whole person studies	Sociology (to study patterns of behaviour related to food)
	Food science/technology (to identify changes in individual preferences for food; sensory qualities)
	Sports science (to identify links between diet and performance)
	Medicine (to study influences of diet on the health of the individual and recovery from illness)
Micro/laboratory studies	Physiology (to understand the role of nutrients in functioning of body systems)
	Biochemistry (to investigate the biochemical role of nutrients in normal and abnormal functioning)
	Molecular biology (to study gene–nutrient interactions)

technologists; sometimes these contain unusual ingredients, which provide nutrients in unexpected amounts (this can be a problem for the nutritionist in giving advice). New processing techniques, such as irradiation, may affect the nutrients in food. New products, specially designed to promote health are now available; these are discussed in Chapter 17.

In modern society, meal patterns have become less rigid and many people no longer eat meals at regular mealtimes. The members of a family may each have an independent meal at different times of the day and the traditional family meal is a rare event.

Concerns about food safety and environmental issues have resulted in changes in dietary habits, the most notable amongst these being the rise in vegetarianism in the UK and the growth of demand for organically grown food. Nevertheless, the great majority of food bought comes from large retail supermarkets that exert a great deal of influence over customer choice.

Health issues have been given a great deal of prominence in the media. Statistics show that populations in Western countries have excess mortality (i.e. death rates) and morbidity (i.e. rates of illness) from many diseases related to diet, such as cardiovascular disorders, bowel diseases and cancers, as well as a high prevalence of obesity and diabetes. At the same time, we are often shocked by images of starvation in other parts of the world where conflict, drought and other disasters have resulted in millions of people suffering acute malnutrition and starvation.

As greater numbers of nutritionists are trained and the discipline becomes more widely studied, knowledge accumulates based on sound evidence. Public health nutrition is now a discipline in its own right, with a specific remit of promoting health through good nutrition. However, as with all scientific research, more questions follow every finding. Consensus is being reached on some of the ways in which diet is involved in Western diseases, and advice can now be based on much firmer evidence. However, new research may cause current advice to be modified. New angles on nutrition research, particularly from the field of molecular biology, are explaining observations made earlier at the whole-body level. Improved methodologies allow more sensitive and appropriate measurements to be made. For example, in the study of energy balance, the use of radioactively labelled water has provided a means of measuring energy expenditure in subjects during their normal lives. This has provided a wealth of information about this important area of nutrition.

The media are very sensitive to public concern, so that news about nutritional findings receives a great deal of publicity. Unfortunately, the style of reporting may distort the scientific detail, so that what is eventually presented by the media may not accurately represent the findings. Moreover, excessive prominence may be given to very minor and insignificant findings, especially if they appear to contradict earlier results. Consequently, rather than being better informed, the public may become confused. It is essential, therefore, that those trained in nutrition have a clear understanding of nutritional issues, and are able to disentangle some of the inaccuracies presented by the media.

WHAT DO PEOPLE EAT?

Different peoples around the world have different dietary patterns, determined by a number of factors. The major factors influencing what is eaten in different cultures are the foods available in that particular culture, traditional practices and beliefs, and any religious prescriptions. The relative importance of these foods is the starting point for many of the published pyramid-shape food guides (Figure 1.1).

The basis of the diet for most people is a core food, referred to as the 'staple', around which the majority of meals are constructed. Without the staple, a meal would not be perceived as a meal. There are usually only a very few core

Activity 1.2

You read the following article in your local paper:

Amazing Weight Loss Breakthrough!!

Doctors at the University of Nirvana have made a revolutionary new discovery, which will change the life of literally millions of people. Volunteers in their laboratories have been eating only three different foods a day and have lost an astonishing 30 lbs in a month!

The secret of their success is eating just one food at each meal. It doesn't matter what food you eat, but it must never be eaten with anything else. So, if you feel like ice cream for breakfast, chocolate for lunch and a steak for dinner – go ahead, the weight will still fall off and you will emerge a slimmer, fitter person.

Doctors claim that anyone can get the same results, as long as they stick to the diet regime of only one food at each meal. They explain that the body needs other foods to help the digestion process. When we eat only one food at a time, food breakdown stops, and so the calories can't pile on!

Results like this have never been obtained before, and it is likely that the whole country will become 'One Food a Meal' crazy.

The scientists do offer a word of caution, however. The weight loss is so astonishing that you should not need to stay on the diet for more than 4 weeks at a time. It may be dangerous if you continue on it for longer than this.

- What effect would you expect this article to have if it were published in the national newspapers?
- What alternative explanations for the findings might there be?
- Why might an article like this be nutritionally dangerous?

Try to find some articles in newspapers or magazines that you feel are misleading and potentially harmful.
- Attempt to identify what it is about the articles that concerns you.
- Try to think of an explanation for the way the article has been written.

Figure 1.1 A pyramid represents the contents of the diet and can be used as the basis of a food guide.

foods in any one culture, sometimes only one. They are generally cereals, or roots and tubers.

Secondary foods are also eaten; these enhance the meal, but are not an essential part of it. They may be endowed with specific properties of their own; for example they may promote strength (protein-rich foods, such as meat) or good health (fruit and vegetables), or they may maintain bodily forces in balance ('hot' and 'cold' foods as in some Eastern cultures). In addition, some secondary foods may be important at particular life stages.

The third category of foods are peripheral foods. These are non-essential, but pleasant to eat. Examples include biscuits, cakes, confectionery, preserves, sauces, puddings and alcoholic beverages. They may also include flavourings and seasonings.

Thus, despite the huge diversity of foods eaten around the world, it is possible to identify common patterns in the foods that people eat. In general, a greater part of the diet comes from the staple in the poorer parts of the world, and the peripheral foods make an excessively large contribution in richer countries. Clearly, the core and secondary foods in any national or cultural diet must supply the essential nutrients in appropriate amounts to sustain life and promote health. Some diets appear to achieve this better than others, as is shown by the fact that mortality rates from diseases that can be attributed to diet are lower in some countries of the world than in others.

HOW IS INFORMATION ABOUT PEOPLE'S DIETS COLLECTED?

To permit any exploration of the role of food in the health and welfare of the whole individual, rather than its biochemical effect at the system or cellular level, it is necessary to investigate what people eat. It is relatively straightforward for individuals to think about their own food intake, and to keep some sort of diary of what they have eaten. Most people can identify foods that they like or dislike, that they eat often or rarely. However, not everyone possesses enough interest in or knowledge about their own food intake to keep a detailed record over a period of time and, for most people, keeping a food record will be quite difficult.

Many of us would also be able to make some statements about the food intake of members of our family, or close friends. However, this information would inevitably be less detailed than our own, as we can rarely know about absolutely everything someone else has eaten. For a nutritionist, trying to find out what people eat poses a number of problems and requires varied approaches.

Population and household information

Information about the diet of a population can be obtained either in a very general way or with progressively more detailed techniques. In many countries, data are collected together in 'food balance sheets', which estimate the amount of food moving into and leaving a country, in much the same way as monetary transactions on a financial balance sheet. This can provide an overview of the theoretical availability of food in a country. Such statistics are collated and published by the United Nations' Food and Agriculture Organization (FAO) for most countries of the world, and are used to provide an overview of food availability.

In Europe, several Household Budget Surveys exist, each providing valuable data about dietary intakes in the specific country. The DAFNE (Data Food Networking) initiative is a collaborative effort across Europe to develop a bank of regularly updated and comparable data in order to assess and monitor trends in dietary patterns.

In the UK, data have been collected by the Household Food Consumption and Expenditure Survey, in particular, the National Food Survey (produced annually by the Ministry of Agriculture, Fisheries and Food) since 1940. This has provided a continuous surveillance of the food coming into households for consumption, together with money spent on food according to

household composition, economic status and geographical location. In 1994, the Survey started to collect data about food eaten outside the home, a reflection of the growing importance of eating out. The National Food Survey in this form ended in March 2001, and has been replaced by a new Expenditure and Food Survey (EFS), which will be published by DEFRA (Department for Environment, Food and Rural Affairs). Information about food consumption, nutrient intakes and food expenditure will, therefore, continue to be collected and published.

A study of this nature, however, cannot tell us the intake of an individual, as all of the data are collected with the household as the unit, without any indication of food distribution within. More information is required on food distribution patterns within households. The EFS will continue to publish information at the level of the household, although individual members will keep their own diaries. It is hoped that this will reduce the incidence of underreporting and increase accuracy.

The use of supermarket till receipts collected over 4 weeks, together with 4-day individual diaries has been used to assess patterns of fat and energy intake and has been shown useful. The involvement of supermarket checkout data to obtain information about population dietary patterns has potential in dietary surveys. Novel ways to collect data continue to be developed.

Individual information

Information on dietary intake of individuals is usually obtained by asking subjects to keep a record of everything they have eaten over a period of time. The level of precision with which this is carried out and the duration of the study have been subject to debate. In general, the more exact the method of measurement tries to be, the less it is likely to reflect the normal, freely chosen diet of the subject.

The exact method used will be determined by the aims of the study. Decisions have to be taken by the researcher to determine the reliability and validity of the methods used. In other words, if the method chosen provides results that can be reproduced on a subsequent occasion, it has a reasonable degree of reliability. A second more difficult question to answer relates to the validity of the information, i.e. how well it measures the subject's intake. Since food and, therefore, nutrient intakes are not constant from day to day for the majority of people, an average intake over a period of time would reflect 'habitual' intakes. The duration over which food intake has to be recorded to obtain a valid measure of habitual intake has been studied and shown to vary for different nutrients. Ultimately, the decision on how long a recording period should be depends on the nutrients to be analysed. For example, for energy and macronutrient intake, Black (2001) reports that a 7-day intake record will provide a result within 15–20 per cent of the true level of intake. For micronutrients, the variability is up to 30–40 per cent for those that are widely distributed in foods, and very large for vitamins, such as A and C, which occur in large amounts in fewer foods. Some of the methods used are discussed below.

The weighed inventory

This is considered to be the 'gold standard' of dietary intake studies. In this method, all the food eaten by the subject during a period, usually 1 week, is weighed and recorded, together with any plate waste. Actual nutrient intakes are then calculated, using data from food composition tables applicable to the particular country (in the UK McCance and Widdowson's tables, published by the Royal Society of Chemistry, are the most widely used – see Food Standards Agency, 2002b). The major drawback of the method is that it requires a considerable degree of motivation and cooperation on the part of the subject. It is quite an intrusive method, which takes time at meals and may thus deter a busy person.

Most subjects tend to underrecord their habitual food intake, possibly because they actually eat less during the study period, or forget/omit to record some of the foods eaten. This seems to be a particular problem in those who are trying to restrain their food intake in some way. Snack foods are often omitted, perhaps because of inconvenience or forgetfulness. Recent work has shown that the fat and carbohydrate intakes are underreported to a greater extent than protein intakes. Food choice may also be altered to facilitate weighing.

Food diaries

In this technique, the food eaten is simply recorded in a notebook, without being weighed. Comprehensive instructions are provided to the subject to explain the procedure. Cooking methods, brand names and recipes are requested. The respondent is asked to provide an estimate of the portion size using household measures, e.g. spoons, cups, units, slices or recording packet weights. The researcher then has the task of quantifying portions eaten. Food models or pictures may help in the quantification of portion sizes. A number of photographic atlases of food portions have been developed and validated in recent years. Other visual images, including those generated by computer may be used in the future, but would also need to be validated. Tables of average portion sizes are available in the UK, based on measurements of typical portions (Food Standards Agency (FSA), 2002a). Database information is available for a large number of typical servings of foods, although they remain only an estimate for each particular subject. A large database, known as DINER (Data Into Nutrients for Epidemiological Research) has been developed as part of the EPIC study, which contains information on over 7000 foods and portion sizes. The food diary method requires that the subject is literate and physically able to write. Alternative ways of recording the size of portion eaten include photographing the meal, and the use of computerized scales with an associated tape-recorder, for example, the PETRA (Portable Electronic Tape Recording Automated) Scales system, which can both weigh and store a description of the meal. In both cases, however, the data still require interpretation and collation by the researcher.

The diary method remains subject to possible changes in the diet by the respondent and failure to record all foods eaten. However, if respondents are adequately instructed, reasonably comprehensive records can be obtained. Generally, women produce more reliable records by this method than men.

A record of foods eaten with no attempt to assess the quantity (a menu record) is a further modification of this approach. Average servings can be used by the researcher and, although the accuracy of individual intake calculation is reduced, this method can provide an overview of dietary patterns.

A simpler and more straightforward approach used increasingly is to compile a food intake record based on food groups, such as those in the Balance of Good Health (FSA, 2001a). This allows an overall profile of the diet to be obtained and the balance to be assessed against a standard desirable pattern.

Food frequency questionnaires

These provide a means of studying intake retrospectively. The use of questionnaires is an inexpensive technique: it can be self-administered by large numbers of people and requires only a short period of time. This tool is often used in epidemiological research. It has the advantage that current diets are not altered. Analysis of the data can be done rapidly using a computerized scoring system. Disadvantages are that the results are culture-specific and a different group may require a new questionnaire. Additionally, individuals with unusual diets within the study group may not fit the predetermined criteria for coding. Even for people with a relatively consistent dietary pattern, it can be quite a complicated task to convert information about a habitual food intake into a frequency over a week, for specific foods. This is complicated further by trying to assess portion sizes of these foods. This type of questionnaire often looks at a subset of foods providing specific nutrients, rather than at the whole diet, and is generally tailored to the aims of a particular study.

In general, questionnaires can give useful information, which may be used to rank individuals within groups into subsets according to intake, rather than to provide precise data on actual intakes.

The diet interview

This technique is widely used by dietitians to obtain a general picture of a person's food intake. It requires a skilled interviewer to elicit an accurate picture of a person's diet history. The time frame is usually 7 days. This can be sufficient to pinpoint potential excesses or deficiencies. The interview may be more or less detailed, depending on the type of information required and its purpose. It usually consists of questions about the daily eating pattern, along the lines of 'What do you usually have for breakfast, mid-morning, lunch, etc.?' It then aims to draw a more precise picture by focusing on the current (or previous) day's intake, by asking 'What did you have for breakfast, mid-morning, lunch, etc. today, or yesterday?' Many people have little awareness of what they eat, so that it may be quite difficult for them to remember even the previous day's food intake. An estimation of portion sizes may also be made, often with the help of food models. A checklist of foods may be used to remind subjects about foods that they do eat, but forgot to mention.

Some of the limitations of a diet history are that it requires both a skilled interviewer and a subject with a reasonable memory. For the latter reason, it is unlikely to be suitable for children and for anyone with a failing memory. It also depends on the subject having a recognized dietary pattern, and a 'usual intake'. In addition, it is time consuming both to complete the interview and to carry out any subsequent analysis of the data collected. Hand-held computers with dietary analysis packages can simplify the process, allowing information from the subject to be entered directly.

A dietary recall interview can be simplified to focus just on the previous 24 hours and obtain a 'snapshot' of a typical intake. This can be done by telephone and need not take more than 15–20 minutes. However, bias is introduced as the day chosen may be atypical. It is also likely that food portion sizes are inaccurate, and the completeness of the record is memory dependent.

Practical issues in dietary survey methods

The way in which food is perceived by the subject may affect what is recorded. This might include perceptions of what their culture group believes they 'should' be eating as well as what the interviewer might expect.

Interaction at a subtle level between an interviewer and subject in the diet history interview may produce varying results when different people carry out the interview with the same subject.

Obtaining dietary intake information from children and adolescents poses particular challenges. With young children, below the age of 8 years, the limiting factors are likely to be knowledge of the names of foods as well as limited attention span and memory. The use of a surrogate reporter may introduce bias. As children become older, the ability to record the food intake increases, but at the same time there may be a greater desire to 'please' the interviewer and accuracy of records may be low. There are no easy solutions to collecting dietary intake data in these age groups, and new or refined survey methods are needed. Some of the problems found in this group include underreporting and non-response, which are also discussed below.

In the last few years, there has been recognition among nutritionists that much of the dietary intake data that are collected contain an element of underreporting. This is confirmed by comparison of energy intake with calculated or measured energy expenditure in many different groups. Measurements of energy expenditure using the doubly labelled water technique are available in some research settings. Biomarkers such as urinary nitrogen levels can also be used to confirm the accuracy of food intake records, although these increase the intrusion of the method, and could reduce compliance.

General findings, for example, based on studies of 77 groups (reported by Black, 2001) show a ratio of energy intake to energy expenditure of 0.83 (when a ratio of 1.0 would be expected). In addition, there is variability between subjects in the extent of misreporting. For 29 per cent of the groups studied, results for energy were within 10 per cent of those for expenditure. In 69 per cent of the groups, energy intake figures were more than 10 per cent below energy expenditure. Only in 2 per cent of the groups were the intake results more than 10 per cent greater than the expenditure results.

In summary, food intakes are usually underreported. This has implications for the calculation of energy intakes, but also nutrient intakes. If nutrient intakes are expressed in relation to the total energy intake, a measure of the nutrient density of the diet can be obtained, expressed as the weight of nutrient/MJ or 1000 Calories. This can then be used for comparison between

Activity 1.3

1 With a partner, try out a diet history interview on one another.
   a Go through all of the times in the previous day when your partner might have eaten something, and ask him/her questions about it.
   b Try to find out how much of everything they ate, how it was prepared, what brand name they had.
   c Did they eat all of it, or were there any left-overs?
2 Reflect on how easily you managed to complete this activity.
   a Did you and your partner have a pattern of eating?
   b How easy was it to assess amounts of food eaten?
   c Did you have the same ideas about what was a small/medium/large serving of a food?
   d Could you remember everything you had to eat 2 days ago, 3 days ago, etc.? How far back would your memory of your diet be reliable?

individuals, even if underreporting has occurred. These findings raise concerns about the accuracy of dietary intake studies, and underline the need for new methods to be developed that can more accurately capture information about individual intakes. Alternatively, more precise techniques for validating the intake records are needed.

STUDIES OF NUTRITIONAL STATUS

These include measurements of:
- anthropometric indicators
- biochemical indicators
- clinical indicators.

Anthropometric indicators

Anthropometric (literally 'measuring man') indicators are basic measurements of the human body. By relating these to standards typical of the test population, any deviations indicate abnormal nutritional status. Measurements commonly used are height and weight; these can be used to calculate the body mass index (BMI):

$$\text{BMI (or Quetelet's index)} = \frac{\text{Weight (in kilograms)}}{[\text{height (in metres)}]^2}$$

The desirable range for BMI is given as 20–25, with values above 30 being associated with obesity. Similarly, values below 18 are indicative of undernutrition.

In children, height and weight results can be compared with standard growth curves (see Chapter 12), which indicate the rate of physical development of a child, particularly when a sequence of measurements is made. In addition, head and chest circumference measures can also be useful in children to indicate rates of growth of the brain and body.

Skinfold thickness measurements at mid-triceps, mid-biceps, subscapular and supra-iliac sites using Harpenden or similar callipers give a surprisingly accurate value for body fat, when used by a skilled person. Figure 1.2 shows the sites for skinfold measurements.

Arm muscle circumference can be calculated by subtracting the thickness of the fatfold from a mid-arm circumference measurement. This can indicate muscle development or wasting, and can be a useful indicator in clinical situations

of change in muscle mass, for example, during illness and rehabilitation.

Waist: hip ratio is increasingly used as an indicator of body fat distribution: the circumference of the waist at the umbilicus and of the hips around the fattest part of the buttocks are used to calculate this ratio. A nomogram may be used, or a simple calculation performed to obtain the ratio. Values above 0.8 in women and 0.9 in men are indicative of a tendency for central fat deposition, and a possible increased health risk. Waist measurements alone have been shown to correlate well with body fatness, and may be used in future as a quick indicator of risk from overweight. Other ratios, such as waist to height, have also been suggested to be equally useful, as they tend to be 'unisex' and, therefore, a single figure can be used as a cut-off point.

Demispan is a measurement of skeletal size, which can be used as an alternative to height measurement, where it is difficult to obtain an upright posture in a subject. Demispan is the distance between the sternal notch and the roots of the middle and third fingers with the arm stretched out at shoulder height to the side of the body. It is particularly useful in elderly people, in whom height might have been lost due to vertebral collapse. The demispan value can then be used to produce two alternative indices

Figure 1.2 Measurement of skinfold for assessment of body fat content. (a) The four commonest sites used are subscapular, supra-iliac, mid-biceps and mid-triceps. Measurements from all four sites are added together for use in formulae to obtain fat mass. (b) For mid-triceps measurement the mid-point of the upper arm is found. (c) The callipers in use. The skinfold is taken lengthways along the arm, grasped firmly between thumb and forefinger, avoiding underlying muscle. The callipers are applied about 1 cm below the operator's fingers and the fold is held throughout the measurement. Three measurements are made and the results averaged.

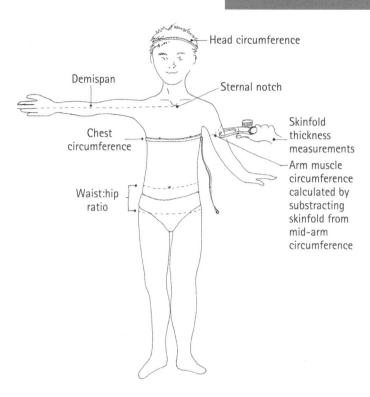

Figure 1.3 Summary of the main methods of anthropometry.

which show good agreement with BMI. These are demiquet, which uses weight/demispan² and mindex which is weight/demispan. The methods of anthropometry are summarized in Figure 1.3.

Biochemical indicators

Biochemical indicators can include assessment of blood and urine samples for levels of a variety of nutrients and/or their byproducts or for levels of nutrient-linked enzyme activities. In addition, analysis may be performed on samples of hair or bone marrow.

Blood (plasma, cells or serum) can provide a great deal of information. Analysis can be used to determine:

- actual levels of a nutrient in relation to expected levels (e.g. vitamin B_{12}, folate, carotenes, vitamin C in white blood cells);
- the activity of a nutrient-dependent enzyme (e.g. transketolase for thiamine);
- the activity of a nutrient-related enzyme (e.g. alkaline phosphatase for vitamin D);
- the rate of a nutrient-dependent reaction (e.g. clotting time for vitamin K);
- the presence of a nutrient carrier or its saturation level (e.g. retinol-binding protein, transferrin (iron)); or
- levels of nutrient-related products (e.g. lipoprotein levels).

Urine samples may be used to monitor the baseline excretion of a water-soluble nutrient or to follow its excretion after a loading dose. Metabolites of nutrients also appear in the urine and their levels can be monitored. Twenty-four-hour urine collections can be assayed for creatinine to indicate muscle turnover rates or for nitrogen content to check protein intakes.

Analyses of bone include bone marrow biopsies, which will show the blood-forming cells, and radiographic examination, which can detect stages of bone development or rarefaction in ageing. Bone densitometry can provide an essential measure of the density of the skeleton.

It is also possible to measure the levels of some trace elements in the hair, although the scientific accuracy of these assays is not proven and, therefore, they should not be relied upon.

A large amount of research is currently directed at finding new and sensitive biomarkers for the activity of nutrients in the body. Developments in molecular biology have opened up possibilities of assessments at gene level to provide much more precise indicators of what role the nutrient is fulfilling and at what levels it needs to be present. A major challenge is to translate *in vitro* findings from laboratory studies to meaningful measures of nutritional status in humans.

Clinical indicators

Clinical indicators are used to detect changes in the external appearance of the body. A number of nutritional deficiencies may cause alterations in superficial structures, although many are non-specific. In addition, changes in appearance may also be unrelated to nutritional state. Signs occur most rapidly in those parts of the body where cell turnover is frequent, such as hair, skin and digestive tract (including mouth and tongue). Therefore, a clinical examination may include the hair, face, eyes, mouth, tongue, teeth, gums, glands (such as the thyroid), skin and nails, subcutaneous tissues (to detect fat thickness, oedema), and the musculoskeletal system (to note bone deformities, ability to walk, muscle wasting). Some internal organs, like the liver, may be felt to note any enlargement. Reflex tests may be performed to test nerve pathways and muscle function. A trained observer will be able to detect many changes in appearance; generally, these are followed up with more specific tests of nutritional status.

WHAT CAN WE LEARN FROM NUTRITIONAL ASSESSMENT?

The techniques described above can be combined to obtain a more detailed picture of the dietary intake and nutritional status of a population. Food intake at the household level has been monitored in the UK for over 50 years in the National Food Survey produced by the Ministry of Agriculture, Fisheries and Food (MAFF). However, this does not collect information about health. In the mid-1980s a new approach was adopted in the UK, with the introduction of a series of studies organized by the Department of Health and MAFF. The first of these was the Dietary and Nutritional Survey of British Adults (commissioned in 1986-87, published as Gregory et al., 1990). This collected information about food intake using 7-day records, together with blood and urine analyses, anthropometry and lifestyle features. The Health Survey for England was set up in 1991 to monitor trends in the nation's health, using a health and socio-economic questionnaire, physical measurements and blood analysis. This is now running continuously and provides an ongoing picture that includes key nutrition-related health indicators.

The National Diet and Nutrition Survey (NDNS) is a cyclical programme, which collects dietary information from surveys of the different age groups in the UK. In this way each subsection of the population should be re-studied every 8 years. Surveys have been published of pre-school children, older people over 65 years, the 4–18 age group; a new survey of adults is due for publication. Other groups, such as vegetarians, people living on a low income and pregnant women are likely to be studied. Monitoring of people's diet is an essential part of the work of the Food Standards Agency, set up in 2000 in the UK. This now has responsibility for commissioning surveys of nutritional intake, as part of its Nutrition Strategy Framework (FSA, 2001b).

Diet is dynamic and, for this reason, ongoing programmes of study and surveillance are necessary, to monitor both what people are eating and the effects of any dietary changes on the patterns of disease.

The NDNS programme aims to:
- provide detailed quantitative information about intakes and sources of nutrients, and the nutritional status of the population;
- measure blood and other indices that give evidence of nutritional status, and relate these to dietary, physiological and social data;
- monitor the diet for its nutritional adequacy;
- monitor the extent to which dietary targets are being met.

In Scotland, both the Scottish Heart Study, which included over 10 000 subjects aged 40–59, and one part of the European MONICA project have provided more specific information about the Scottish diet.

Other countries approach the monitoring of nutrition in similar ways. In the USA, the National Health and Nutritional Examination Survey (NHANES) collects data about food intakes, anthropometric indices, blood pressure and blood levels of minerals and vitamins. Surveillance of the diets of populations occurs in Australia, Canada and several European countries. Cross-population studies are also performed; the SENECA (Survey in Europe on Nutrition and the Elderly, a Concerted Action) study is one such example.

HOW IS THE INFORMATION GOING TO BE USED?

The declared purpose of any nutritional surveillance programme is to identify links between diet and disease, and thereby to formulate policy and advice aimed at minimizing the risk of disease, by altering the diet.

All countries have food policies that relate to the provision of a safe food supply, and that incorporate a wide range of measures relating to production, taxation, trade, politics and social and consumer issues. In some cases these may run counter to health policies, for example, by the promotion of fats, dairy produce and meat. These policies may also concentrate on legislation about pesticide residues, additives or food processing. Incorporating a nutrition policy into a food policy is, however, more problematic as there may be conflicting interests between food producers and the health professionals. Where nutrition is supported at government level, it is necessary for the government to facilitate the nutrition policy by changes to legislation, taxation, food labelling or other measures. Without such changes, a nutrition policy might not be workable. It is, therefore, important that government policy-making is informed by good-quality nutrition surveillance information, and that appropriate policy decisions are made.

The UK Food Standards Agency works with the Department of Health to improve the health of the UK population through encouraging and facilitating the adoption of a healthy balanced diet. The FSA has put forward its plans in the Nutrition Strategic Framework to enable it to achieve the following objectives.

- Secure a sound evidence base for action to promote a healthy diet.
- Develop appropriate means of informing the general public.
- Identify and address barriers to changing dietary behaviour.
- Evaluate and monitor the effectiveness of the action taken.

In order to achieve these objectives, the FSA is working with many other key players, including the Scientific Advisory Committee on Nutrition (SACN), which has replaced Committee on Medical Aspects of Food Policy (COMA), government departments including Health and Education, the food industry and the scientific community. Their work will build on many of the goals already achieved since the publication of 'The health of the nation' white paper, which set out specific health goals for England to be achieved within a decade (DoH, 1992). These related to heart disease and stroke, accidents, mental health, sexual health and cancer. A Nutrition Task Force (NTF) was set up to discuss ways in which the targets relating to nutrition could be achieved, using all the parties involved in the food chain to form 'healthy alliances'.

One of the major aims of the NTF was to produce a simple and easy to understand National Food Guide to provide a basic tool for teaching the elements of a balanced healthy diet. This was to be available to all educators, at whatever level, so that a consistent message was given from all sides. The National Food Guide (the Balance of Good Health) was developed, tested and eventually launched in 1994 (HEA, 1994). This is still used in the UK and has recently been reissued by the FSA as the Balance of Good Health; it is discussed more fully in Chapter 3. The NTF set in train a great number of initiatives and, as a consequence, nutritional issues are now much more to the fore in the national health agenda. The FSA now has the responsibility for taking these forward into the first decade of the twenty-first century. There is more information about food policy in Chapter 18.

SUMMARY

1 Nutrition is a very broad discipline. It may be of interest to people from a variety of backgrounds, who can also make useful contributions to its knowledge base.

2 There has been a huge increase in interest in nutrition in the last decade and people want to be better informed.

3 To be informed about nutrition, it is necessary to know what people eat and how his can be measured. The advantages and disadvantages of these methods are important to consider.

4 The dietary information must be supplemented by information about health. Both of these need continual updating, as neither remains static.

5 This information is used in making policy decisions about dietary advice to improve health.

STUDY QUESTIONS

1 Which methods of obtaining information about food intakes would you use in each of the following examples, and for what reason:

   a A study to identify groups in a population who have a high, or low, intake of dietary fibre (non-starch polysaccharide; NSP).

   b An investigation into iron intakes in a group of children who do not eat meat.

   c A comparison of food intakes between two populations who have different disease patterns.

   d A pregnant woman who needs advice about her diet.

2 Discuss with a colleague the benefits and disadvantages of adding specific nutrients to manufactured foods. Do you think this practice would help or hinder the work of a nutritionist?

3 What factors, apart from nutrition, might play a role in the health of a population? How could these be taken into account in results of nutritional assessment?

4 Perform a small survey among your acquaintances and friends to discover:

   a what they understand by the term nutrition;

   b how relevant to their health and well-being they consider their food intake to be;

   c if they would consider changing their diet to improve their health.

Draw some conclusions from your findings.

REFERENCES AND FURTHER READING

Bassey, E.J. 1986: Short report: demispan as a measure of skeletal size. *Annals of Human Biology* 13(5), 499–502.

Beaglehole, R., Bonita, R., Kjellstrom, T. 1993: *Basic epidemiology*. Geneva: WHO.

Beghin, I., Cap, M., Dujardin, B. 1988: *A guide to nutritional assessment*. Geneva: WHO.

Bingham, S.A., Gill, C., Welch, A. et al. 1994: Comparison of dietary assessment methods in nutritional epidemiology: weighed records v. 24 hr. recalls, food-frequency questionnaires and estimated-diet records. *British Journal of Nutrition* 72, 619–43.

Bingham, S.A., Welch, A.A. McTaggart, A. et al. 2001: Nutritional methods in the European Prospective Investigation of Cancer in Norfolk. *Public Health Nutrition* 4(3), 847–58.

Black, A.E. 2001: Dietary assessment for sports dietetics. *British Nutrition Foundation Nutrition Bulletin* 26, 29–42.

Cade, J., Thompson, R., Burley, V. et al. 2002: Development, validation and utilisation of food-frequency questionnaires – a review. *Public Health Nutrition* 5(4), 567–87.

Colhoun, H., Prescott-Clarke, P. (eds) 1996: *Health survey for England 1994*. London: HMSO.

DoH (UK Department of Health) 1992: *The health of the nation. A strategy for health in England*. London: HMSO.

Food Standards Agency 2001a: *The balance of good health*. London: FSA.

Food Standards Agency 2001b: *Your food – farm to fork*. London: FSA.

Food Standards Agency 2002a: *Food portion sizes*, 3rd edn. London: The Stationery Office.

Food Standards Agency 2002b: *McCance and Widdowson's the composition of foods*, 6th summary edn. Cambridge: The Royal Society of Chemistry.

Gregory, J., Foster, K., Tyler, H. et al. 1990: *The dietary and nutritional survey of British adults*. London: HMSO.

HEA (Health Education Authority) 1994: *Introducing the National Food Guide: The balance of good health. Information for educators and communicators*. London: Health Education Authority.

Livingstone, M.B.E., Prentice, A.M., Strain, J.J. et al. 1990: Accuracy of weighed dietary records in studies of diet and health. *British Medical Journal* **300**, 708–12.

Livingstone, M.B.E., Robson, P.J. 2000: Measurement of dietary intake in children. *Proceedings of the Nutrition Society* **59**, 279–93.

Margetts, B.M. Nelson, M. 1997: *Design concepts in nutritional epidemiology*, 2nd edn. Oxford: Oxford University Press.

Nelson, M., Haraldsdottir, J. 1998: Food photographs: practical guidelines II. Development and use of photographic atlases for assessing food portion size. *Public Health Nutrition* **1**(4), 231–8.

Ransley, J.K., Donnelly, J.K., Khara, T.N. et al. 2001: The use of supermarket till receipts to determine the fat and energy intake in a UK population. *Public Health Nutrition* **4**(6), 1279–86.

Trichopoulou, A., Naska, A. (eds) 2001: The DAFNE initiative. Assessment of dietary patterns across Europe using household budget survey data. *Public Health Nutrition* **4** (5B).

Welch, A.A., McTaggart, A., Mulligan, A.A. et al. 2001: DINER (Data Into Nutrients for Epidemiological Research) – a new data-entry program for nutritional analysis in the EPIC-Norfolk cohort and the 7-day diary method. *Public Health Nutrition* **4**(6), 1253–65.

2

WHAT ARE THE INFLUENCES ON EATING HABITS?

The aims of this chapter are to:

❏ discuss the reasons for eating and possible mechanisms controlling eating;
❏ describe food habits;
❏ explore the factors influencing food choice, the interactions between them and how they change;
❏ help the reader understand how their own food habits are determined.

On completing the study of this chapter, you should be able to:

❏ describe the physiological and metabolic signals that determine food intake;
❏ discuss how social and cultural influences play a part in modifying basic physiological mechanisms;
❏ analyse your own food habits, and show how these have developed and are influenced currently;
❏ recognize the importance of individuals' particular food habits and appreciate how these may be resistant
·to change.

Activity 2.1

Before studying this chapter, spend a little time thinking about:

■ why you eat;
■ what you eat;
■ what are some of the reasons for choosing the particular foods.

You may find that this is a surprisingly difficult task. We are generally quite unconscious of our reasons for eating and choosing particular foods. Only when we have a basic framework with which to study these influences can we begin to gain insight into our own behaviour related to food.

Most people, if asked why they eat, would respond with 'to stay alive' or 'because of hunger'. Both of these are appropriate answers: the body has a physiological need for food and, when deprived for even a short period of time, a sensation of hunger is experienced. This is a normal physiological response, which is designed to balance the output and storage of nutrients with their input from food.

In addition, however, people eat for a number of other reasons. In the West, eating is a matter of habit because food is usually widely available, often at all hours of day or night. There are also socially accepted 'mealtimes', when there is an expectation of eating, regardless of hunger, and there are social norms associated with eating, which define what behaviour is and is not acceptable.

Food provides us with sensory satisfaction, it is (usually) pleasant to eat, and this aspect of certain foods can induce people to eat when they have no physiological need to do so.

We have a very personal relationship with food. It is something we deliberately take into our body and which becomes part of us. This can have very profound meanings for some people, but for everyone it implies that there are psychological influences on eating.

Each of these influences on eating will be discussed in turn, to demonstrate that even something as basic as supplying the body with the energy for its survival can involve more than an understanding of physiology.

REASONS FOR EATING

Physiological need

Signals relating to all of the processes involved in the initiation and cessation of eating are integrated and organized by the brain. These controlling mechanisms have been studied mainly in experimental animals. This is because humans are more complicated, with many cultural and social conventions, which influence food intake, and which can override the physiological mechanisms. A schematic diagram of the various components of the control mechanism integrated by the brain is given in Figure 2.1.

In an individual whose weight remains constant, there is evidently a balance between the input of food and its metabolism and energy output. Consideration of the various stages of the process helps to identify where control mechanisms could be operating.

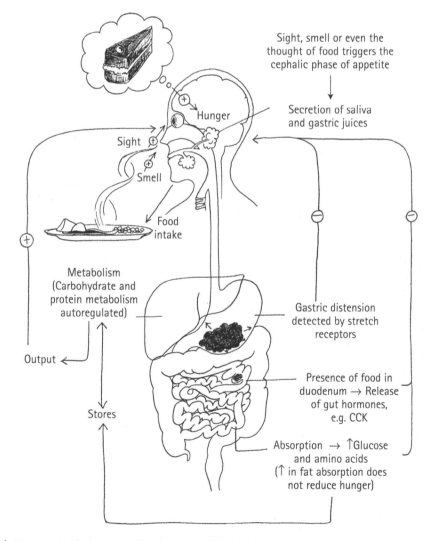

Figure 2.1 Physiological factors controlling hunger and food intake.

Sensory signals

The sight, smell or even thought of food triggers the cephalic phase of appetite, which stimulates hunger and prepares the digestive tract for the ingestion of food by secretion of saliva and gastric juices. When eating starts, the food stimulates the senses of taste and touch (via the texture and consistency of the food). Variety in the sensory properties of foods offered in a meal can further stimulate eating, whereas a meal that contains only one item rapidly leads to satiation. This is the sensation that stops food intake at a meal and is associated with a feeling of fullness.

Pre-absorptive information

Ingested food causes gastric distension. This is detected by stretch receptors, which send signals to the brain. The presence of food and early digestion products in the duodenum causes the release of a large number of gut hormones, some of which have been shown to inhibit food intake. The most extensively studied of these is cholecystokinin (CCK), which has been shown to produce satiety in many animal species, including humans. CCK is stimulated particularly by the presence of protein and fat digestion products in the duodenum. The presence of residual protein in the stomach at the start of a meal has a restraining effect on food intake, and particularly on the intake of protein. Newly discovered peptides, such as PYY and ghrelin signal to the brain that the stomach is full (Wilding, 2002). Satiety is described as the sensation that delays the next food intake, thus affecting the interval between meals.

Ingestion of liquids, even those containing macronutrients, is less well regulated by these mechanisms than ingestion of solids.

Post-absorptive signals

All of the digestion products have been proposed as regulators of food intake. Fluctuations in blood glucose level and, therefore, its availability to the cells of the nervous system and brain, were originally believed to be the cornerstone of feeding behaviour regulation. Carbohydrate-rich meals suppress further intake for between 1 and 3 hours after eating. This may be associated with the period during which insulin levels are raised after a meal. This is the glucostatic theory of food intake. However, it cannot satisfactorily explain control of eating in all situations.

A further theory, the lipostatic theory, proposes a relationship between body fat reserves and eating behaviour, such that an increase in stored fat would reduce intake. It is only recently, however, that a mechanism to support this has been identified.

Leptin is a relatively recently discovered (in 1994) protein, released principally from adipose tissue as well as other tissues. Because it is released at one site and acts at a distant site, it fulfils the criteria of a hormone. Amounts produced reflect the size of the fat store in both humans and animals. Leptin release from adipose tissue is also influenced by levels of feeding, such that fasting results in a rapid fall in leptin secretion and levels rise again on refeeding. In addition, exposure to cold inhibits leptin release. Leptin secretion from adipose tissue is also influenced by several other hormones. Release is stimulated by insulin, glucocorticoids, oestrogens and cytokines (released as part of immune reactions). The major inhibitors of leptin release are adrenaline and noradrenaline, mediated by the sympathetic nervous system. One of the functions of leptin is to act in the hypothalamus, where it causes the release of a number of neuropeptides, including neuropeptide Y. This has a potent action to inhibit food intake. In obese humans and animals, leptin receptors have a low sensitivity, resulting in poor recognition of the size of fat stores and, therefore, dysregulation of food intake.

Further regulation of food intake may occur via the activity of lipoprotein lipase, an enzyme found in adipose tissue.

Amino acid levels also have an effect on feeding behaviour, with shifts in plasma and brain concentrations of particular amino acids causing changes in intake. There is competition between different amino acids for uptake across the blood–brain barrier; consequently, an elevation of one amino acid may inhibit the uptake of others. The importance of some amino acids lies in their role as precursors for brain neurotransmitter substances; these may be the effectors of changes in feeding behaviour.

Metabolism

The blood levels of metabolites are regulated by the liver and peripheral tissues, which remove them from the circulation and may also have an effect on feeding behaviour.

It is becoming clear that metabolism of the energy-providing nutrients is regulated with different levels of precision. Alcohol, as a potential toxin, must be oxidized completely and removed as quickly as possible. Its metabolic regulation is perfect and all alcohol is completely metabolized.

The capacity of the body to store carbohydrate and protein is limited, and blood levels of glucose and amino acids are carefully controlled. It is now believed that under normal circumstances very little carbohydrate is actually converted to fat. The conversion of carbohydrate to fat is very inefficient, with approximately 25 per cent of the potential energy wasted as heat. Metabolism of both glucose and amino acids is thought to 'autoregulate' to match the intake level.

Fat metabolism, however, exhibits no such 'autoregulation', probably because of the large capacity for fat storage in the body. Therefore, fat metabolism does not correlate well with fat intake and there is no evidence that fat oxidation adjusts when intake increases. Consequently, one can conclude that fat intake plays a smaller role in the control of food intake than do either carbohydrates or proteins. This may provide an explanation for the 'fattening' effects of high-fat diets, which can be consumed without any consequent change to fat oxidation. Also evidence from feeding studies of diets where fat content has been covertly increased shows that a change in fat levels has no effect on satiety and subsequent food intakes. This means that such diets are easy to consume leading to 'passive overconsumption', and may be a significant contributory factor in obesity.

Integration by the brain

Early research identified hunger and satiety centres in the hypothalamus; these could be artificially stimulated or destroyed, resulting in starvation or overeating. The function of these centres was thought to be the maintenance of adequate levels of energy-providing nutrients in the blood. The dietary macronutrients, carbohydrates, fats and proteins, were the primary candidates for these regulatory factors. It is now clear that this is an oversimplified picture. The brain receives information from receptors and metabolites about the whole feeding process, from the initial thought about food to the final metabolism of its breakdown products. Changes in plasma concentrations of nutrients resulting from metabolism in the liver and peripheral tissues are also monitored. A number of these have been mentioned in the earlier sections. In particular, leptin levels are believed to be important, through their action on neuropeptide Y, causing inhibition of food intake. Low levels of leptin are thought to cause a number of adaptive changes to minimize weight loss, including increased food intake. In addition, levels of serotonin, which promotes feelings of satiety, are influenced by the amounts of tryptophan crossing the blood-brain barrier. By these means, food intake and metabolic processes can be regulated to match the body's needs. This complex integration occurs in the brain, probably by appropriate changes in the levels of neurotransmitters.

In addition, it has been proposed that unconscious reflex pathways are established, particularly during childhood, whereby the body 'learns' the metabolic consequences of particular eating patterns and responds accordingly. If such reflexes are not established, perhaps due to erratic eating behaviour in childhood, then control mechanisms remain less efficient. Much remains to be learned about the complex control of eating.

Habit as an influence on eating behaviour

In parts of the world where food is readily available, intake could occur at any time of day or night. Most people do not eat continuously, but usually at fairly clearly defined 'mealtimes', with 'snack times' interspersed between them. This behaviour has become a habit, and many Westerners believe that they should have three meals a day together with two or three snacks, with the main meal either in the middle of the day or in the evening (see Figure 2.2). In other societies, especially among the poor, fewer meals are eaten, maybe only one or at most two

Figure 2.2 Habit influences eating behaviour.

within a day. Therefore, it appears that there is no physiological need to eat so frequently, although it will be necessary to eat to satiation when mealtimes are infrequent. If eating is more continuous, the sensations of satiety or hunger may never be experienced. The brain, therefore, lacks the necessary input to recognize these, which may result in poor regulation of eating behaviour at some point in life.

What is the difference between meals and snacks?

A snack is an eating occasion where just one type of food is eaten, perhaps accompanied by a drink, and might include biscuits, chocolate or sandwiches, for example. Often this is eaten in an informal setting, or perhaps in the street, or while travelling. In the last 20 years, more informal eating has been taking place, as lifestyles become more flexible. In some instances, all of the food taken during the course of a day may be classified as 'snacks', with perhaps as many as ten or more being consumed. This is particularly prevalent among young people, and causes concern to nutritionists as some of the snack foods eaten are low in micronutrients, but may contain substantial amounts of fat and/or sugar.

However, not all snack foods are nutritionally poor: sandwiches, fruit, nuts and drinks, such as milk or fruit juice, can provide useful nutrients.

A meal generally contains a selection of different separate items, usually eaten with utensils (although in some cultures this is not usual), and takes some time to prepare and to eat. Traditionally, this would be eaten in a designated eating place, for example, at a table. More flexible lifestyles, however, mean that meals now may be eaten in more informal settings, perhaps from a tray while watching the television, or in the street out of the packaging in the case of fish and chips or a burger. Because it includes more items, a meal is more likely to contain a greater number of nutrients, although there are still meals which can be nutritionally very poor.

There needs to be a degree of organization of mealtimes in a society that operates by the clock. Chaos would ensue if in every office, classroom and business organization people wandered off to eat whenever they felt like it. Some accepted schedule is essential, both from the consumers' and from the cooks' point of view. It could be argued that rigorous timing of meals is introduced too early in life. Some infants in the first months of life are still fed 'by the clock', usually 4-hourly. Feeding 'on demand' gives the infant the opportunity to be fed when actually hungry, although it does introduce a level of unpredictability into the mother's life.

Some people eat just because food is available. They are unable to resist the desire to eat, and are apparently less sensitive to their own internal cues about needing food than to external signals. Others may deliberately avoid food or eat in very small amounts, disregarding their internal signals and gauging what they eat by external cues related to the size of the plate, what other people are having or what they think is an appropriate amount for them.

Both of the above types have developed particular habits that control their eating, which are usually more powerful than the physiological need. In the extreme, these can result in disordered eating – both overeating, or bingeing, and compulsive dieting, or perhaps a cycling between these two extremes. These are discussed further in Chapter 8.

Figure 2.3 Psychological need as a trigger to eating.

Psychological need

Eating is a pleasurable activity, and can satisfy some of our internal needs. Boredom provides a major incentive to eating and may fill many empty hours for people. Depression or anxiety can also make people turn to food for comfort. This is believed to stem from the reassurance given by food provided by parents to children, linking positive feelings about parental care and love with the food. It is important that the 'food as comfort' response is not made too frequently, as it is likely to result in overweight, often with associated emotional problems (see Figure 2.3).

We may also offer food to people to comfort them; for example, a child who has fallen and been hurt may be cuddled and then offered something to eat (often a sweet or biscuit). After a funeral, people may come together to share food. This acts as a comforting gesture for both those providing the food, as well as those eating it. If we remember that provision of food is linked with loving and caring, it is easy to see how rejection of the food by the intended recipient can be hurtful and painful. This happens with young children who are learning about food, but can become manipulative and cause their carers

considerable hurt. They may use food rejection to express feelings of anger, jealousy or insecurity, or to gain attention. Children who have to follow a special diet for health reasons may be particularly at risk of this type of behaviour. Using food as a weapon can become a habit maintained into adult life. Sometimes this weapon is turned against the self, in situations where food intake is chaotic (see Chapter 8).

Sensory appeal

The way in which a food stimulates our senses by its appearance and smell, taste and texture may also increase our desire to eat it. Most people claim that the taste of the food is the prime consideration, although for adolescents the appearance also rates highly.

The visual appeal of the food, although important to attract the eye, can be quite deceptive, however, and gives no indication of nutritional value. Most sighted people would be very wary of accepting and eating a food they could not see. Our expectations of the taste of a food are prepared by its appearance – we expect an orange-coloured drink to have a sweet, citric taste; anything else might lead to rejection. The food industry is well aware of the importance of the 'correct' visual stimulus and uses a range of colorants to produce an acceptable finished appearance. However, the numbers of these are less than they were 10–20 years ago as consumers become more concerned about safety aspects, and are increasingly prepared to buy foods with a more 'natural' colour (see Figure 2.4).

The smell of the food must also meet our expectations. We use this to detect if food has 'gone off' and we are enticed to eat by pleasant aromas. We can recognize many foods purely from their smell. Smell and taste interact to produce the flavour of the food; if the sense of smell is lost; for example, when suffering from a cold, food may seem tasteless. The number of taste buds is highest in children, who have them on the insides of the cheeks and throat, as well as over the surface of the tongue. These begin to decrease from adolescence and are considerably reduced by the age of 70.

Figure 2.4 Sensory appeal as a trigger for eating.

Children's food preferences and choices are driven primarily by taste. Relative to adults, children have a preference for very sweet taste, and avoid bitter tastes. The liking for intense sweetness declines into adolescence, more so in girls than boys. There is also a link between energy density and sweetness, and this is believed to be a means by which intake of high-energy foods is assured to support growth and development in children. Once adulthood is reached, the need for such energy-dense foods is reduced, and the liking for intense sweetness tends to disappear. The taste acuity for the bitter taste also declines, and adults accept bitter tastes more readily. There is also a move to less energy-dense foods, which are often those associated with a healthier diet, with increasing age. Taste perception can change in certain circumstances: pregnant women, surgical patients and people with cancer all report an altered ability to taste certain foods. It has been suggested that zinc status plays a role in this. Unusual appetites for particular foods may also develop. People can become accustomed to a particular taste if this is perceived to be an advantage. The bitter tastes found in beer, quinine (in tonic water) and coffee appear to be an acquired taste for many people, although some find them unpleasant all their lives.

The texture and taste of the food in the mouth provide us with the pleasurable aspects of eating. The feel of the food in the mouth can include its texture, temperature and even any pain it produces. We expect particular foods to be presented at a certain temperature (e.g. ice cream or hot tea). Extremes of temperature can cause pain to the mouth and teeth. Chilli contains a chemical substance (capsacin), which irritates the nerve endings, triggering pain. Some substances can cause a local anaesthetic effect in the mouth – chewing coca leaves (widespread practice in parts of South America) has this effect; its purpose is to dull the hunger sensation among peoples who have little food.

Food technologists can measure optimal levels of various sensory characteristics (such as sugar content, aroma, water content, temperature), which are associated with the highest level of pleasure. These are aptly named 'bliss points'. These are not fixed forever and can become modified if the diet changes, although the initial alteration to the diet will be associated with a reduction in pleasure. For example, an individual who normally takes two spoonfuls of sugar in their tea probably will have that concentration of sugar as their 'bliss point'. Cutting out sugar will result in a reduction in 'bliss'. In time, the subject is likely to adapt to the newer taste, the level of 'bliss' is restored at a lower sweetness, and drinking tea with the original level of sugar will no longer be acceptable. This sequence will apply to other changes made to the diet that have sensory implications, including cutting down fat or salt intakes.

Variety also encourages us to eat. Studies on both animals and humans have shown clearly that, when offered a variety of food, total intake is greater than when just a single food is offered. Thus, it is possible to make rats overweight by offering them a 'cafeteria diet', containing chips, burgers, crisps, chocolate, etc., rather than ordinary rat pellets; they eat more of the mixed diet. Humans will also overeat when offered something new; for example, having apparently eaten their fill of a main course, many people will still manage to have a dessert afterwards. It has also been noted that more food is eaten when meals are accompanied by wine and taken in a social setting. These factors occurring together can promote an unconscious overconsumption.

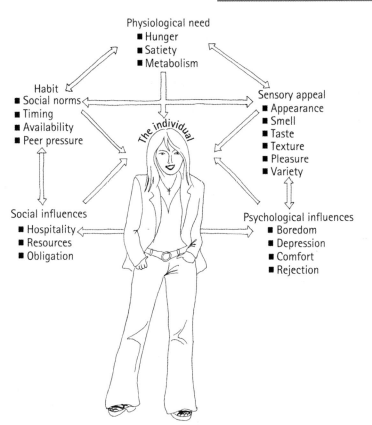

Physiological need
■ Hunger
■ Satiety
■ Metabolism

Habit
■ Social norms
■ Timing
■ Availability
■ Peer pressure

The individual

Sensory appeal
■ Appearance
■ Smell
■ Taste
■ Texture
■ Pleasure
■ Variety

Social influences
■ Hospitality
■ Resources
■ Obligation

Psychological influences
■ Boredom
■ Depression
■ Comfort
■ Rejection

Figure 2.5 Why do we eat?

Overweight is much less common in communities around the world where only a few foods appear regularly in the diet – it seems that monotony imposes its own limits on eating. On the other hand, organizing food into different courses, with different flavours, seems to enhance the food intake.

Social influence

Food may also be used in a social context to please or displease others. Offering food or drink is recognized as a gesture of hospitality, and refusal may be interpreted as rejection. This may extend to the obligation to eat food that is not wanted or even disliked, to avoid offending the giver. This may be a particular problem for visitors to other countries, who may be presented with unknown or even unacceptable food, yet feel obliged to consume it.

In situations where food is scarce, or budgets are very restricted, wasting food may be socially unacceptable, and individuals may feel it necessary to eat everything provided. The opposite may also apply – waste may be quite acceptable where food supplies are plentiful, or where left-over food can be put to other uses, such as feeding pigs or poultry.

All of these influences and some of their interrelationships are summarized in Figure 2.5.

FOOD HABITS

So far, we have learned that the primary reason for eating is to satisfy our hunger, but that what and when we eat can also reflect who we are, the society we live in, our upbringing and how we perceive ourselves. We can define food habits as the typical behaviour of a particular group of people in relation to food. They provide an important signal of the identity of the group. They will determine food choice, as well as eating times and numbers of meals, size of portions, methods of food preparation and

Activity 2.2

Using your experience, try to identify which of the factors given in Figure 2.5 are likely to be most important for the following people:

a yourself

b a pre-school-age child

c a mother with young children

d a teenage girl/boy

e an elderly woman, living on her own.

Account for your answers.

who takes part in the meal. Food habits are a product of the environmental influences on a culture and, in general, are resistant to change.

Some of the components of an individual's food habits are shown in Figure 2.6.

Acquisition of food habits

The acquisition of food habits is largely unconscious, since they are acquired at a young age from parents, which incidentally ensures transmission between generations. The strongest influence on a child in its acquisition of food habits is generally its mother, who is likely to be the most closely involved with the provision of food. Children learn what is acceptable as food, and what is not. Foods that are associated with good times are often preferred to those that do not have these connotations. We may remember particularly foods that we ate on holiday and seek these out to help relive happy memories. Children are dependent on the food practices and beliefs of the adult caregivers; this may

restrict a child's opportunities to try many foods, if they are not part of the adult's food choice. In addition, some foods may be seen as inappropriate for children and, therefore, not offered.

After the initial socialization within the home environment, children learn more food practices from other people, or institutions outside the home. A major force may be the school, where behaviour is learned from other children, as well as through the food provided in school meals and tuck shops, and more formal teaching about food in lessons. All of these will broaden the child's view of food and will affect the food practices.

Later still, other people may influence food habits as different views are encountered with a widening social circle. Foreign travel also provides experience of different food habits.

Changing food habits

Although food habits are resistant to change, they are not static. Change may come from within the culture. For example, the increase in female employment in the West has resulted in a dramatic increase in the availability of convenience food. Fewer households now eat meals prepared from basic ingredients on a regular basis. Weekday meals in particular are composed to a great extent of convenience items, with perhaps the addition of a home-prepared vegetable or starchy staple (such as rice or potato). The prevalence of microwave ovens, together with widespread ownership of freezers, has meant that meals can be ready in minutes, and that even quite young children can prepare themselves

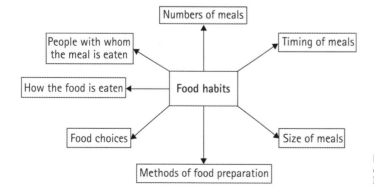

Figure 2.6 Some of the main components of a person's food habits.

something hot to eat with little risk of accident. The consequence of this has been that, in many families, mealtimes are no longer taken together. Instead, individual members of the family may eat at times convenient to themselves, often heating up different meals in the microwave. In addition, around 30 per cent of meals eaten are likely to be consumed away from home, in work or school canteens, cafes, fast-food outlets, restaurants or in the car. The National Food Survey (Department for Environment, Food and Rural Affairs (DEFRA), 2001) showed that on average three meals per week were eaten outside the home (not from the home food supply), and this represents 30 per cent of the expenditure on food.

Another source of change is the increase in the availability of information about world cookery. Examples of the cuisine of different cultures are found in restaurants, supermarkets and as cookery programmes on the television, and the wide availability of many exotic ingredients makes it possible for these 'foreign' dishes to be included into traditional food habits. Many books describe how to prepare these dishes.

The media are also responsible for changing food habits. This may occur through the following.

- Advertising and the promotion of new food products (although the information given here may be biased).
- Programmes or articles that aim to increase people's knowledge about food, perhaps in the context of nutrition and health.
- Providing role models in the form of characters in programmes and advertising. These contribute a subtle force towards change in food habits by the food they eat and the attitudes they express. Some of the messages put forward are not necessarily conducive to health; for example, there is believed to be a prevailing message that only thin women are healthy and attractive, which causes often disastrous changes to food habits among the female population.

Food habits may have to change when an individual suffers from an illness requiring dietary alteration for its management. The difficulty of changing food habits is best seen in such subjects, who often struggle to maintain dietary changes, even when there are very good health reasons for doing so.

Nutrition educators and health promoters aim to change food habits towards a healthier balance. This is a very complex process because of the multi-faceted influences on food habits. Different influences may be at work in determining what is eaten from day to day or even from meal to meal. A further factor is the strength of the attitude of the subject towards food and healthy eating. If they are ambivalent about either of these, change may be difficult to bring about. Finally, the subjective recognition that change is needed to the diet is a powerful influence in determining whether it is undertaken.

Therefore, an educator may need to consider the strength of the subject's belief:

- that food and healthy eating are important;
- that these can influence their individual health in a beneficial way;
- that making changes to food and eating has a high priority amongst factors that influence food choice.

Studies have identified many barriers to making changes towards healthy eating that are more prevalent amongst those subjects who make fewer changes. In the study by Margetts et al. (1998), these included:

- a perception that there is a lack of clear messages about healthy foods;
- a belief that the tastiest foods are the ones that are 'bad';
- confusion about what to eat;
- difficulty of eating healthy food away from home;
- costs of healthy eating;
- lack of concern about what is eaten.

In addition, changes towards healthier eating are less likely to be found among younger, lower income groups and those who smoke. This emphasizes that dietary change is closely linked to other lifestyle indicators in complex ways.

Food choices

Within the context of a culture's food habits, each individual makes their own, personal food choices, which are likely to be different from those of anyone else. There are many ways to study individual food choices, and much has been written about them. There are still areas of uncertainty, however, and research into determinants of food choice, especially within family groups, is ongoing. Viewpoints may be anthropological, economic, physiological or administrative, political, psychological or sociological, as well as nutritional. The following is a nutritional perspective on food choice.

In very broad terms, people can only choose from the range of food available to them; thus, factors that determine food availability are important. Given a range of foods, an individual will not necessarily choose to eat all of them. The choice will depend on what is acceptable to them, personally. Hence the two main determinants of food choice are availability and acceptability. The main factors influencing these are shown in Tables 2.1 and 2.2.

Availability
Physical/environmental factors
In the West, this factor is less important now than it was 20 or more years ago. Food preservation, storage and distribution around world markets are so efficient that it rarely matters whether the

local area produces a food or not. It can generally be imported from elsewhere. This creates a uniformity of foods available, and there is concern that many interesting varieties of locally produced foods are being lost, or remain available only in a speciality market. Differences exist, however, in what food is available to buy in a locality. This will be dependent on factors such as population density and, therefore, the number of shops in the vicinity, and ease of access, which will determine the cost of transporting food into the area. The perishability of a food will also determine the range over which it can be transported. For these reasons, rural areas in most countries generally have a smaller range of food available than urban areas.

However, in places not reached by the world market, where locally grown produce is eaten, physical factors such as type of soil, rainfall or transportation are important determinants of what food is actually available. Perishability of food and the means of preservation available will also determine how long food can be kept. Thus, for a subsistence family in a developing country, physical factors are extremely important determinants. Their access to the local market and the range of foods available there will have a major impact on the food they eat.

TABLE 2.1 Factors influencing the availability of foods			
Physical/environmental	**Legislative**	**Economic**	**Food handling**
Locality (soil/climate)	National/international laws	Money	Access to shops
Transport/marketing		Budget priorities	Cooking skills
Distribution costs	Health recommendations	Cost of foods	Knowledge
Perishability		Significance of foods	Cooking facilities
		Variety	Time available

TABLE 2.2 Factors influencing the acceptability of foods		
Cultural	**Physiological**	**Social/psychological**
National identity	Physiological need	Status (of self/of foods)
Culture group	Hunger/satiety	Group identity
Core, secondary and peripheral foods	Appetite/aversion	Communication
Meal patterns	Sensory appeal	Ritual
Religious ideology	Personal preference/choice	Emotional support
Taboos/prohibitions	Therapeutic diets	Reward/punishment

Legislative factors

Government legislation aims to ensure that food available for purchase is of a suitable quality and has not been adulterated. There is also agricultural policy, which regulates the prices received by the producers of crops. Trade agreements and sanctions may operate at particular times between different countries. In addition, the UK, as a member state of the European Union, is subject to Europe-wide laws relating to food and agricultural production. All these factors will influence the type of food available for sale in shops and its exact composition, especially in terms of additives and minimum standards of composition.

In recent years, the labelling of foods has become more explicit, with more information about the nutritional composition appearing on the label. This is to be applauded as an important means of educating people about nutrition, as well as providing useful information for anyone who wishes to understand more about the food they eat. European laws on labelling affect products marketed in the UK.

Legislation has also been needed to control the introduction of some of the new foods resulting from developments in food technology. Recent introductions in Britain have included irradiated foods, items produced from research in genetic engineering and foods containing synthetic substitutes (e.g. for fat). In addition, there is a growing market in 'functional foods'. All have been the subject of safety testing, and have needed to obtain government approval before being marketed.

Economic factors

The cost of food is a major determinant of what people perceive as available to them; it ranks only after taste in general surveys of influences on choice. Within the range of foods available to them, people can only eat what they can afford, or choose to afford. The second point is important, since it brings into consideration the priorities that exist in spending money. The annual National Food Survey shows that in 2000 (DEFRA, 2001) on average people in Britain spent 9.5 per cent of their budget on food, although this is less among the better off, and can be much more (up to 30 per cent or more) among lower income groups. Even though the percentage of income spent is higher, the amount of money spent is actually less; in 2000, households in the lowest income group spent 15 per cent less than the UK average on food and drink. People see their food budget as one of the more flexible items in their expenditure; other expenses such as fuel, rent, cigarettes and alcohol may take priority. When income is small and food budget cuts are made, food distribution within the family may change, food treats may still be bought and the children's likes and dislikes attended to. The variety of foods eaten becomes smaller and the diet becomes more monotonous. These issues are discussed further in Chapter 13.

Food handling

If food is available and there is money with which to buy it, bringing it home and preparing it for eating remain as possible areas of difficulty. Getting to the shops and bringing food home may be a major problem, especially for families with no car, older people or those with disabilities. This will determine where the shopping is done, how often and the sorts of foods that can be bought and carried home. Many supermarkets in Britain have moved to peripheral locations outside towns, which makes shopping easier for the car-owning customers who spend a lot of money, but very difficult for those families living further away, without transport. These then rely on the local shops, which inevitably keep less stock, thereby restricting choice.

Once the food is in the kitchen, most of it has to be prepared in some way for eating. This will depend largely on the knowledge and skill of the cook, facilities and time available. Cooking skills are variable; it has been suggested that fewer people now know how to cook. This has been attributed to the escalating reliance on pre-prepared convenience foods, which eliminate the need for cooking skills. Often the only skill required is the ability to open a packet or can and heat the contents. Some foods can even be eaten cold out of the packaging in which they were bought. In families where cooking does take place, the complexity of the preparation of the food will reflect the cook's personal experience of food and cooking, education, interest and time available.

Acceptability

Cultural factors

Each cultural group possesses its own typical food selection patterns. These may be similar to those of related cultural groups, but are unlikely to be the same. Even within a relatively small country such as the UK, there are different regional foods, such as haggis in Scotland, laver bread in Wales and jellied eels in London. However, all these groups also share similar 'British' food choices, such as fish and chips or roast beef. It is not just the choice of food that may vary between the cultures, but also the way in which it is cooked, the seasonings and flavourings used and the way it is served.

Traditional foods confer a sense of identity and belonging. This is very deeply held, since for most people it derives from the socialization process in childhood, discussed earlier. The strength and persistence of this cultural identity may be illustrated by two examples. First, when people holiday in another country, many will seek out foods with which they are familiar. Although they may be prepared to try the local dishes, it is often with a sense of curiosity and a preconceived idea that they will be strange. More importantly, when people emigrate to another country for long-term settlement, they often suffer a sense of alienation or difference from the adopted environment. They may adopt the host country's style of dress and speak the language, but the food that is eaten in the privacy of their home may remain very traditional. This provides a link with the homeland and support in an alien environment.

If in addition to providing a cultural identity, the food is also associated with religious beliefs, traditional food habits may persist longer still. Studies on migrants to Britain show that first-generation members adhere strongly to traditional food practices. With the second generation, these practices are less widespread, unless they are associated with religious prescription. Conflict may arise between the generations as a result. Short-term migration does not, however, bring about changes to the diet, with evidence pointing to a reluctance to include host-country foods and an adherence to traditional foods, even if they are hard to find.

The types of foods that may be served to form a meal are culturally determined. People may classify foods in different ways: for example, into 'sweet' and 'savoury', or 'healthy' and 'less healthy', 'snack food' (or 'junk food') and 'proper meal'. Nutritionists categorize foods more systematically in terms of their main nutritional role in the diet. Currently, most Western countries use five food groups: cereal/grain (or starchy) foods, fruit and vegetables, meat and meat substitutes, milk and dairy produce, fatty and sugary foods. An appropriate amount of each group should be eaten to provide a nutritionally balanced diet.

Foods can also be described in terms of their place in the diet, as core, secondary or peripheral foods (Table 2.3).

As well as providing the accepted norms for what can be eaten, cultural identity will also determine what should not be eaten. Each culture has clearly defined ideas about what is 'food' and 'non-food'. In many instances, these distinctions have arisen for sound reasons, including scarcity of a particular plant or animal, or its potential harmfulness. In addition, there may be prohibitions on particular foods at certain times of life, particularly in infancy and during pregnancy. Many cultures have prohibitions associated with pregnancy, based on beliefs about possible effects on the fetus. Although generally harmless, some may restrict intakes of foods, such as meat or other useful sources of iron, for which needs are increased in pregnancy. It is also believed by some that eating a particular mixture of foods around the time of conception can influence the gender of the embryo.

A taboo that occurs in most world cultures is that against cannibalism, but even this deep-rooted taboo is not universal. There are records throughout history of people reverting to cannibalism in times of severe hardship, such as wartime siege, or following an air crash in an inaccessible region, as well as some cases of murder followed by cannibalism.

Many world religions also forbid the eating of particular foods completely or at special times. These include a prohibition on pork among Muslims and Jews, and on all animals

TABLE 2.3	Core, secondary and peripheral foods	
Core foods	**Secondary foods**	**Peripheral foods**
The most important foods in the diet – the staple of the region (normally a cereal or a root)	Enhance the meal, but not essential	Non-essential, but pleasant to eat
Usually one or two foods only (in Britain: bread/cereals and potatoes)	May have specific perceived properties (e.g. protein-rich, healthy, promoting balance, suitable for particular ages/ conditions in life)	Special occasion foods, e.g. eaten at festivals, celebrations (e.g. turkey at Christmas or Thanksgiving, birthday cake)
Tend to appear in most meals	May include meat/fish, vegetables, pulses, fruit	Food with special properties, e.g. bedtime drinks
Nutritionally, a source of carbohydrate, some protein and a range of minerals and vitamins		May include biscuits, cakes confectionery, alcoholic drinks, exotic fruit, sauces, drinks, e.g. tea/coffee

Activity 2.3

Make a list of your food intake over the previous few days. For each food, identify to which of the categories in Table 2.3 it belongs.
- Which of the categories appears most frequently?
- Are your meals made up of all three categories?
- What about your snacks?

among the Hindus. These are considered further in Chapter 13.

Physiological factors

Appetite is associated with memories of particular foods, and is the desire for a specific food or foods. In animals, there is some evidence that such desires for particular foods are linked to a specific nutritional need. This is very difficult to demonstrate in humans and has, therefore, not been proven. The opposite is an aversion to a specific food; this is often linked to an unpleasant memory of that food or an experience associated with it.

Personal preferences for foods are usually linked to a liking for the sensory attributes of the food, which contribute to the pleasure of eating it. Liking a food is frequently given as the main reason for choosing it; however, people will eat foods they feel neutral about, or even dislike in certain circumstances, for example, to please others. Most people select their food from a relatively small number of items that appear frequently in their diet. New foods may be tried on occasions, often as a result of advertising or promotion of the product in the media. The wealthier members of society include more variety in their choices than those on a low income. Compared with traditional hunter–gatherer societies, who would eat a wide range of wild products from the land at different seasons, our Western diet is quite limited.

Children are considered to be the age group most reluctant to diversify their diet, with some individuals eating so few foods that they threaten their nutritional status.

Because of the importance of personal preference in making food choice, it is important that individuals are allowed to exercise some control over what is eaten. Loss of control can lead to loss of appetite. This can be a reason for poor intakes in hospitalized patients or residents in other institutions, where menus are centrally determined, perhaps repetitive and little choice is offered.

The need to follow a special diet for therapeutic reasons will affect personal food selection, and is a further area where loss of control and self-determination may cause problems with compliance. This is a particular problem in adolescents, who may refuse to comply with dietary restrictions, as part of the maturing process. Food selection may be deliberately restricted in those wishing to control their weight: eating behaviour becomes inhibited, and less food than is required to alleviate hunger may be eaten. Also, specific food groups (the 'fattening foods') may be avoided, while others are eaten in their place (the 'slimming foods'). If the inhibition of intake is broken, for a number of reasons, food intake may become excessive, resulting in binge eating, until the inhibitory influence is restored. This pattern of restrained eating appears to exist, to a greater or lesser extent, in up to 80–90 per cent of women in Western society. In some it results in clinically recognized conditions of anorexia or bulimia nervosa.

Special diets may be adopted for moral or ideological perspectives, and these will impose constraints on individual food choice. Of these, the vegetarian diet has become the most prevalent in Britain in recent years. The extent to which people stop eating all animal produce varies, and some of those claiming to be vegetarian may still actually consume some animal foods, even white meat as well as fish, eggs, cheese and milk. Reasons for choosing this diet may stem from abhorrence of the killing of animals (and the methods used), and concern about the exploitation of animals reared in cramped conditions for food. More recent publicity about aspects of food safety related to foods of animal origin, such as beef, chicken, eggs and milk, has convinced others that avoiding these foods may be healthier (see Chapter 13 for further discussion).

Whatever the rationale for the special diet, the individual's freedom of choice is restricted. It makes the person different from the rest of their culture group (this may be one of the objectives!). Consequently, it may create barriers to the sharing of food, causing alienation and possibly avoidance of social eating situations, or lack of compliance with therapeutic diets. Giving as much freedom of choice as possible within the constraints of a special diet will help the individual to regain their self-determination and enhance compliance.

Choosing to follow a 'healthy' diet is a positive choice made by an increasing number of people. This has arisen from the recognition that many of the diseases prevalent in Western society may have a dietary origin. The understanding of these links may not be very accurate and even confused, as may also the understanding of what constitutes a 'healthy' diet. A common belief is that eating too much fat causes heart disease in men, or that too much chocolate will make women fat. Thus, one or two aspects of current dietary guidelines may be adopted, while others are ignored. Only a tiny percentage of the population manage to achieve all of the dietary guidelines, and the idea of a 'whole-diet' approach to healthy eating has not been widely recognized. The concept of 'healthiness' also becomes blurred by food safety issues, including concerns about additives in foods, genetically modified products, food that is not fresh, ready-made foods containing unknown ingredients and possible contamination by microorganisms, such as *Listeria* or *Salmonella.*

Social/psychological influences

Although our own physiological needs and wants are important determinants of what we find acceptable to eat, we are nevertheless also influenced in our actions by the prevailing social conditions, as well as our own psychological make-up.

Food and the way it is presented can be used to express status in society. The most obvious distinction is that between having and not having food. The wealthy generally have access to more and varied food, while the poor have less choice and are more likely to go hungry. In some societies, it is a sign of wealth and status to be obese.

Individual foods may also have differing status: those that are more expensive or difficult to get, such as grouse, venison or caviar, will be perceived as being high status. On the other hand, foods such as tripe or pig's trotters may be equally unusual, but because of their association with low-income diets, have a low status. Everyday foods, such as potatoes, sausages and baked beans, will also have relatively low status. The status of foods may change with time, depending on how they are valued. For example, in the nineteenth century, brown bread was considered coarse and fit only for the lower classes; now it is seen as healthy and desirable in the diet, and its status has increased considerably.

What is eaten in particular circumstances is likely to reflect the assumed status of the food. When eating alone, it does not matter what we eat, and people may 'treat' themselves to combinations of foods that they would not eat in company. As soon as food is eaten in company, value judgements are made on the basis of the foods. The status of the foods served reflects the implied status in which the diners are held. Thus, the type of food shared in a meal implies more than satisfying a physiological need. Sharing food with others is very symbolic: it confirms previously established links, and a sense of mutual identity. There is also powerful peer pressure in food selection.

Relationships within groups of people are confirmed in the sharing of food: usually the most powerful or most important members of the group are served first. This not only confirms their superiority, but allows them to choose the prime parts of the meal.

The food preferences of men and women often differ; in most cultures men consume more meat and women consume more fruit and vegetables. Women tend to eat more of the foods that are regarded as 'healthy'. It is suggested that these differences are associated with the traditional gender roles, which still exist in society. Women remain in charge of the food-related activity; therefore, they tend to know more about food. Information about healthy diets tends to be seen more by women, as it features in women's magazines, or in leaflets available from supermarkets or in doctors' surgeries. However, despite this greater knowledge, or level of information, decisions about what is eaten are shown to be dictated in many families by the men and children, rather than the women. Studies of changes in food intake on marriage show that both partners make some adjustments,

with husbands adopting more of the wives' habits initially, but reverting to their original habits in time. Nevertheless, married men tend to have healthier diets than single men.

Differences have also been reported in the way food is eaten, with men taking gulps and mouthfuls, whereas women nibble and pick. As a consequence of this, it is suggested that some foods are more appropriate for women (such as fish or fruit) and other foods for men (red meat, bread).

Food can be a powerful means of communication. A box of chocolates given as a present is perhaps the most widely used example of food acting as a token of affection. Some may find it easier to give the chocolates than to put into words what they are feeling. A cup of tea is a typically British answer to a difficult social situation, when words are hard to find. A family eating a meal together is sharing not only food, but the affection they feel for each other. Rejecting the meal in this situation can, therefore, be a very potent dismissal of the love being offered. Reciprocal invitations to meals or parties by both adults and children strengthen the social bonds. Children may exchange small items of food, such as sweets, to communicate their friendship.

A special form of communication by means of food exists in the ritual use of food. Many religions use foods as offerings to their deities. Christians use bread and wine. The end of the growing season and the harvest are marked in many communities by a festival, with a sample of the crops being offered in thanksgiving, often to the poorest members of the community.

Certain life events are marked by specific ritual meals – baptismal feasts, wedding breakfast, the funeral wake. Group membership may also be marked by rituals involving food or drink; for example, the pre-wedding ritual of stag night and hen party, where the men and the women separately undergo a 'rite of passage', usually involving large amounts of alcohol.

Food represents security from the earliest age, so that in times of stress it can form an important support. Anxiety can provoke eating as a means of coping with tension, although in some individuals stress can result in a loss of appetite and an inability to eat. Anxiety may also lead to feeding others, for example, anxious mothers may overfeed their children to relieve their own anxiety about them. Abnormal eating patterns have also been linked with uncertainty about a person's role or position in society. It has been suggested that both overweight and anorexia nervosa may originate from a dissociation between the socially desirable body image and that with which the individual feels psychologically at ease.

In the case of obesity, it is argued that overeating occurs as a deliberate attempt to add substance to the body (generally female) in an effort to cope with the demands of the world. In anorexia nervosa, the body size is deliberately reduced to escape from the pressures of society on the adult female, and return to the child shape.

SUMMARY

1 Eating is regulated by the brain, which integrates many afferent signals coming from external and internal sources. This allows food intake to be matched to metabolic needs. However, this regulation is more efficient for some components of the diet than for others.
2 Apart from the physiological need to eat, food intake is also regulated by psychological needs, social influences, the sensory satisfaction obtained from eating, and by habit.
3 What is eaten is also influenced by many factors that determine both the availability of food and its acceptability to the individual.
4 Despite many differences between cultures in actual foods eaten, influences on eating and food choice are similar.
5 The interaction of influencing factors may be a key determinant in achieving dietary change.

STUDY QUESTIONS

1 What information is available to the brain to allow food intake to be regulated? Consider the macronutrients in the diet and discuss how precise this regulation is for each one.
2 The sensory appeal of food in very important. Give examples of some situations where:
   a sensory properties may not be detected by the eater;
   b additional care needs to be taken to enhance sensory appeal.
3 Consider the food habits of members of your family or your immediate friends.
   a Have they changed in the last 10 years?
   b If so, can you account for any changes?
   c If they have remained the same, what have been the major factors maintaining this consistency?

4 Suggest ways in which government action could influence food habits. What barriers to change might this encounter?
5 What might be the nutritional consequences of a diet composed entirely of:
   a core foods
   b secondary foods
   c peripheral foods?
6 In what ways can the following influence food habits:
   a travel
   b education
   c multi-ethnic societies?

REFERENCES AND FURTHER READING

Blundell, J.E., Halford, J.C.G. 1994: Regulation of nutrient supply: the brain and appetite control. *Proceedings of the Nutrition Society* 53, 407–18.

Burnett, C. 1994: The use of sweets as rewards in schools. *Journal of Human Nutrition and Dietetics* 7, 441–6.

Charles, N., Kerr, M. 1988: *Women, food and families*. Manchester: Manchester University Press.

Cotton, J.R., Burley, V.J., Weststrate, J.A. et al. 1994: Dietary fat and appetite: similarities and differences in the satiating effect of meals supplemented with either fat or carbohydrate. *Journal of Human Nutrition and Dietetics* **7**, 11–24.

Craig, P.L., Truswell, A.S. 1994: Dynamics of food habits of newly married couples: who makes changes in the foods consumed? *Journal of Human Nutrition and Dietetics* **7**(5), 347–62.

DEFRA, 2001: *National Food Survey 2000 Annual report on food expenditure, consumption and nutrient intakes*. London: The Stationery Office.

Margetts, B.M., Thompson, R.L., Speller, V. et al. 1998: Factors which influence 'healthy' eating patterns: results from the 1993 Health Education Authority health and lifestyle survey in England. *Public Health Nutrition* **1**(3), 193–8.

Mennell, S., Murcott, A., van Otterloo, A.H. 1992: *The sociology of food: eating, diet and culture*. London: SAGE Publications.

Stubbs, R.J., Harbron, C.G., Murgatroyd, P.R. et al. 1995: Covert manipulation of dietary fat and energy density: effect on substrate flux and food intake in men eating ad libitum. *American Journal of Clinical Nutrition* **62**(2), 316–29.

Weststrate, J.A. 1996: Fat and obesity. *British Nutrition Foundation Nutrition Bulletin* **21**, 18–25.

Wilding, J.P. 2002: Neuropeptides and appetite control. *Diabetic medicine* **19**, 519–27.

Wood, R.C. 1995: *The sociology of the meal*. Edinburgh: University Press.

BASICS OF A HEALTHY DIET

The aims of this chapter are to:

❏ review the development of ideas about healthy eating;
❏ describe the basis and application of dietary reference values;
❏ discuss the dietary goals that have been put forward, and some of the dietary planning tools and mechanisms that are available to assist with constructing a diet.

On completing the study of this chapter, you should be able to:

❏ explain the fundamental ideas about healthy eating and the goals that have been developed;
❏ understand the significance of dietary reference values and be able to use them appropriately;
❏ use a dietary planning guide to evaluate diets;
❏ understand and show how to make use of information available on food labels in constructing a diet;
❏ evaluate information given in pamphlets about healthy eating;
❏ explain the health implications of alcohol consumption.

In Chapter 2 the factors affecting food habits and food choice were discussed. The choice of foods offered to people in Western societies is enormously diverse, with novel foods being developed by food technologists. However, instead of making it easier for us to choose what to eat according to our particular desires at a specific time, the increased variety makes it more difficult. Consequently, many people cope with the huge selection, often over 6000–9000 different items in a major supermarket, by consistently selecting only a very narrow range of foods.

In addition, many people are increasingly concerned with improving their health, and consumers wish to make food choices that will help in this. Various views are put forward to support particular dietary choices; the most polarized are those between plant-based or meat-based diets. There is now a substantial body of evidence to support the view that, where food is abundant, increasing the intake of plant-based foods, in particular fruit and vegetables, can help to reduce the incidence (i.e. the number of new cases in a given time period in a population) of chronic disease. However, the exact proportions of meat-based and plant-based foods in the diet that might support optimal health are impossible to determine. Epidemiological evidence does, however, support the view that diets based largely on plant foods are most associated with health and longevity, where food supplies are adequate. It is thus particularly important to provide some guidance for people to be able to select foods that will help to maintain their health.

A HEALTHY DIET – WHICH FOODS TO CHOOSE?

If we are interested in and committed to taking care of ourselves and others, the 'healthiness' of our selection of food needs to be considered. However, 'healthiness' is not the only feature we look for in our food. Most of us would be very reluctant to eat an unfamiliar food just because we were told it was healthy; the property of healthiness would be included in the general consideration of the food in deciding whether or not to include it in the diet.

However, food that constitutes a 'healthy diet' is in the main not very different from that which makes up a less healthy diet – it is the balance of the parts making up the total meal or diet that is important. As has been said elsewhere in this book, there are no 'bad' foods; it is their place in the general picture of the diet that is important. Some foods provide only a very narrow range of nutrients, perhaps even just one. If such foods comprise a substantial part of the daily intake, the consumer will run the risk of not meeting nutritional requirements for a range of nutrients. The greater the range of foods, the less likely are there to be 'gaps' in the nutrient intake, and the more likely it is that the consumer will meet the nutritional needs.

We are attracted by variety in foods, and would find a diet containing just one or two foods very monotonous. This might result in a smaller intake of the foods. The converse is also true: when presented with a variety of foods, we move from one to another and are likely to eat more. The appearance of a tempting

dessert after a filling meal can readily override feelings of satiety, simply because of the novelty aspect!

Selecting several foods is, therefore, beneficial for our nutrient intake. Traditional meal patterns can help us to decide on combinations of foods to make up meals, as well as what foods to have at specific points of our day. The pattern of core, secondary and peripheral foods discussed in Chapter 2 serves as a general guide. It must be recognized that there is increasing variation in this pattern. It is possible that, in future generations, meals may be quite different, although there are also signs of a 'traditionalist revival', which may take us back to the old-established food patterns.

A HEALTHY DIET – HOW MUCH TO EAT?

In addition to deciding what foods to eat, each person makes a decision about the quantity to consume. From experience we have learned what is an adequate serving size for us and this obviously varies between individuals.

Our ability to assess how much of a food we would like to eat relies on learned responses established during our childhood and added to whenever a new food has been introduced. The sensations arising from the stomach when a particular serving size has been eaten will be remembered and will help to determine our behaviour in the future. Other reflex pathways, linked to the metabolic consequences of the meal, may also be part of the regulatory process. It is believed that this type of learning is an important component of the control of food intake (as discussed in Chapter 2).

The variability of 'normal' serving sizes between individuals is a dilemma for those studying food intakes in populations. There is no such thing as an 'average' serving size, which would apply to everyone. However, for the sake of expediency, such a measure is quoted and used in many contexts. However, in relation to this 'average', it is recognized that different people will also have 'large' and 'small' servings. Interpretations of these are also subjective and, therefore, variable.

Activity 3.1

Make a list of foods that you usually eat during the course of a week. Divide them up into four columns: foods eaten at breakfast, lunch, evening meal, and snack foods.

■ Is this easy to do? If so, you have got strong ideas about what foods are appropriate at what times, and in what meals. If you found it quite hard to do, this may be because you have a much 'freer' food structure, and the items in your diet may serve several roles.

■ Check with a partner how easy their list was to write into columns.

■ Finally, check how much agreement there is between your list and your partner's – do you consider the same foods as appropriate at particular times?

Activity 3.2

1 *Observation*: During the next few days, use any opportunities you may have to observe people at mealtimes. Notice whether the amounts of food items they consume are similar to or greater/smaller than you would choose.

2 *Quantitative assessment*: If you have access to dietary or household weighing scales, make measurements of the typical serving size that you select of everyday foods. Ask members of your family or your colleagues/friends to do the same. Collate the information from as many different people as possible.
   ▪ How much variation do you find?
   ▪ Are portion sizes for some foods more variable than others?
   ▪ Can you offer explanations for this?
   ▪ What are the health implications of people's different concepts of 'appropriate' serving size?

Dietitians try to resolve this issue by using replica foods, which generally represent the 'average' serving. Patients may then indicate whether the amount they would consume is similar to this or different. There is always, of course, the tendency to claim that one's intake follows the average.

WHAT ARE THE FEATURES OF A 'HEALTHY' DIET?

This question is likely to produce a number of different responses from people, depending on their level of interest in nutrition and their understanding of the principles of health.

Answers will fall into one or several of the following categories.
▪ Eating more or less of particular foods.
▪ Eating more or less of particular nutrients.
▪ Eating specific foods that are believed to have 'healthy' properties. (This may include taking nutritional supplements or eating organically produced food.)

▪ Adopting particular diet-related practices, as well as lifestyle changes.
▪ Having a 'balanced diet'.

Each of these will be discussed in turn to consider how well they answer the question of what are the features of a healthy diet.

Eating more or less of particular foods

This response derives from the belief that there are 'good' foods and 'bad' foods, and that we should eat less of the latter and more of the former. Unfortunately, it is not a straightforward matter to classify foods in this manner; individual foods are less important than the way in which they are combined in diets. However, foods that contain a lot of fat or sugar, or those which have been extensively refined or processed, are likely to be of less value in a complete diet, since they reduce the nutrient density. This means that the remaining foods in the diet must contain more of the micronutrients to compensate.

This can be a particular problem in people who have relatively small appetites, or who are sedentary and, therefore, have low energy needs, since their potential intake of the more nutritious foods in the diet will be limited.

Eating more or less of particular nutrients

This has been one way in which advice about healthy eating has been promoted. In many countries, initial dietary guidelines included advice to eat less fat (especially saturated fat), reduce salt and increase dietary fibre. It is not surprising, therefore, that these are now repeated by consumers as the central principles of healthy eating.

However, people eat foods and not nutrients. Foods (with a very few exceptions) are not simply a source of one nutrient and, therefore, reducing the intake of a certain group of nutrients by excluding particular foods from the diet may have consequences for other nutrients also found in those foods. For example, if milk and dairy products are excluded because of their fat content, this can have serious implications for intakes of calcium and riboflavin.

The corollary of this is that some foods contain a nutrient in quite large amounts. If this is not made explicit, the intake of that particular food may not be altered. For example, ordinary hard cheese (such as Cheddar cheese) is recognized by most people as a source of protein and calcium, important for growing children and for bones. However, it is also very rich in fat. In listing sources of fat, many people would omit to mention cheese, and will continue to eat it often in quite large amounts. If changes are made only to the most obvious sources of fat, such as the spreading fats, cooking oils and full-fat milk, but other sources including cheese, pastries, biscuits and cakes are not reduced, then the overall impact on total fat intakes will be small.

As a consequence, more recent dietary guidelines have moved away from this focus on nutrients and have reverted to giving advice on foods that should be included in the diet, together with advice about quantities.

Eating specific foods that are believed to have 'health-promoting' properties

There is a perception that only certain foods are healthy, and they should be included in the diet. Linked to this is the belief that, when these foods are present, it does not matter what else the diet contains. Thus, in practice, an individual might be eating all the wrong proportions of macronutrients, but believes the diet is healthy because it includes a high-fibre breakfast cereal and semi-skimmed milk. Clearly there is some confusion here. A single food or two cannot make a diet healthy, although they can begin to redress an unbalanced diet.

Another example in this category is the inclusion of nutritional supplements to correct deficiencies in the food consumed. Although the nutritional content may well be improved by the supplements, especially in terms of the micronutrients commonly found in supplements, the balance of macronutrients may still be unhealthy. Again the consumer has a mistaken perception that they are eating healthily.

Including 'organically' grown products in the diet may reduce the level of chemical additives and contaminants consumed, but again does not necessarily make the diet nutritionally better balanced.

The remedy for an unbalanced diet that contains unhealthy proportions of the macronutrients and perhaps inadequate amounts of the micronutrients lies in a change in the foods consumed, and an alteration in the proportions of the different food groups. Improving an imperfect diet can be likened to dealing with a plumbing problem in the house, such as a leaking pipe. It can be dealt with by putting a bucket underneath, and living with the problem; this parallels the taking of supplements or adding one or two 'healthy foods' to the diet. Alternatively, the householder can call in the plumber and have the pipe mended. Similarly, an individual can obtain nutritional advice, either from a dietitian or nutritionist, or from information booklets, and change their diet for the better. In the long term, the latter will clearly be the more satisfactory solution.

Adopting particular dietary practices or lifestyle changes

A whole range of behaviours may be included here. Some diet-related examples, which are suggested by people as 'healthy eating', might include:

- eating regularly
- having breakfast
- cutting down on convenience or junk foods
- eating home-cooked foods
- drinking water
- losing weight
- planning what to eat
- eating organic food
- eating less meat (especially red meat)
- eating more fish/fruit/vegetables.

(A survey of your friends and family would produce many more.)

Lifestyle changes might include:

- taking exercise
- not eating late at night
- giving up smoking
- reducing alcohol intake
- becoming vegetarian.

Although the latter are not strictly ways of obtaining a healthy diet, they may be perceived as part of the healthy lifestyle, which includes diet. This is most clearly seen amongst people who become vegetarian, who often make changes not only to dietary intake but also to many other aspects of life, frequently adopting a more 'environmentally sensitive' lifestyle.

It is not being suggested here that to eat healthily one should adopt a vegetarian diet, although this is a belief held by some. Diets can be healthy (and also unhealthy) whether they contain meat and animal products, or not.

Eating a 'balanced' diet

Although this can be an appropriate definition of what is meant by healthy eating, it is imprecise and, as such, is open to many interpretations. Over the last 40–50 years, the concept of a balanced diet has changed. Its earlier interpretation was of a diet that provided the macronutrients in sufficient amounts to prevent deficiency, with protein often seen as a priority. There was a belief that, if the macronutrients were adequate, then the micronutrients would 'take care of themselves'. This may have been true when the diet contained mostly food close to its natural state, with few processed and manufactured foods on the market.

More recently, it was realized that simply meeting the requirements for macronutrients does not lead to good health, as evidenced by the high rates of 'Western diseases', such as coronary heart disease, cancer as well as obesity. Clearly, something was wrong with this approach.

It is only in the last decade that the 'balance' concept has been clarified to show suggested proportions of different food groups to be included in the diet. This aims to meet both macronutrient and micronutrient needs, as well as achieving a balance of nutrients that could promote health. This has, therefore, involved a change in the concept of 'a balanced diet', which has perhaps not been recognized by everyone. In addition, levels of energy expenditure have fallen, so that energy intakes need to be less. It then becomes even more important to make sure that what is eaten has the appropriate balance of other nutrients.

In the UK, the Ministry of Agriculture, Fisheries and Food (MAFF) produced *Eight guidelines for a healthy diet* in 1990. These were intended to be an update on diet and health for people with some knowledge of nutrition, to give guidance on the balanced diet. The guidelines were as follows.

1 Enjoy your food.
2 Eat a variety of different foods.
3 Eat the right amount to be a healthy weight.
4 Eat plenty of foods rich in starch and fibre.
5 Don't eat too much fat.
6 Don't eat sugary foods too often.
7 Look after the vitamins and minerals in your food.
8 If you drink, keep within sensible limits.

These were supported by a number of additional information leaflets about food labelling and food safety. These guidelines are now still current in the UK, following their re-issue in 1998.

Similar dietary guidelines exist in other countries and are reviewed regularly. In the USA, there is a 5-yearly review. The most recent in-depth scientific review resulted in an expansion of the guidelines from seven to ten. These are intended for children from age 2 years and healthy adults. The new 2000 Dietary Guidelines for Americans are as follows (Johnson, 2000).

- Aim for a healthy weight.
- Be physically active each day.
- Let the pyramid guide your food choices.
- Eat a variety of grains daily, especially whole grains.
- Eat a variety of fruits and vegetables daily.
- Keep foods safe to eat.
- Choose a diet that is low in saturated fat and cholesterol and moderate in total fat.
- Choose beverages and foods that moderate your intake of sugars.
- Choose and prepare foods with less salt.
- If you drink alcoholic beverages, do so in moderation.

A comparison with the UK guidelines shows a great deal of common ground, as would be expected, as both derive from the scientific base that supports advice on healthy eating.

WHAT NUTRIENTS ARE NEEDED, AND IN WHAT AMOUNTS?

In practice, the majority of people have no idea about the actual quantities of nutrients they require each day, and yet most manage to obtain approximately sufficient amounts to maintain adequate health. Whether their health is as good as it could be (i.e. 'optimal') is a matter for debate.

Nutritionists require more specific information on which to base scientific and reasonable advice. The starting point for these figures is the nutritional requirement.

Nutritional requirement

Each individual uses or loses a certain amount of each nutrient daily; this amount must, therefore, be made available to the tissues either from the daily diet or from the body stores of that nutrient. If the nutrient is taken from body stores, it must be replaced at a later stage, otherwise the stores will gradually become depleted and the person will be totally reliant on their daily intake. Eventually, a deficiency state might develop, if the intake is insufficient.

The amount of each nutrient used daily is the physiological requirement. It is defined as the amount of a nutrient required by an individual to prevent signs of clinical deficiency. This amount varies between individuals; it could differ from day to day due to different levels of energy expenditure. It may also alter with the composition of the diet owing to changes in efficiency of absorption or utilization of nutrients.

There are, however, a number of inherent problems with this definition. First, it is argued that this approach, based as it is on the very least amount needed to survive without developing a deficiency, leaves no margin of safety. Consideration could be given to the provision of a nutrient store to act as a reserve in time of physiological stress or reduced intake. Second, it gives no guidance on how to determine the requirement for nutrients for which there is currently no recognized clinical deficiency. This applies to fats (except essential fatty acids) and sugars. Third, there are no universally agreed criteria of when clinical deficiency exists. This is because a clinical deficiency reflects one end of a continuum, making it difficult to define precisely, as indicated in Figure 3.1.

It is cumbersome to obtain individual values for each nutrient requirement. One solution is to look at the average requirements of groups of similar people and to define a reasonable

Adequate intake

Intake low

Stores replete

Stores being used; levels falling in circulation

Stores depleted/ levels of enzyme (or active form) falling

Enzyme/active form levels low/ signs of clinical deficiency

Figure 3.1 The stages of development of a clinical deficiency. This is a general guide to the progression from adequacy to deficiency. In some cases, the biochemical end-point may be very difficult to identify or there may be no specific signs associated with deficiency.

minimum level. The age of the child is taken as a basis for defining 'similar' children; for pregnant women, the stage of pregnancy is taken as the common basis; for other groups of the population, age and gender are common criteria. This is the approach used by the Panel on Dietary Reference Values of the Committee on Medical Aspects of Food Policy, which produced the most recent set of data for the UK in 1991 (DoH, 1991). This Panel derived information about nutritional requirements in a number of ways. These included:

- measures of the actual intakes of particular nutrients in populations that are apparently healthy;
- the intakes of nutrients that are required to maintain balance in the body;
- amounts of a nutrient needed to reverse a deficiency state;
- amounts needed for tissue saturation, normal biochemical function or an appropriate level of a specific biological marker.

The appropriate method has to be selected for each nutrient, taking into account its metabolic activity, mode of excretion, storage in the body and the availability of suitable biochemical indicators. None of the criteria used in determining the level of requirement is deemed perfect, but is the best available with the current state of knowledge.

DISTRIBUTION OF NUTRITIONAL REQUIREMENTS IN A POPULATION

When measurements of requirements are obtained from a sufficiently large population, the results are assumed to follow a typical 'normal' distribution curve. This indicates that, for the majority, the requirement is around the mean for the group, but some have higher requirements and some lower values. If the group is sufficiently large, then half will fall above the sample mean and half below it; this is simply a property of the distribution and not something peculiar to nutrition or requirements.

FROM REQUIREMENTS TO DIETARY REFERENCE VALUES

Having established the range of nutritional requirements for a particular nutrient, it is

LRNI: Lower reference nutrient intake
EAR: Estimated average requirement
RNI: Reference nutrient intake
SD: standard deviations

Figure 3.2 The normal distribution curve of nutrient requirements in a population and levels used for setting dietary recommendations.

necessary to define more precisely what would be an adequate level of intake to meet these requirements. Several options might be available (Figure 3.2). Setting the level at a point A, which is above the range of individual requirements, would ensure that everyone's needs were met but might pose a risk in terms of excessive intakes, if the nutrient was harmful in large amounts. There would also be cost implications – should people be encouraged to buy so much food to meet this high level? An alternative might be to set the level at point B, which is the mean. By definition, this would imply that this level of intake would be sufficient for half of the population, but would be inadequate for the other half. This would not be satisfactory for most nutrients. However, point B, which is defined as the estimated average requirement (EAR), is used as the reference value for energy intakes. This is because it would clearly be undesirable to advise people to consume a level of energy that was above the needs of most of the population. In addition, the reference values are actually intended for use by groups. Within a group, there will be some whose energy needs are above and some below the EAR. If the food provided, or consumed, contains an amount of energy that reaches the EAR, and the individuals eat to appetite, then one can assume that their energy needs are being met. If the mean energy provided or consumed lies below the EAR, this suggests that some of the group may not be reaching their EAR and, conversely, a mean intake above the EAR implies an excessive intake of energy amongst some members of the group. However, judgements about individuals cannot be made by comparison with the EAR figure, as this is a group mean.

In practice, for the majority of nutrients, the Panel followed the pattern of previous committees and used a point that is towards the upper end of the distribution curve of nutritional requirements, at the mean + 2 standard deviations. Because of the particular properties of this type of distribution curve, this point (C) covers the requirement figures for 97.5 per cent of the population. It could be argued that this leaves 2.5 per cent of the population outside the limits and, therefore, at risk of an inadequate intake. However, in practice, it was felt that an individual would not have extremely high requirements for all nutrients, and it was thus unlikely that anyone would consistently fail to meet requirements across the range. Eating to satisfy appetite would be likely to ensure adequate intake.

Therefore, to summarize, point C was identified as the reference nutrient intake (RNI). In addition, the Panel identified point D, at the lower end of the requirement range. This represents the mean − 2 standard deviations, and covers the requirements of only 2.5 per cent of the population, who fall below this level. Again, it is possible that there are some people who have nutritional requirements consistently below this point and who may, therefore, meet their needs at this level of intake. However, it is more probable that, if someone is consuming an intake as low as this, they are not meeting their nutritional requirement. This point has been called the lower reference nutrient intake (LRNI). It effectively represents the lowest level that might be compatible with an adequate intake.

The dietary reference value (DRV) tables (published by the UK Department of Health as Report 41; DoH, 1991), therefore, provide three distinct figures for the majority of nutrients: the LRNI, EAR and RNI, which can be used as a yardstick to give a guide on the adequacy of diets. The Panel chose a new name for these figures, moving from the recommended daily amount (RDA), which was used previously. It was felt that

this name had been too prescriptive, suggesting that the amounts given referred to what individuals must consume. The corollary of this was that intakes that fell below the RDA were deemed to be deficient.

In setting the dietary reference values with a range of figures, the Panel intend the range to be used and, therefore, to provide more flexibility in assessing dietary adequacy. In addition, the DRV tables contain other data on dietary requirements for fats and carbohydrates, and some micronutrients for which little information was available.

Fats and carbohydrates

The approach to dietary requirements based on deficiency is not appropriate for nutrients having no specific clinical deficiency. Consequently, in the past, no RDA figures were set for fats and carbohydrates. There is now considerable public health interest in fat and carbohydrate intakes, and a desire for guidance on intake levels. The DRV Panel used their judgement, therefore, based on research evidence of health risks at particular levels of intake, to arrive at population average figures for the components of dietary fats and carbohydrates as well as nonstarch polysaccharides. Rather than giving absolute figures, the DRV values are expressed in terms of the percentage of total energy, which ideally should come from the various components (Table 3.1). To provide further guidance, individual minimum and maximum values are cited for some of the components.

Some micronutrients

In the case of some of the micronutrients, insufficient data were available to establish a normal distribution of requirements and thence derive values for LRNI and RNI. In these cases, the Panel, wishing to give guidance, have provided a 'safe intake' figure, which is considered to be sufficient to fulfil needs, but is not so high that there is a risk of undesirable effects.

In the USA, a similar approach has been adopted in the revision of the Recommended Daily Allowances that had been set in 1989. Since 1998, the National Academy of Sciences has constituted a number of expert panels to prepare a comprehensive set of reference values

TABLE 3.1	Dietary reference values for fat and carbohydrate for adults, as a percentage of daily total food energy intake (excluding alcohol)		
	Individual minimum	**Population average**	**Individual maximum**
Saturated fatty acids		11	
Cis-polyunsaturated fatty acids		6.5	10
n-3	0.2		
n-6	1.0		
Cis-monounsaturated fatty acids		13	
Trans-fatty acids		2	
Total fatty acids		32.5	
Total fat		35	
Non-milk extrinsic sugars	0	11	
Intrinsic and milk sugars		39	
Total carbohydrate		50	
Non-starch polysaccharides (g/day)	12	18	24

From DoH, 1991. Crown Copyright is reproduced with the permission of Her Majesty's Stationery Office.

for nutrient intakes for healthy US and Canadian populations. A number of reports have presented Dietary Reference Intakes (DRI) for vitamins and some minerals. These parallel the DRV figures published by DoH (1991) in the UK. The DRI includes a number of values as follows.

- Recommended dietary allowance (RDA), which covers the needs of most individuals in a particular life stage and gender group.
- Estimated average requirement (EAR), which represents the mean requirement of the individuals in a population.
- Adequate intake (AI) represents an amount for a nutrient that is believed to satisfy needs, but for which there is insufficient evidence to describe the full range of reference intakes.
- Tolerable upper intake level (UL) – the highest level of a nutrient intake that is likely to pose no risk of adverse health effects for almost all individuals in the general population. As intake increases above UL, the risk of adverse effects increases.

Although the figures presented in the US tables are not always the same as those in the UK, they provide similar guidance on the range of nutrient intakes compatible with health.

If the UK tables are compared with those produced by the Food and Agriculture Organization/ World Health Organization (FAO/WHO) or by other countries, differences both in the range of nutrients listed and the amounts advised are found. This implies two things. First, there are differences in needs between peoples of certain countries, as a result of differing lifestyles and perhaps different genetic make-up of the population. Therefore, when tables of reference values are used, they should be those relating to the country in question. Second, opinions differ between the committees drawing up the tables in different countries as to the safety margins that should be added to the figures. As a result, final figures also differ. This does not mean that some are more 'correct' than others; it reflects differences in emphasis and serves to underline the uncertainty surrounding such figures. It is important to remember that these figures are never an 'absolute' when their uses are considered. They are basically the 'best judgement' based on the physiological and nutritional data available at the time.

Practical applications

For individuals

It is important to remember that the DRV tables are not designed for use to judge individual nutritional intakes for their adequacy. They should rather be applied to groups of healthy individuals. However, since in practice they are used to assess individual diets, some words of caution are necessary.

Figure 3.3 shows the results of a riboflavin intake study in a large group of boys. Three boys in this group (boys A, B and C) were found to have intakes of A, B and C mg respectively.

The following conclusions can be drawn from the results:

■ With an intake of A mg, we can be fairly sure that boy A is not reaching his nutritional requirement for riboflavin, since it falls at the level of the LRNI. He may already be showing signs of clinical deficiency, such as dermatitis. If not, he should be investigated, and given advice on increasing his riboflavin intake.

■ Boy B's riboflavin intake, of B mg, is below the EAR for the group. However, this does not necessarily imply that he is receiving an inadequate intake. He may simply be a child with a low individual requirement. On the other hand, if he is not growing normally or showing signs of ill-health, his needs are probably not being met and his intake should be increased.

■ At first sight, boy C's intake of C mg seems to be quite adequate, as it almost reaches the RNI; it is quite likely that this is the case. However, the possibility could exist that he has a very high requirement, which is not being met by the current intake, even though it appears quite high. It can only be assumed that his intake is sufficient, if there is no evidence of inadequacy.

Figure 3.3 Distribution of riboflavin intakes in a population of 12-year-old boys.

Most people are unlikely to consume an amount of each nutrient to match the requirement exactly. However, it is probable that those with higher needs consume more than those whose needs are lower. The higher the correlation of intake and needs, the lower the risk of deficiency there is in any one individual. Unfortunately, the information about individual needs is not available and judgement must be used. The higher the intake level (i.e. the closer it is to the RNI), the lower the risk that it is inadequate. On the other hand, levels approaching the LRNI level are likely to carry a high risk of being inadequate.

Thus, a firm statement about an individual diet is only possible when the intake falls outside the range of RNI to LRNI. Nevertheless, the DRV Panel estimated that the risk of deficiency is about 15 per cent with an intake at the EAR, and falls to negligible levels when the intake approaches the RNI. However, it rises sharply at low levels of intake, approaching 100 per cent at the LRNI.

For groups of individuals

Group mean intakes eliminate the intra-individual variability and, therefore, allow more confident interpretation of results. When a group mean exceeds the RNI, the likelihood of many members of the group having intakes substantially below the RNI is small. Means around or below the RNI suggest that there are some members of the group whose intake may be inadequate. The lower the mean with respect to the RNI, the greater the chance that some members have an inadequate intake. This use is particularly important in evaluating dietary survey data.

For dietary planning

DRVs are used, for example, in institutions in planning diets for groups of individuals. In these cases, the RNI should be taken as the target (except for energy). Similarly, if a dietary prescription for an individual is being planned, then the RNI should be the target, since there is no other information about the actual needs of the individual.

Food labelling

Traditionally, food labelling has used the RDA value previously published in the UK. This corresponds to the current RNI level and is, therefore, sufficient or more than sufficient for 97.5 per cent of the population. In using this figure on food labels, the manufacturer may underestimate how much of the requirement for an individual is actually being supplied.

For example, suppose a food label claims that the food product provides, in a typical serving, 100 per cent of the RNI (or RDA) for vitamin C. Using the DRV figure, we can discover that it, therefore, supplies 40 mg. However, for an adult woman, the LRNI is only 10 mg, and the EAR is 25 mg. Therefore, for an individual whose needs are low, say 15 mg, this food product will actually supply 260 per cent of the actual needs. This is quite different from the claim of 100 per cent. As a result of such discrepancies, the Panel suggested that it would be better if EAR values were used in food labelling. However, the DRV figure does provide a reference point for the fortification of foods, and for the development of new food products.

The Institute of Grocery Distribution (IGD) in the UK has proposed a set of Guideline Daily Amounts (GDA) for use in food labelling. These are based on the predicted daily consumption of an average consumer eating a diet conforming to UK DRV (DoH, 1991) recommendations. The agreed GDA are as follows.

	Men	Women
Calories	2500	2000
Fat (g)	95	70
Saturated fat (g)	30	20

These figures are being used in some labelling in the UK, and help the consumer to see more simply how much fat and saturated fat the food contains as a part of the target daily intake.

Additional labelling directives operate in the UK, related to EU rulings, which use RDA as the basis for guidance. The RDA figures are EU agreed, and are not necessarily the same as the UK RNI or EAR figures. Thus, several yardsticks are in operation, each providing somewhat different information to the consumer.

DIETARY PLANNING

It is important that those who use figures from the dietary reference value tables should understand how they have been derived and, therefore, what are their uses and limitations. In practice, however, this is not always possible and, therefore, a means to translate the scientific information contained in the DRV tables into more accessible format is needed.

Meal planning tools

Many countries in the West have used meal selection guides for a number of years to help their consumers with healthy eating. Food guides provide a framework to show how foods can be combined together in a day's eating to provide an overall intake, which contains the appropriate range of nutrients. They achieve this by:

■ grouping together foods that provide (generally) similar nutrients, and that may be interchangeable in the diet;

■ making a quantitative statement about the number of 'servings' of foods from each group to be taken daily.

Food guides were first devised in the USA. They first appeared in 1916 and consisted of five food groups – milk and meat, cereals, vegetables and fruits, fats and fat foods, sugars and sugary foods. Further developments occurred between the 1940s and 1970s, with changes to the number and components of the groups used. Such changes reflected an increase in the understanding of the role of diet in health and disease prevention. In particular, more guidance was given about the consumption of fat, sugar and alcohol in the later guides than their earlier counterparts.

Most countries that have developed such a food guide use either the concept of a pyramid or a circle to illustrate that there are various components making up a whole diet. The most recent version of the USA Food Guide is a pyramid (Figure 3.4). This indicates that the foods in

Figure 3.4 The USA Food Guide pyramid: a guide to daily food choices. (Adapted from The Food Guide Pyramid. US Department of Agriculture/US Department of Health and Human Services.)

the groups at the base of the pyramid should be present in the greatest amounts and 'support' the diet. Progressive layers above this should be consumed in smaller amounts. By implication, those at the top (fats, oils and sweets) should be used sparingly, and are the least important components of the diet. The Guide indicates the numbers of servings as a range; individuals with lower nutritional needs (e.g. children) should take the lower number of servings. The Guide also does not apply to infant feeding.

Note also that the Guide does not imply that any single food is essential in the diet, no food alone provides all the necessary nutrients. What is important, however, is to include variety in the diet. In this way, shortcomings in one food are likely to be compensated by an adequate intake in another food. In 1999, a Food Guide adapted for children aged 2–6 years was published in

the USA. The nutritional messages are the same as those in the original Food Guide Pyramid. However, the foods pictured are those commonly eaten by children in this age group. In addition, the words used are shorter and the illustrations show active children, in an attempt to promote the importance of physical activity. Most children in the USA have been found not to meet the guidelines depicted in the Pyramid, especially with respect to the grains, fruit and dairy groups. This is resulting in concern about nutritional intakes, especially of sugars, saturated fats and very low calcium intakes. In addition, the rising prevalence (i.e. the numbers of people affected in the population) of overweight and obesity, that now affects over 20 per cent of children in the USA has led to this initiative, in an attempt to influence eating habits at a young age.

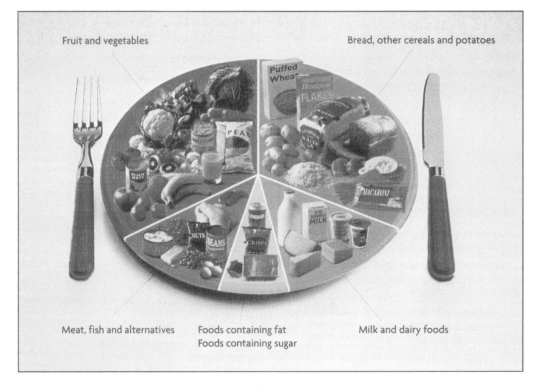

Fruit and vegetables

Bread, other cereals and potatoes

Meat, fish and alternatives

Foods containing fat
Foods containing sugar

Milk and dairy foods

Figure 3.5 The UK National Food Guide: the Balance of Good Health. (From Food Standards Agency 2001: *Balance of good health: information for educators and communicators.* London: Food Standards Agency.) Reproduced by kind permission of the Food Standards Agency.

In the UK, a National Food Guide (the Balance of Good Health) was launched for the first time in 1994 (Figure 3.5). The design is a tilted plate incorporating five food groups in the following proportions.

Segment size as per cent of whole plate	
Bread, other cereals and potatoes	33
Fruit and vegetables	33
Meat, fish and alternatives	12
Milk and dairy foods	15
Fatty and sugary foods	8

The nutritional details of the groups used in the Balance of Good Health are presented in Table 3.2.

The emphasis in the UK Guide is on foods, rather than nutrients, and shows the importance of considering the diet as a whole rather than concentrating on specific foods that may be 'good' or 'bad'. The format was selected after extensive consumer research, which considered a number of possible designs and tested preference for them amongst consumers and their performance as nutrition education tools.

The purpose of the Balance of Good Health is to allow all nutrition educators to provide a consistent message and thereby to reduce the confusion about the creation of a balanced diet. It is, therefore, intended that the Guide should be used widely to provide simple messages of balance and proportion of the food groups in a practical way. In addition, the Guide is intended to be sufficiently flexible to allow choices based on personal preferences and dietary habits, and to take into account availability, costs, cultural norms and ethnic diets. It is, therefore, not intended to be prescriptive.

As with any other food planning guide, the Balance of Good Health does not take into account the needs of those on special diets, infants and children under 5 years, or frail elderly people. Individuals in these groups may need to

TABLE 3.2   Nutritional details of the five groups in the UK National Food Guide (the Balance of Good Health)

Name of food group	Composition of food group	Key nutrients found in group
Bread, other cereals and potatoes	All breads made with yeast and other breads Cereals, including wheat, oats, barley, rice, maize, millet and rye together with products made from them, including breakfast cereals and pasta Potatoes in the form usually eaten as part of a meal (but not as a snack, e.g. crisps)	Carbohydrate NSP Vitamin B complex Calcium Iron (Recommend: ■ low-fat methods of cooking, and sauces/dressings, spreads ■ high-fibre varieties to maximize micronutrients)
Fruit and vegetables	Fresh, frozen, chilled and canned fruit and vegetables Fruit juices Dried fruit *Not included*: potatoes, pulses, nuts	Vitamins C, E and carotenes (antioxidant vitamins), folate Minerals: potassium, magnesium, trace minerals Carbohydrate NSP Majority are low in energy
Meat, fish and alternatives	Carcass meats, meat products (but not pastries and pies) Fish and fish products Poultry Eggs Pulses and nuts	Protein B vitamins (especially B_{12}) Minerals: phosphorus, iron, zinc, magnesium NSP (from pulses only) Long-chain polyunsaturated fatty acids (in oily fish) Meat and its products may be significant contributors to fat intake (low-fat alternatives available)
Milk and dairy foods	All types of milk Yoghurt Cheese	Protein Calcium Fat-soluble vitamins (except in low-fat varieties) B vitamins (riboflavin, B_{12}) *Not included*: butter and eggs
Fatty and sugary foods	Butter, margarine, fat spreads, oils and other fats Cream Crisps and fried savoury snacks Cakes, pastries, biscuits Chocolate and sugar confectionery Sugars and preserves Ice cream Soft drinks	Energy Fat Sugar Essential fatty acids Fat-soluble vitamins

NB: The Guide does not include composite dishes: these should be allocated to groups according to their main ingredients.

pay greater attention to the nutrient density of the foods consumed if their intakes are small.

The Guide also aims to help in achieving the dietary guidelines originally published by the UK Government in 1990 in the form of the *Eight guidelines for a healthy diet* (MAFF, 1990). The re-issue of these incorporates the Balance of Good Health as an illustration of how the two can be used in conjunction.

HOW TO USE THE BALANCE OF GOOD HEALTH

The Guide is concerned with the proportions of the foods in the diet. The simplest way to use the Guide, therefore, is to calculate the proportion of the total daily diet provided by foods from the different food groups in terms of numbers of servings eaten during the day. Some concern has been expressed that the definition of a 'serving' or 'portion' is not made explicit. However, it

should be remembered that for any one individual, servings of particular foods are consistent over time; it is the contribution of each of these servings to the whole diet that is important.

Figure 3.6 illustrates how the Guide can be applied to assess an individual diet. It is also possible to identify the shortcomings of the diet in this way, and use it as the basis for remedial advice. Adding together the numbers of servings gives the following percentages of the total:

Bread/cereal group	6 servings	= 30 per cent
Fruit and vegetables	4 servings	= 20 per cent
Meat and alternatives	4 servings	= 20 per cent
Dairy foods	2 servings	= 10 per cent
Fats and sugars	4 servings	= 20 per cent

It is, therefore, possible to see how this day's intake complies with the Balance of Good Health. Clearly, there is not quite enough of the bread and cereals group, far too little fruit and vegetables and rather too much of the remaining

Figure 3.6 Example of a day's food intake and the numbers of servings from the Balance of Good Health.

Activity 3.3

Now carry out a similar exercise on your own food intake. You may have already kept a record of a typical day, or several days' food intake. Make an assessment of the proportions of your diet coming from the various groups.
■ What groups are overrepresented?
■ Are some underrepresented?
Use the Balance of Good Health to suggest alternatives in the diet that could make the balance better.

three groups. In this way, it is possible to focus on which parts of the diet need attention and make suggestions for replacing foods.

A CONSISTENT MESSAGE

One of the main objectives of the Balance of Good Health is to provide a consistent message for all consumers about a balanced diet. There is evidence of confusion about a number of issues related to healthy eating. These can be found among many consumers as well as in the media, advertising and the catering industry. In particular, confusion exists in relation to intakes of specific nutrients or groups of nutrients. These include fat, complex carbohydrates and sugars, salt, alcohol and antioxidant nutrients. In addition, specific constituents of food, such as additives, or techniques used in food processing, for example, irradiation, cause concern and are linked to 'healthy eating'. Organic foods are generally perceived as being 'healthy', even when their nutrient composition is similar to that of non-organically produced foods. Exotic ingredients or foods are sometimes credited with exceptional nutritional properties; and (often unfounded) claims about 'live' yoghurt, honey, herb drinks and new 'functional foods' all add to the confusion of the consumer.

NUTRITION INFORMATION

There are numerous booklets and leaflets now available to the consumer produced by food companies, retailers, hospital trusts and many other organizations. How should these be viewed and what is the quality of the information they contain? Many of them are sound and very informative. Some, however, can be misleading, often not by what they actually include, but by judicious omission of key points.

When reading nutrition information leaflets, ask yourself the following questions.
■ Is the dietary advice being offered compatible with a balanced diet, as described by the Balance of Good Health?
■ Is the advice stressing the importance of one nutrient or food, to the exclusion of or in preference to others?
■ Is a particular product or brand being promoted?
■ Is there bias in the advice being given because of other interests that the sponsor of the leaflet may have?
■ Does the leaflet promise unrealistic outcomes?
■ Does the advice suggest that you buy products that you have never used before?
■ Is the advice being given appropriate to you and your lifestyle?
■ Is the leaflet written by a registered nutritionist or dietitian?
■ Is scientific evidence being quoted, including references to reputable sources of information?
■ Is there an address from which further information can be obtained?
If you can be satisfied that the evidence is balanced and unbiased, then the leaflet is likely to be worthwhile and can be a useful source of information. However, biased leaflets should not be used, as these simply add to the confusion.

It is simply not true that nutrition professionals are continuously changing their views and advice, as the media claim. Scientific debate is an important way of moving knowledge forward, and without it a subject stagnates and becomes dated. New ideas and fresh approaches are essential to continually check that our theories can be supported and that the advice we give is based on sound empirical evidence. The majority of nutrition experts do agree on the basic advice about healthy eating. Where there may be disagreement, it may reflect particular interests of the parties involved or relate to issues where the literature also conflicts.

THE QUESTION OF ALCOHOL

The consumption of alcohol is not discussed in the basic guidance on a balanced diet, as it is not an essential component of the diet and does not feature in all diets. Yet the consumption of alcohol is prevalent, with estimates suggesting that almost 90 per cent of the population in the UK consume alcohol at some time each year. Alcoholic beverages are consumed as part of many social activities, but consumption can also become excessive and result in physical, psychological and social harm to the individual as well as those around them. Economic estimates suggest that health and other problems related to alcohol consumption, including time away from work, represent a heavy financial burden. However, there is also very substantial revenue to the Government from the taxes levied on alcoholic beverages.

Published recommendations relating to alcohol generally adopt the perspective of limiting the intake rather than actively promoting consumption.

In order to quantify amounts of alcohol drunk from a variety of different sources, a standard 'unit' of alcohol has been developed. In the UK, this is equivalent to 8 g or 10 mL of ethanol. This amount of ethanol is found in the following measures of common drinks:

- ■ ½ pint of standard-strength beer (284 mL)
- ■ 1 measure of spirit (25 mL)
- ■ 1 glass of wine (125 mL).

Many other drinks are on the market that do not fit exactly into these categories and it can be difficult, without adequate labelling, to identify exactly how many units are present in a drink.

The definition of a unit differs between countries, and in the USA, equals 12 g of alcohol.

Benchmarks for safe levels of intake of alcohol have been published, using the concept of a unit. These are that men should not exceed 3–4 units per day and women should not exceed 2–3 units per day. In addition, there should be some drink-free days during the week. These benchmarks were introduced in 1995 to replace older guidelines that stated safe intakes to be 21 units and 14 units per week for men and women, respectively. There has been an increase in binge drinking, especially among young people, and amounts of this order were being consumed in one night. This was clearly not a safe intake, and the advice to spread alcohol consumption over a greater period of time was introduced as a consequence.

With progressively higher intakes, there is a greater risk of harm occurring. Consequences of excessive alcohol consumption include damage to every system of the body, including the liver, digestive system, heart, brain and nervous system. In addition, nutritional intake is likely to be affected and chronic overconsumption is associated with a number of specific nutritional deficiencies. Even at moderate intakes, it is likely that alcohol contributes to the total energy supply and this may result in weight gain. Social consumption of alcohol accompanying meals has been shown to be associated with a larger food intake as well as the consumption of higher levels of fat.

However, moderate alcohol consumption has also been linked to beneficial effects, particularly in protection against coronary heart disease. There is a J-shaped relationship between overall mortality and alcohol consumption, with abstainers and heavier drinkers having higher mortality rates than those seen in moderate drinkers. Maximum health advantage for coronary heart disease lies at levels of intake between 1–2 units per day. The reasons for the shape of this curve are still not agreed. In addition, the J-shaped relationship is now known to apply predominantly to men over the age of 35 years and women after the menopause, with benefits increasing in older age groups. The level at which no harm is caused by alcohol also increases with age, so that the young drinker is most at risk. Mortality risk is increased in young drinkers at levels of alcohol consumption normally considered to be 'safe'; this may be associated with accidents and injury rather than the long-term physical damage caused by alcohol itself.

On a population basis, there is no recommendation to increase alcohol consumption, for although abstainers might benefit from a small amount of alcohol, the extra harm that could ensue from increased drinking among heavier consumers would not translate into an overall improvement in health.

SUMMARY

1 Eating healthily is not a matter of adding specific 'health-giving' foods to the diet, using specific food preparation techniques, avoiding additives or taking nutritional supplements. None of these will make the diet healthy.
2 Choosing a healthy diet involves knowing what mixtures of foods to select and in what quantities.
3 Adequate amounts of food must be consumed to meet nutrient requirements. These are expressed as Dietary Reference Values and cover the needs of most of the population.
4 The Food Guides show how a balanced diet can be created, by choosing from a wide range of foods, in appropriate quantities.
5 Alcohol intake can be beneficial to health when taken in small to moderate amounts. Benefits are more likely in middle-aged and older people.

STUDY QUESTIONS

1 A number of commonly eaten foods are perceived as being 'healthy' or 'unhealthy'.
   a Compile a list of approximately 20 foods that you consider fulfil these criteria.
   b Ask a number of friends to define the foods as 'healthy' or 'unhealthy'.
   c State whether different people choose the same foods or whether there are differences (e.g. by age, gender).
   d Account for the perceptions about these foods.

2 For what nutritional reasons might a vegetarian diet be considered 'healthier' than an omnivorous diet?
3 Explain why a nutritional deficiency state can be difficult to define precisely. What different end-points are used to delineate deficiency?
4 Distinguish between an individual's nutritional requirement and the reference nutrient intake for a particular nutrient (e.g. vitamin C).
5 Explain why an intake below the level of the RNI may be nutritionally adequate.

REFERENCES AND FURTHER READING

Achterberg, C., McDonnell, E., Bagby, R. 1994: How to put the Food Guide Pyramid into practice. *Journal of the American Dietetic Association* 94, 1030–5.

DoH (UK Department of Health) 1991: *Dietary reference values for food energy and nutrients in the United Kingdom.* Report on Health and Social Subjects No. 41. Report of the Panel on Dietary Reference Values of the Committee on Medical Aspects of Food Policy. London: HMSO.

DoH (UK Department of Health) 1995: *Sensible drinking.* The Report of an Inter-Departmental Working Group. London: HMSO.

Fairweather-Tait, S.J. 1993: Optimal nutrient requirements: important concepts. *Journal of Human Nutrition and Dietetics* 6, 411–17.

Hunt, P., Gatenby, S., Rayner, M. 1995: The format for the National Food Guide: performance and preference studies. *Journal of Human Nutrition and Dietetics* 8, 335–51.

Institute of Grocery Distribution 1995: *Voluntary nutrition labelling guidelines to benefit the consumer.* Watford: Institute of Grocery Distribution.

Johnson, R.K. 2000: The 2000 Dietary Guidelines for Americans: foundation of US nutrition policy. *British Nutrition Foundation Nutrition Bulletin* **25**, 241–8.

MAFF (Ministry of Agriculture, Fisheries and Food) 1990: *Eight guidelines for a healthy diet.* London: Food Sense.

Mela, D.J. 1993: Consumer estimates of the percentage energy from fat in common foods. *European Journal of Clinical Nutrition* **47**(10), 735–40.

Nestle, M. 1999: Animal v plant foods in human diets and health: is the historical record unequivocal? *Proceedings of the Nutrition Society* **58**, 211–18.

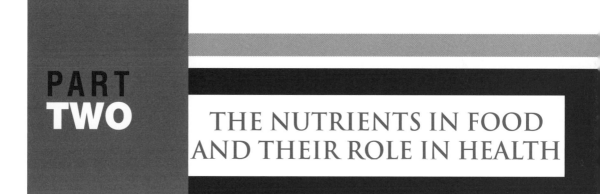

PART
TWO

THE NUTRIENTS IN FOOD AND THEIR ROLE IN HEALTH

CHAPTER
4

PROTEINS

The aims of this chapter are to:

❏ describe the composition and nature of proteins and identify protein-providing foods in the diet;
❏ show how proteins are digested and metabolized;
❏ identify the role of proteins in the body;
❏ discuss the concept of indispensable amino acids and how this is reflected in measurement of protein quality;
❏ explain the need for protein at different ages and in health and disease.

On completing the study of this chapter you should be able to:

❏ describe the basic structure of proteins and explain how they are altered by cooking;
❏ describe the process of protein digestion;
❏ explain the significance of indispensable amino acids and how foods may be combined to provide an appropriate balance;
❏ discuss the role of proteins and amino acids in the body, in health and disease, and the consequences of protein deficiency;
❏ explain the needs for protein at different stages of life and in trauma.

The word 'protein' is derived from the Greek and means 'holding first place'. Proteins are essential in the structure and function of all living things; without them no life can exist. Their importance, however, lies principally in the amino acids of which they are composed.

Some people associate protein with strength and muscle power, and perceive meat as being the most valuable source of protein. This view is only partly true; proteins are an essential component of muscles, but this is only one of their many functions in the body. Meat is a source of protein, but so also are many other foods, both of plant and animal origin. There is nothing special about protein from meat.

There are millions of different proteins – plant, animal and human – but all are built up from the same 20 amino acids. The particular sequence and number of amino acids contained in a protein determine its nature. With 20 different amino acids to choose from, and chains

which include perhaps several hundred different amino acids, the variety is almost endless. There are over three million ways of arranging amino acids in the first five places of a chain alone. The variety of proteins that exists is far greater than that of carbohydrates and fats. However, each protein has its own particular sequence of amino acids, which is crucial for its properties and functions. If even one amino acid is missing or misplaced in the chain, the properties of the protein will alter. The sequence of amino acids is controlled by the genetic machinery of our cells, encoded in the DNA and RNA chains. This critical relationship between the number of units contained and function does not apply in the case of carbohydrates: they may contain more or fewer of the particular component unit (usually a monosaccharide) without significant changes in properties.

The majority of the amino acids originate from plants, which are able to combine nitrogen from the soil and air with carbon and other substances to produce amino acids. These are then built into proteins by plants. Humans obtain their proteins either directly by eating plants, or by eating the animals (and their products), which have themselves consumed the plants. This does not mean that our bodies contain exactly the same proteins as plants and animals. The proteins we eat are broken down into their constituent amino acids and are rebuilt, or some new amino acids are first made, before new proteins are made in our bodies. Our bodies are able to make some amino acids from others, but there are certain amino acids (called essential, or indispensable) that cannot be synthesized by the body and which must, therefore, be supplied by the diet. This is shown in Figure 4.1.

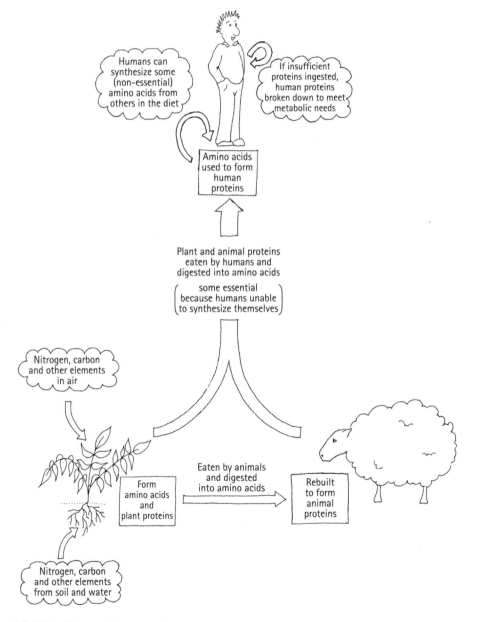

Figure 4.1 Origin of human dietary protein.

It is our need for these amino acids that makes it vital that we have adequate amounts of protein in our diet. If an individual fails to eat sufficient amounts of protein, the body's own structural proteins are broken down to meet metabolic needs for repair. In addition, other protein-requiring functions also fail, with resulting illness and possible death. To judge the needs of an individual for protein, therefore, it is important to understand how proteins are used in the body and the magnitude of the daily turnover.

AMINO ACIDS – THE BUILDING BLOCKS

Amino acids are relatively simple substances. All have the same basic structure: a carbon (known as the α carbon), with four groups of atoms attached to it:

- an amino group ($-NH_2$)
- an acid group ($-COOH$) always present
- a hydrogen atom ($-H$) and
- a fourth group, which varies between different amino acids and characterizes each one. This is the side-chain, identified as $-R$ in the 'generic' formula of an amino acid:

Varying group
Provides diversity of structure and function between amino acids and the proteins they form

The simplest amino acid is glycine, in which the side-chain R is an H atom. Thus, the formula for glycine is:

(It is worth comparing this with the formula for the simplest fatty acid, namely acetic acid: it is clear that the difference between these is small, with one of the H atoms in the fatty acid,

replaced with an NH_2 group to produce the amino acid.)

It is possible to compare the next fatty acid with the next amino acid, and see that again an H has been replaced by an NH_2 group:

Propionic acid   Alanine

The nature of the side-chain will determine some of the properties of the amino acid and of proteins that contain a high proportion of these acids. Side-chains may be aliphatic (open chain structure) or aromatic (i.e. unsaturated ring structure), acidic or basic (Table 4.1).

Except in the case of glycine, in which the α carbon has two H atoms attached, all other amino acids have four different groups attached to the α carbon. This implies that the molecule so formed can exist as two optically active isomers that are the mirror image of one another: D and L forms. This also occurs in monosaccharides, as discussed in Chapter 6. The majority of amino acids in nature exist in the L form; however, some D amino acids do exist in foods, and a few can be metabolized by the body. Generally, metabolic reactions in the body distinguish between L and D forms of amino acids and D forms are used less well. Some transamination of D-methionine and D-phenylalanine can take place to their respective L forms.

When amino acids combine to form proteins, they do so through the $-NH_2$ group of one amino acid reacting with the $-COOH$ group of the adjacent amino acid, splitting off H.OH (water) in the process. The link is known as a peptide link, and the proteins thus formed are known as polypeptides, or peptide chains. The polypeptide backbone does not differ between different protein

TABLE 4.1 The amino acids classified according to the nature of their side-chains

Aromatic amino acids	Aliphatic amino acids		Acidic amino acids and their amides	Basic amino acids
Phenylalanine	Glycine		Aspartic acid	Lysine
Tyrosine	Alanine		Asparagine	Arginine
Tryptophan	Valine	(branched-	Glutamic acid	Histidine
	Leucine	chain amino	Glutamine	
	Isoleucine	acids		
	Serine	(OH in side-		
	Threonine	chain)		
	Cysteine	(S groups in		
	Cystine	side-chain)		
	Methionine			
	Proline			

chains, it is the side-chains (R–) that provide the diversity.

A chain of amino acids may be written as:

When the whole chain is put together in three-dimensional space, the R– side-chains have to fit together without colliding with one another. Some are attracted to each other; some are repelled. Side-chains consisting of only carbon and hydrogen tend to come together, for they exclude water. Side-chains with oxygen or –NH$_2$ groups will mix with water, so these tend to occupy adjacent places. Thus, the nature and location of the side-chains within a polypeptide chain will determine its arrangement. It will fold or coil in an attempt to bring together compatible side-chains. In addition, other weaker bonds (e.g. hydrogen bonds) also form to provide further levels of organization of the protein structure. These will determine the strength and rigidity of the protein as well as dictating its final shape. Proteins with different roles in the body will have different shapes, most appropriate to their function. Their shape may, for example, be thread-like, helical or globular.

In addition, the shape of the protein may be altered by changes in its environment, such as heat or pH change, which affect its stability. Once the change in shape has passed a certain point, the protein is said to be denatured. This means that specific properties of the protein, such as antibody or enzyme activity, are lost. However, the nutritional value remains unchanged, as the amino acids themselves are still present and unchanged.

Cooking processes cause denaturation of protein – the change from raw to cooked forms is something with which we are familiar. For example, there is a noticeable difference between a raw and cooked egg, or the curdling of milk in the presence of acid or bacteria in the production of many dairy products. These changes occur because of the loosening of the weaker bonds holding the protein in shape so that its natural shape is lost, and some of the molecules rearrange themselves in new positions. Usually, cooking or food preparation processes do not affect the basic peptide bonds.

PROTEINS IN FOOD

The overall proportions of amino acids in plant foods are different from those needed by humans; those in foods of animal origin are more similar. Many different sources of protein exist, the main ones in the British diet being

TABLE 4.2	Sources of protein		
Food	Protein (g/100 g)	Protein (g/average serving)	Energy from protein (%)
Wholemeal bread	9.4	3.4	17.3
White bread	7.9	2.8	14.4
Cornflakes	7.9	2.4	8.4
Boiled rice	2.6	4.7	7.5
Semi-skimmed milk	3.4	6.8	29.5
Yogurt, low fat	4.2	5.3	21.5
Cheese, Cheddar type	25.4	10.2	24.4
Egg	12.5	6.3	34.0
Beefburger	28.5	25.7	34.7
Beef, stewed	15.1	39.3	44.4
Roast chicken	27.3	27.3	61.7
Pork chop	31.6	44.2	49.2
Cod in batter	16.1	29.0	26.1
Peanuts, salted, roast	24.5	6.1	16.2
Peanut butter	22.6	4.5	14.9
Baked beans	5.2	7.0	24.8
Peas	6.0	4.2	35
Potatoes, boiled	1.8	3.2	10
Cheese and tomato pizza	14.4	33.1	20.8

Data calculated from Food Standards Agency (2002a, 2002b).

meat, milk, bread and cereals. However, protein can also be provided by other animal products, such as eggs, dairy produce (cheese and milk-based desserts) and fish. Plant foods that are useful sources of protein include all cereals and their products (including pasta and breakfast cereals), legumes, nuts and seeds. For many people of the world who follow vegetarian diets, the plant foods are the only sources of protein; clearly they can provide an adequate supply of protein. Roots and tubers do not have a high protein content but, if they constitute a substantial proportion of the diet, this protein can make an important contribution.

Table 4.2 shows the amounts of protein contained in a range of foods. However, since some of the protein sources do not contain all of the amino acids needed by humans, it is important that a range of protein sources is eaten to allow small amounts in one food to be compensated with another source. This is discussed further later in this chapter in the section on protein quality.

DIGESTION AND ABSORPTION OF PROTEINS

Proteins must be digested in order to release the amino acids of which they are composed so they can enter the body pool and be used for cell growth, repair or protein synthesis. The chemical linkages between amino acids are all peptide bonds, yet a number of different peptidases are needed to cleave these bonds because of the differing nature of the side-chains on the amino acids adjacent to the bonds. Therefore, a single type of peptidase could not split a protein chain into its constituent amino acids in the same way that a single lipase or amylase can split fat into fatty acids or starch to glucose. Several different peptidases act on the proteins of our foods, each attacking bonds adjacent to particular side-chains on the amino acids. Other enzymes attack bonds at the ends of the peptide chain, taking off single amino acids, one after the other.

In the stomach, hydrolysis of the protein takes place by the action of the hydrochloric acid secreted there. This denatures the protein and allows the peptides to be attacked. In addition, the acid also activates the enzyme pepsinogen into its active form of pepsin. This enzyme attacks a range of peptide bonds and, therefore, is able to split the long protein chain into a series of shorter, polypeptide chains.

On passing from the stomach, the polypeptides are further digested by enzymes secreted from the pancreas and activated in the duodenum. These include trypsin, chymotrypsin, collagenase, elastase and carboxypeptidase. These enzymes are able to split the chain at specific peptide bonds, as well as removing end amino acids. Final digestion is completed by enzymes located in the brush border of the small intestine, including aminopeptidases and tripeptidases. These split the remaining peptides into single amino acids, or pairs of amino acids, which are absorbed and finally hydrolysed to amino acids in the intestinal mucosal cells.

There are a number of specific carrier molecules that transport the products of protein digestion across the intestinal mucosa into the bloodstream. Separate carrier systems have been identified for the basic, neutral and dicarboxylic amino acids and there is competition between the individual amino acids for the carrier. In addition, there are carriers for small peptides. The process is summarized in Figure 4.2.

It is worth pointing out that ingestion of supplements, which may contain several amino acids of the same chemical type, will result in competition for absorption. Thus, the amino acid present in greatest concentration will be absorbed preferentially, but the absorption of the others may be impaired. This may result in unbalanced amino acid absorption. Further, absorption of amino acids and peptides from natural, protein-containing foods occurs more quickly and efficiently than that from an equivalent mixture of free amino acids.

In general, protein digestion is extremely efficient, and up to 99 per cent of ingested protein is absorbed as amino acids. In young infants, however, whole antibody proteins secreted in maternal milk are absorbed from the gut. These give protection against infections, particularly during the first days of life, when colostrum is secreted by the mother's mammary glands. Colostrum is rich in immunoglobulins, which confer immunity to the child. It is also possible that proteins from cows' milk or wheat flour may, if given at this time of life, set up antibody production in the infant. This occasionally causes subsequent 'food intolerance' or 'food allergy' (see Chapter 16).

Most of the amino acids pass into the bloodstream from the intestines, and travel to the liver in the hepatic portal vein. Some pass into

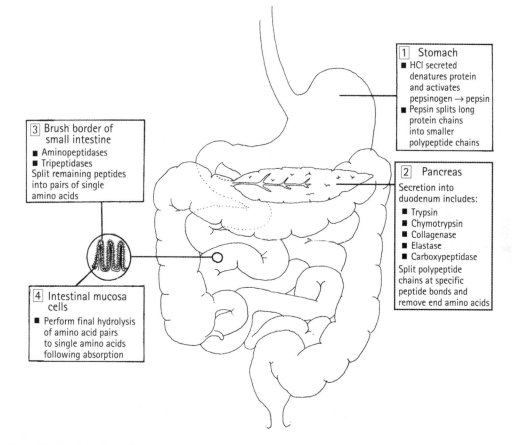

3 Brush border of small intestine
- Aminopeptidases
- Tripeptidases
Split remaining peptides into pairs of single amino acids

4 Intestinal mucosa cells
- Perform final hydrolysis of amino acid pairs to single amino acids following absorption

1 Stomach
- HCl secreted denatures protein and activates pepsinogen → pepsin
- Pepsin splits long protein chains into smaller polypeptide chains

2 Pancreas
Secretion into duodenum includes:
- Trypsin
- Chymotrypsin
- Collagenase
- Elastase
- Carboxypeptidase
Split polypeptide chains at specific peptide bonds and remove end amino acids

Figure 4.2 Digestion of proteins.

the liver cells, others go on to the general circulation. The liver is thought to monitor the absorbed amino acids and to adjust their rate of metabolism according to the needs of the body. A small number of amino acids remain in the cells of the intestinal mucosa, for synthesis of protein and other nitrogen-containing compounds. Glutamine is thought to promote cell division in the gastrointestinal mucosa, and is used by the intestinal cells as a primary source of energy. It is particularly important in times of trauma to maintain gut integrity.

AMINO ACID METABOLISM

The cells of the body are able to synthesize the carbon skeleton and add the side-chains of 12 of the 20 amino acids, using amino groups from other amino acids; these are the dispensable (or non-essential) amino acids. However, there are eight amino acids that cannot be made by the body in this way and, therefore, have to be supplied in the diet. These are called the indispensable (or essential) amino acids.

They are leucine, isoleucine, valine, lysine, tryptophan, threonine, methionine and phenylalanine. Histidine is also indispensable for children, and also, in some circumstances, for adults. It has been proposed that this classification is too rigid, as it is recognized that some amino acids may become indispensable in certain circumstances (Table 4.3).

TABLE 4.3	Amino acids that may become indispensable under certain circumstances
Amino acid	**Situation when it may become indispensable**
Cysteine and tyrosine	In the neonate
	May also spare methionine and phenylalanine
Arginine	In urea cycle disorders
	Metabolic stress
Taurine	In neonates and during growth
	Prolonged parenteral nutrition
Glutamine	May be needed in trauma, cancer and patients with immune deficiencies

The body is able to convert many amino acids from one to another. It does this by the process of transamination, which involves moving an amino group from a donor amino acid to an acceptor acid (called a keto acid), which in turn becomes an amino acid.

The remnants of the donor amino acid (the carbon skeleton) are then utilized in other metabolic pathways, usually to produce energy or in the synthesis of fatty acids. Alternatively, they may themselves receive an amino group, and be reconverted to an amino acid.

Amino acids may also be broken down by the process of deamination, in which the amino group, having been removed, is incorporated into urea in the liver, and eventually excreted via the kidneys in urine. The amount of urea excreted daily is a useful indicator of the rate at which protein turnover is taking place, and can also be used to calculate the protein needs of an individual. The remaining carbon fragment can be converted to pyruvate and then glucose, in which case the amino acid is known as 'glucogenic'. Alternatively, if it leads to the formation of acetyl coenzyme A, and then ketone bodies or fatty acids, the amino acid is called 'ketogenic'.

Several amino acids are both glucogenic and ketogenic, meaning that their carbon skeletons can give rise to both glucose and fats. Only the amino acids leucine and lysine are purely ketogenic, and cannot be used to make glucose.

These exchanges allow the body to make maximum use of its protein supplies, both from the diet and from that which is recycled within the body (see Figure 4.3).

The amino acid pool

The amino acid pool contains amino acids obtained from protein in the diet and the amino

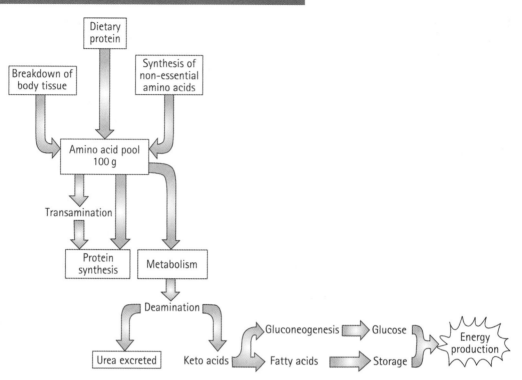

Figure 4.3 Summary of amino acid metabolism.

acids released from breakdown of cells and general metabolic processes of renewal in the body. From this pool, the cells of the body can take the amino acids they need to produce the proteins they require. If the pool does not contain the appropriate amounts needed, a cell has two possible options:

■ it can simply make less of the protein it requires, limited by the amino acid present in least amounts; or

■ it can break down some of its own protein to release the amino acids it requires for synthesis.

Obviously neither of these alternatives is the ideal solution; in both cases less protein than required is present in the cell, either because some was broken down to make new protein or because too little was synthesized. If this situation continues, there will be a deterioration of function. It is, therefore, important that the amino acid pool is adequate for the body's needs. This also means that it must contain the indispensable amino acids in the right proportions, so that synthesis can take place. If one of these amino acids is in

short supply at the time that it is needed, perhaps because the diet did not contain much, then synthetic reactions will be restricted to an extent determined by this amino acid. This is then termed the limiting amino acid, and this concept is used later in the chapter in the discussion of protein quality.

The total size of the amino acid pool has been estimated at 100 g, including the plasma and smaller amounts in the tissues. It principally contains dispensable (non-essential) amino acids, since the indispensable amino acids are used rapidly or, if present in excess, are deaminated. The pool represents the balance of the flux between the incoming amino acids (from diet and tissue breakdown) and the use of amino acids for synthesis of proteins or for deamination and energy production. It has been estimated that the total amount of protein turnover in a day is in the region of 250–300 g; this is greater in infants and less in the elderly. The balance is regulated by the needs of the body and the size of the pool. If the pool becomes too large, then more deaminating enzymes will be activated and amino acids will be broken down and their nitrogen excreted as urea. The carbon skeletons will be used for energy or to synthesize fat.

Since the body has no means of storing excess protein or amino acids, eating more protein than the body requires results in breakdown of amino acids, with the production of fatty acids, glucose and urea, and heat. Since we generally live in warm houses and wear appropriate amounts of clothes, this excess heat is not used for maintaining body temperature, but is largely dissipated as waste heat.

If insufficient protein is eaten, the body has to use its own 'endogenous' protein to provide the amino acids needed for the pool and, therefore, to maintain normal protein turnover. In time, the tissue proteins will be seen to waste, and the ability of the body to maintain all of the functions requiring protein will deteriorate. Eventually, a state of protein deficiency will occur.

If insufficient energy sources are being supplied to the body in the form of carbohydrate or fats (even if protein intake appears adequate), then protein will be degraded and used for energy, since the body's first priority is to meet its energy requirements from whatever source is available. When this happens, the amino acids are converted to glucose (a process known as gluconeogenesis) and used for energy. This means that they are no longer available for synthesis. This is a wasteful use of protein by the body and is seen to an extreme extent in untreated diabetes mellitus, as well as in situations of physiological trauma (such as fever, burns, fractures or surgery), especially if food intake is reduced. The consequences are a decline in muscle bulk as well as reduced levels of plasma proteins, enzymes and constituents of the immune system. Thus, for amino acid use to be optimal, the energy needs must also be satisfied, preferably from fat and carbohydrate sources, which are, therefore, described as 'sparing' protein.

The greatest part of amino acid metabolism takes place in the liver; other sites, however, include the skeletal muscle and, to a lesser extent, the heart, brain and kidneys. Muscle is the main site of metabolism of the branched-chain amino acids (leucine, isoleucine and valine), and produces large amounts of glutamine and alanine, which can be used for energy in fasting or other emergencies. The kidneys are also an important site of amino acid metabolism, including gluconeogenesis, and production of ammonia from glutamine, which is essential for the maintenance of acid–base balance. In addition, the kidneys are responsible for ridding the body of nitrogenous waste from protein catabolism.

The brain has transport systems for the uptake of neutral, basic and dicarboxylic acids, and there is competition between amino acids for the carrier systems. Several of the amino acids act as neurotransmitters or as their precursors:

- glycine and taurine are believed to be inhibitory neurotransmitters;
- aspartate is thought to be an excitatory neurotransmitter;
- tryptophan is the precursor of serotonin (5-hydroxytryptamine), an excitatory neurotransmitter;
- tyrosine is used in the synthesis of dopamine, noradrenaline and adrenaline (the catecholamines);
- a number of neuropeptides are found in the brain; these have a wide range of functions, including regulating hormone release, endocrine roles and effects on mood and behaviour.

Thus, changes in uptake of amino acids or varying levels in the brain can have diverse effects.

Control of protein metabolism

Amino acid and thus protein metabolism is under the control of the endocrine system. Recent evidence suggests that the body has a well-defended system for metabolic adaptation, which protects essential functions and internal homeostasis. This is necessary in the face of varying protein intakes and changing internal demands. Protein synthesis is promoted by insulin, which facilitates the uptake of amino acids into tissues. On the other hand, glucagon, catecholamines and glucocorticoids have the opposite effect, and promote protein degradation. Growth hormone is an anabolic agent for protein. However, the exact effects of these hormones may vary between tissues and at different levels of nutrient intake.

For example, the effect of insulin on peripheral tissue uptake of amino acids is maximal for the branched-chain amino acids, but minimal for tryptophan. Thus, after a carbohydrate-containing meal, which stimulates insulin release, the uptake of tryptophan into tissues, including the brain, is increased, as competing amino acids are no longer present. This is believed to stimulate serotonin synthesis in the brain and may be responsible for the drowsiness experienced after carbohydrate ingestion. This also contributes to a reduction in food intake.

USES OF PROTEINS

Proteins serve a large number of functions in the body. Some are key components in structure, some are enzymes, hormones or buffers, others play a part in immunity, transport of substances round the body, blood clotting and many other roles (see Figure 4.4 for a summary).

Body composition

Protein is a key component of the structure of the body. Each cell contains protein as part of the cell membrane and within its cytoplasm. Muscles, bones, connective tissues, blood cells, glands and organs all contain protein. This protein is synthesized during growth, repaired, maintained and replaced during life, and forms a source of amino acids that can be drawn on in emergencies, although at the expense of the tissue it comes from. Only the brain is resistant to being used as a source of amino acids for emergency use. Thus, the protein in our body structure is not static, but a dynamic constituent that is in a state of continuous flux.

Formation of enzymes

Almost all enzymes are proteins and thus proteins are instrumental in facilitating most of the chemical reactions that occur in the body. This includes the digestion of nutrients (including protein), the regulation of energy production in cells and the synthesis of all the chemical substances found in the body. Enzymes are essential to normal life.

Homeostasis

The physiological mechanisms of the body aim to maintain a constant internal environment in the face of continued changes that might disturb it. This is achieved by the action of various proteins operating in specific ways.

Hormones

Many of these consist of amino acids. They act as the messengers carried in the circulation, and control the internal environment; for example, by regulating metabolic rate (thyroid hormones), blood glucose levels (insulin, glucagon), blood calcium levels (parathyroid hormone, calcitonin), the digestion process (secretin, cholecystokinin) (CCK) and response to stress (adrenaline).

Acid–base balance

Proteins act as buffers in the circulation by accepting or donating H^+ ions and thereby maintaining a fairly constant pH in the blood and body fluids.

Fluid balance

Because of their size and inability to leak through the walls of the blood vessels, proteins in the plasma exert an osmotic effect that holds

Figure 4.4 Summary of uses of protein.

fluid within the circulation. This prevents excess pooling of body fluids in the tissue spaces. A reduction in the levels of albumin and globulin causes oedema as a result of loss of fluid from the circulation into the tissue spaces.

Immunity

Proteins play a key role in the function of the immune system. They are needed for normal cell division to produce the cellular components. In addition, the antibodies and other humoral agents that are released are composed of amino acids. Thus, a protein deficiency will result in defective immune function. This is seen clearly in children suffering from protein–energy malnutrition, who have an increased susceptibility to infection as a result of poor immune function. There is good evidence that certain amino acids may have a more specific role in immunonutrition. Among those being studied, glutamine, which is a precursor for glutathione, improves gut barrier function and may be an essential nutrient for a number of immune system cells. Glutamine has been described as conditionally essential in critically ill patients, when there is trauma or physiological stress. Other amino acids that have been studied in similar situations include arginine and taurine.

Transport

Many of the substances that need to be carried around the body from either the digestive system or stores to sites of action cannot travel in the blood alone, usually because they are insoluble or potentially harmful. When these substances are attached to proteins, particularly albumin or globulins, transport is facilitated. The level of carrier protein present at any time may determine the availability of the particular substance to the tissues. Haemoglobin is a transporting protein, serving to carry oxygen in the body. In this case, it is the ability of the haemoglobin molecule to take up a large amount of oxygen that provides the advantage over oxygen transport simply in solution by the blood. Reduced availability of haemoglobin (either because of iron or protein deficiency) will affect the provision of oxygen to the tissues.

In addition, transport proteins also carry substances across cell membranes; for example, during absorption in the digestive tract. As well as facilitating transport, proteins may also bind with some constituents of the body to provide a safe method of storage; for example, iron is stored in association with ferritin.

Blood clotting

Several proteins found in plasma play an essential role in blood clotting, including prothrombin and fibrinogen. Failure to synthesize these (for example, in deficiency of vitamin K, which acts as a cofactor) will result in prolonged bleeding times.

Other functions

Although not its primary role, protein can serve as a source of energy when insufficient carbohydrate and fat are available to meet the body's needs. Proteins also form the major components of the hair and nails, as well as the structural framework of bones.

It is also important to note that non-protein nitrogenous compounds are produced from some of the amino acids. Glycine is used in haem, nucleic acid and bile acid synthesis. Other examples include the use of tryptophan to make nicotinic acid and tyrosine in catecholamine synthesis.

NITROGEN BALANCE

An overall indicator of protein metabolism in the body is the nitrogen balance, which is the difference between nitrogen intake and nitrogen output. When the balance is positive, protein is being retained in the body, indicating tissue synthesis. A negative nitrogen balance occurs when there is a net loss of protein from the body, either because there is catabolism or because protein or energy intakes are insufficient to meet the daily needs (see Figure 4.5).

When nitrogen intake and output are in equilibrium, then protein is neither being gained nor lost. Nitrogen balance studies do not, however, tell us where the protein is being stored or catabolized, or what its functions are. Not all nitrogen

Figure 4.5 Components of nitrogen balance.

flux relates to protein: there is some metabolism of non-protein nitrogen taking place, and some retention of nitrogen may represent increases in this fraction rather than in protein content. However, it is generally assumed that the nitrogen (N) in Western diets is largely of protein origin, and the conversion factor of $N \times 6.25$ is used to convert between nitrogen and protein content. This implies that all proteins contain 16 per cent nitrogen; in reality the amount of nitrogen in proteins varies between 15.7 per cent in milk and 19 per cent in nuts.

Losses of nitrogen can occur from the body via a number of routes. Faecal loss of nitrogen represents unabsorbed dietary nitrogen together with residual nitrogen from the digestive juices and mucosal cells shed into the tract. In health, these losses are small. Nitrogen is lost in the urine in the form of urea (mostly), ammonia, uric acid and creatinine. The urea content reflects dietary intake and, therefore, decreases as protein intake falls. Creatinine levels are relatively constant, as these are related to the muscle mass, and represent its daily turnover. In addition, nitrogen is lost daily in skin cells, hair, nails, sweat and saliva and, although it is possible to measure these by meticulous study, in practice, a constant figure is used.

Balance studies carried out when the diet is devoid of protein are used to indicate the obligatory losses of nitrogen. Values obtained in such studies give an average obligatory protein loss of 0.34 g/kg body weight for adults (or 55 mg of nitrogen/kg body weight).

Nitrogen balance studies have been criticized as imprecise for a number of reasons. These include:

- overestimation of intake;
- incomplete estimation of losses – gaseous nitrogen loses are usually uncounted (breath and colonic gases);
- uncertainty about adaptation to changes in protein intake.

However, despite these shortcomings, there is still a role for nitrogen balance data until newer methodologies are sufficiently reliable and robust. These include the use of tracer-labelled amino acid oxidation studies. The most commonly used isotope is ^{13}C, with measurement of labelled CO_2 excretion. These studies allow factorial assessments of metabolic demands, efficiency of utilization and requirement. However, it is still problematic to arrive at information relating to whole-body protein turnover.

PROTEIN QUALITY

If a protein is to be useful to the body, it should supply all of the indispensable amino acids in appropriate amounts. If this is not the case, any synthesis that is required can only take place by breaking down existing proteins. Alternatively, limited synthesis may take place until all of the amino acid present in least amounts has been used up. The body cannot synthesize incomplete proteins, therefore, synthesis is limited by this amino acid. Such an amino acid is termed 'limiting', and the protein from which it comes would be described as having low quality. How can this be quantified?

Milk or egg proteins have traditionally been used as the 'reference proteins', as their amino acid pattern most nearly conforms to that of total body protein. Most recently, the amino acid pattern of human milk has been set as the standard against which all other proteins can be judged for their efficiency of meeting human needs.

Different sources of protein have been shown to match the required amino acid pattern to varying extents, and combining different plant foods, for example, makes it possible to obtain the necessary amino acids from several sources and achieve an overall balance (Table 4.4).

TABLE 4.4	The use of complementary foods to make up for limiting amino acids in some plant foods		
Plant food	**Limiting amino acid**	**Useful complementary food**	**Example of meal**
Grains (or cereals)	Lysine, threonine	Legumes/pulses	Beans on toast
Nuts and seeds	Lysine	Legumes/pulses	Hummus (chickpeas with sesame seeds)
Soya beans and other legumes/pulses	Methionine	Grains; nuts and seeds	Lentil curry and rice
Maize	Tryptophan, lysine	Legumes	Tortillas and beans
Vegetables	Methionine	Grains; nuts and seeds	Vegetable and nut roast

Populations have naturally been doing this for generations; there is nothing new about it and many traditional dishes reflect this.

In addition, it is possible to complement protein foods of plant origin with foods derived from animals to compensate for the limiting amino acid. In particular, milk and its products provide good complementary protein to partner the plant foods. Examples of such traditional mixtures include bread and cheese, macaroni cheese, rice pudding, cereal and milk.

Measuring protein quality

Chemical score

This compares the amount of each indispensable amino acid in the test protein with the amount of this amino acid in the reference protein; the chemical score is the value of this ratio for the limiting amino acid:

$$\text{Chemical score} = \frac{\text{Amount of amino acid in test protein (mg/g)}}{\text{Amount of amino acid in reference protein (mg/g)}} \times 100$$

The reference scoring pattern for the most frequently limiting amino acids was developed by the FAO/WHO/UNU (1985):

Amino acid	Reference score (mg/g protein)
Leucine	19
Lycine	16
Threonine	9
Valine	13
Methionine + cystine	17

The calculation does not take into account the digestibility of the protein and is, therefore, a very theoretical value. Digestibility is particularly an issue for many plant-based diets and some cereals, for example, millet and sorghum, and needs to be considered especially for children in developing countries.

Biological value

The biological value (BV) of a protein is a measure of how effectively a protein can meet the body's biological need. To make this measurement, the test protein is fed to an experimental animal as the sole source of protein, and the nitrogen retention and loss are measured. The greater the nitrogen retention, the more of the protein has been used. (Remember that, if a protein cannot be used because it contains limiting amino acids, it cannot be stored and, therefore, is broken down and the nitrogen excreted as urea.)

$$BV = \frac{\text{Nitrogen retained} \times 100}{\text{Nitrogen absorbed}}$$

or more precisely:

$$BV = \frac{\text{Dietary nitrogen} - (\text{urinary nitrogen} + \text{faecal nitrogen}) \times 100}{\text{Dietary nitrogen} - \text{faecal nitrogen}}$$

For egg protein, BV is 100; and for fish and beef the value is 75. It is generally agreed that a BV of 70 or more can support growth, as long as energy intakes are adequate.

For both BV and chemical score, the result for a single food is of relatively little relevance because most people consume a mixture of foods in their daily diet.

Millward (1999) reports that ongoing research into the adequacy of protein intakes in diets around the world has shown that, even with revised amino acid scoring methods, the problem of inadequate protein or severely limiting amino acids is not as widespread as commonly assumed.

PROTEIN REQUIREMENTS

Requirement figures for protein are calculated on the basis of nitrogen balance studies, which estimate the amount of high-quality milk or egg protein needed to achieve equilibrium. The safe level of protein intake was established by FAO/WHO/UNU (1985) as 0.75 g/kg body weight per day. In addition to nitrogen balance results, increments were included for growth in infants and children, calculated from estimates of nitrogen accretion. In pregnancy, protein retention in the products of conception and maternal tissues was calculated and, for lactation, the protein content of breast milk in healthy mothers was used to obtain the reference value.

Uncertainty is expressed about the accuracy of these balance studies because they give results that are considerably higher than minimum nitrogen losses in adults on protein-free diets. Also the duration of the studies may not be sufficient for adaptation to occur. Finally, it is unclear how the amount of energy given to the subjects affects the results.

Figures recommended in the UK (DoH, 1991) for adults are calculated on the basis of 0.75 g protein/kg body weight per day. Values obtained using reference body weights for adults are shown in Table 4.5. Current intakes in the UK are considerably higher than the values recommended here. The National Food Survey (DEFRA 2001) shows that the mean daily total protein intake was 67 g, of which 41.1 g was of animal origin. This intake represents 147 per cent of the mean RNI for protein and, even in the largest households, the intake is well above the mean RNI at 117 per cent.

TABLE 4.5	Dietary reference values for protein for adults	
Gender/age	Estimated average requirement (g/day)	Reference nutrient intake (g/day)
Males		
19–50 years	44.4	55.5
50+ years	42.6	53.3
Females		
19–50 years	36.0	45.0
50+ years	37.2	46.5

From DoH, 1991. Crown copyright is reproduced with the permission of Her Majesty's Stationery Office.

Major food groups providing protein were shown to be:

Milk products and cheese	21.3 per cent of total
Meat and meat products	32 per cent
Cereals and cereal products	26 per cent

It is assumed that, in the UK, there is a sufficient variety of different protein sources to eliminate concerns about protein quality. However, for those individuals whose diet contains a considerable amount of unrefined cereal and vegetable, a correction for digestibility of 85 per cent is to be applied.

Report 41 (DoH, 1991) suggests that it is prudent to avoid protein intakes that are in excess of an 'upper safe limit' of 1.5 g/kg per day, suggesting that such high intakes may contribute to bone demineralization and a decline in kidney function with age. It has been found that there is a linear relationship between increases in animal protein intake and calcium loss in the urine, although the relationship with bone demineralization is still unclear. More recent evidence has largely failed to support concerns about effects of high protein intakes on kidney function, unless there is pre-existing renal disease. A number of cross-sectional studies in the USA and Britain have shown an inverse relationship between protein intakes and blood pressure and stroke. However, the possible mechanisms involved are yet to be discovered, and intervention studies have been unable to replicate these effects.

Finally, it should be noted that those individuals with high energy needs, such as athletes, consuming a typical Western diet, are likely to ingest protein in excess of this 'upper safe limit', unless they make adjustments to the balance of macronutrients in their diet. This should preferably be achieved through consuming more carbohydrate, rather than more fat, but may be impractical in terms of the volume of food required.

Many questions remain to be resolved and new issues are continually being raised in this field. Some of these are briefly discussed below.

- Newer research on individual amino acids suggests that requirement figures for indispensable amino acids may need to be increased and, therefore, the safe level of protein intake may need to be revised upwards. Given the prevalence of undernutrition in the world, such a revision would have enormous implications in terms of global food policies.

- The distinction between essential and nonessential amino acids may become less clear-cut, as studies have shown that there is some potential for amino acid synthesis from urea residues, by the colonic bacteria. Factors that might influence this synthesis and availability to the host may need to be considered in the future.

- It is already clear that needs for specific amino acids vary between individuals and at different times of life and conditions. The ability to cope with these life situations may also depend on optimal amino acid availability and the presence of other nutrients.

PROTEIN DEFICIENCY

Insufficient protein intake is a problem for many people of the world, especially the poor in many countries. It is rarely their only nutritional problem; the diet is likely to be low in energy and fat, and may contain marginal amounts of many nutrients. In addition, there are likely to be social, economic and environmental problems, which increase the likelihood of infection and reduce the availability of health care. Low levels of educational achievement are also likely to be found in these societies owing to a lack of opportunity.

Children are most likely to suffer from protein deficiency in a complex picture of protein-energy malnutrition, which can take a number of different forms. Classically, the two main forms are marasmus and kwashiorkor; there is considrable debate as to whether these are separate conditions or two ends of the spectrum of the same condition. They have been seen to occur in the same village and even in the same child at different times, suggesting a common cause. The child exhibits growth failure, in particular, a slowing of linear growth, resulting in stunting (Figure 4.6). Usually the child is miserable and

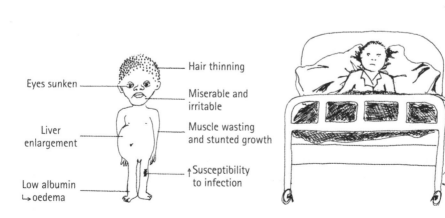

Figure 4.6 Example of cases of protein deficiency.

irritable. There is likely to be liver enlargement, possibly oedema, changes to the hair and skin; the eyes may be sunken and also show signs of vitamin A deficiency. Susceptibility to infection is increased, and the coexistence of infection and malnutrition may precipitate death.

The exact causes of this clinical picture are unclear. Low protein intake can result in many of the signs, with low albumin levels resulting in oedema. It is possible that an imbalance of amino acids may be responsible, as the syndrome does not occur in wheat-growing areas, but is common where cassava, yams, maize and plantain are the staple. Most recently, it has been suggested that food contaminated with moulds may be responsible, or that a lack of antioxidants prevents the body coping appropriately with the free radicals produced by toxins or infections.

Treatment involves restoring the nutritional status of the body, while treating infections, electrolyte imbalances and hypothermia, all of which may be present in a sick child with protein-energy malnutrition. In addition, the whole family may need to be educated about nutrition and health to provide long-term improvement and to prevent the condition recurring.

Protein deficiency as part of more generalized malnutrition also occurs in the community and particularly in hospitalized patients in Britain. When pre-existing illness, poor appetite, surgical or medical treatment and prolonged hospitalization coincide, there is the likelihood that insufficient nutrients will be consumed. Thus, although the process may not necessarily start as protein deficiency, if food intakes are minimal, protein catabolism will quickly follow.

In addition, the catabolic response to trauma also increases protein breakdown, contributing to the negative nitrogen balance. Particularly vulnerable are overweight patients, in whom adiposity masks muscle wasting. Negative nitrogen balance may persist for some time before action is taken. Reports published during the last 20 years have indicated a prevalence of malnutrition in hospital patients ranging from 20 to 50 per cent in different studies. Several policy documents have been produced during this time and nutrition teams established in many hospitals.

It is recognized that undernutrition has major implications on the clinical outcome for the patient. These include:

- increased post-operative complications and poor wound healing;
- increased risk of pressure sores;
- poor immune response and increased susceptibility to hospital infections;
- reduced muscle strength, weakness, immobility, inability to cough;
- apathy and depression;
- reduced quality of life;
- prolonged hospital stay;
- increased mortality.

In addition to these, there are increased economic implications for the hospital.

The causes of undernutrition may be disease-related or arise for social or psychological reasons. In addition, they may have their origins in hospital services, routines and procedures. The latter may include the food provided, the timing of meals in relation to other procedures, and the facilities and help available for eating. The dietetic and catering services can address some of these, others need to be addressed at the ward level. Protocols should be in place to identify and manage patients at risk of undernutrition. The Better Hospital Food project (DoH, 2000), launched in 2001 in the UK aims to improve meal provision, through greater choice and flexibility so that food can be provided to suit patient need and preferences, and ensure adequate nutrition.

It is important, therefore, that patients are weighed regularly and that assessments of nutritional status are made, such as grip strength, mid-arm muscle circumference or plasma albumin levels. Suitable provision and help with oral consumption of foods or supplements is needed and more vigorous nutritional support via other routes when necessary. Careful monitoring of at-risk hospital patients is necessary, with all of the medical team needing an awareness of the potential problem. Increasing knowledge and awareness of the importance of nutrition as treatment among doctors is seen as a cornerstone for any improvements. This has been addressed by the Royal College of Physicians (2002), but will take time to come into effect at ward level.

SUMMARY

1 Proteins are composed of combinations of amino acids, creating an enormous diversity of proteins.
2 Twenty different amino acids occur in proteins. The body uses these very efficiently, and is able to convert some of the amino acids into others. However, eight of them cannot be made in the body, and must be provided in the diet; they are the indispensable amino acids. At certain times, for example, in young children, or in stress and trauma, other amino acids may become indispensable.
3 Proteins fulfil a great many functions in the body, acting as hormones, enzymes, carriers and maintaining homeostasis.
4 Dietary sources of protein may be of animal or plant origin. The ability of the body to make full use of the amino acids supplied depends on the energy intake and the pattern of the amino acids in the protein. An inadequate amount of one amino acid may limit the usefulness of the whole protein, unless it is combined with a complementary source, which provides the limiting amino acid.
5 Protein requirements are based currently on nitrogen balance studies.
6 Intakes of protein in the UK are above the reference nutrient intake (RNI) in healthy adults. The hospital patient may, however, be at risk of protein deficiency, which may compromise recovery.

STUDY QUESTIONS

1 Draw a flow diagram to show the movement of amino acids within the amino acid pool when the body has adequate supplies of protein. Show how this changes when protein is in short supply.
2 Explain why a protein deficiency might result in:
   a oedema
   b an increased susceptibility to infection.
3 It has been suggested that Western diets contain excessive amounts of protein.

a Keep a record for 1 week of how many times you eat protein-rich food. Use the information in Table 4.2 to help you.
b Are your sources of protein mostly from animal or plant foods, or a combination of both of these?
c Can you identify combinations of different protein sources in your meals, such as those discussed in the chapter?
d Compare your results with those of others in your group. What do you find?

REFERENCES AND FURTHER READING

DEFRA (UK Department for Environment, Food and Rural Affairs) 2001: *National food survey 2000. Annual report on food, expenditure, consumption and nutrient intakes.* London: The Stationery Office.

DoH (UK Department of Health) 1991: *Dietary reference values for food energy and nutrients in the United Kingdom.* Report on Health and Social Subjects No. 41. Report of the Panel on Dietary Reference Values of the Committee on Medical Aspects of Food Policy. London: HMSO.

DoH (UK Department of Health) 2000: *The NHS plan: a plan for improvement, a plan for reform.* London: Department of Health.

FAO/WHO/UNU 1985: *Energy and protein requirements.* Report of a joint FAO/WHO/UNU Expert Consultation. WHO Technical Report No. 724. Geneva: WHO.

Food Standards Agency 2002a: *Food portion sizes*, 3rd edn. London: The Stationery Office.

Food Standards Agency 2002b: *McCance and Widdowson's The composition of foods*, 6th summary edn. Cambridge: Royal Society of Chemistry.

Jackson, A.A. 2003: Human protein requirement: policy issues. *Proceedings of the Nutrition Society* 60, 7–11.

Lennard Jones, J.E. 1992: *A positive approach to nutrition as treatment.* London: Kings Fund Centre.

McWhirter, J.P., Pennington, C.R. 1994: Incidence and recognition of malnutrition in hospita *British Medical Journal* **308**, 945–8.

Millward, D.J. 1999: The nutritional value of plant-based diets in relation to human amino acid and protein requirements. *Proceedings of the Nutrition Society* **58**, 249–60.

Royal College of Physicians 2002: *Nutrition and patients, A doctor's responsibility.* London: Royal College of Physicians.

Scrimshaw, N.S., Waterlow, J.C., Schurch, B. (eds) 1996: Protein and energy requirements symposium. *European Journal of Clinical Nutrition* **50** (suppl. 1).

Waterlow, J.C. 1995: Whole body protein turnover in humans – past, present and future. *Annual Review of Nutrition* **15**, 57–92.

CHAPTER
5

FATS

The aims of this chapter are to:

❑ describe the nature and characteristics of fats important in human nutrition;
❑ explain the importance of the essential fatty acids;
❑ discuss the role of fat in the diet and trends in fat consumption;
❑ study the transport of fats in lipoproteins;
❑ discuss the role of fat in the body;
❑ discuss the part played by adipose tissue in metabolism.

On completing the study of this chapter you should be able to:

❑ discuss the nature of various fats in the diet and the nutritional importance of the different types;
❑ discuss the advantages and disadvantages of fat in the diet;
❑ describe the current levels of fat intake in the UK;
❑ discuss the importance of omega-3 fatty acids in the body;
❑ explain the role of adipose tissue;
❑ understand the general importance of fat in the body and its role in health.

All living cells contain some fat in their structure, since fatty acids are essential components of cell walls and intracellular membranes. In addition, mammals and birds store fat throughout the body, especially between the muscles, around internal organs and under the skin. Many fish have fat stored exclusively in the liver, but in the oily fish (like herring and mackerel) it is present throughout the flesh. In the plant kingdom, fats are found in the fruits of various plants such as olives, maize, nuts and avocados. Plants manufacture fats by photosynthesis, the same process that they use to make carbohydrates. Animals use or store the fat they ingest, or can synthesize fat from surplus energy taken in as carbohydrates or proteins. This does not generally apply in humans under normal circumstances. Advice on healthy eating encourages us to reduce our intake of certain types of fats and increase others. Names such as cholesterol, polyunsaturates, omega-3s are used by food manufacturers and can be very confusing for many people. To be able to understand the rationale and the details of this advice, it is necessary first to understand the nature of fats, and how this is related to their behaviour in the body. Only then can we interpret the advice both for ourselves and others.

WHAT ARE FATS?

Fats are substances that are insoluble in water, but soluble in organic solvents like acetone. In addition, fats are greasy in texture and are non-volatile. When we think about fats in the diet, most people make a distinction between fats, which are solid at room temperature, and oils, which are liquid. Chemically, however, these two groups are similar; the major attributes that produce the differences in solubility are size of the molecule and types of bonds present. To the chemist and biochemist, all of these compounds are 'lipids'. In nutrition, the most important lipids are triglycerides (or triacylglycerols), which constitute over 95 per cent of the fat we consume. In addition, there are phospholipids, sterols and fat-soluble vitamins in the diet and body tissues. If we consider an average fat intake of 100 g per day, this would be made up as follows:

90–95 g	triglycerides
4–8 g	phospholipids
1 g	glycolipids
350–450 mg	cholesterol

There are also other lipids in nature that are not important in nutrition.

Like carbohydrates, lipid molecules contain carbon, oxygen and hydrogen atoms linked in a specific and unique way. The simplest lipids are the neutral fats (triacylglycerols or triglycerides).

Triglycerides

These are the building blocks of most fats in the body. Structurally, they are made up of a backbone of glycerol to which three fatty acids are attached. Glycerol is a very simple molecule. When a fatty acid combines with glycerol, the linkage occurs between the –OH group in the glycerol and the –COOH group of the acid by esterification, with the loss of a molecule of water.

Glycerol

Fatty acid

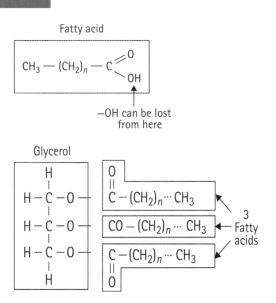

Usually three different fatty acids are attached to the glycerol molecule, creating a huge diversity of triglycerides.

Triglycerides are readily broken down and resynthesized. A fatty acid can also be removed from the glycerol molecule by de-esterification, which occurs during the digestion of fats. Resulting products are diglycerides and monoglycerides, containing two or one fatty acid, respectively. Fatty acids can be replaced on glycerol molecules by re-esterification. These two processes create particular triglycerides to meet the specific needs of the body.

Fatty acids are chains of carbon atoms with hydrogens attached in the form of methylene ($-CH_2$) groups. At one end of the chain is a methyl group ($-CH_3$), and at the other end an acid group ($-COOH$). The simplest of the fatty acids is acetic acid with the formula $CH_3.COOH$; thus, the chain is only two carbons long. Most naturally occurring fatty acids contain even numbers of carbons in their chain, normally ranging from 4 to 24 carbons. Thus, the basic formula for a fatty acid is $CH_3.(CH_2)_n.COOH$, where n is any number between 2 and 22.

Fatty acids with six or fewer carbons may be described as 'short chain', those containing 8–12 carbons are 'medium-chain', and those in which the chain is 14 carbons or more are 'long-chain' fatty acids. The human diet contains mostly long-chain fatty acids, with less than 5 per cent coming from those having fewer carbons. The most commonly occurring chain lengths are 14 and 16.

No fat consists of a single type of triglyceride. In butter, for example, the main fatty acids attached to glycerol are butyric, oleic and stearic acids, although there are 69 different fatty acids actually present.

It is the identity of the fatty acids present within a triglyceride that determines its physical characteristics. Thus, a triglyceride made up predominantly of short-chain fatty acids is likely to be a hard fat, whereas one consisting of long-chain fatty acids will have a lower melting point, and may even be an oil at room temperature. In addition, the proportions of saturated and unsaturated fatty acids present will also affect its hardness.

Types of fatty acids

Fatty acids occurring in nature can be divided into three categories:
- saturated fatty acids;
- monounsaturated fatty acids with one double bond; and
- polyunsaturated fatty acids with at least two double bonds.

In a saturated fatty acid, the carbon atom holds as many hydrogens as is chemically possible; it is said to be 'saturated' in terms of hydrogen. In an unsaturated fatty acid, there are one or more double bonds along the main carbon chain, known as ethylenic bonds. Each double bond replaces two hydrogen atoms. If there is just one double bond, the acid is monounsaturated, if two or more double bonds are present, the fatty acid is polyunsaturated.

Implications of unsaturation

The location of double bonds in a polyunsaturated fatty acid is not random. Multiple double bonds are separated by a methylene group, as follows:

$$— CH = CH — CH_2 — CH = CH —$$

If the location of the first double bond is identified, the remainder can be predicted from this. A system of nomenclature has been devised that classifies unsaturated fatty acids into families, according to the position of the first double bond. These are the omega (also known as n-) families: 3, 6 and 9. The families of the common fatty acids are given in Table 5.1, together with the number of carbon atoms and, in the case of the unsaturated fatty acids, the number of double bonds present. Fatty acids from one family cannot be converted into another family, any interconversion can only occur within the same family.

Where double bonds exist, there is a possibility of cis or trans geometric isomerism, which affects the properties of the fatty acid. Most naturally occurring forms are the cis isomers, in which the hydrogen atoms are on the same side of the double bond. Figure 5.1 shows the structural arrangement of different fatty acids types. In cis configurations, the molecule is folded back, kinked or bent into a U-shape. In this arrangement, fatty acids pack together less tightly, increasing, for example, the fluidity of membranes. When the hydrogen atoms are arranged on opposite sides of the double bond in trans configuration, the molecule remains elongated and similar to a saturated fatty acid. This allows the trans fatty acid molecules to pack more tightly together, and raises the melting point of the fat. To the consumer, this means that the fat is harder.

Trans fatty acids are produced as a result of processing and are thus found in products containing hardened fats, such as hard margarine, pastries, biscuits and meat products. In addition, trans fatty acids are produced during transformations by anaerobic bacteria in the rumen of sheep and cows, so that some trans fatty acids may be found in meat and products from these animals, such as milk and dairy products. Evidence is accumulating that trans fatty acids have adverse effects in the body and this is discussed further in Chapter 14.

A further consequence of unsaturation, particularly in polyunsaturated fatty acids, is that the spare electrons are highly reactive

TABLE 5.1 Classification of fatty acids by saturation, chain length and family

Type of fatty acid	Name	Number of carbon atoms: double bonds (fatty acid family)
Saturated	Butyric acid	4
	Caproic acid	6
	Caprylic acid	8
	Capric acid	10
	Lauric acid	12
	Myristic acid	14
	Palmitic acid	16
	Stearic acid	18
	Arachidic acid	20
Monounsaturated	Palmitoleic acid	16:1
	Oleic acid	18:1 (*n*-9)
	Eicosenoic acid	20:1 (*n*-9)
	Erucic acid	22:1 (*n*-9)
Polyunsaturated	Linoleic acid	18:2 (*n*-6)
	Alpha-linolenic acid	18:3 (*n*-3)
	Arachidonic acid	20:4 (*n*-6)
	Eicosapentaenoic acid (EPA)	20:5 (*n*-3)
	Docosahexaenoic acid (DHA)	22:6 (*n*-3)

Note: In the shorthand system used in the table, the number of carbon atoms precedes the colon, the number of double bonds follows. The allocation to specific fatty acid families occurs on the basis of the position of the first double bond in the molecule, counting from the methyl end. Thus in the *n*-3 family, the first double bond occurs on the third carbon from the methyl end, in the *n*-6 and *n*-9 families, these occur on the sixth and ninth carbons, respectively.

Figure 5.1 Spatial configuration of saturated, *cis* and *trans* unsaturated fatty acids.

and vulnerable to oxidation. In the presence of free radicals, such as 'singlet' oxygen or reactive hydroxyl groups, the double bonds can be attacked, leading to the formation of lipid oxides or peroxides. These change the properties of the fat, and may lead to malfunction and disease. Free radicals arise in the body as part of normal metabolic processes and can thus readily attack polyunsaturated fatty acids. The resulting products are themselves highly reactive, triggering a chain reaction and producing more highly reactive products. The body has a complex defence mechanism against such reactions in the form of antioxidants, which exist both intracellularly and extra-cellularly, and whose function is to react with the free radicals and thus inactivate them. There is more discussion about antioxidants in Chapter 14.

Essential fatty acids

Although the body can synthesize most of the fat it requires, it has been known since the early part of the twentieth century that certain of the polyunsaturated fatty acids cannot be synthesized and must be supplied in the diet. If they are excluded, a deficiency syndrome will develop, which in animals has been shown to include retarded growth and skin lesions, such as dermatitis. This deficiency can also occur in humans. Consequently, these fatty acids are known as 'essential fatty acids'. Occasionally, you will find them referred to as 'vitamin F'.

The essential fatty acids are linoleic (18:2, n-6) and alpha-linolenic (18:3, n-3) acids. Vertebrates lack enzymes to introduce double bonds at the n-3 and n-6 position, and cannot, therefore, synthesize members of these fatty acid families. However, if acids containing these double bonds (i.e. the essential fatty acids) are provided in the diet, other members of the family can then be produced by a series of desaturation (adding a double bond by removing hydrogen) and elongation (adding two carbon atoms) reactions:

Moreover, there is competition between the fatty acid families for the enzymes involved, with the result that a predominance of one family (e.g. n-6 acids) in the diet can limit the synthesis of some of the larger members of the n-3 family. For this reason, both n-6 and n-3 fatty acids should be supplied in sufficient amounts in the diet.

An intermediate product in the conversion of linoleic acid to arachidonic acid (n-6 family), is gamma-linolenic acid (GLA). This is supplied in quite large amounts by some unusual plant oils, particularly evening primrose oil, borage and blackcurrant seed oils. Many claims are made for the beneficial effects of these oils, especially evening primrose, although there does not currently appear to be an identified role for GLA.

More recently, interest has focused on the n-3 fatty acids contained in fish oils. These supply very long chain n-3 acids, such as eicosapentaenoic and docosahexaenoic acids, which are not made in large amounts in the body. They are particularly important in the development of the nervous system and retina in young infants, and a dietary source is needed in very early life. The ability to convert the smaller n-3 acids to EPA and DHA does exist in the young infant, but probably is not sufficiently active to produce adequate amounts.

Normally, breast milk produced by mothers consuming mixed diets would supply sufficient amounts of DHA, but formula-fed infants may receive inadequate quantities, and some milks are now being formulated with additional long-chain polyunsaturated fatty acids. Pre-term babies are particularly vulnerable to receiving insufficient amounts of these, and again need to obtain a fortified feed to ensure their intake.

Diet ⟶ 18:2 (n-6) ⟶ 18:3 (n-6) ⟶ 20:3 (n-6) ⟶ 20:4 (n-6)
Linoleic acid   Gamma-linolenic acid   Dihomo-gamma-linolenic acid   Arachidonic acid

Diet ⟶ 18:3 (n-3) ⟶ 18:4 (n-3) ... 20:5 (n-3) ⟶ 22:6 (n-3)
Alpha-linolenic acid   Eicosapentaenoic acid (EPA)   Docosahexaenoic acid (DHA)

(Note: Some of the intermediate acids have been omitted from the n-3 series, for clarity.)

The relative proportions of *n*-6 and *n*-3 acids in the Western diet have changed in the last 30 years for a number of reasons.

- There has been an increase in the consumption of vegetable oils, such as corn and sunflower oil as a result of healthy eating initiatives, to replace the traditional consumption of butter and other animal fats.
- Total intakes of meat from ruminant animals (beef and lamb) that are a source of *n*-3 fatty acids, have fallen. Furthermore, the *n*-3 acid content of the meat has also declined as the animals are fed less on grass and more on alternative concentrates to maximize production.
- Consumption of oily fish (and total fish) has been declining over this period, resulting in lower intakes of *n*-3 acids.

Consequently, there is concern that insufficient quantities of *n*-3 acids can be synthesized in the body, as there is too much competition from the *n*-6 acids. This has potential implications for the metabolic products derived from these acids and their effects in the body. There may be consequences within membranes throughout the body, as well as effects on neurotransmitter functions in the brain and on mood.

Evidence from a number of studies across Europe indicates that the ratio of *n*-6 to *n*-3 acids is approximately 6:1. Proposals have been made in the USA and Europe that the intake of *n*-3 acids should increase, without any further increases in *n*-6 acids, to reduce this ratio. Strategies to achieve this and safety considerations need to be considered.

Further discussion of the possible beneficial effects of *n*-3 fatty acids is to be found in Chapter 14.

Conjugated linoleic acid (CLA)

A group of isomers of linoleic acid, containing different geometrical double bond configurations, have become of interest. The double bonds are conjugated or contiguous, rather than methylene-separated, as they are in linoleic acid. The two double bonds can be in carbon positions 8 and 10, 9 and 11, 10 and 12, or 11 and 13. Each of the double bonds can also be in the *cis* or

trans configuration, and this results in a number of possible isomers. The most studied of these is C18:2 c9t11 isomer. This isomer has also been called rumenic acid, as it is predominantly produced in the rumen of cows and sheep. The main dietary sources of this acid are, therefore, dairy products and meat from ruminants. CLA has been reported to have anticarcinogenic, anti-atherogenic and immune-modulating potential, although the mechanisms are unclear. Body weight gain, with reduced fat mass and increased protein, has been shown in mice. CLA appears to be safe at doses up to ten times those normally found in the diet. Research into its bioavailability and potential benefits of naturally occurring or supplemented CLA is ongoing.

Other lipids

Besides triglycerides, important lipids in nutrition are phospholipids and sterols. Phospholipids are closely related to triglycerides, as they contain a glycerol backbone and two fatty acids. However, the third fatty acid is replaced by a phosphate group and a base. The commonest phospholipid, lecithin (also called phosphatidylcholine), contains choline as the base. It is widely distributed in cell membranes throughout the body and is also a component of the surfactant in the lungs, which facilitates breathing by reducing surface tension in the alveoli. Other bases found in phospholipids include serine, inositol and ethanolamine.

All phospholipids serve an essential function in the body, as their structure contains both a hydrophobic (water hating) and a hydrophilic (water loving) area. This allows them to associate with both lipid and aqueous compounds in the body, and to serve as an emulsifying agent, allowing these two dissimilar parts to coexist. Their role is particularly important in cell membranes, and high concentrations are found in the brain and nervous system. Sphingomyelin is a phospholipid occurring in the myelin sheath of nerve fibres. All the phospholipids can be synthesized in the body and are, thus, not essential in the diet.

Sterols are ringed structures containing carbon, hydrogen and oxygen. The most prevalent example of this group in animals is cholesterol (Figure 5.2), which is a waxy substance that can be synthesized by the body from acetyl coenzyme A. The main site of synthesis is the liver, although all cells of the body can make it. The human body typically contains about 100 g of cholesterol, of which 7 per cent is found in the blood, and the remainder distributed in all cells of the body. Here, cholesterol plays a number of roles:

- maintenance of the structure and integrity of cell membranes;
- regulation of the fluidity of cell membranes;
- facilitation of the communication between the cell and its environment, including transport across the membrane;
- limiting the leakage of Na and K ions across the membrane;
- synthesis of bile acids, which are needed for fat absorption;
- synthesis of hormones, including the sex hormones, steroids and vitamin D.

In the diet, cholesterol is only found in foods derived from animals. Plant foods contain phytosterols, the most important being beta-sitosterol, which is found in nuts, cereals and fats and oils. Vegetarian diets are low in cholesterol, unless they include some animal products, like milk and eggs. Body cholesterol levels in an individual are kept fairly constant, with synthesis decreasing as dietary intake increases and vice versa. Absorption of cholesterol is variable, ranging from 15 to 60 per cent of dietary intake. Large intakes of phytosterols may inhibit cholesterol absorption and this has been utilized in a number of functional products developed to lower cholesterol levels. Cholesterol is excreted from the body in the faeces, having been secreted into the digestive tract in the bile produced by the liver.

Levels of cholesterol in the blood are partly genetically determined, so that effects of dietary intake may be quite variable. Plasma cholesterol levels in some individuals respond minimally to changes in dietary intake of cholesterol, while in others the response is much greater. Raised blood cholesterol levels are a major risk factor in the development of cardiovascular disease and, for this reason, a great deal of research has been undertaken to discover the factors which affect them. These are discussed further in Chapter 14.

FATS IN THE DIET

Nutritionists may describe fats in the diet as 'visible' or 'invisible' fats (see Figure 5.3). Visible fats are those that can be clearly seen in our food; these include the spreading fats, cooking oils and the fat around pieces of meat. As this fat is obvious, the consumer can quite readily make an effort to reduce it – by using less spread on bread, by not using oil in frying and by trimming the fat off meat.

Visible fats

Invisible fats

Figure 5.2 Chemical structure of cholesterol.

Figure 5.3 Sources of visible and invisible fats.

Invisible fat is more difficult to remove. This is the fat that is often integral in a food product, for example, the fat in egg yolk, the fat contained within tissues in meat and fish, in nuts and, particularly, in processed and manufactured foods, such as sausages, burgers, pies, biscuits, cakes, pastries and chocolate. It is clearly more difficult to reduce this fat – it involves either changing the product by making it with less fat or simply eliminating the food from the diet. Some success has been achieved by food producers in promoting lower fat milk and dairy products, and lower fat versions of some processed foods. A major difficulty is that the consumer often does not appreciate how much fat is contained in a food, because it cannot be seen. Moreover, the labelling of foods may be often confusing, with essentially meaningless slogans, such as 90 per cent fat free or 30 per cent less fat, providing no information about how much fat we are actually eating.

Some examples of the fat contents of selected foods are given in Table 5.2.

Trends in intakes of fats

Historical records suggest that fat intakes in many parts of Europe increased quite markedly at the start of the twentieth century, rising from a level of around 20 per cent of the total energy in the late nineteenth century, to values around 30 per cent by the 1920s. Studies from this era are not necessary comparable with today's methods, but they do indicate a rapid increase over a relatively short time. Expressed as a percentage of the total energy intake, fat intake has risen steadily since data have been collected by the National Food Survey. Levels in the 1940s were around 34 per cent of total energy. Throughout the 1950s and 1960s, they rose to reach 41 per cent and continued at a slower rate to reach 43 per cent by the mid-1980s. Levels

TABLE 5.2 Fat contents of selected foods per 100 g, per average serving portion and as per cent energy from fat			
Food	Fat (g/100 g)	Fat (g/average serving)	Energy from fat (%)
Cheddar cheese	34.9	14.0	75.5
Cottage cheese	4.3	2.2	38.3
Boiled egg	10.8	5.4	66
Milk: full-fat	3.9	7.8	53.2
Milk: semi-skimmed	1.7	3.4	33.2
Milk: skimmed	0.2	0.4	5.6
Cream: single	19.1	5.7	89.1
Cream: double	53.7	16.1	97.4
Butter/soft margarine	82.2	8.2	99.4
Low-fat spread	37.6	3.8	92.7
Beefburger	23.9	21.5	65.3
Beef pie	19.4	28.1	56.3
Lean beef, roast	6.3	5.7	28.1
Cheese and tomato pizza	10.3	23.7	33.5
Digestive biscuit	20.3	2.6	39.2
Rich fruit cake	11.4	8.0	29.9
Doughnut with jam	14.5	10.9	38.9
Chocolate bar	30.7	16.6	53.1
Potato chips	6.7	11.1	31.9
Baked potato with skin	0.2	0.4	1.3

Data calculated from Food Standards Agency (2002a, 2002b).

have gradually been falling since this time, and in 2000, the Department for Environment, Food and Rural Affairs (DEFRA) (2001) found that fat contributed 38.2 per cent of total energy intake. It is worth noting that carbohydrate intakes have mirrored this trend, with an initial fall, followed by a rise in the percentage of energy from carbohydrate. The implications of these changes for health are discussed in Chapter 8.

It is important to remember that the figures discussed above reflect the percentage of energy from fat in the total energy intake. The actual amount of fat consumed has been decreasing, as noted by successive National Food Survey reports. There has been a greater reduction in fat intakes in the higher than in the lowest income group, so that fat intakes are now marginally greater in this latter group. The data are shown in Table 5.3. On average, the difference in fat intake between social groups, regions and families within the UK is relatively small. Much greater differences are seen if culturally different societies are compared.

One should remember, however, that there has been a progressive trend towards eating outside the home, which is more frequent in Group A than Group D households. Therefore, the recorded intakes do not include all of the food consumed by individuals. Eating out was measured for the first time in 1994, and the National Food Survey reports show that foods eaten out have a higher percentage fat content than those eaten at home.

In addition to changes in the total fat intake, there has also been an alteration in the balance of the saturated, monounsaturated and polyunsaturated fatty acids in the diet. The changes reported by DEFRA (2001) in the percentage of energy from the main groups of fatty acids are shown in Table 5.4. These values reflect trends in food consumption patterns, with a decline in the consumption of whole milk, butter, margarine and lard, and increases in the intake of oils and spreads made from vegetable oils. Many of these changes have been prompted by advice on healthy eating in the last two decades and the response of food manufacturers.

TABLE 5.3	Trends in total fat (g) and energy (Calories) intakes, per person per day, showing mean population figures and intakes in the highest (Group A) and lowest (Group D) income groups studied by the National Food Survey (DEFRA, 2001). The figures do not include confectionery and soft or alcoholic drinks					
Year	Population mean		Group A		Group D	
	Fat (g)	Energy (Calories)	Fat (g)	Energy (Calories)	Fat (g)	Energy (Calories)
1950	101	2474	109	2542	97	2379
1960	115	2630	120	2600	106	2540
1970	121	2600	124	2520	108	2470
1980	106	2230	106	2150	105	2240
1990	86	1870	86	1710	86	1890
2000	74	1750	68	1600	75	1720

TABLE 5.4	Percentage of energy from the main groups of fatty acids		
Year	Saturated fatty acids	Monounsaturated fatty acids	Polyunsaturated fatty acids
1972	19.3	15.9	4.3
1980	18.9	16.0	4.6
1990	16.7	15.3	6.7
2000	15.0	13.5	6.9

Sources of fat in the British diet

Table 5.5 shows the main sources of fat and fatty acids in the British diet, based on data from the National Food Survey 2000 (DEFRA, 2001). There have been some advances in the breeding and particularly butchering of animals in the last decade, so that new analyses of meat available in the UK show reductions in the fat content of lamb, beef and pork, with the greatest reductions achieved in pork. To an extent it has also been possible to alter the fatty acid composition of the fat in meat by manipulating the types of fats fed to animals. This is more successful in non-ruminants, such as pigs and poultry, than in ruminants, as these tend to saturate fat by bacterial action in their rumen.

Sources of essential fatty acids

The parent acid of the *n*-6 polyunsaturated fatty acid (PUFA) family, linoleic acid occurs in meat, eggs and nuts (walnuts, brazil nuts, almonds and peanuts). It also occurs in seeds used for oils and spread, such as sunflower, soya, corn, sesame and safflower. The parent of the *n*-3 PUFA family, alpha-linolenic acid is found in dark green, leafy vegetables and meat from grass-fed ruminants. Oils derived from nuts and seeds are also a source of this acid (as well as the nuts themselves). Examples include walnuts, peanuts, almonds, soya, rapeseed and linseed. The longer members of the *n*-3 family are found in oil-rich fish, such as sardines, pilchards, salmon, trout, herrings, mackerel and fresh (not canned) tuna.

Cod liver oil is also a rich source, although not a common component of the diet.

Activity 5.1

Look at a number of foods that are claimed to have less fat, such as sausages, cheesecake, bacon, burgers, salad dressings. Work out how much fat there is in a typical serving, or per 100 g.

- Is it less than in the comparable 'normal fat' product?
- How much less is it?
- How many fewer grams of fat will you eat by substituting this food in your diet?

Activity 5.2

Various spreads, margarines and butters contain different amounts and proportions of fatty-acid types. Prepare a chart of the ones commonly found in your local supermarket or grocery store, and compare the percentages of total fat, proportions of different types of fatty acids and the amount of fat per serving, or per 100 g in each. You can also include some cooking oils in this survey.

- Which type of spread appears to have the lowest fat content?
- Does this spread also have the lowest content of saturated fatty acids?
- What are the implications of your results for someone trying to eat less fat?

TABLE 5.5	Sources of fat and fatty acids in the British diet (calculated from DEFRA, 2001)			
Food group	**Percentage of contribution to total**			
	Fat	**Saturated fatty acids**	**Monounsaturated fatty acids**	**Polyunsaturated fatty acids**
Fats and oils	26	21	28	41
Butter	6	10	5	1.5
Spreads/oils	16	6.5	18.5	34
Meat and meat products	22	22	28	15
Milk, dairy and cheese	17	28	14	4
Cereals and cereal products	16	17	16	16

Why do we eat fat?

People who are culturally accustomed to eating fat, such as the populations of the Western world, find that food with a significantly reduced fat content is unpalatable. This is because Westerners are used to the way that fat enhances the palatability of food. Food containing fat creates a particular 'mouthfeel', a feeling of creaminess and smoothness when taken into the mouth, which is related to the presence of fat emulsions in a food.

Activity 5.3

Compare the sensations in your mouth after a mouthful of skimmed milk (very low fat), normal fat milk, single cream and double cream.

In addition, fat enhances the flavour of foods, as many of the substances responsible for 'flavour' and 'odour' are volatile fatty substances, originating from the lipid in the food. Adding fat to a food can, therefore, enhance its sensory appeal. For example, frying or roasting foods (such as potatoes) produces flavours that cannot be obtained by boiling the same food. Hence the popularity of potato chips (French fries). Aromas associated with oranges or coffee are also oil-based. Sometimes the presence of these fat-based smells can be very unpleasant in a kitchen; cooking oil that has been used several times, and thus contains a number of fat oxidation products, releases a very unsavoury smell.

Fat is a concentrated source of energy. It supplies 37 kJ/g (9 Calories/g), which is more than any other macronutrient. It has the advantage that a large amount of energy can be consumed in a relatively small volume of food. This may be important for people with a small appetite or those whose energy needs are very high, such as athletes or those undertaking other strenuous activity. In addition, it can be helpful when patients are being fed by a tube, where a smaller volume of feed is an advantage.

However, the disadvantage of the high energy concentration is that it becomes very easy to overconsume energy – a small amount of fat-rich food can provide unexpectedly high fat intakes. The converse of this is that, where people have very little fat in their diet, they have to consume large volumes of food to meet their energy needs. For children, in particular, this volume may be unobtainable and this may be one of the contributory factors to undernutrition in developing countries. Adding a small amount of oil to a traditional starchy rural diet can make a great deal of difference to overall energy intake.

As well as supplying energy in the diet, fats also provide a vehicle for other essential nutrients, in particular, the fat-soluble vitamins and the essential fatty acids. The absorption of fat-soluble vitamins from the digestive tract depends on the presence and normal digestion/absorption of fats. Thus, people on low-fat diets may be at risk of insufficient intake of these vitamins. (See Figure 5.4 for a summary of these points.)

DIGESTION AND ABSORPTION OF FATS

Fat digestion is uncomplicated. One type of lipase (a fat-splitting enzyme) can split the link between glycerol and any fatty acid. A small amount of lipase, called lingual lipase, is produced in the mouth. This is probably of greatest importance in infants, as it is particularly active in the breakdown of milk fats. Milk digestion is also facilitated in breast-fed infants by the presence of a lipase in the milk itself.

The main process of fat digestion starts in the stomach, where the churning action breaks it down into a coarse emulsion. The emptying of fats from the stomach into the duodenum causes the release of several hormones called

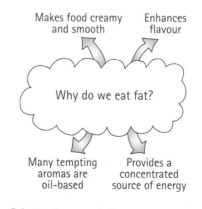

Figure 5.4 Why do we eat fat?

enterogastrones, which inhibit further stomach emptying. In this way, the release of fats for digestion in the intestine is slowed down, and a fat-rich meal stays in the stomach for longer, creating satiation. The main lipase is that from the pancreas, which splits fats in the jejunum into a mixture of fatty acids and glycerol, together with some monoglycerides.

However, fats are not soluble in the watery mixture of the small intestine and would normally aggregate into large droplets. These need to be split up into tiny droplets by emulsifying agents, which are both fat and water soluble. In the gut, this is carried out by the bile acids, which emulsify the fat and enable lipase to act. Bile acids are made in the liver from cholesterol, concentrated and stored in the bile ducts and gall bladder, and then secreted into the duodenum when the food enters from the stomach. Partly split fats and free fatty acids aid the bile salts in emulsifying the neutral fats. The bile acids that have been used in fat digestion are reabsorbed in the ileum, and pass in the blood to the liver, where they act as a stimulus for their resecretion into the bile. They, thus, undergo what is termed an enterohepatic circulation. Interference with this circulation will alter the level of bile acids and their precursor, cholesterol. The bile salts that return to the liver act as an inhibitor to further synthesis from cholesterol. If fewer return to the liver, then more synthesis of bile salts from cholesterol can occur, thus lowering the level of cholesterol in the blood.

Phospholipids are also broken down by removal of their fatty acids, by the action of the enzyme phospholipase. Cholesterol esters in the diet are hydrolysed by esterases to remove the fatty acid and so release cholesterol for absorption.

Once the fats have been split into their constituents, they merge into tiny spherical complexes, known as micelles, which diffuse easily into the intestinal cell (or enterocyte). Once inside the enterocyte, the fat digestion products are reassembled into triglycerides, although not the same as the original ones in the diet. These are then coated with phospholipids and apolipoproteins to produce chylomicrons. This 'envelope' provides a means of stabilizing lipids in an aqueous environment, such as the circulation. In addition to the triglycerides, the chylomicrons also contain other fat digestion products, such as cholesterol and fat-soluble vitamins. Too large to diffuse into the blood capillaries of the gut wall, the chylomicrons pass into the lacteals of the lymphatic system, and eventually enter the bloodstream at the thoracic duct in the neck, where the lymphatic system drains into the blood. Fat digestion is summarized in Figure 5.5.

Some smaller fatty acids, containing 4–10 carbon atoms, are able to pass into the blood capillaries in the gut, and so are absorbed directly into the hepatic portal vein, where they attach to plasma albumin and are transported to the liver. These types of fatty acids have the advantage of being a little more water soluble; they are, therefore, not so dependent on emulsification by the bile for their digestion. In some patients, where there is a fat digestion problem owing to a lack of bile, introducing short-chain fats into the diet may be a temporary way of adding dietary fat, which would otherwise not be tolerated. The two ways in which fat digestion products enter the body are summarized in Table 5.6.

Fat digestion is normally very efficient, with 95 per cent of ingested fat being absorbed. However, in some instances digestion and/or absorption will be defective. If fat is undigested or unabsorbed, it will appear in the faeces. This produces a characteristic faecal appearance, with waxy stools, which tend to be foul smelling and, because they float, are difficult to flush away. This condition is called steatorrhoea. Unabsorbed fats will remove other fat-soluble components from the body, in particular, the fat-soluble vitamins, and chronic steatorrhoea may be associated with a specific vitamin deficiency.

Causes of steatorrhoea may include:

■ failure to produce lipase as a result of pancreatic insufficiency, or problems with the production or secretion of bile;
■ gallstones, which can block the secretion of bile into the gut;
■ inefficient absorption of fat due to defects in the surface of the small intestine, which may be flattened or inflamed; and
■ ingestion of mineral oils, such as liquid paraffin, as a laxative.

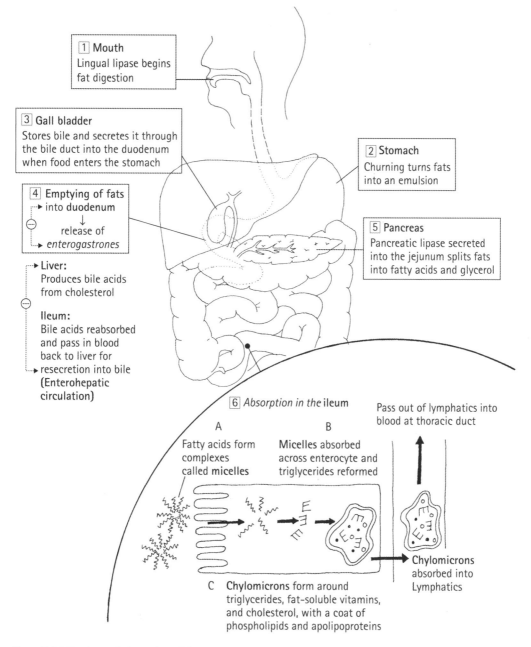

1 Mouth
Lingual lipase begins fat digestion

3 Gall bladder
Stores bile and secretes it through the bile duct into the duodenum when food enters the stomach

2 Stomach
Churning turns fats into an emulsion

4 Emptying of fats
→ into duodenum
↓
⊖ release of
↳ *enterogastrones*

5 Pancreas
Pancreatic lipase secreted into the jejunum splits fats into fatty acids and glycerol

Liver:
Produces bile acids from cholesterol

⊖

Ileum:
Bile acids reabsorbed and pass in blood back to liver for
→ resecretion into bile
(Enterohepatic circulation)

6 Absorption in the ileum

Pass out of lymphatics into blood at thoracic duct

A
Fatty acids form complexes called **micelles**

B
Micelles absorbed across enterocyte and triglycerides reformed

Chylomicrons absorbed into Lymphatics

C **Chylomicrons** form around triglycerides, fat-soluble vitamins, and cholesterol, with a coat of phospholipids and apolipoproteins

Figure 5.5 Digestion and absorption of fats.

TRANSPORT OF FATS IN THE BODY

Because of their hydrophobic nature, fats have to be carried around the circulation in association with hydrophilic substances, otherwise they would separate out and float on the surface of the blood, like the cream from the milk. Chylomicrons, which facilitate the entry of digested fats into the circulation, are one example of such an association. These are the largest and lightest of a group of aggregates collectively known as lipoproteins. Lipoproteins are classified according to their density and can be separated by ultracentrifugation of a blood sample. At one end of the range are the large light chylomicrons, then, arranged in decreasing size, come very low density, low-density and high-density lipoproteins, usually referred to by their acronyms VLDL, LDL and HDL.

Fats in the blood are carried in lipoproteins, irrespective of whether they have originated from the diet or been synthesized in the body. In both cases, the triglyceride and cholesterol esters are coated with a shell of phospholipid and apolipoprotein. The apolipoprotein provides an 'identity tag' by which the body cells recognize the particular type. The lipoproteins are not constant in their composition: they are dynamic particles, which release and pick up their constituents as they travel around the body.

However, it is possible to describe the typical composition of each type, as shown in Table 5.7. It can be clearly seen that the chylomicrons contain predominantly triglycerides and are thus very low in density. The major constituents of VLDLs are also triglycerides. LDLs contain mostly cholesterol and are its major carriers in the body. HDLs are predominantly made up of

protein, with smaller fat contents than the other types. This accounts for their high density. There is also a difference in size, with the chylomicrons being the largest and the HDL the smallest of the particles.

Chylomicrons start to appear in the blood within 30 minutes of eating a fat-containing meal, with a peak after approximately 3 hours. They cause an increase in plasma lipid levels, and serum samples taken during this time have a milky appearance because of this. Some chylomicrons may continue to enter into the blood after a fat-rich meal over a period of up to 14 hours.

As chylomicrons circulate in the blood, fats are removed from them by specific lipoprotein lipases in the blood vessel walls, especially in the liver, skeletal muscle and adipose tissue, and free fatty acids and glycerol are released. The body uses these products for particular metabolic processes needed at the time. This may involve fuelling muscle contraction or perhaps being stored in the adipose tissue for subsequent use. Chylomicrons may also pass some of their free cholesterol to HDLs.

The remnants of the chylomicrons are eventually broken down in the liver and used to make

TABLE 5.6	Summary of fate of fat digestion products
Short-chain fatty acids Medium-chain fatty acids Glycerol	Absorbed directly into hepatic portal vein

Triglycerides (reconstituted from
   long-chain fatty acids and
     monoglycerides)
Cholesterol
Phospholipids
Fat-soluble vitamins
	Made into chylomicrons; absorbed into lacteals,
	carried via lymphatic system into the blood

TABLE 5.7	Typical compositions of lipoprotein particles (as per cent)			
	Triglyceride	Cholesterol	Phospholipid	Protein
Chylomicrons	90	5	3	2
VLDL	60	12	18	10
LDL	10	50	15	25
HDL	5	20	25	50

other lipoproteins. The liver cells synthesize fat (endogenous fats) brought in from fatty acids; cholesterol is also synthesized. Eventually, the fats made in the liver are packaged as VLDLs and exported into the rest of the body.

As the VLDLs travel through the body, lipoprotein lipase removes their triglycerides, in much the same way as for chylomicrons. Both chylomicrons and VLDLs contain the apolipoprotein apo-CII, which activates lipoprotein lipase. As they lose triglycerides, the VLDLs become smaller and the proportion of cholesterol in them increases. Thus, they are transformed into LDLs.

One other transformation also occurs. This is the loss of some of the apolipoprotein, so that the remaining 'identity tag' is that of the LDLs. This is apolipoprotein B_{100} (apo-B_{100}) and is vital for the normal metabolic functioning of LDLs.

The function of LDL is to act as the major carrier of cholesterol, taking it to the tissues where it is needed in cell membranes or for synthesis of metabolites, such as steroid hormones. Specific receptors for apo-B_{100} are present on cell surfaces. These allow the LDLs to attach to the cell, and the whole LDL–receptor complex is taken into the cell, where it is broken down by enzymes. The activity and number of receptor sites can vary, thus controlling cholesterol uptake by cells. In the genetically determined condition familial hypercholesterolaemia, subjects lack the LDL receptor, resulting in high circulating levels of LDLs.

HDLs are responsible for the removal of spare or surplus cholesterol as well as apolipoproteins from cells and other lipoproteins; this is known as reverse cholesterol transport. When cholesterol is picked up by the HDLs, it quickly becomes esterified, which allows it to be taken into the hydrophobic core of the lipoprotein. In this way, the outer layer of the HDL maintains a diffusion gradient for more cholesterol to be picked up. This system allows cholesterol to be removed from the tissues and taken to the liver. This completes the lipid transport cycle (Figures 5.6 and 5.7).

Because LDLs and HDLs are so intimately involved with cholesterol transport, they are believed to be closely associated with the development of atheroma and particularly of heart disease. Consequently, factors influencing the circulating levels of LDLs and HDLs have been extensively studied. It is believed that they are influenced by a number of factors, including

Figure 5.6 Exogenous lipid transport.

Figure 5.7 Endogenous lipid transport and metabolism.

genetics, hormone levels, age, gender, smoking, exercise and diet. One such gene, which appears to be particularly important, is that for apolipoprotein E (APOE). Several variants have been identified, which account for a proportion of the variation in LDL levels within a population. Variants may also determine the response of lipoprotein levels to changes in dietary factors and the rate of clearance from the circulation.

Factors affecting lipoproteins are discussed in more detail in Chapter 14.

FUNCTION OF FAT IN THE BODY

In considering the role of fat in the body, it is important to recognize that fat occurs throughout the body, as part of the structure of every cell membrane, as well as being found in discrete areas as adipose tissue. Fat is essential in body composition and, as such, has many diverse functions in the body. These are:

- structure
- storage
- metabolism.

It should be remembered, however, that these categories are not separate and distinct from one another and there is considerable overlap between them.

Structure of membranes

The structure of biological membranes consists of lipid molecules that are often associated with other residues, such as phosphate groups or carbohydrates, together with cholesterol and proteins. The exact nature of the membrane is very dependent on the types of fatty acids present, varying with their length, degree of saturation and spatial arrangement. In addition, various fats occur on the surface of the skin and contribute to its waterproof properties. Some of these fats are quite unusual, containing chains with odd numbers of carbon atoms, branched chains and double bonds in unusual locations. Free fatty acids, which are thought to have bactericidal properties, may also be present.

Storage – the adipose tissue

The body is able to store fat as an energy reserve, in specialized cells, called adipocytes, which are found in adipose tissue. Adipocytes make up only about half of the total cell numbers within adipose tissue; fibroblasts, macrophages and vascular tissue are other important components. Adipose tissue plays a major role in metabolism (discussed below). Two types of adipose tissue have now been identified – the predominant form, white adipose tissue (WAT) and brown adipose tissue (BAT), which occurs in much smaller amounts. Brown adipose tissue differs from WAT in several respects, most noticeably in having many more mitochondria, blood capillaries and nerve fibres than the white tissue. This type of fat is much more widespread in newborn animals, and provides a means of heat generation at this critical stage of life, before shivering mechanisms develop. It used to be thought that brown fat then disappeared, but more recent research suggests that small amounts persist into adult life, and may play a part in generating heat as a means of ridding the body of surplus energy.

The WAT cells store fat as a single droplet, which fills almost the entire cell contents, pushing the remaining organelles to the very edges of the cell. The fat stored in the body is a reflection of the type of dietary fat; thus, an individual eating a diet rich in polyunsaturated fats will have more of these in their adipose tissue. On the other hand, a person who has small fat stores and consumes little fat will have adipose tissue fats that are more typical of fat synthesized in the body containing mainly palmitic, stearic and oleic acids.

The number of fat cells has been estimated at about 5×10^{10} in a mature adult. There has been considerable debate about the means of expansion of fat stores. This can occur by hyperplasia, which is an increase in cell number, or by hypertrophy, which is an increase in size of existing cells. It had been believed that adipocyte numbers were set in early infancy, and would remain at this level for life, but this is now known to be incorrect. The size of adipocytes is related to their fat stores, so these will vary with the flux of fat into and out of stores. As fat stores increase, it is postulated that new cells are formed from preadipocytes already present in the body. Whether adipocytes can be lost on reduction of fat stores is still under debate, although there is evidence that apoptosis (programmed cell death) can occur, but the significance of this in individuals is unknown.

It has also become clear that adipose tissue depots to an extent may be self-regulatory, and that depots in various parts of the body respond differently to physiological demands. In particular, there are differences between fat stored in the abdominal region and that in the thighs and buttocks. The fat adjacent to lymph nodes is proposed as having an important role in supporting the immune system, and may become much larger in chronic inflammatory states at the expense of other fat depots, resulting in changes in body fat distribution. This has been noted in HIV infection and Crohn's disease.

The ability to store fat as an energy reserve offers an additional benefit, that of insulation and protection. Adipose tissue covers some of our more delicate organs, such as the kidneys, spleen, spinal cord and brain, to protect them from injury. This protective fat is used less readily as fuel in a fasting individual. Most of the fuel-storing adipose tissue is found under the skin, as subcutaneous fat. Here it also provides insulation to facilitate the maintenance of body temperature. In hot climates, this can be a disadvantage, with overweight individuals sweating readily to lose heat. On the other hand, sufferers from anorexia nervosa, who have little subcutaneous fat, will feel cold even on a warm day, and will dress in several layers of clothing both to provide extra warmth, but perhaps also to disguise their extreme thinness. The body also stores fat-soluble vitamins in its adipose tissue.

Metabolic roles

Meeting the energy needs – fat metabolism

The provision of energy is probably the most commonly recognized function of fats. Fat is an energy-dense fuel; more than twice as much energy is provided per gram of stored fat than can be obtained from each gram of carbohydrate or protein. This means that our bodies can store a large amount of reserve energy in a relatively small volume. If our major stores of energy were in the form of carbohydrate, we would either have much smaller reserves or weigh much more!

The storage and release of energy from adipose tissue is under continuous hormonal control, mainly by insulin and noradrenaline. It has been proposed that the adipose tissue is an essential buffer in the body to regulate fats whose levels vary with intermittent food intake. This buffering action can fail, e.g. in obesity or in conditions of too little body fat, resulting in metabolic abnormalities, such as insulin resistance (see below).

Fat storage

The adipocytes extract triglycerides from passing lipoproteins by the action of the enzyme lipoprotein lipase (LPL). This enzyme is activated by insulin and is, therefore, most active in the postprandial phase (after meals). The triglycerides are broken down by LPL, taken into the adipose tissue cell and then reassembled into new triglycerides for storage. The storage and release of fat is a dynamic process, with a continuous flux of fats into and out of the cells. A great deal of fat storage occurs after meals, when there are increased numbers of chylomicrons and VLDLs in the circulation. In theory, fat may be synthesized from carbohydrate, but this happens only in exceptional circumstances of extremely high carbohydrate intakes and is very inefficient. Other sites in the body can also make fat, in particular, the liver and mammary gland during lactation. However, the liver does not normally store significant quantities of fat; a liver loaded with fat is generally diseased. The mammary gland is able to synthesize shorter chain fatty acids, with lauric and myristic acids predominating (C_{12} and C_{14}).

Fat utilization

The body uses stored fat as its major energy supply, releasing non-esterified fatty acids (NEFA) into the circulation under the influence of noradrenaline released by the sympathetic nervous system. At most levels of activity, fat provides a significant proportion of the energy used. It is only when we exercise very intensively (e.g. running the 100 metres sprint) that all the energy comes from carbohydrate, since fat cannot be metabolized sufficiently quickly (see Chapter 16). The lower the level of activity, the greater the proportion of energy that comes from fat. However, some glucose continues to be used for metabolism as the brain, nervous system and red blood cells require it. Under normal circumstances, glucose levels are maintained by hormones such as insulin, adrenaline and cortisol, which ensure that sufficient is present to fuel these essential tissues and organs. If there is no supply of glucose entering the body, organs such as the liver are capable of making glucose from protein residues and glycerol from fat breakdown (see Figure 5.8).

Fat breakdown to supply ATP occurs by the successive splitting of acetic acid molecules from the ends of long-chain fatty acids. These acetic acid molecules then enter the same common pathway that serves carbohydrate metabolism. For complete oxidation, some carbohydrate must be present. If there is no glucose or glycogen,

Figure 5.8 The role of adipose tissue in metabolism.

then acetic acid molecules combine in pairs to form ketone bodies. Once formed, ketone bodies are sent to the peripheral tissues, where they can be converted back to acetyl coenzyme A and used in the normal Krebs (or citric acid) cycle. A mild rise in ketone body production (ketosis) will occur whenever fat mobilization occurs, for example, during moderate exercise, overnight fast and conditions associated with low food intake, such as acute gastroenteritis or the nausea and vomiting of early pregnancy. A more severe type of ketosis causing mental confusion or coma, as well as physiological changes (muscular weakness and overbreathing), may occur in severe states of these kinds and also in diabetes mellitus. In this case, insulin lack prevents normal glucose entry into cells and thus glucose oxidation. Symptoms associated with mild ketosis include lethargy, headache and loss of appetite. These are very general, however, and may be caused by many other factors.

If we fast, the body rapidly metabolizes body fat. Initially, there is also rapid breakdown of lean tissue as the body uses protein residues to maintain blood glucose supplies. After a number of days, however, the brain and nervous system adapt to the use of ketone bodies for energy, and survival using fat stores becomes possible. Inevitably, a fatter person will be able to survive longer than one with limited fat stores at the outset.

Link with glucose metabolism – insulin resistance

Research on the metabolic changes that occur in overweight and obesity has identified close links between amounts of adipose tissue and sensitivity to insulin and, therefore, glucose metabolism.

- Sensitivity to insulin has been shown to decrease with increasing levels of body fat, even at relatively normal body mass index (BMI) levels.
- Insulin normally inhibits the release of NEFA from adipose tissue, but in obesity this response is reduced per unit of fat mass. However, because there is more stored fat, the total amount of NEFA released is actually increased.

- The removal of triglycerides (as chylomicrons or VLDL) from the circulation by the action of LPL may also be depressed by reduced sensitivity of this enzyme to insulin.
- The overall consequence is a chronically raised level of circulating fats (lipaemia), which deposit in a number of tissues, including liver and skeletal muscle. This suppresses glucose utilization by muscle, stimulates the production of glucose in the liver and stimulates insulin release. High levels of NEFA may also damage the pancreatic β-cells that secrete insulin. Thus, there is interference with the normal insulin-mediated glucose disposal, owing to a failure of the buffer capacity of the adipose tissue (see Figure 5.9).

Adipose tissue and metabolic regulation

Adipose tissue is now recognized as having a role as a source of many metabolic regulators, with more factors still being discovered. The most important of these has been leptin, discovered in 1994, which is produced predominantly by adipose tissue, but has also been shown to be secreted by other organs like the stomach, mammary gland and placenta. Leptin receptors are also found in adipose tissue but are principally sited in the hypothalamus. Leptin has been shown to interact with neuropeptides in the brain to inhibit food intake. It also plays a role in energy expenditure, probably via BAT, and is a signal to the reproductive system in sexual maturation. Leptin release is under the control of the sympathetic nervous system.

There are many other factors released by adipose tissue with diverse actions and some as yet unidentified.

- Proteins involved in lipid and lipoprotein metabolism include LPL and cholesteryl ester transfer protein, important in accumulation of cholesteryl ester in WAT.
- Proteins that play a role in blood pressure regulation and blood clotting are also secreted, and may be a link with disorders of these processes in obesity.
- Immune function is also influenced by secretory products from the adipose tissue, including cytokines (most notably tumour necrosis factor α (TNFα)) and complement system

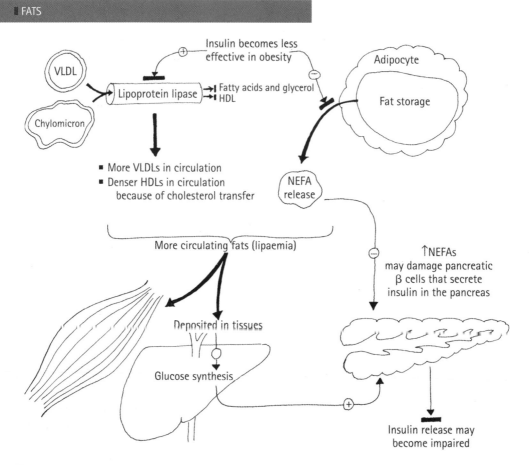

Figure 5.9 Aspects of insulin resistance.

products. The cytokines in turn appear to have a regulatory role in various aspects of adipose tissue function. The immune system uses up to 15 per cent of the body's resting metabolic rate, and it may be that the close relationship between adipose tissue energy stores and the immune system is a means of ensuring that adequate energy can be provided when the immune system is under stress. TNFα inhibits fat storage and would, therefore, make fatty acids immediately available.

■ Metallothionein is a stress response protein that acts as an antioxidant, and may protect fatty acids in adipose tissue from damage by free radicals during high rates of oxygen utilization.

Steroid metabolism

Cholesterol is essential in the body. It is the precursor for the synthesis of the steroid hormones, which includes those produced in the adrenal gland, as well as the sex hormones. It is also a prerequisite for the formation of vitamin D in the skin. In addition, cholesterol is used in the manufacture of bile salts in the liver, which, as we saw earlier in this chapter, are vital in the normal digestion of dietary fats. The bile salts can be reabsorbed from the lower gut and reused by the liver. Some, however, can be trapped in the faeces and removed from the body. In this case, more bile salts have to be synthesized from cholesterol. Adipose tissue is a major site for storage of cholesterol.

Many of the steroid hormones are converted to their active form in the tissue. This includes formation of oestradiol from oestrone, testosterone from androstenedione and oestrogens from androgens. The last of these can form an important source of female hormones in overweight individuals, which may have positive benefits in terms of maintaining bone health after the menopause, but also negative consequences in increasing the risk of hormone-dependent tumours.

Essential fatty acids

There are two major metabolic roles for the essential fatty acids. The presence of essential fatty acids in the membranes of cells and their organelles contributes to the stability and integrity of these membranes. Signs of deficiency include changes in the properties of membranes, particularly increases in permeability. These are accompanied by reduced efficiency of energy utilization and, therefore, poorer growth. The n-3 acids are of particular importance in the membranes of the nervous system and brain, as well as the retina. Docosahexaenoic acid (22:6) is particularly concentrated in the retina, and levels increase in the fetal brain and retina in the later stages of pregnancy. Development continues in early childhood, and a supply of these long-chain fatty acids is essential to optimize neurological development.

In addition, essential fatty acids are the precursors of a family of bioactive compounds called eicosanoids, which act as metabolic regulators in a number of key functions. Two major pathways for eicosanoid production exist. Prostaglandins, prostacyclins and thromboxanes are made by the cyclo-oxygenase pathway, and leukotrienes are produced by the lipoxygenase pathway. Eicosanoids are derived from fatty acids with 20 carbon atoms. Thus, the majority originate from arachidonic acid (20:4), which is a member of the n-6 fatty acid family and is produced in the body from the essential fatty acid, linoleic acid. However, some are produced from eicosapentaenoic acid (20:5), which is a member of the n-3 family, made in the body from the essential fatty acid, alpha-linolenic acid. It is believed that a predominance of n-6 acids in the body may prevent the formation of eicosanoids of the n-3 series. Prostaglandins and other eicosanoids are very potent substances; therefore, they are produced at the site of action and very quickly inactivated. They are made from essential fatty acids contained in the phospholipids of cell membranes. Thus,

although they may be described as 'hormone-like', they do not circulate in the blood in the same way. Their release is triggered by a variety of physiological stimuli, including hormones, such as adrenaline, antigen–antibody reactions and mechanical damage or injury.

Prostaglandins have a range of diverse functions, such as:

- lowering of blood pressure;
- blood platelet aggregation;
- diuresis;
- effects on the immune system;
- effects on the nervous system;
- rise in body temperature;
- stimulation of smooth muscle contraction;
- gastric secretion.

Some members of the eicosanoids have opposing actions. For example, prostacyclins are produced in the endothelial lining of the arterial wall and are powerful inhibitors of platelet aggregation, as well as causing the artery walls to relax. They, therefore, lower blood pressure. In contrast, thromboxanes are produced in the platelets, where they stimulate aggregation and cause contraction of the blood vessel wall, thereby increasing blood pressure. It is, therefore, important that these two eicosanoids are normally balanced, to prevent major changes in circulatory function. Leukotrienes, on the other hand, are pro-inflammatory.

The different fatty acid families give rise to different series of eicosanoids. Those produced from the n-3 family have less powerful effects on platelet aggregation and vasoconstriction (haemodynamic functioning) and on inflammation than do the n-6 derived eicosanoids. This is believed to be the explanation for the potential benefits of fish oils rich in n-3 acids in relation to heart disease. This is discussed further in Chapter 14.

Increasing the levels of n-3 fatty acids in the body has also been shown to displace some of the n-6 acids from cell membranes of white blood cells. As a consequence, less pro-inflammatory eicosanoids are produced as part of the immune response. In addition, n-3 acids may affect other parts of the immune response, such as cytokine activation. These effects are of potential benefit in chronic inflammatory conditions, and supplementation with fish oils has been shown to reduce symptoms in subjects with rheumatoid arthritis. There are potential benefits also in asthma, psoriasis and Crohn's disease, although more research is needed in these areas.

HOW MUCH FAT SHOULD WE HAVE IN THE DIET?

For many nutrients, the answer to such a question would entail a consideration of the prevention of deficiency of the particular nutrient. However, in the case of fat, there is no recognized deficiency state that develops from the absence of fat in general. The only problem arises from an absence of the essential fatty acids. It should, therefore, be possible to set levels for guidance on intake of these fatty acids, in order to prevent deficiency. Evidence of the need for essential fatty acids comes from reports of linoleic acid deficiency in children and in clinical situations in adults. The dietary reference values report (DoH, 1991) recommends that linoleic acid should provide at least 1 per cent of total energy and alpha-linolenic acid at least 0.2 per cent. This amounts to between 2 and 5 g of essential fatty acids daily, which can be readily achieved from a serving of fish, seed oil used in cooking or green leafy vegetable. Since the publication of this Report, there has been more interest in the possible health benefits of n-3 fatty acids and the implications of the ratio of n-6 to n-3 fatty acids. There are no firm recommendations on a desirable ratio at the time of writing, but it has been proposed that linoleic acid (n-6) should comprise a maximum of 3 per cent of energy intake and total n-3 acids should be 1.3 per cent of energy. Thus, the ratio of n-6 to n-3 fatty acids should be between 2:1 and 3:1. Specific interest has focused on the diets of pregnant women, where the status of long-chain polyunsaturated fatty acids is correlated with those in the baby. The importance of n-3 acids for neurological development in the fetus and infant has been discussed earlier in this chapter, and women whose diets contain high levels of n-6 acids, or minimal amounts of n-3 acids may be unable to supply their baby with adequate levels of n-3 acids, either via the placenta, or in breast milk. Premature infants may be especially at risk, although term babies also need an adequate supply. The addition of long-chain fatty acids to formula milk is now permitted by European and UK legislation, to improve intakes in infants. There is a need for more research in this area.

The recommended levels of total fat and the distribution of this fat into saturated, monounsaturated and polyunsaturated fats is based on our knowledge of intakes in populations and evidence on the incidence of disease in these populations, i.e. an optimum health approach. The main diseases that are considered in advice on fat are atherosclerosis and cancer, and much of the guidance on fat intakes aims to reduce the incidence of these diseases. Consequently, recommended levels in the UK are that total fatty acid intake should average 30 per cent of dietary energy including alcohol. Of this, 10 per cent of total energy should be provided by saturated fatty acids, 12 per cent by monounsaturated fatty acids, an average of 6 per cent from polyunsaturated fatty acids and 2 per cent from *trans* fatty acids. When calculated as total fat (including glycerol), these figures amount to 33 per cent of total dietary energy including alcohol, or 35 per cent of energy from food.

Further discussion of the rationale for these figures and the links with atherosclerosis, coronary heart disease and cancer can be found in Chapters 14 and 15.

SUMMARY

1 The diet contains saturated and unsaturated fatty acids, arranged in triglycerides of varying composition. The nature of the fatty acids influences the physical characteristics of the dietary fat. In addition, the diet contains small amounts of cholesterol and phospholipids.

2 Fat intakes in the UK have fallen in absolute terms in the last 40 years, but in relation to the total energy intake, levels remain at about 40 per cent of food energy. The majority of fat intake comes from fats, oils, meats and meat products.

3 Fats increase the palatability of the diet and can contribute to overconsumption of energy, because of the high energy content per unit weight.

4 Digestion of fats requires the presence of bile from the liver. Failure of fat digestion results in steatorrhoea.

5 Fat is transported in the circulation in the form of lipoproteins, which vary in their content of triglycerides and cholesterol.

6 Essential fatty acids are specifically needed in the diet in small amounts for membrane structure and synthesis of eicosanoids.

7 Stored fat is an important energy reserve and serves to insulate and protect the body. It also has important regulatory roles in metabolism and as a secretory organ for a number of bioactive factors.

8 Advice for the population in general is to reduce total fat intakes.

STUDY QUESTIONS

1 Both gamma-linolenic acid and alpha-linolenic acid contain 18 carbon atoms and three double bonds. In what ways are they different and why is this important?

2 What are the functions of the phospholipids and how does this relate to their structure?

3 Suggest some explanations for the finding of the National Food Survey that food eaten outside the home has a higher fat content than that eaten at home. What do your explanations imply about promotion of healthy eating?

4 Find out, by discussion, why people enjoy having fat in their diet. Do the reasons you obtain agree with those given in this chapter?

5 Under what circumstances might you expect an essential fatty acid deficiency to occur?

REFERENCES AND FURTHER READING

British Nutrition Foundation 1999: n-*3 fatty acids and health*. Briefing paper. London: British Nutrition Foundation.

DEFRA 2001: *National Food Survey 2000 Annual report on food expenditure, consumption and nutrient intakes*. London: The Stationery Office.

DoH (UK Department of Health) 1991: *Dietary reference values for food energy and nutrients in the United Kingdom*. Report on Health and Social Subjects No. 41. Report of the Panel on Dietary Reference Values of the Committee on Medical Aspects of Food Policy. London: HMSO.

DoH (UK Department of Health) 1994: *Nutritional aspects of cardiovascular disease*. London: HMSO.

Food Standards Agency 2002a: *Food portion sizes*, 3rd edn. London: The Stationery Office.

Food Standards Agency 2002b: *McCance and Widdowson's The composition of foods*, 6th summary edn. Cambridge: Royal Society of Chemistry.

Frayn, K.N. 2001: Adipose tissue and insulin resistance syndrome. *Proceedings of the Nutrition Society* 60, 375–80.

Galli, C., Simopoulos, A.P., Tremoli, E. (eds) 1994: Effects of fatty acids and lipids in health and disease. *World Review of Nutrition and Dietetics* 76, 1–149.

Macdiarmid, J.I., Cade, J.E., Blundell, J.E. 1994: Dietary fat: grams or percentage energy? Analysis of the dietary and nutrition survey of British adults and the Leeds high fat study. *Proceedings of the Nutrition Society* 53, 232A.

Morton, G.M., Lee, S.M., Buss, D.H. et al. 1995: Intakes and major dietary sources of cholesterol and phytosterols in the British diet. *Journal of Human Nutrition and Dietetics* 8(6), 429–40.

Pond, C. M. 2001: Long-term changes in adipose tissue in human disease. *Proceedings of the Nutrition Society* 60, 365–74.

Roche, H.M., Noone, E., Nugent, A. et al. 2001: Conjugated linoleic acid: a novel therapeutic nutrient? *Nutrition Research Reviews* 14, 173–87.

Sanderson, P., Gill, J.M.R., Packard, C.J. et al. 2002: UK Food Standards Agency *cis*-monounsaturated fatty acid workshop report. *British Journal of Nutrition* 88, 99–104.

Trayhurn, P., Beattie, J.H. 2001: Physiological role of adipose tissue: white adipose tissue as an endocrine and secretory organ. *Proceedings of the Nutrition Society* 60, 329–39

Wise, A., McPherson, K. 1995: The relationship between individual beliefs and portion weights of fat spreads. *Journal of Human Nutrition and Dietetics* 8(3), 193–200.

The aims of this chapter are to:

❏ describe the carbohydrates that are important in human nutrition, including simple and complex carbohydrates;
❏ review the digestion and absorption of carbohydrates;
❏ consider the desirable levels of carbohydrate in the diet;
❏ study the health implications of dietary carbohydrates.

On completing the study of this chapter, you should be able to:

❏ discuss the different types of carbohydrates in the human diet and explain their relative importance;
❏ explain how different carbohydrates differ in their absorption, and the practical implications of this;
❏ identify health aspects of both simple and complex carbohydrates, and the associated guidelines on dietary intakes of the various types;
❏ discuss the implications of sugar consumption with respect to dental health.

Carbohydrates are a group of substances found in both plants and animals, composed of carbon, hydrogen and oxygen in the ratio of 1:2:1. The name 'carbohydrate' was first used in 1844 by Schmidt, but the sweet nature of sugar had already been recognized for many centuries. It is said that sugar was extracted as early as 3000 BC in India; Columbus is credited with introducing sugar cane into the New World in the fifteenth century, and in the sixteenth century Elizabeth I is reported to have had rotten teeth owing to excessive consumption of sugar.

Foods providing carbohydrates are the cheapest sources of energy in the world. For many small farmers in developing countries, they provide not only the main food, but also a source of income for the family. In terms of the world commodity trade, carbohydrate-containing foods, predominantly cereals, represent a major part. In addition, we find foods containing carbohydrates pleasant and attractive to eat, especially those that contain sugars.

In modern times, carbohydrates have tended to be dismissed as of little importance in the diet, supplying only energy. In addition, carbohydrates have been reputed to contribute to a number of diseases including dental caries, diabetes, obesity, coronary heart disease and cancer, although some of these links are not proven. Some scientists suggest that, if sugar was a newly discovered food, with a major role as a food additive to increase sweetness, then it probably would not obtain a safety licence and would be banned. However, since the early 1980s, nutritionists have recognized the importance of complex carbohydrates in our diet, and these have been promoted as a major source of energy and nutrients in our diets, in preference to fat.

SOME DEFINITIONS

The empirical formula for carbohydrates is $C_n(H_2O)_n$. The simple forms of carbohydrates are the sugars, which are generally present as single

Figure 6.1 Structural formulae for three simple sugars.

units called monosaccharides, or as double units called disaccharides. Chains of simple sugars with 3–10 units are termed oligosaccharides. When the sugars are combined together in longer and more complex chains, they form polysaccharides. In addition, the diet may also contain sugar alcohols, which are hydrogenated sugars, for example, sorbitol.

Most of the carbohydrates in the diet come from plants. They are synthesized from carbon dioxide and water, under the influence of sunlight, by the process of photosynthesis. The disaccharide sucrose accumulates as the major product of photosynthesis in the chloroplast. Germinating seeds can also convert fat and amino acids into sugar. All plant cells are also able to convert glucose and fructose into sucrose.

Monosaccharides

Monosaccharides are the simple sugars. Each molecule usually consists of four or five or, most often, six carbon atoms, generally in a ring form. In the hexoses, the six-carbon monosaccharides, which are the commonest in the diet, the ring contains one oxygen atom and all but one of the carbon atoms, the remaining carbon, hydrogen and oxygen atoms being located 'above' or 'below' the ring (Figure 6.1). It is important to note that glucose can exist in two isomeric forms: D-glucose and L-glucose (known as stereoisomers). However, only D-glucose is used in the body. Fructose and galactose are the other nutritionally important monosaccharides; they can also exist as stereoisomers. All three are six-carbon monosaccharides, or hexoses ('hex' meaning six, '-ose' is the standard ending used for

carbohydrates). Fructose and galactose have the same empirical formula as glucose, but differ in the way the atoms are arranged in the ring. Other arrangements are possible, and are found in various plant and bacterial carbohydrates.

Glucose (also called dextrose) is the main carbohydrate in the body, although it only constitutes a small part of dietary carbohydrate intake. It is present in honey, sugar confectionery, fruit and fruit juices, vegetables, some cakes, biscuits and ice cream. It is a fundamental component of human metabolism, being an 'obligate fuel' (i.e. essential under normal circumstances) for a number of organs, most notably the brain. Consequently, levels of glucose in the blood are controlled within narrow limits by a number of hormones.

Traditionally, fructose (also called laevulose) has not been present in large amounts in the human diet. Naturally occurring sources include honey, fruit and some vegetables. In recent years, high fructose corn syrup has increasingly been used as a sweetening agent in beverages and processed foods. This is derived from the hydrolysis of starch obtained from corn, initially to glucose and then by subsequent conversion to fructose. The syrup thus produced is inexpensive and has almost entirely replaced sucrose in products such as soft drinks, canned fruit, jams, jellies, preserves and some dairy products. The major advantages of this syrup are that it does not form crystals at acid pH, and it has better freezing properties than sucrose. These changes are making fructose one of the major simple sugars in the Western diet.

After absorption, fructose is transported to the liver, where it is metabolized rapidly. The

Glucose + glucose   Maltose

Figure 6.2 The condensation of two molecules of glucose to form maltose. First an OH group from one glucose and an H atom from another glucose combine to create a molecule of H_2O. Then the two glucose molecules bond together with a single O atom to form the disaccharide maltose.

products can include glucose, glycogen, lactic acid or fat, depending on the metabolic state of the individual.

Galactose is not usually found free in nature, being part of the lactose molecule in milk. However, fermented milk products may contain some galactose that has been released. Once absorbed into the body, galactose may be incorporated into nerve tissue in growing infants or, if not required, it is transformed either into glucose or glycogen for storage. In lactating (breastfeeding) women, galactose is synthesized from glucose and included as lactose in the milk secreted by the mammary glands.

Other monosaccharides occasionally found in foods include xylose and arabinose in white wine and beer, mannose in fruit, and fucose (a methyl pentose sugar) in human milk and bran.

Sugar alcohols may also be present in food. The three most commonly found are sorbitol, mannitol and xylitol. They are absorbed and metabolized to glucose more slowly than the simple sugars. This confers the advantage of a slower rise in blood glucose levels, which is why 'diabetic' foods are sometimes sweetened with sorbitol. Although the rate of absorption is slower, the amount of energy they ultimately provide is the same as from the simple sugar, so they are of no benefit where energy reduction is required. However, the sugar alcohols are useful in reducing dental caries, since they are not fermented by the bacteria in the mouth and, therefore, do not contribute to acid production. For example, xylitol has been shown in a number of studies to have a cariostatic (caries-preventing) effect when included in chewing gum or candies.

The slow rate of absorption of the sugar alcohol can, however, result in diarrhoea if large amounts are consumed in a short time.

Disaccharides

Disaccharides are formed when monosaccharides combine in pairs. Those of importance in nutrition are sucrose, lactose and maltose. In each case, a molecule of water is lost when the two constituent monosaccharides combine, in a condensation reaction. This is illustrated in Figure 6.2, showing the formation of maltose.

Sucrose (sometimes called invert sugar) is the commonest and best known disaccharide in the human diet. It is formed by the condensation of glucose with fructose. It is obtained from sugar beet or sugar cane, both of which contain sucrose as 10–15 per cent by weight of the plant. The juice extracted from these plants is purified and concentrated, and the sucrose is crystallized out and removed. Byproducts of this process include molasses, golden syrup and brown sugar. Sucrose is also contained in honey and maple syrup. Naturally occurring sucrose is also found in fruit, vegetables and some cereal grains. Sucrose is added to a great many manufactured foods, both sweet and savoury.

Lactose (milk sugar) is present in the milk of mammals. In the West, most of the lactose is provided by cows' milk and its products. In addition, any foods that contain milk powder or whey, such as milk chocolate, muesli, instant potato, biscuits and creamed soups, will contain some lactose. It is also found in human milk. Lactose consists of glucose and galactose.

Activity 6.1

Look at a range of different manufactured products in the supermarket or grocery shop. Identify all the different names used to describe added sugars. Compare them against the list given below.

Sugar	Sucrose	Brown sugar	Invert sugar
Glucose	Sorbitol	Laevulose	Lactose
Mannitol	Polydextrose	Corn syrup	Caramel
Honey	Molasses	High fructose corn syrup	
Maple syrup	Dextrose	Fruit sugar	Maltose
Fructose	Dextrin		

How many of the foods that you looked at contain more than one of the above forms of sugar?

Maltose (malt sugar) is mainly found in germinating grains, as their starch store is broken down. Its major source is sprouted grain, such as barley or wheat used in the manufacture of beer. The 'malt' produced by the sprouting is then acted on by yeasts to produce the familiar fermented product. Small amounts of maltose may also be found in some biscuits and breakfast cereals and in malted drinks. Maltose consists of two glucose units.

Oligosaccharides

Oligosaccharides contain less than ten monomer units to make up the molecule. They are present in a number of plant foods including leeks, garlic, onions, Jerusalem artichokes, lentils and beans. Generally, these sugars are considered to be of minor nutritional significance. However, both the galactosyl-sucroses (raffinose, stachyose and verbascose) contained in legume seeds and the fructosyl-sucroses in onions, leeks and artichokes are resistant to digestion in the upper gastrointestinal tract. Consequently, they pass largely unchanged into the colon, where fermentation occurs, resulting in the production of volatile fatty acids and gases and causing flatulence. This can be uncomfortable and may discourage the consumption of these foods. Nevertheless, there are health benefits from this

fermentation, and oligosaccharides have been studied and developed as possible components of prebiotics or functional foods, which provide a food source for colonic bacteria (see Chapter 17).

Polysaccharides

Polysaccharides contain many (more than ten) monosaccharide units arranged in straight or branched and coiled chains. These may be made up of hexoses, pentoses or a mixture of these, sometimes with other constituents, such as uronic acid.

Traditionally, a distinction has been made between polysaccharides that are digestible, and therefore 'available', such as starch, and the 'unavailable' indigestible forms, such as cellulose, hemicelluloses and lignin, which were also termed 'dietary fibre'. In recent years in the UK, these have been more clearly differentiated into:

- starches; and
- non-starch polysaccharides (NSPs).

Both of these groups of polysaccharides are of plant origin, comprising the store of energy in the plant and its structural framework, respectively. A comparable carbohydrate store in animals is in the form of glycogen, but its content in the diet is negligible.

Starch

Starch consists of linked glucose units arranged in either straight or branched chains. Amylose is the straight-chain form of starch. It contains several hundred glucose molecules linked by alpha-glucosidic bonds between carbons 1 and 4 of adjacent glucose molecules. The linkage is formed by a condensation reaction, with the loss of a molecule of water. The branched-chain component of starch, amylopectin, contains some alpha bonds between carbons 1 and 4, with additional bonds linking carbons 1 and 6, at intervals, to produce side-branches. In this way, amylopectin may contain thousands of glucose units in one polysaccharide unit (see Figure 6.3). Most of the common starchy foods such as potatoes, cereals and beans contain approximately 75 per cent amylopectin and 25 per cent amylose. The presence of a large amount of amylopectin allows the starch to form a

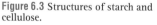

Figure 6.3 Structures of starch and cellulose.

stable gel with good water retention. Along with naturally occurring starches in foods, such as cereals, roots, tubers and pulses, food processing may add two further forms of starch into the diet. These are extruded starch products, such as savoury snacks and breakfast cereals, and modified starches, which are added to foods as emulsifiers and stabilizers.

Processed starches

In general, the processing of starchy foods makes them more attractive for human consumption. For example, the grinding of wheat grains to make flour makes it possible to produce bread, cakes, biscuits, etc. Such rigorous processing disrupts the starch granules, releasing amylose and making it readily available to digestive enzymes, and thus increases digestibility.

However, if moist starchy foods are heated and then cooled, the sols formed by amylose and amylopectin during the heating stage will become gels on cooling, which retrograde on further cooling into insoluble precipitates. Amylose gels retrograde more readily than amylopectin gels, so their relative proportions are an important determinant of the physical properties of the cooked food. Some retrograded starch can still be digested, albeit more slowly. In particular, the retrograded amylose particles are especially resistant to digestion and form an important part of the starch that escapes digestion in the small intestine.

Resistant starch is the name given to the components of dietary starch that are resistant to the normal enzymatic digestion process in the small intestine. They originate in three possible ways.

- The physical structure of the food may prevent access to digestive enzymes if the starch is surrounded by fat, or is in large lumps owing to inadequate chewing. Once these barriers are removed during digestion, the starch can be broken down.
- The nature of the cell walls around the starch granules may impede digestion. Walls in cereals may be partly broken down by milling and grinding, in potatoes by mashing, but the cell walls in legumes are thicker and constitute a more resistant barrier. When starchy foods are eaten with little disruption of cell walls, digestion will be slowed.
- Where the starch has become retrograded by heating and cooling, the enzymes are no longer able to break the bonds. This starch will travel undigested into the colon, where, together with the non-starch polysaccharides in dietary fibre, it plays a positive, beneficial role in health.

Non-starch polysaccharides

For many centuries the belief has been held by some that the non-digestible part of our diet derived from plant foods can have an influence on health. In the early 1970s the concept of 'dietary fibre' and its relationship with disease was more clearly developed. Interest was awakened by reports that the low prevalence in rural Africa of some intestinal disorders common in the West could be associated with the high intakes of dietary fibre. Further, diverticular disease of the colon, generally treated with a fibre-depleted diet, was found to improve greatly when a diet rich in dietary fibre was given. Evidence was also presented that dietary fibre might reduce the risk of other 'Western diseases', such as coronary heart disease and diabetes. These ideas were very attractive and were enthusiastically received because they were offering new explanations for the aetiology (i.e. the factors contributing to its causation) of some common diseases.

The 'fibre hypothesis', which was developed from these ideas, broadly stated that:

- a diet rich in foods containing plant cell wall material (i.e. unrefined plant foods, including cereals, vegetables and fruits) is protective against 'Western diseases'; and
- a diet that is depleted of such materials may in some cases cause 'Western diseases' or in others be a factor facilitating their development.

Unfortunately, the term 'dietary fibre' is misleadingly simple. The original definition included all material undigested by the endogenous secretions of the human digestive tract. This collective term covered a number of very diverse compounds, all having their origin in plants, but having different physiological and physical properties, and probably varying effects in the body. As a result, general statements about the properties of 'dietary fibre' might not apply for certain constituents. A further problem arises with the analysis and quantification of 'dietary fibre' in foods, to allow proper scientific study. One of the initial methods of analysis (Southgate method), included unavailable carbohydrate but also lignin and some resistant starch. A number of other methods for the measurement of fibre have been used in different parts of the world, giving quite different results in any single commodity and increasing confusion.

In 1990, the British Nutrition Foundation Task Force recommended that the term 'fibre' should become obsolete and much more precise terminology, based on accurate analytical methods, be used. The Englyst method determines non-starch polysaccharides by a component analysis method using gas–liquid chromatography. In this way, it is possible to separate starch, resistant starch and NSP, and to define the physical and chemical properties of the various complex carbohydrates in the diet. The method also allows the soluble and insoluble fractions of NSP to be separated and quantified. From this, the specific biological effects will be more readily identified. However, it is important to recognize that results from studies may not be directly comparable, if different analytical methods have been used to quantify the dietary fibre.

A further complication is that this terminology is not widely accepted; the USA and some European countries continue to use 'dietary fibre',

analysed by an enzymatic/gravimetric method (Association of Official Analytical Chemists; AOAC, 2000), which includes lignin and resistant starch. The results obtained by AOAC are termed 'total dietary fibre'. Food composition tables in the UK (Food Standards Agency, 2002) provide NSP values for all foods where these are available. There is additional information available about AOAC values for a smaller number of foods. It is recommended that these are used in food labelling to provide harmonization across Europe.

Although the term 'high-fibre diet' is actually rather meaningless scientifically, it represents a concept understood by the public and as such will, therefore, be used at relevant points in the text.

Constituents of NSP

Non-starch polysaccharides include a number of polymers of simple sugars, together with uronic acid. They are broadly divided into cellulose and non-cellulosic polysaccharides. Their relationship to total carbohydrate in the diet is summarized in Figure 6.4.

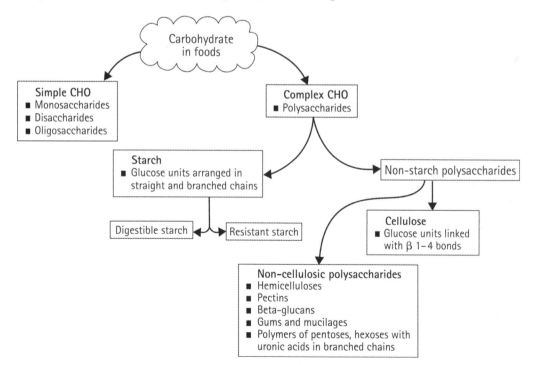

Figure 6.4 The relationship of non-starch polysaccharides (NSPs) to other sources of carbohydrate (CHO).

Cellulose is the principal component of cell walls in plants. It is made up of glucose units, linked by beta 1–4 linkages, which are resistant to digestion. It has a very stable crystalline structure, which gives it low reactivity (see Figure 6.3).

The non-cellulosic polysaccharides comprise hemicelluloses, pectins, beta-glucans, gums and mucilages. The sugars they contain include arabinose, xylose, mannose, fucose, glucose, galactose and rhamnose. Those NSPs that contain predominantly cellulose tend to be insoluble; an increasing content of uronic acids increases solubility. Wheat bran and, therefore, whole grain wheat products contain a high proportion of insoluble NSP and only traces of uronic acids. Cereals such as oats and barley, however, are particularly good sources of beta-glucans, which are water-soluble polymers of glucose. Fruit and vegetables, in general, have more uronic acids and pectin in their NSPs, and thus a higher proportion of soluble fibre than cereals.

Gums and mucilages are generally found in the human diet as a result of manufacturing processes. Gums are extracted, for example, from the acacia tree or the Indian cluster bean, and are used as thickeners, stabilizers and emulsifiers by the food industry. Mucilages from algae and seaweeds are also used by the food industry as stabilizers and thickeners.

The soluble and insoluble NSP contents of some common foods are shown in Table 6.1. It should be noted, however, that the separation into soluble and insoluble fractions is not chemically very distinct and depends on the method of extraction used.

The National Food Survey (DEFRA, 2001) found that the British diet contained 12.6 g of NSP per day, with a range of 5–19 g and 7–25 g reported in men and women, respectively. Vegetarians and vegans tend to have greater intakes of NSP. Mean values of NSP intake for the USA are 15 g/day, with a higher intake recorded in men. Other urban populations in affluent countries are reported to have similar intakes, but slightly higher intakes have been recorded in rural populations. This probably reflects a greater energy intake, related to higher energy expenditure levels. In the UK, the NSP is provided by:

Cereals and cereal products	47%
Vegetables and potatoes	36%
Fruit	11%

DIGESTION OF CARBOHYDRATES

The purpose of digestion is to make all dietary carbohydrates into small units (mostly of glucose)

TABLE 6.1	Non-starch polysaccharide (NSP) content of some common foods, showing soluble and insoluble fractions		
Food	Total NSP (g/100 g)	Soluble NSP (g/100 g)	Insoluble NSP (g/100 g)
White bread	1.5	0.9	0.6
Wholemeal bread	5.8	1.6	4.2
Weetabix	9.7	3.1	6.6
Oatcakes	5.9	3.5	2.4
Rice, white	0.2	Trace	0.2
Apples	1.6	0.6	1.0
Bananas	1.1	0.7	0.4
Peanuts	6.2	1.9	4.3
Baked beans	3.5	2.1	1.4
Lentils	1.9	0.6	1.3
Potatoes	1.2	0.7	0.5
Carrots	2.5	1.4	1.1

Adapted from Englyst et al. (1988). Reproduced with kind permission of Blackwell Science Ltd.

which can be absorbed across the mucosal wall of the digestive tract and used by the cells in metabolism. Digestion is brought about by both physical and chemical means. Biting and chewing in the mouth, and churning by the stomach, ensure that pieces of food are broken down into a semiliquid chyme, so that enzyme action can occur.

Sugars

The diet contains simple sugars not only of different sizes but also in different physical states. Some are consumed in their natural state, contained within the cells of the food plant. These include all the simple sugars found in fruits and vegetables. We eat them with the cell walls and other plant material with which they are associated. Eating them often requires a certain amount of effort in biting, chewing and digestion. These sugars have been termed 'intrinsic', and are generally considered to have little or no undesirable effects on our health.

In addition, the diet also contains sugars which are free, that is, extracellular or not contained within cells. These come from milk, where the lactose is free in solution, from honey, which contains free fructose and glucose, and from the large number of foods that contain added sugars. These sugars are 'unpackaged' and readily available both for bacterial action in the mouth, and for rapid absorption and metabolism. The name 'extrinsic sugars' has been given to this group. Those present in milk are not considered to cause detrimental effects to health. However, the 'non-milk extrinsic sugars', which include sucrose, corn syrup and synthetic fructose in recipes and manufactured foods and drinks, have potentially damaging effects for health. These will be considered in more detail later in the chapter.

Whether sugars are intrinsic or extrinsic will determine how much cellular breakdown has to take place before they are released. Apart from this, the simple monosaccharides require no digestion before being absorbed. Disaccharides, such as lactose and sucrose, require to be split by their specific enzymes, lactase and sucrase, into monosaccharides before they can be absorbed. These enzymes are to be found in the brush border of the mucosal cells of the duodenum and upper jejunum. Studies of the process of digestion show that the digestion of sucrose and lactose is virtually complete in the small intestine.

However, some individuals lack the enzyme lactase and are thus unable to complete the digestion of this sugar. This may arise for two different reasons. The most common is 'primary lactase non-persistence', which is a normal disappearance of lactase from the mucosal cells after infancy. This occurs in many ethnic groups around the world whose customs do not include the use of milk beyond infancy. Caucasians are one of the few groups who continue to produce lactase throughout life; even so, the ability to digest lactose declines with age. In the UK, lactase non-persistence has been recorded in 55 per cent of ethnic Indians and 82 per cent of ethnic Afro-Caribbeans. If milk is consumed by someone with lactase non-persistence, the lactose remains in the intestines, attracting water and causing a feeling of distension, abdominal discomfort and diarrhoea. These signs result from fermentation of the lactose by intestinal bacteria, producing large amounts of gas and acid. Milk derivatives such as yogurt, in which the lactose has been fermented, do not cause these problems. In addition, small amounts of milk may be tolerated if introduced gradually. The use of probiotic preparations that contain milk-fermenting bacteria can also facilitate tolerance to milk.

Lactase deficiency may also arise as a secondary condition, resulting from damage to the intestinal mucosa by some other disease process, such as malnutrition, HIV infection and parasitic infestations. Deficiencies of sucrase may also occur, but these are rare.

Starch

In the mouth, salivary amylase (ptyalin) acts on cooked starch granules. It is not clear how far this digestion progresses and whether there are differences between people who eat their food very quickly and those who chew each mouthful thoroughly. It is also possible that this early breakdown of starch in the mouth may make a significant difference to overall digestibility. The enzyme travels down to the stomach, mixed with

TABLE 6.2 Classification of starch according to digestibility

Type of starch	Example of occurrence	Probable digestion in small intestine
Rapidly digestible	Freshly cooked starchy food	Rapid
Slowly digestible	Mostly raw cereals	Slow but complete
Resistant		
Physically inaccessible	Partly milled grains and seeds	Resistant
Resistant granules	Raw banana and potato	Resistant
Retrograded	Cooled, cooked potato, bread and cornflakes, savoury snack foods	Resistant

From Englyst, H.N. and Kingman, S.M. 1990: Dietary fibre and resistant starch: a nutritional classification of plant polysaccharides. In: Kritchevsky, D., Bonfield, C., Anderson, J.W. (eds), *Dietary fibre*. Reproduced with kind permission of Plenum Press Publishing Corporation, New York.

chewed food. It is now thought likely that, protected by starch and some of its degradation products, salivary amylase continues to be active until the chyme reaches the small intestine.

Here, pancreatic amylase continues the breakdown of starch, acting on 1–4 linkages in both raw and cooked starch. Amylose in starch is degraded to mainly maltose and maltotriose, with small amounts of glucose produced; amylopectins are broken to oligosaccharides by the time the chyme reaches the distal part of the duodenum.

Digestion is completed by oligosaccharidases bound to the surface of the brush border cells; these are substrate specific and liberate glucose as the end-product of the digestion process.

Some starch is resistant in varying degrees to digestion by amylases. A classification of the digestibility of starch has been proposed (see Table 6.2). It must be remembered, however, that digestibility is variable and probably dependent on the composition of the meal.

Also the nature of starch granules varies from one food to another, some being more susceptible to the action of amylase than others. Most readily digested are the starches of most cereals, sweet potato and tapioca. Starch from raw potato and unripe banana is resistant, but cooking of the potato and ripening of the banana increases digestibility. Starch in peas, beans and yams is most resistant to digestion by amylase. Dietary oligosaccharides, found in onions, garlic and leeks, artichokes, beans, peas and some cereals are not broken down or absorbed in the small intestine, and pass further along the bowel together with resistant starch (although they are not starch molecules).

Resistant starches that escape digestion in the small intestine become available for fermentation in the colon by the bacterial flora. The result of this process is an increase in faecal mass owing to the multiplication of the bacteria, production of short-chain fatty acids (acetic, propionic and butyric acids) and a decrease in colonic pH. In addition, CO_2, H_2 and some CH_4 are produced. These contribute to a sensation of bloating and flatulence. It has been estimated that between 20 and 30 per cent of the potential energy contained in the resistant starch becomes available to the body in the form of short-chain fatty acids absorbed from the colon. Figure 6.5 summarizes the digestion of carbohydrates.

Non-starch polysaccharides

In the mouth, high-fibre foods generally require more chewing. This slows down the process of eating and stimulates an increased flow of saliva. The saliva contributes to the volume of the swallowed food bolus. Once in the stomach, the fibre-rich food tends to absorb water and the soluble component starts to become viscous. Both of these changes delay stomach emptying. In the small intestine, the soluble fibre travels slowly because of increased viscosity; this prolongs the period of time available for the absorption of nutrients. The fibre may also bind some divalent ions in the small intestine, making them unavailable for absorption at this point.

SUGARS

Mouth
- Intrinsic sugars are released through biting and chewing
  and
- Churning by the
Stomach

Monosaccharides require no further digestion
  but
- for disaccharides
  e.g. lactose
  sucrose
Brush border of duodenum and jejunum
- Digestive enzymes secreted (lactase and sucrase)

digestion impaired by
Lactase deficiency
Two types:
- Primary lactase non-persistence
  – disappearance of lactase from mucosal cells after infancy
- Secondary lactase deficiency
  – due to damage of mucosa by disease, e.g. malnutrition, HIV infection, parasitic infections
  ↓
If milk is consumed, lactose remains in intestines
  ↓
Distension
Discomfort
Diarrhoea

STARCH

Mouth
- Salivary amylase begins digestion
- Chewing allows the enzyme to be combined with the food
- Amylase continues to be active until the food reaches the small intestine

Pancreas
- Secretes pancreatic amylase into the small intestine
- This acts on 1–4 linkages
  Amylose
  ↓
  Maltose + maltotriose (and some glucose)
  Amylopectin
  ↓
  Oligosaccharides
Brush border of duodenum
- Secretes oligosaccharidases
  Oligosaccharides
  ↓
  Glucose

Digestion escaped by
Resistant starch
- This becomes available for fermentation in the colon by bacterial flora
  ↓
  Bloating and flatulence

Non-starch polysaccharides
These are not digested by enzymes, but aid the digestion and absorption of other nutrients by slowing down passage of food through the gut

Figure 6.5 Digestion of carbohydrates.

Once in the large intestine, the soluble fibre becomes a food source for the growth and multiplication of the bacterial flora. The consequences of this are exactly the same as described above for resistant starch. Thus, both resistant starch and soluble NSPs contribute to increasing bulk in the large intestine, and the production of fatty acids and gases.

Insoluble fibre, which has reached the colon largely unchanged, swells by water holding, and adds further to the volume of the colonic contents. The faeces, therefore, are both bulkier and softer because of the increased water content.

ABSORPTION OF CARBOHYDRATES

After digestion, the resulting monosaccharides are absorbed from the gut lumen across the mucosa into the blood by one of three mechanisms:

- simple diffusion;
- facilitated diffusion; or
- active transport.

The latter two processes allow faster absorption of the simple sugars than could be achieved by simple diffusion alone. This becomes particularly important in the later stages of absorption, as concentrations in the gut lumen fall. Active transport involves the breakdown of ATP and the presence of Na$^+$.

Absorption of sugars causes a variable rise in blood sugar. When given individually, glucose and maltose produce the greatest increase, followed by sucrose, lactose, galactose and fructose. The effects are not necessarily the same when these sugars are consumed as part of a meal. The level of glucose in the blood rises to a maximum in about 30 minutes and falls to fasting levels after 90–180 minutes. The rate of rise to the maximum and the rate of fall vary with the nature of the meal, and are related to the digestion rates occurring in the small intestine and the speed of release of glucose.

It is possible to measure the relative effects of different carbohydrate foods on the blood sugar level. The rise in blood glucose following ingestion of a portion of a test food containing 50 g of available carbohydrate is compared with the effect on blood glucose of a 50 g available carbohydrate portion of a standard, such as glucose or white bread. Comparison of the areas under the two glucose curves obtained produces a 'glycaemic index' (Figure 6.6).

The glycaemic index of a large number of foods has been determined. Glycaemic responses vary between individuals, but the ranking of response to different foods can be predicted from the standard results. Foods grouped according to their glycaemic index are shown in Chapter 16.

$$\text{Glycaemic index} = \frac{\text{Area shaded in vertical lines}}{\text{Area shaded in horizontal lines}} \times 100$$

Figure 6.6 Rise in blood glucose after eating, and the calculation of glycaemic index.

Activity 6.2

- Why might diets with a low glycaemic index be beneficial in diabetic subjects?
- What foods should be recommended?
- Why might diets with a low glycaemic index help to promote satiety?
- In what ways might diets with low glycaemic index be beneficial in endurance athletes?

Diets with a low glycaemic index have been shown to have various health benefits, including reduction of blood lipids and improved blood glucose control in diabetic subjects. They also enhance satiety and increase athletic endurance. More research is needed to increase the evidence base on relationships between glycaemic index and health, in specific conditions and for the general population. There are moves to introduce labelling of products with their glycaemic index, although there needs to be public education about the significance of this measure before any such initiative.

By definition, we would not expect the non-starch polysaccharides to be absorbed. However, these compounds do not travel through the digestive tract completely unchanged. Physical breakdown and bacterial fermentation are the main changes that alter both the soluble and insoluble fibres as they pass through the digestive tract. Some of the fatty acids released as a result of fermentation are absorbed and provide usable energy.

Figure 6.7 Metabolism of carbohydrates.

METABOLISM OF CARBOHYDRATES

In discussing carbohydrate metabolism in the body, it is simplest to consider glucose, fructose and galactose. These travel in the bloodstream from the small intestine to the liver, where they are stored as long chains of glucose units in the form of glycogen. The liver stores one-third of the body's total glycogen (about 150 g). The remainder of the glucose may pass on to the muscles, where it is also stored as glycogen. Storage of glycogen is encouraged by insulin, the hormone produced by the β cells of the pancreas. Liver glycogen is readily transformed back into glucose whenever the blood sugar level falls below about 4 mmol/l. Thus, glucose can continue to supply energy to the brain,

central nervous system and other organs whether the person has eaten or not. The glucose from the blood passes into these tissues where it is oxidized and energy is released by means of one of several pathways (glycolysis, tricarboxylic acid cycle, hexose monophosphate pathway), depending on circumstances. A number of vitamins are needed to achieve this oxidation, most notably thiamin, riboflavin and nicotinic acid. Insulin is also needed to facilitate the entry of the glucose into tissues (see Figure 6.7). Muscle glycogen is not used to maintain blood sugar levels, rather its role is to provide energy directly for muscle contraction.

Glycogen is stored in association with water and is a bulky way of storing energy. Thus, the body only contains enough glycogen to provide energy for relatively short periods of time, although new research suggests that glycogen stores are well controlled. Longer term energy stores are maintained in the form of fat and, as a last resort, as protein. If we take in more carbohydrate than we need, the body will use the glucose to fill its glycogen stores and then could convert the remaining glucose into the more permanent storage form – fat. Unlike the limited storage capacity for glycogen, the body can store unlimited amounts of fat. In practice, this does not occur in humans to any significant extent and carbohydrate metabolism is stimulated to utilize the excess carbohydrate. As a consequence, energy from fat is not used and fat may be stored. Fat synthesis from carbohydrate only occurs when extremely large amounts of carbohydrate are consumed over a period of days.

WHY DO WE NEED CARBOHYDRATES IN THE DIET?

From the above discussion, it is clear that carbohydrates are an important source of energy for the body, providing glucose for immediate use and glycogen reserves (see Figure 6.8). All the cells of the body require glucose and some, such as the brain, nervous system and developing red blood cells, are 'obligatory' users of glucose. We are able to make some glucose from proteins and fats in the process of gluconeogenesis. This enables the body to survive when the glycogen stores are depleted and no carbohydrate has been eaten. Almost all the body's amino acids (those

known as glucogenic) and the glycerol part of triglycerides (about 5 per cent of the weight of fat) but not the fatty acids can be converted to glucose. However, using protein to make glucose is potentially harmful, since tissue protein may be broken down. This happens in starvation both in the early stages before the body adapts to using more fats for essential energy, and in the final stages when body fat stores have been depleted, and the body's structural protein is being used for energy.

A further problem arises when there is insufficient carbohydrate available to complete fat metabolism. In the absence of carbohydrate, acetyl coenzyme A accumulates and condenses to form ketone bodies. This state, known as ketosis, is associated with mild disturbances of cellular function and is an early indication of insufficient carbohydrate availability in the body. So, even though glucose can be produced from non-carbohydrate sources, the processes are inefficient and potentially harmful, and indicate a specific need for carbohydrate in the diet to supply energy.

Carbohydrates are also used in the synthesis of various metabolically active complexes. Glycoproteins are important components of cellular membranes, in particular on the extracellular surface. They are also found as circulating proteins in blood or plasma. Glycolipids, such as sphingolipids and gangliosides, have roles at receptor sites on cells and in synaptic transmission.

Mucopolysaccharides have important water-holding or binding properties in many sites of

Figure 6.8 Why do we need carbohydrates in the diet?

the body; they occur in basement membranes and in intercellular cement and form an integral part of cartilage, tendon, skin and synovial fluid. Disorders of mucopolysaccharide metabolism have been associated with a number of disease states. Little is currently known about the influence of dietary sugars on these compounds or on specific quantitative requirements.

HOW MUCH CARBOHYDRATE SHOULD WE HAVE?

The intake of dietary carbohydrate must not only be sufficient to provide the necessary energy for the survival of the body, but must also contain sufficient specific sugars to allow the synthesis of essential complex molecules. However, this is difficult to quantify; it is much easier to calculate the amount of protein needed by the body to maintain nitrogen balance, and the amounts of fat to supply the essential fatty acids.

The only true requirement for carbohydrates that current knowledge has identified is for the prevention of ketosis. Estimates of the minimum amount of carbohydrate needed by an adult are in the range of 150–180 g carbohydrate per day. This does not necessarily need to be supplied entirely from the diet: 130 g could be synthesized by gluconeogenesis, with the remaining 50 g provided exogenously from food. The total figure represents 29 per cent of the total energy expenditure.

Studies on pregnant rats indicate that a minimum amount of carbohydrate, up to 12 per cent of glucose, is needed to sustain pregnancy and lactation and avoid high mortality rates in the offspring. This points to other specific requirements for synthesis of carbohydrate-containing complexes.

In the UK, the recommendations made about carbohydrates use an 'optimum' intake approach, which includes an amount sufficient to: prevent ketosis; avoid starvation but not induce obesity; avoid adverse effects on the large intestine, and on lipid and insulin metabolism; and to avoid caries. In addition, the intake should contribute to an enjoyable diet. The sources of carbohydrate should be as unprocessed as possible, as any increase in the degree of processing is linked with

possible adverse effects. The dietary reference values report suggests that:

- dietary carbohydrate should supply 50 per cent of energy;
- sugars not contained within cellular structures (the non-milk extrinsic sugars) should constitute no more than 10 per cent of the energy; and
- the balance should be made up from complex carbohydrates and other sugars, such as those in fruits and milk.

Dietary guidelines published in other countries on the whole adopt a similar approach to sugar intake with a level of approximately 10 per cent being recommended. Some scientists believe that such a low level is not achievable alongside the goal to lower fat intakes. Studies of the British diet have shown that a reciprocal relationship exists between intakes of fat and refined sugars, and that lowering the sugar intake is likely to cause an increase rather than the desired reduction in the intake of fats. This highlights one of the dilemmas associated with looking at individual nutrient components of the diet to compile 'whole diet' guidelines.

The National Food Survey 2000 (DEFRA, 2001) showed the reciprocal trend in carbohydrate and fat intakes in the UK over the past 60 years, with a decreasing percentage of the energy from carbohydrate being accompanied by an increased percentage from fat. Recently, this trend has reversed and, currently, carbohydrate percentage is rising, as fat percentage falls. The most recent survey showed that carbohydrates provided 46.6 per cent of total energy. The total intake of carbohydrates was 218 g from household food, which contained 131 g of starch and 87 g of total sugars (including 47 g of non-milk extrinsic sugars). A further 21 g of carbohydrate was consumed from foods eaten outside the household. These figures show that the proportions of carbohydrates consumed in the UK do not match the dietary guidelines.

CARBOHYDRATES AND HEALTH

There is a great deal of confusion surrounding the links between carbohydrates and health.

Activity 6.3

Perform a small survey, asking your friends and family what they believe about carbohydrates, in relation to health. Is there a difference in answers according to the gender of the respondent or their age?

When you have completed the study of the following section, return to your answers and check how many correct opinions were expressed.

Opinions about carbohydrates include the following:

- 'they are fattening';
- 'they provide instant energy';
- 'they are bad for the teeth';
- 'they are essential to life".

In order to evaluate these views, it is necessary to distinguish between the various types of carbohydrates in the diet, since each behaves differently in the body.

Health aspects of sugars

In general, moderate amounts of sugar in the diet give us pleasure without harming health. It is only when amounts eaten become large and possibly displace more nutrient-dense items from the diet that there is potential for harmful effects. Their concentration in the mouth has potential to damage the teeth and the rate at which the digestion products of sugars enter the blood can have consequences for metabolism. Each of these possible health consequences will be evaluated.

Do they supply 'empty calories'?

This term implies that sugars provide nothing but energy, as they contain no other nutrients. Intrinsic sugars eaten in association with cell wall material are slowly released during digestion. It is not easy to consume large amounts of intrinsic sugars, as they come packaged along with plant cell wall materials, for example, in fruit. In this case, intrinsic sugars are associated with other nutrients, such as vitamin C, carotene and potassium. The non-milk extrinsic sugars, in particular sucrose (but also other simple sugars

added during food manufacture), can be present in some foods, such as sugar confectionery or soft drinks, where they might be the only nutrient. In this case, sugar would supply only energy. If the sugar is present in large concentrations in only a small volume of food, large amounts can be consumed without our being aware of it. In an active individual whose daily energy needs are perhaps 12.6 MJ (3000 Calories), large amounts of sugar may make little difference to the overall nutrient content of the diet. This is because many other foods are being eaten to provide the necessary energy. Several studies, both in children and adults, have shown that when a high sugar intake is part of a high energy intake, micronutrient intakes are not compromised. However, in someone who has only a small energy requirement perhaps of 6.3 MJ (1500 Calories), a high intake of sugar would allow little space in the rest of the diet for nutrient-rich foods. In this case, the diet may well be short of essential micronutrients.

Nevertheless, a subject with a small appetite should not be prevented from eating sugar, as small amounts might enhance the palatability of the diet and might encourage a greater overall food intake. This is particularly applicable to older people or those with illnesses affecting appetite.

Does sugar lead to overweight?

Worldwide studies tend to show that obesity in a population rises as sugar intake increases. However, this is an oversimplification, since the relationship may not be causal. In general, fat intakes are much better correlated with the occurrence of obesity than are sugar intakes. Epidemiological surveys of different populations have repeatedly observed an inverse relationship between reported sugar consumption and the degree of overweight.

It is also possible to show that removing sugar from the diets of volunteers causes weight loss and, if sugar is unknowingly substituted by artificial sweeteners (thus leaving the sweet taste), energy intake is reduced and not compensated by an increase in other foods. These results imply that including sugar in the diet inflates the energy intake.

Further information comes from studies on the satiating effects of carbohydrates. After consumption, digested carbohydrates can influence a number of physiological mechanisms involved in satiety. These studies show that, although the sensory characteristics of sweet carbohydrates encourage consumption at the outset, carbohydrates later act as effective appetite suppressants, reducing hunger ratings and subsequent food intake.

On balance, therefore, it seems that sugars are not a major culprit in the development of overweight. It should be remembered that 1 g of carbohydrate provides 16 kJ (3.75 Calories), compared with 37 kJ (9 Calories) per gram of fat, 17 kJ (4 Calories) per gram of protein and 29 kJ (7 Calories) per gram of alcohol.

Dental caries

Although the 1980s saw a fall in the incidence of tooth decay in many parts of the UK, this decline has stopped, and incidence is again increasing. Caries in early childhood affects one in ten of all 3–4 year olds in the UK. There is regional variation, and in Scotland, 50 per cent of children aged 3.5–4.5 years had experienced caries. In 30 per cent of these it had extended into the dental pulp. Extensive evidence suggests that the most important dietary factors in the causation of dental caries are simple sugars. In the surveys mentioned, there was a higher incidence of caries in children who used a sweetened comforter. In older children, a study of 12-year-olds in England found that 50 per cent had no decay.

Numbers of decayed teeth continue to increase into adulthood, with averages from surveys in the UK reported to be:

16–24 years	10.8 decayed, missing or filled teeth
25–34 years	16.0
35–44 years	19.0

These figures demonstrate that caries is a problem for all age groups, but may also reflect the recent improvement in dental health among the younger adults, compared with the older group shown here.

Teeth are generally covered in a layer of plaque made up of bacteria (*Streptococcus mutans* is the prevailing species) and sticky polysaccharides. The dietary sugars provide the substrate for the multiplication of oral bacteria and the production of acid as a fermentation product. The acid causes a fall in pH within 5–10 minutes; as the pH reaches a critical value of 5.4, the tooth enamel begins to demineralize. Fortunately, buffers in the saliva work to restore normal pH level, generally within 30 minutes of the consumption of sugar. However, if sugar consumption occurs at frequent intervals, the teeth are exposed for prolonged periods of time to the low pH, resulting in damaging demineralization and the development of caries (see Figure 6.9).

The evidence comes from a number of different types of study.

- Observations of the rate of dental caries in a population and its relationship with sugar consumption show a close correlation. This

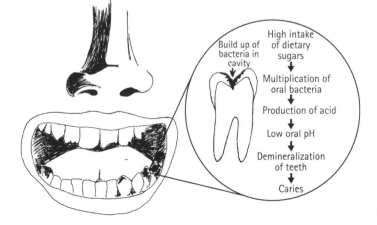

Figure 6.9 Development of dental caries and the role of diet.

applies when different countries are compared or when comparisons are made at different times in the same country. From these data it has been possible to show that, on a population basis, an increase in the average daily intake of sugar by 20 g/day is associated with one extra decayed/missing/filled tooth.

- Studies on isolated communities have shown that, where sugar consumption is negligible, dental caries is unknown. Introduction of sugar into the diet is accompanied by increased incidence of tooth decay.
- Intervention studies, in which sugar intake is manipulated, both in terms of quantity and timing of consumption, have shown a clear relationship with dental caries.
- Most recently, studies in which oral pH has been measured following consumption of sugar-containing foods and drinks show the rapid fall in pH that follows sugar intake and that results in dissolution of the tooth enamel. Experiments in animals confirm the pivotal role of sugars in the process; artificial sweeteners in foods are not associated with development of decay. Studies of plaque microorganisms in culture provide further evidence of their ability to generate acids from sugar substrates.

All of these studies confirm that the most cariogenic (caries-causing) sugars are the non-milk extrinsic sugars, which are present on the tooth surface without cell walls. Also relevant are the concentration of the sugar, the period of contact and the frequency of consumption. Thus, a low concentration that passes through the mouth very quickly will have much less effect than a concentrated source of sugar present in a sticky form that remains in the mouth for a long time. A further factor is the amount of saliva produced to wash away the sugar remnants and buffer the acid. More saliva flows at the end of a meal than when a small sugary snack is eaten. Thus, less damage will be caused to teeth if sugar is consumed with meals. Glucose and fructose are fermented at a similar rate to sucrose, but their overall impact on dental health is less as they are consumed less often and in smaller amounts.

In contrast, starch is poorly fermented by the oral bacteria and is, therefore, less acidogenic. Cooked staple starchy foods, such as rice, potatoes and bread are, therefore, of low cariogenicity. Uncooked starch is of very low cariogenicity, but also is rare in human diets. Some foods contain cooked starch together with substantial amounts of added sugars. These will be cariogenic to the same extent as a similar quantity of sucrose.

Recommended intakes of sugar for dental health

Twenty-three national expert committees around the world have set targets for the intake of added sugars, the average being 10 per cent or less of energy intake. This is also the recommendation made by the UK Dietary Reference Values Report (DoH, 1991).

The dose–response relationship between caries and extrinsic sugar consumption shows that sugar levels should not exceed 60 g/day for adults and teenagers. For younger and pre-school children, these intakes should be proportionately reduced. Thus an intake of 30 g/day would be advised for a pre-school child. In addition, the European guidelines state that sugar consumption should be no more than four occasions per day. Above this frequency, there is an increased risk of dental caries.

Advice relating to reducing caries risk from sugar consumption was compiled by the Committee on Medical Aspects of Food Policy in their report on 'Dietary sugars and human disease' (DoH, 1989). The main points are summarized as follows.

- The consumption of non-milk extrinsic sugars should be decreased and replaced by fresh fruit, vegetables and starchy foods.
- Those providing food for families and communities should seek to reduce the frequency with which snacks are consumed.
- For infants and young children, simple sugars should not be added to bottle feeds; sugared drinks should not be given in feeders where they may be in contact with teeth for prolonged periods; dummies or comforters should not be dipped in sugars or sugary drinks.
- Schools should promote healthy eating patterns both by nutrition education, and by

providing and encouraging nutritionally sound food choices.

■ Elderly people with teeth should restrict the amount and frequency of consumption of non-milk extrinsic sugars because their teeth are more likely to decay owing to exposure of tooth roots and declining salivary flow.

■ When medicines are needed, particularly long term, 'sugar-free' formulations should be selected by parents and medical practitioners.

■ Dental practitioners should give dietary advice, including reduction of non-milk extrinsic sugar consumption, particularly to those who are prone to dental caries. To facilitate this, the teaching of nutrition during dental training should be increased.

Diabetes mellitus

Evidence linking diabetes mellitus with carbohydrate consumption and especially sucrose consumption is far from conclusive. Non-milk extrinsic sugars, because of their rapid rate of digestion and absorption, can result in a rapid increase in blood glucose and high levels of insulin. However, restriction of sugar intake may form part of the management of diabetic patients. Non-insulin-dependent diabetes mellitus, which develops more commonly in older people, is linked with overweight and it can thus be supposed that excessive intake of any source of energy may increase the risk of its developing. A diet rich in complex carbohydrates and containing non-starch polysaccharides is recommended in the management of diabetes.

Metabolic consequences of sugar intake

When sucrose is fed to subjects at levels of 18–33 per cent of total energy intake, a number of changes occur in the serum profile. It is believed that these result from a rapid influx of sugars into the circulation. The changes include:

■ increased fasting plasma triglycerides in men and post-menopausal women;

■ decreased HDL cholesterol;

■ increased fasting insulin levels.

It is suggested that these effects are particularly noticeable in a subsection of the population, possibly about 15 per cent, who are deemed 'carbohydrate-sensitive'. These changes in serum lipids and insulin have all been associated with disease, although a direct casual link with sugars is not proven. Diseases that may be implicated include coronary heart disease, diabetes, gallstones, hypertension and kidney stones.

Other consequences for health

A number of other conditions have been linked with a high sugars intake, although the evidence on these is scant. People who suffer from Crohn's disease have consistently been reported to have a history of a high sucrose intake, compared with controls. Although a precise mechanism is as yet unproven, it is possible that sugars in high concentrations may affect intestinal permeability and damage the mucosal wall, leading ultimately to gastrointestinal disease. There is also a suggested relationship between sugars and hyperactive, criminal or delinquent behaviour.

There is a widespread belief that ingestion of glucose or a carbohydrate-rich food can improve intellectual performance. This is difficult to evaluate as there are many aspects of mental function that can be measured and the effects of glucose are not consistent. However, reaction time tests, information processing, word recall and memory tests have all been shown to improve after a glucose drink. Variations in glucose control may also affect mental function. The evidence for these results and mechanisms mediating the findings, however, remain elusive.

Summary

The present household intake of total sugars in the UK amounts to 87 g/head per day (DEFRA, 2001) and includes 47 g of non-milk extrinsic sugars (NMES). The food groups contributing to total and NMES intakes are shown in Table 6.3. These figures do not include the additional 20 g of NMES consumed outside the home, from soft and alcoholic drinks and confectionery.

Overall, 22 per cent of total energy comes from sugars, although there are substantial differences between the age groups. For instance, breastfed and bottle-fed infants may obtain 40 per cent of their total energy from sugars. This gradually declines to 26–29 per cent among pre-school children and 19–25 per cent in older children. Levels of intake among adults fall between

TABLE 6.3	Food groups contributing to total and non-milk extrinsic sugars (NMES) intakes (DEFRA, 2001)	
Food group	Contribution to total sugars (%)	Contribution to NMES intake (%)
Cereals and cereal products	24	29
Sugars and preserves	21	40
Fruit	19	13
Milk and milk products	19	–

17 and 21 per cent of energy, although studies on unemployed adults found levels up to 25–28 per cent of total energy intake coming from sugars.

At these levels of intake, it is unlikely that sugars increase the risk of cardiovascular disease, high blood pressure or diabetes. There is also no sound evidence that sucrose causes behaviour problems. However, people with sugar intakes in excess of 200 g/day should replace some with starchy food. Finally, sugars can contribute to obesity and overweight, as can almost any other food, if consumed in excess of energy needs. People who are trying to reduce their weight should reduce their sugar intake as well as their total food intake.

Health aspects of starch

For many years, starchy foods had a bad nutritional image. This started to change in 1977, when the McGovern Report (Select Committee on Nutrition and Human Needs, 1977) recommended that complex carbohydrates should be increased to compensate for the reduction of fat needed to cut heart disease rates. Starchy foods have many nutritional advantages. Foods such as potatoes, bread and other cereal products, nuts, pulses and seeds provide not only complex carbohydrate in the form of starch, but also non-starch polysaccharides and other nutrients, such as protein, iron and the vitamins B and E.

Starchy foods had a reputation for being 'fattening' and were often the first items to be cut out of weight-reducing diets. In fact, they have a lower energy density and a higher satiety value than most foods with a significant fat content. For example, a plate of potatoes or of rice contains the same amount of energy as four average biscuits, yet most of us can imagine the difference in the feeling of fullness produced. Increasing the consumption of starchy foods can reduce the proportion of fat in the diet.

An economic advantage of starchy foods is that they are inexpensive. Where people have to live on a low income, they can be very valuable nutrient-rich foods.

During passage through the digestive tract, the products of starch digestion are released slowly. Consequently, the effects on blood sugar levels are small and these foods tend to have a lower glycaemic index. It is for this reason that starchy foods are particularly advantageous in the management of diabetes. Resistant starch present in starchy foods has properties similar to those of non-starch polysaccharides and, therefore, shares some of the health benefits of this group of carbohydrates.

In the UK, the average domestic consumption of starches amounts to 131 g/person per day (DEFRA, 2001). This represents 28 per cent of total energy intake. The major food sources of starch are:

Cereals and cereal products	74% of total
Potatoes	10% of total

Intakes of starchy foods are almost 50 per cent higher in men than women. This may reflect the prevailing belief among women that starchy foods are 'fattening'; however, it may also reflect the higher total energy intake of men. The dietary reference values report (DoH, 1991) suggests that starchy foods should comprise 37 per cent of the total energy intake. It can thus be seen that, in general, the UK diet is lacking adequate amounts of complex carbohydrates.

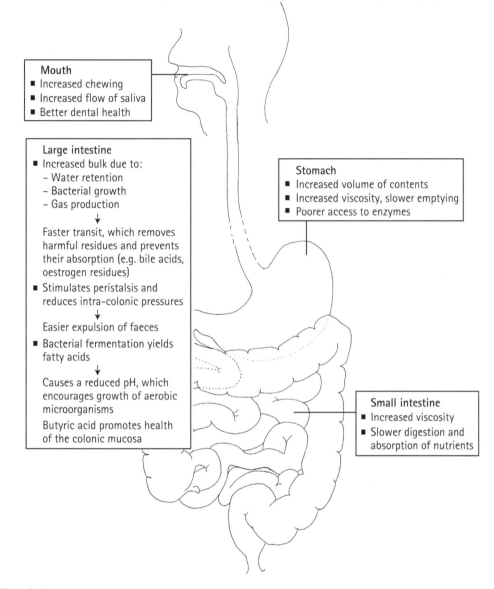

Figure 6.10 Summary of the effects of non-starch polysaccharides in the digestive tract.

Health aspects of non–starch polysaccharides

Figure 6.10 summarizes the effects of non-starch polysaccharides on the digestive tract. From this, it is possible to consider the proposed health benefits of NSPs.

In the mouth, the presence of NSP can promote dental health. This may be the result of the physical effects indicated in the figure, as well as the different foods eaten on a higher fibre diet.

The presence of NSPs in the stomach can contribute to the sensation of satiety, and possibly help in weight maintenance. The increased viscosity resulting from soluble NSP slows emptying from the stomach. The association of nutrients with cell wall material results in a longer digestion process, before nutrients are liberated.

In the duodenum, the viscous contents move slowly and release their nutrients over both a longer time and a greater length of the gut. This means that the rise in blood levels of nutrients is prolonged and attains lower peaks. The major application of this rests in the management of diabetes, where better control of blood sugar levels can be achieved. Both soluble and insoluble sources of NSP can play a role. It has been suggested that between meals blood glucose levels may be regulated by insoluble NSP intake, although further research is required.

Most of the effects of NSPs occur in the large intestine. Bowel contents are increased in volume by a number of mechanisms. This facilitates propulsive contractions of the large intestine and reduces the transit time. As a result, less pressure is needed to move the bowel contents. This is believed to be of benefit for a number of bowel disorders, including constipation and diverticular disease. (In diverticular disease, there are small pockets, or hernias, formed in the mucosa of the colon, which may become inflamed. It is thought that high pressure in the bowel may contribute to their formation.) It has also been proposed that regular consumption of an NSP-rich diet may reduce the risk of appendicitis, and may be of benefit in some cases of irritable bowel syndrome.

If intakes are low, the converse effects are seen, with small volumes of bowel contents, which move slowly and allow harmful residues to persist. Some metabolites may be absorbed and have metabolic consequences (e.g. on cholesterol metabolism). The increased pressure generated in moving bowel contents may damage the colonic mucosa. Finally, the alkaline pH encourages growth of anaerobic bacteria, which are associated with the production of more harmful metabolites, including some carcinogens.

Unabsorbed NSP has the facility to bind other substances. This is the result of charged particles on its surface as well as the mesh-like structure, which can physically trap other molecules. Consequently, possibly harmful metabolites or residues can be eliminated from the bowel with the NSP residues. This includes bile salt metabolites, cholesterol, drug and hormone residues, and possible carcinogenic byproducts from the diet. While these are still present in the bowel, their concentration may be reduced because of the greater water content associated with the NSP. Thus, NSP may be of benefit in

prevention of gallstones, coronary heart disease and various cancers.

Although many of these mechanisms appear possible, it is difficult to obtain conclusive evidence of the preventive role of NSP in many diseases. This is mainly because:

- an increased intake of NSP is often associated with other 'healthy' aspects of the diet, such as lower fat intakes;
- many of the diseases mentioned take many years to develop; therefore, studies need to be prolonged;
- the diseases may be multifactorial in origin and NSP may be only one of several factors involved; and
- techniques to measure NSP intakes accurately are still being developed.

Nevertheless, epidemiological data do suggest that in populations where NSP (or fibre) intakes are higher, bowel disorders are less. It is on this basis, especially in relation to constipation, that the dietary reference value report (DoH, 1991) makes the recommendation that NSP intakes should be on average 18 g/day, with an individual range from 12 to 24 g/day. This would increase the average stool weight by 25 per cent to a level of 100 g/day. Population studies indicate that, at higher stool weights, there is a reduced risk of bowel cancer, gallstones and diverticular disease.

In addition to these effects, there is consistent evidence that an increase in the NSP intake of the diet, without an increase in energy, is associated with a modest weight loss. This may average 1.9 kg over 3.8 months, and is of a similar magnitude to those observed when percentage of fat is reduced in the diet. The effects are noted with consumption of high-fibre foods or fibre supplement. The exact mechanism contributing to the effect is unclear, but may be a composite net result from: energy dilution in the food, extra chewing required, gastric distension, gastric emptying, and nutrient absorption rates and caloric excretion in faeces. On this basis, it is suggested that an increase in fibre intakes, in line with recommendations, could make an important contribution to weight management.

Foods that provide fibre (or NSP) are the wholegrain cereals, fruits and vegetables, and it is recognized that many other nutrients and non-nutritional factors are also provided beside the NSP content. For this reason it is difficult to attribute effects of a diet rich in these foods solely to its fibre content. However, many studies do show that wholegrain cereal intakes are linked to lower incidence of chronic diseases and it is probable that some of this effect is related to fibre intakes. For example:

■ a significantly lower risk of mortality from heart disease in a number of cohorts, is linked to the regular consumption of at least one serving of wholegrain cereal per day;

■ at least one daily serving of wholegrain cereal is associated with a reduced risk of cancer, especially gastrointestinal cancer, probably through direct effects in the bowel or through a role in weight control;

■ evidence from population-based and clinical studies suggests that regular consumption of wholegrain cereals in the diet may be an effective way of lowering the risk of developing Type 2 diabetes, through better glycaemic control.

In summary, there are many advantages to be gained from an adequate intake of NSP. These may be effected directly by the consequences of NSP in the digestive tract, or by some of the associated nutrients and other phytochemicals, which are associated with NSP in foods. Following dietary guidelines to eat more starchy carbohydrate foods and fruit and vegetables will ensure adequate levels for health.

SUMMARY

1 Carbohydrates may be classified by size and by digestibility.

2 The simple sugars are readily digestible, and are important in the diet as a source of energy and for the manufacture of carbohydrate complexes necessary for the structure and function of the body.

3 Excessive intakes of simple sugars (in amounts greater than 200 g/day) are undesirable. However, amounts smaller than this do not specifically and uniquely cause overweight or diabetes. Dental caries, however, is linked to the intake of simple sugars, especially if eaten at frequent intervals. Nevertheless, the Dietary Reference Value report recommends a maximum of 10 per cent of energy from non-milk extrinsic sugars.

4 Starches may be digestible or resistant. The digestible starches release glucose more slowly than do simple sugars. In addition, food sources of starch generally contain other nutrients. Starches are, therefore, considered to be desirable in the diet. Resistant starch escapes digestion in the small intestine but is fermented by bacteria in the large intestine. This is believed to be of benefit to health.

5 Non-starch polysaccharides can be classified as soluble or insoluble. The soluble NSPs contribute to viscosity in gut contents, and slow the absorption of nutrients. The insoluble NSPs retain water and increase bulk in the large intestine. Both forms have beneficial effects for health, both within the digestive tract and for general metabolism.

STUDY QUESTIONS

1 a Draw up a table to compare the sources and properties of intrinsic and extrinsic sugars.
   b How do these sources of sugars differ in their metabolic effect in the body?

2 a Account for the variable digestibility of starch from different sources in the diet.
   b Why are starchy foods encouraged in the diet?

3 Healthy eating advice recommends a reduction in the intake of non-milk extrinsic sugars to 10 per cent of total energy.

   a What changes in the diet would be needed to achieve this?
   b What effect might these changes have on other components of the diet?

4 a Suggest practical and realistic ways in which an increase in starchy carbohydrates intake might be promoted.
   b What other benefits might follow from the changes you suggest?

REFERENCES AND FURTHER READING

Ahrens, U. (ed.) 1998: *Oral health, diet and other factors.* British Nutrition Foundation Task Force Report. London: British Nutrition Foundation.

Association of Official Analytical Chemists 2000: *Official methods of analysis,* 17th edn. Gaithersburg, MD: AOAC.

Blaak, E.E., Saris, W.H.M. 1995: Health aspects of various digestible carbohydrates. *Nutrition Research* 15(10), 1547–73.

Bolton-Smith, C., Woodward, M. 1995: Antioxidant vitamin adequacy in relation to consumption of sugars. *European Journal of Clinical Nutrition* 49(2), 124–33.

Conning, D. (ed.) 1993: *Biological functions of carbohydrates.* London: British Nutrition Foundation.

DEFRA 2001: *National Food Survey 2000 Annual report on food expenditure, consumption and nutrient intakes.* London: The Stationery Office.

DoH (UK Department of Health) 1989: *Dietary sugars and human disease.* Report on Health and Social Subjects No. 37. Report of the Panel on Dietary Sugars. Committee on Medical Aspects of Food Policy. London: HMSO.

DoH (UK Department of Health) 1991: *Dietary reference values for food energy and nutrients in the United Kingdom.* Report on Health and Social Subjects No. 41. Report of the Panel of Dietary Reference Values of the Committee on Medical Aspects of Food Policy. London: HMSO.

Englyst, H.N., Bingham, S.A., Runswick, S.A. et al. 1988: Dietary fibre (non starch polysaccharides) in fruits, vegetables and nuts. *Journal of Human Nutrition and Dietetics* 1, 247–86.

FAO (Food and Agriculture Organization) 1998: *Carbohydrates in human nutrition.* Report of a joint FAO/WHO Expert Consultation. Rome: FAO.

Food Standards Agency 2002: *McCance and Widdowson's The composition of foods,* 6th summary edn. Cambridge: Royal Society of Chemistry.

Howarth, N.C., Saltzman, E., Roberts, S.B. 2001: Dietary fibre and weight regulation. *Nutrition Reviews* 59(5), 129–39.

Jackson, A.A. 1992: Sugars not for burning. In Eastwood, E., Edwards, C., Parry, D. (eds) *Human nutrition: a continuing debate.* London: Chapman & Hall, 82–99.

Naismith, D., Nelson, M., Burley, V. et al. 1995: Does a high-sugar diet promote overweight in children and lead to nutrient deficiencies? *Journal of Human Nutrition and Dietetics* 8(4), 249–54.

Richardson, D.P. 2000: The grain, the wholegrain and nothing but the grain: the science behind wholegrain and the reduced risk of heart disease and cancer. *British Nutrition Foundation Bulletin* 25, 353–60.

Select Committee on Nutrition and Human Needs, United States Senate 1977: *Dietary goals for the United States* (McGovern Report). Washington, DC: US Government Printing Office.

Sheiham, A. 2001: Dietary effects on dental disease. *Public Health Nutrition* 4(2B), 569–91.

CHAPTER
7

The aims of this chapter are to:

❑ discuss the components of energy balance: energy intake and energy output;
❑ study energy intake and how it can be measured;
❑ study energy output and its component parts;
❑ consider the different requirements for energy in various individuals in different activities.

On completing the study of this chapter, you should be able to:

❑ describe the amounts of energy obtained from different macronutrient sources;
❑ identify different ways in which energy intake can be measured;
❑ discuss the components of energy output and their relative contribution to the total.

Energy is the essence of life – without it, we could not survive. We need energy for all the basic physiological functioning of the body, particularly at cellular level in active transport pumps, but also more apparent functions, such as breathing, digestion and excretion. The most energy-demanding organ is the brain. In addition, our muscles require energy to function – the heart to keep blood circulating to all the tissues, and our skeletal muscles to maintain posture, balance and mobility. For any activity, whether to do with our occupation, leisure or sport, more energy must be supplied. Even when we are asleep we are using energy. Also, in the early years of life and during pregnancy, additional energy is required for growth.

This energy has to be provided from the macronutrients in our food, which are broken down to their constituent parts by digestion and metabolized in the tissues. Some of the energy will be used immediately (according to an oxidative hierarchy – see Chapter 8) and some stored. If more is eaten than is needed, there is a net increase in the body's energy content and the size of the stores increases. Conversely, if the current energy needs are greater than the intake

of energy, then some will have to be provided from stored energy. These are the fundamentals of energy balance.

UNITS OF MEASUREMENT OF ENERGY

Two different units of measurement have been used in nutrition to quantify energy, reflecting the development of understanding of this subject. Traditionally, energy was perceived as heat and measured in calories, where one calorie of heat raised the temperature of 1 mL of water through 1°C. Measurements of energy in nutrition were in units of 1000 Calories, or kilocalories (often shown as kcalories or Calories for simplicity).

The unit preferred by nutritionists today is the kilojoule (or megajoule for larger amounts of energy), which is the SI unit for the measurement of energy. The joule was originally defined as the amount of energy exerted when a force of 1 newton was moved through a distance of 1 metre. Like the calorie, it is a small unit (1 Calorie = 4.18 joules), and so normally appears as the kilojoule (kJ = 1000 joules), or the megajoule (MJ = 1000 kJ) in nutrition.

The Calorie is still widely used by the public, appears on food labels, and underpins most weight control diets. For this reason, it has been very difficult for nutritionists to move entirely to the SI measurement of energy. Food labelling in the UK, however, shows energy contents in both units.

It is interesting to note that the unit of electrical energy consumption, the watt, is also linked to the joule. Something using electrical energy at 1 joule/second is using 1 watt of electricity. The rate of energy use of a typical man, 11 MJ (or 2600 Calories) per day, is about 100 joules/second, or 100 watts. Feel the heat given out by a 100 watt light bulb, and remember that you are giving out that much heat yourself!

ENERGY INTAKE

This is the first part of the energy balance equation and includes a study of both the quantity of food eaten by an individual, as well as its energy content. The determinants of when and how much food people eat are discussed in Chapter 2, and you are recommended to refer to this section to consider the physiological basis of food intake.

Energy content of foods

Different foods provide different amounts of energy for a given weight. This is determined by their content of macronutrients. Carbohydrate, fat, protein and alcohol in a food contribute to its energy content. The micronutrients, vitamins, minerals and water do not contribute to energy. In order to study energy intake, the nutritionist has to know the energy content of foods that may be eaten, digested, absorbed and then oxidized in the body. Various methods have been developed to obtain these values.

Bomb calorimeter

In a laboratory, the amount of energy contained in a food is determined with a bomb calorimeter (Figure 7.1). This is a steel vessel with a tight-fitting stopper. It is filled with oxygen under pressure and a weighed amount of the food is

Figure 7.1 The bomb calorimeter.

placed into the crucible within. The whole apparatus is sunk in a water bath of known volume and temperature. The food is ignited electrically and burns explosively as the energy held in the chemical bonds is released in the form of heat. The heat of combustion is measured from the rise in water temperature.

An alternative measurement is to determine the amount of oxygen used during the combustion, since this is converted to carbon dioxide and water in combining with the carbon and hydrogen molecules of the food.

Examples of heats of combustion obtained from a bomb calorimeter are:

	kJ/g	Calories/g
Starch	17.2	4.1
Glucose	15.5	3.6
Fat	39.2	9.37
Protein (egg)	23.4	5.58

These represent the gross energy of the food, which is greater than the true quantity of energy obtained by the cells of the body for a number of reasons. Small amounts of the potential energy are lost during the processes of digestion and absorption, which are not 100 per cent efficient, even in health. Estimates suggest that digestion rates are as follows:

Carbohydrates	99%
Fats	95%
Protein	93%

TABLE 7.1	The energy conversion factors used in the current UK food composition tables	
	kJ/g	Calories/g
Protein	17	4
Fat	37	9
Carbohydrate (available monosaccharide)	16	3.75
Alcohol	29	7

In illness, the losses may be substantially greater owing to vomiting, diarrhoea and inefficient digestion and absorption.

Proximate principles

The amount of energy that the body receives from a food, called the metabolizable energy, can be calculated from values known as 'proximate principles'. These are based on extensive, meticulous experimental work, some of which dates back to the early years of the twentieth century. Such was the accuracy of this work that few changes have had to be made to the values obtained with the more sophisticated techniques now available. The proximate principles provide a value for the amount of energy that is available for metabolism from each macronutrient contained in a food. Thus, after analysing a food to determine its content of fat, protein, 'available' carbohydrate (starch and sugars) and alcohol, it becomes possible to calculate the amount of energy provided for each 100 g of the food. These are the figures that appear in the food composition tables used in the UK (Food Standards Agency, 2002b) shown in Table 7.1.

The contribution to metabolizable energy from non-starch polysaccharides is discounted in the calculation of energy used in the food tables, although they are partially fermented in the large bowel to short-chain fatty acids by bacteria. Thus, the calculated metabolizable energy may be slightly lower than the true value, if some energy is obtained from non-starch polysaccharides. On the other hand, a diet rich in non-starch polysaccharides may interfere with the absorption of some of the other macronutrients, thereby reducing the metabolizable energy obtained.

On balance, the effects may actually cancel each other out.

In addition, there may be losses of metabolizable energy in illness. For example, in poorly controlled diabetes, energy in the form of glucose is lost in the urine; in nephrotic syndrome, large amounts of protein, another potential source of energy, are excreted.

This method allows us to calculate the amount of energy the body can derive from any combination of the macronutrients, in effect, therefore, any food. Using this approach, it is also then possible to find out what proportion of the total energy taken in has actually been provided by the individual macronutrients. Dietary guidelines are generally formulated in these terms. Data for selected foods are shown in Table 7.2.

Most foods do not contain the ideal proportions of the macronutrients as given in dietary guidelines. It is the combination of different foods within a complete diet that determines whether the balance of the diet is right. For this reason, it is misleading to speak of 'bad' foods and 'good' foods in terms of the proportions of energy they supply from the macronutrients. All foods can be useful, when combined with others in a mixed diet. However, if a diet contains too many foods that all have a similar pattern of energy provision, perhaps containing high percentages of energy from fat, then the total diet risks being too high in fat. It is, therefore, only an overdependence on particular types of food, resulting in a diet which is a long way from that suggested by dietary guidelines that might be termed 'a bad diet'. It should be remembered, however, that even such a diet can be redeemed by including foods that redress the balance of macronutrients.

TABLE 7.2	Percentage of energy from carbohydrate, protein and fat in selected foods		
Food	Total energy content of 100 g serving (kJ)	Energy (%) from		
		Protein	Fat	Carbohydrate
Wholemeal bread	922	17	10	73
Cornflakes	1601	8	2	90
Boiled rice	587	8	8	84
Milk, semi skimmed	195	30	32	38
Cheese, Cheddar type	1725	25	75	0
Butter/margarine	3042	1	99	0
Low-fat spread	1519	7	91	2
Egg, boiled	612	35	65	0
Beef stew	570	45	42	13
Chicken, roast	742	63	37	0
Baked beans	355	25	6	69
Peanuts	2491	17	79	5
Peas	291	35	11	54
Potatoes, boiled	306	10	1	89
Chocolate	2177	6	52	42

Data calculated from Food Standards Agency (2002a, 2002b).

Diet surveys

Information about the energy content of foods can be applied in a practical way to assess energy intakes of groups of the population. Usually this is performed using survey techniques. Many such studies have been undertaken, using the methodologies described in Chapter 1. However, it must be remembered that it is very difficult to obtain accurate information about what people actually eat. In recent years, it has become clear that, in most surveys of food intake, the subjects have underreported their consumption levels. For example, the 'Dietary and nutritional survey of British adults' (Gregory et al., 1990) found the mean energy intakes of the subjects to be 10.2 MJ (2450 Calories) in the men and 7.02 MJ (1680 Calories) in the women. These figures are low compared with the dietary reference values. In fact, when dieters and those who were unwell were excluded from the sample, 40 per cent of the women and 27 per cent of the men were calculated to have an energy intake that was less than 1.2 × basal metabolic rate. This clearly provides insufficient energy for any significant amount of activity as part of the daily lifestyle, and is unlikely to be the true picture. In the light

Activity 7.1

Susan has a diet that provides her with a total of 8.8 MJ (2100 Calories) per day, but wishes to know if it contains the appropriate proportions of the macronutrients in line with dietary guidelines. On analysis, the nutritionist finds that the diet contains:

Carbohydrate	200 g
Protein	95 g
Fat	100 g
Alcohol	10 g

The energy obtained from these macronutrients can, therefore, be calculated and expressed as a percentage of the total amount of energy in the diet.

Carbohydrate: $200 \times 16 = 3.2$ MJ. Therefore, per cent of total is $3.2/8.8 \times 100 = 36\%$.

Protein: $95 \times 17 = 1.6$ MJ. The % of total is $1.6/8.8 \times 100 = 18\%$.

Fat: $100 \times 37 = 3.7$ MJ. The % of total is $3.7/8.8 \times 100 = 42\%$.

Alcohol: $10 \times 29 = 0.29$ MJ. The % of total is $0.29/8.8 \times 100 = 3\%$.

Check these figures against the dietary guidelines (Chapter 3), and draw some conclusions about Susan's intake.

Activity 7.2

Using your own diet record, calculate the percentage of the energy in your diet coming from the different macronutrients.

■ How do your figures compare with the dietary guidelines?

■ Can you identify particular foods in your diet that are contributing to an especially high/low intake of one of the macronutrient groups?

Compare your results with those of other students; if possible, produce a table of results for a whole group.

■ How similar are the results?

■ Which macronutrient is the most variable?

■ What difference does including alcohol in the total energy intake make to the individual macronutrient percentages? (Check in the dietary reference values report (DoH, 1991) to see how the guidelines vary when alcohol is included or excluded.)

Activity 7.3

Compare the figures given below from the National Food Survey for the proportions of the dietary energy provided by the macronutrients with those given in Chapter 3 as part of the dietary reference values for the UK.

Which nutrients are overrepresented?

Now look at how the total energy intake is made up from the major food groups.

■ How does this compare with the Balance of Good Health recommendations? (See Chapter 3 for details.)

■ Can you identify the food/food groups that are consumed in excessive amounts, and those that need to be increased?

■ What would happen to the total intake of energy and of other nutrients if one of the groups was omitted completely from the diet? (Look at each group in turn when considering your answer.)

of evidence on the prevalence of overweight and obesity in the population, it was concluded that these values must be an underestimate of the true intakes.

Results from the 2000 National Food Survey (DEFRA, 2001) report that the total amount of energy consumed per person was 1878 Calories (including household food and food eaten out). The percentages of the total energy supplied by the different macronutrients (excluding alcohol) were:

Carbohydrates	46.6
Protein	14.6
Fats	38.2

Contribution from food groups

It is also possible to obtain information from the National Food Survey (DEFRA, 2001) about how the major groups of foods contribute to our overall energy intake. The percentages of total energy intake from each of the groups are:

Cereals and cereal products	33
(Including bread 7; biscuits, cakes 9)	
Meat and meat products	14
Fats and oils	10
Vegetables (including potatoes)	10
Milk, dairy and cheese	13
Soft/alcoholic drinks and confectionery	7

All other food groups contribute less than 10 per cent of the total energy.

Careful inspection of these figures shows that the majority (about 80 per cent) of the energy in the UK diet is actually obtained from staple foods, such as bread, cereals, pasta, potatoes, meat, fruit and vegetables. Of the remainder, 10 per cent is supplied by foods that contain only fat (fats and oils), and nearly 10 per cent by foods that contain only simple carbohydrate (sugars), such as sugar, soft drinks and confectionery. These are the foods that could be termed 'empty energy'. The majority of energy in the diet is accompanied by micronutrients.

ENERGY OUTPUT

The second part of the energy balance equation relates to the usage of energy by the body in performing its various functions and activities.

Figure 7.2 The components of energy output.

The components of energy output or expenditure have been studied extensively and will be considered in turn (see Figure 7.2). They are:

- basal metabolic rate;
- thermogenesis (related to food intake);
- physical activity;
- growth (at certain stages of life).

Measurement of energy output

The body converts the energy of food into ATP with an efficiency of approximately 50 per cent, with the remaining energy being lost as heat. When the ATP itself is used by the body to do work a further loss of heat occurs, equal to approximately 50 per cent of the energy in the ATP. Finally, the work itself generates heat. In this way, it can be seen that a body's total heat production gives a measure of the amount of energy that has been used.

Because of this, it is possible to use calorimetry, or the measurement of heat, to quantify the amount of energy expenditure. If heat is measured directly, the technique is known as direct calorimetry. However, in many cases, it is not practical to do this, and an indirect approach is used, based on the utilization of oxygen. This is valid because the rate of oxygen consumption is proportional to the amount of ATP synthesis, and each mole of ATP synthesized is accompanied by production of a given amount of heat. It is thus reasonable to use measurements of oxygen consumption to calculate heat production within the body.

It is possible to see from the chemical equations for the oxidation of carbohydrates and fats how much oxygen is used and how much carbon dioxide is produced.

Glucose oxidation:
$$C_6H_{12}O_6 + 6O_2 \rightarrow 6H_2O + 6CO_2$$
$$+ 15.5 \, kJ/g \text{ of energy}$$

Starch oxidation:
$$(C_6H_{10}O_5)_n + 6nO_2 \rightarrow 5nH_2O + 6nCO_2$$
$$+ 17 \, kJ/g \text{ of energy}$$

Fat oxidation:
e.g. glyceryl butyro-oleostearate (the main fat in butter)

$$C_3H_5O_3.C_4H_7O.C_{18}H_{33}O.C_{18}H_{35}O + 60O_2$$
$$\rightarrow 43CO_2 + 40H_2O + 39 \, kJ/g \text{ of energy}$$

It can be seen that, for carbohydrate oxidation, the volume of carbon dioxide produced equals the volume of oxygen used. When fat is oxidized, however, the volume of carbon dioxide produced is about 70 per cent of the volume of oxygen consumed. These values are usually expressed as a fraction: CO_2 produced/O_2 consumed, known as the respiratory quotient (RQ). The RQ for carbohydrates is 1.0, and for fats averages 0.71 (different fats have slightly different values). The non-nitrogenous portions of proteins are, on the whole, intermediate in composition between fats and carbohydrates and, for protein, the RQ is usually given as 0.83.

The RQ value can be used to discover the amount of energy production for each litre of oxygen consumed, since this is also predictable from the equation. Normally, the body uses a mixture of substrates for its metabolism, and the metabolic mixture being used can be determined from a measurement of RQ. Thus a value close to 0.7 suggests that mainly fats are being metabolized; conversely, a value close to 1.0 would indicate carbohydrate-fuelled metabolism. In practice, the usual metabolic mixture provides an RQ of around 0.8.

In summary, if one can determine oxygen usage and/or carbon dioxide production, it is possible to calculate the amount of energy released during metabolism. With information about both oxygen and carbon dioxide, it is

TABLE 7.3	Energy yields obtained from the oxidation of different substrates			
Nutrient	Oxygen consumed (litres/g)	Carbon dioxide produced (litres/g)	Respiratory quotient	Energy equivalent (kJ/kcal per litre of oxygen)
Starch	0.829	0.829	1.0	21.2/5.06
Glucose	0.746	0.746	1.0	21.0/5.01
Fat	2.019	1.427	0.71	19.6/4.69
Protein	0.962	0.775	0.81	19.25/4.66

TABLE 7.4	The effect on energy yield of different metabolic mixtures and respiratory quotient (RQ)		
RQ	kJ per litre of oxygen	Energy (%) derived from	
		Carbohydrate	Fat
0.71	19.6	1	99
0.75	19.8	16	84
0.80	20.1	33	67
0.85	20.3	51	49
0.90	20.6	68	32
0.95	20.8	84	16
1.00	21.1	100	0

possible to derive the actual RQ that applies. However, if only one of the gases has been measured, an RQ of 0.8 is assumed (as this represents the average metabolic mixture). It is estimated that not adjusting for the actual RQ probably introduces an error of 3–4 per cent, which is generally acceptable for most purposes.

Tables 7.3 and 7.4 provide the RQ and oxygen utilization values used in these measurements.

Direct calorimetry

The original human calorimeter was designed by Atwater and Rosa in 1905. This was the size of a small room, and contained a bed and stationary exercise bicycle. The walls were well insulated to prevent any heat loss, and all heat dissipated by the subject was transferred to circulating water in the walls of the chamber. Increases in water temperature could be measured, and these represented the subject's heat loss.

In addition, the gases flowing into and out of the chamber could be analysed, giving additional information about the subject's metabolism. Such calorimeters are still in use today. The

major difference lies in the methods by which the heat output is measured in the walls of the chamber; modern calorimeters use microchips and computers for this. There is also a reduction in size, with some modern calorimeters being the size of a phone booth or even smaller.

The major drawback of the human calorimeter (apart from its cost) is that it only allows a limited amount of activity, and is thus not usable for 'real-life' measurements.

If the calorimeter is large, the length of time taken for any changes in heat to be measurable is longer. At a minimum, a calorimeter of 1.6 m^3 provides a response in 3 minutes; one with a size of 20 m^3 takes 2 hours to show a response. The accuracy of measurements with a direct calorimeter is of the order of 1–2 per cent.

Indirect methods
Respiratory gas analysis
The principle of indirect calorimetry is based on the relationship between oxygen use and carbon dioxide production, described above. To apply this, the method used must be able to measure

either or possibly both of the gases over a period of time. Equipment used for this purpose ranges from the large and stationary to more portable versions. Obviously stationary equipment can only be used when subjects are resting; more mobile activities require portable equipment.

Originally, the respiration chamber itself was used, with the gases inspired and expired by the subject sampled and analysed. More recently, a hood or small plastic tent is placed over the recumbent subject to collect the gases, which these days pass straight into automated analysers linked to computer printouts, to provide instant data. This type of measurement is useful in hospital patients who may be confined to bed. The equipment must be mobile and moved to the bedside.

Mobile equipment has largely been of the 'backpack' variety, worn by the subject during physical activity. The necessary link between the equipment and the subject's respiratory system has been by way of a corrugated tube, mouthpiece and nose clip. This is not especially comfortable, and can both limit the duration of the measurement and affect the normal pattern of breathing.

Isotope methods

Alternative approaches have been developed in recent years. The most significant of these is the doubly labelled water technique, using stable isotopes of hydrogen and oxygen (^2H and ^{18}O). The subject drinks a small volume of labelled water. The hydrogen equilibrates in the body water pool (producing hydrogen-labelled water), the oxygen in both the water (as oxygen-labelled water) and in the carbon dioxide pools. Thus, the ^{18}O is contained in both the carbon dioxide and water, and the ^2H is contained only in the water; therefore, the labelled oxygen is lost from the body faster than the hydrogen.

The rates of loss of the isotopes are generally measured in a series of samples of body fluid, such as urine, over a period of days (up to 21). The difference between the rates of loss of the two isotopes, therefore, represents the loss of carbon dioxide, and can be used to calculate carbon dioxide and, hence, heat production. In turn, this can be used to derive energy expenditure.

Several assumptions are made with this technique, most notably about isotope fractionation in the body. In addition, as oxygen usage is not measured, the RQ has to be estimated. However, if a concurrent food intake record is kept, then an RQ value from the intake can be calculated, assuming there is energy equilibrium.

This technique provides a useful, safe and non-intrusive way of measuring carbon dioxide turnover, and hence metabolism over periods of time. As a result, a large amount of information has been derived in recent years about energy expenditure in groups of subjects that previously have been difficult or unethical to study, such as the elderly, pregnant and lactating women, and young infants and children.

Measurements of 24-hour energy expenditure can be made by a relatively novel isotope technique, the bicarbonate–urea method. The technique uses the isotope dilution principle. Labelled CO_2, given subcutaneously as bicarbonate, is diluted by endogenous CO_2; the extent of this dilution is measured by the isotope activity in urinary urea, produced over a 24-hour period. This allows the CO_2 produced in the body to be calculated, and energy expenditure found using values for the energy equivalent of CO_2.

Other methods

A number of other techniques have been used to measure energy expenditure, including:

- activity diaries;
- heart rate monitoring;
- skeletal muscle recording (electromyography);
- pedometers (to record movement);
- energy intake studies for subjects in energy balance.

All of these give less reliable results, but may be of value when groups of subjects are being studied, to provide more general data.

Some of the methods listed above can provide estimates of the intensity of exercise or patterns of activity during a period of exercise that may provide useful additional information. Activity diaries are prone to omissions, especially of small habitual movements, that may be important over a 24-hour period, and may over-report structured or intense activity.

Application of measurements of energy expenditure

In the case of individuals in hospital, it is often vitally important to know the exact amount of energy required by the body. For example, patients who are being fed intravenously have little opportunity to regulate their intake according to appetite. Their clinical state, for example, after major surgery, or the treatment being administered may have a dramatic impact on their metabolism, and energy needs may be as little as 50 per cent of those calculated, or up to 150 per cent of this value. There is, therefore, a serious risk of underfeeding or overfeeding, if exact energy expenditure is not known. This is particularly a hazard in overweight and obese patients, in whom layers of adipose tissue may mask a significant loss of lean tissue.

COMPONENTS OF ENERGY OUTPUT

Basal metabolic rate

The single largest component of a person's daily energy output is the basal metabolic rate (BMR). In a sedentary individual it may represent 65–70 per cent of total energy expenditure. BMR is defined as 'the sum total of the minimal activity of all tissue cells of the body under steady state conditions'.

This generally means that BMR is measured when no digestion or absorption of food is taking place (at least 12 hours after eating), and in a subject who is in a state of physical and mental relaxation. If measurements are made within a shorter time interval after a meal, the value obtained is called the resting metabolic rate, as it will be somewhat higher than the true BMR. The greater part of the energy is used in driving the osmotic pumps that maintain the differences between extracellular and intracellular fluids, and for the synthesis of proteins and other macromolecules. Only about 10 per cent of the total basal energy is used for internal mechanical work, including the functioning of the heart, respiratory system and digestive tract. Tables of BMR values generally give figures as Calories or kilojoules per kilogram body weight, per hour. As a general rule, the BMR for men averages 4.2 kJ (1.0 Calories) per minute and for women 3.75 kJ (0.9 Calories) per minute. Metabolism in subjects during deep sleep (called minimal metabolic rate), may be 5–10 per cent lower than BMR.

Various factors, both external and internal, can affect the BMR of an individual, and these are now considered (see Figure 7.3).

Body weight

Since basal metabolism reflects the energy needed to sustain the function of the body, it is

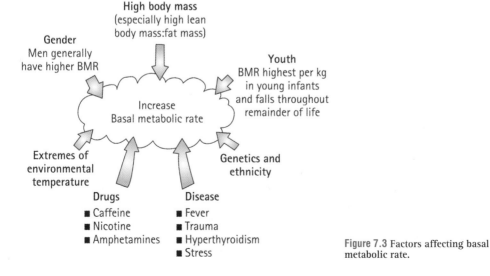

Figure 7.3 Factors affecting basal metabolic rate.

clear that the larger the body, the greater will be the BMR. Weight is thus a critical determinant of BMR. Measurements on many subjects confirm this relationship. However, the two major components of body weight make a different contribution to the total BMR, with lean body mass being considerably more metabolically active than fat mass. The metabolic activity of lean tissue is relatively constant between individuals, so if BMR is expressed as kilojoules or Calories per kilogram of lean body mass only, the result is similar for all individuals. It is the proportion of fat mass in the total body weight that modifies the final figure.

Gender

The BMR for women is lower than that for men because of differences in the proportions of body fat to lean. In women, the body fat content is, on average, 10 per cent higher than in men, with a consequently lower lean mass and thus lower BMR. This gender difference is apparent by the age of 2 years.

A further aspect is the energy demand made on the mother's body during pregnancy and lactation to support the growth of the fetus. Changes occur to the maternal BMR to allow for a more efficient use of energy, and these are described more fully in Chapter 11.

Age

The BMR (per kg) is highest in young infants and falls throughout the remainder of the life cycle. The decline is relatively slow in children and adolescents, in particular, but once adulthood has been reached, there is a gradual progressive decline of approximately 2 per cent per decade after the age of 30 years. This is related to the amounts of metabolically active tissue present at different ages, as well as the rapid rates of growth in early infancy and adolescence. It is also higher in young infants because of the need to maintain body temperature. As people age and become more sedentary, the amount of lean tissue declines, with a parallel fall in BMR. However, if a person retains a high level of activity, the decline in BMR with age is much smaller as the lean tissue mass is more effectively preserved.

A failure to acknowledge and adapt to the declining energy needs may, in a proportion of the population, explain the increase in body weight that tends to occur in the middle years of life.

Disease

Both diseases and their treatments may have an influence on the BMR. Since the thyroid hormones are regulators of the metabolic rate, undersecretion or oversecretion by the thyroid has a major influence on metabolism. Fever and trauma tend to increase metabolism. Stress can also increase energy expenditure in the short term. Various drugs or pharmacological agents have an effect on metabolism and many increase the rate, for example, caffeine, nicotine and amphetamines. Some drugs, such as beta blockers and antidepressants, may reduce metabolism. Undernutrition also depresses metabolic rate.

Measuring BMR in people who are ill may, therefore, not give accurate results, if confounding factors are not allowed for. BMR may vary at different stages of the disease; thus, the point in its time course when BMR is measured could be important. Anxiety, blood transfusions, effect of pre-test treatments or feeding regimes may all influence the outcome of a BMR measurement. In translating the BMR result into a total energy expenditure, it should also be remembered that a bedridden patient will have a much lower level of physical activity, so that energy requirements overall may be less than in health, even if BMR is elevated.

Other factors

There are a number of other factors that may have an influence on metabolism, including genetics, climate and ethnicity. These are all difficult areas to study and, although some examples of differences arising from genetic or ethnic variation have been reported, other studies fail to show such differences. Most Westerners respond to changes in climate by adjusting their clothing and the level of heating or air-conditioning in their environment. When people are prevented from doing so, then metabolism is seen to increase both at low and at high environmental temperatures.

Thermogenesis

As mammals, including humans, are warm-blooded, our bodies need to generate heat to maintain body temperature (thermoregulatory thermogenesis). This requires energy and will be a variable aspect of our energy balance. Mostly, we exist in environments at a comfortable, or thermoneutral, temperature so that little extra energy is used to keep warm, although before the widespread introduction of central heating into homes, it is probable that more energy was used to maintain body temperatures. Eating affects energy expenditure because the body uses energy in eating, digesting and absorbing the food, transporting the nutrients and incorporating them into the cells. It represents the inefficiency of the body's processing of its food intake. This is usually called the 'thermic effect' of food or 'diet-induced thermogenesis'. In the past, this was known as 'specific dynamic action' of food, and was thought to derive specifically from proteins. However, all the macronutrients of the diet contribute to this heat production, although fats contribute least and proteins the most. It varies between individuals and also between meals of different size and composition, but as a general guide is believed to amount to 10 per cent of the total energy eaten in a meal. Thus, if a meal containing 3 MJ (750 Calories) is eaten, the amount of energy available to the body for use will be 10 per cent less than this. Thermogenesis also occurs as a result of cold exposure, hormonal state or drug intake, although these are difficult to quantify.

Physical activity

This is the aspect of our total energy expenditure over which we have most control. We can choose to undertake a range of different activities during the course of a typical day, walking to work or school, taking part in sports, having hobbies for our spare time that involve movement. On the other hand, we can drive or take the bus to work, we can sit during our break and lunch hours and, on returning home, spend the evening in front of the television. Clearly, such contrasting lifestyles will be associated with different levels of energy output.

It has been shown by careful measurements that the amount of energy expended in activity is related to the size of the body being moved and, consequently, to the BMR. Therefore, two individuals, both weighing 60 kg, will expend a similar amount of energy performing the same task. In contrast, a person weighing 100 kg will use twice as much energy in a given task as a 50 kg person. This is an important finding, as previous calculations of energy expended in activities made no reference to the size of the person performing them. Many figures have been derived that quantify the average amount of energy used, in relation to the BMR, for specific activities. These are known as physical activity ratios (PARs), which represent the energy costs of activities. In the USA, these are called METs (metabolic equivalents), and this acronym is also seen in many training and fitness contexts in the UK. By expressing these in terms of the BMR, one value for each activity can then be applied to all individuals regardless of age, size or gender, since these will already have been taken into account in the calculation of the BMR itself.

In deriving the PARs, some generalizations have to be made. A certain amount of activity is common to most people; this includes the general 'personal maintenance' activity associated with washing, dressing, preparing and eating food and generally moving about from room to room in the home environment. It is assumed that this makes similar demands on the body for all individuals, and a factor of 1.4 is attributed to it. The period of sleeping has a PAR of 1.0; it is assumed that during this period there is no increment above BMR. Various occupational activities may also be grouped together, based on the usual and average amount of physical activity involved. In addition, the PAR values make no judgement about the intensity with which the work is carried out and, if it continues for a period of time, whether rest periods are taken. Some examples are shown in Table 7.5.

CALCULATION OF ENERGY EXPENDITURE

In order to calculate total energy expenditure, it is necessary to obtain a figure for the BMR.

TABLE 7.5 PARs for calculation of energy expenditure

Activity	PAR
Lying at rest/sleeping	1.0
Quiet sitting activities (e.g. reading, TV)	1.2 (range 1.0–1.4)
Active sitting activities (e.g. driving, playing piano)	1.6 (range 1.5–1.8)
Stationary standing activities (e.g. ironing, laboratory work, washing-up)	1.6 (range 1.5–1.8)
General mixed standing/sitting (e.g. personal activities, washing, dressing, eating)	1.4
Activities involving moving about (e.g. cleaning, tidying, cooking, bowling)	2.1 (range 1.9–2.4)
Walking, average speed, making beds	2.8 (range 2.5–3.3)
Gardening, playing table tennis	3.7 (range 3.4–4.4)
Walking quickly, dancing, swimming	4.8 (range 4.5–5.9)
Jogging, football, tennis	6.0

From DoH, 1991. Crown copyright is reproduced with the permission of Her Majesty's Stationery Office.

Various equations, such as the du Bois and Harris–Benedict equations, have been derived to facilitate this, based on experimental measurements of BMR in subjects. Most widely used at present are those derived by Schofield, based on measurements made on over 10 000 subjects, and derived as regression equations from the plots of results. These, together with some more recent data on elderly subjects, are used in the dietary reference values report (DoH, 1991), and were the basis of the FAO/WHO/UNU (1985) recommendations on energy intake.

The equations for adults are given below (DoH, 1991).

Figure 7.4 Summary record of daily activity.

	BMR	
	MJ/day	Calories/day
Males		
18–29	0.063W + 2.896	15.1W + 692
30–59	0.048W + 3.653	11.5W + 873
60–74	0.0499W + 2.930	11.9W + 700
Females		
18–29	0.062W + 2.036	14.8W + 487
30–59	0.034W + 3.538	8.3W + 846
60–74	0.0386W + 2.875	9.2W + 687

W = body weight (kg).

Example of calculation of energy expenditure

Bill is aged 40, and weighs 70 kg. His BMR is calculated as follows: $(0.048 \times 70) + 3.653 = 7.01$ MJ/day. Therefore, his hourly BMR = 7.01/24 = 292 kJ/hour.

He recorded his daily activity pattern and the summary is shown in Figure 7.4. Energy expenditure is, therefore, calculated as follows, with the appropriate PAR values, and using his hourly BMR.

	Duration (hours)	× PAR ×	BMR/ hour =	Energy used (kJ)
Sleeping	7	1.0	292	2044
Driving	2	1.6	292	934
Personal activities	3	1.4	292	1226
Watching TV	3	1.2	292	1050
Playing football	1	6.0	292	1752
Sitting at work	8	1.2	292	2803
Total				9809 = 9.8 MJ

Thus, Bill expended 9.8 MJ in the course of this day.

In comparison with his BMR, which is 7.01 MJ, it is possible to calculate his physical activity level (PAL) throughout the day. This represents the amount of extra energy that he expended, above his BMR, and is calculated as energy expenditure/BMR, i.e. 9.8/7.01 = 1.4. This means that, over the day, he used 40 per cent more energy than that simply needed for his BMR.

This is a very average figure for a relatively sedentary population, typical of the UK, and forms the basis for the estimated average requirements for energy, given in the dietary reference values report and summarized in Table 7.6.

Activity 7.4

Keep a record of your own activities for two periods of 24 hours. They need not be consecutive, but should represent differing levels of your own activity. Find your body weight and use this to calculate your BMR. Then construct a chart similar to the worked example above, to allow you to calculate your total energy expenditure over the 2 days. Work out the ratio of your total energy expenditure with respect to your BMR: this is your physical activity level.

■ Is there anything that surprises you about the results for the 2 days you have chosen – for example, is the difference between them more or less than you expected?

■ Which component of your daily activity has made the largest contribution to the total – is it your BMR, or a particular activity?

■ If you had a period of strenuous exercise, what proportion of the total did this constitute? Is this more or less than you expected? For what period of time would you need to continue this level of exercise for it to equal half of your BMR expenditure?

■ Did you have different periods of sleep during the two recorded days? Did this make a difference to your output?

■ Compare your results with those of others. What differences can you find? Can you account for them?

TABLE 7.6	EAR for energy for adults in megajoules per day (Calories/day)	
Age (years)	Males	Females
19–50	10.60 (2550)	8.1 (1940)
51–59	10.60 (2550)	8.0 (1900)
60–64	9.93 (2380)	7.99 (1900)
65–74	9.71 (2330)	7.96 (1900)
75+	8.77 (2100)	7.61 (1810)

From DoH, 1991. Crown copyright is reproduced with the permission of Her Majesty's Stationery Office.

SUMMARY

1 Energy balance represents the relationship between energy intake and energy output.
2 Energy intake is the metabolizable energy of foods, generally calculated from the proximate principles. Dietary surveys tend to underestimate energy intakes.
3 Energy output comprises basal metabolic rate, thermogenesis and physical activity.
4 Basal metabolic rate is influenced by a number of factors, including age, gender and body weight.
5 Energy expenditure in activity is related to the basal metabolic rate and can be calculated by the use of factors known as physical activity ratios. The overall daily energy expenditure can be compared with the BMR in the form of the physical activity level.

STUDY QUESTIONS

1 Distinguish between and account for any differences in the yield of energy from a food when:
   a it is combusted (burned) in a bomb calorimeter;
   b its constituents become available for use at cellular level in the body.
2 Would a diet with a low fat content (e.g. 15 per cent of energy from fat) be appropriate for:
   a healthy child with an average (not large) appetite;
   b an elderly, housebound person.
   Explain your viewpoint.

3 Including the energy from alcohol in calculating the contribution from each macronutrient to the total energy intake can make important differences to the results. Comment on the following cases:
   a Harry: total energy intake = 12.8 MJ fat 33 per cent, protein 15 per cent, carbohydrate 40 per cent, alcohol 12 per cent;
   b Alex: total energy intake = 10.6 MJ fat 40 per cent, protein 12 per cent, carbohydrate 48 per cent;
   c Sam: total energy intake = 15 MJ fat 28 per cent, protein 13 per cent, carbohydrate 34 per cent, alcohol 25 per cent.

REFERENCES AND FURTHER READING

Conway, J.M. (ed.) 1995: Advances in human energy metabolism: review of current knowledge (Symposium). *American Journal of Clinical Nutrition* 52(5), 1033–75.

DEFRA 2001: *National Food Survey 2000 Annual report on food expenditure, consumption and nutrient intakes.* London: The Stationery Office.

DoH (UK Department of Health) 1991: *Dietary reference values for food energy and nutrients for the United Kingdom.* Report on Health and Social Subjects No. 41. Report of the Panel on Dietary Reference Values of the Committee on Medical Aspects of Food Policy. London: HMSO.

FAO/WHO/UNU 1985: *Energy and protein requirements.* Report of a joint FAO/WHO/UNU Expert Consultation. WHO Technical Report No. 724. Geneva: WHO.

Food Standards Agency 2002a: *Food portion sizes,* 3rd edn. London: The Stationery Office.

Food Standards Agency 2002b: *McCance and Widdowson's The composition of foods,* 6th summary edn. Cambridge: Royal Society of Chemistry.

Gibney, G.R. (2000): Energy expenditure in disease: time to revisit? *Proceedings of the Nutrition Society* 59, 199–207.

Gregory, J., Foster, K., Tyler, H., Wiseman, M. 1990: *The dietary and nutritional survey of British adults.* London: HMSO.

Schofield, W.M., Schofield, C. James, W.P.T. 1985: Human nutrition. *Clinical Nutrition* 39C (suppl.), 1–96.

Scrimshaw, N.S., Waterlow, J.C., Schurch, B. (eds) 1996: Protein and energy requirements symposium. *European Journal of Clinical Nutrition* 50 (suppl. 1).

Westerterp, K.R. 1999: Body composition, water turnover and energy turnover assessment with labelled water. *Proceedings of the Nutrition Society* 58, 945–51.

CHAPTER 8

ENERGY BALANCE

The aims of this chapter are to:

❏ discuss the concept of energy balance and review its components;
❏ describe the situations where energy intake and output are not in balance;
❏ study the components of body composition and the ways it is measured;
❏ consider the health risks of excessive and low body weight, and how to bring about weight change.

On completing the study of this chapter, you should be able to:

❏ explain the changes in energy balance that contribute to weight loss or weight gain;
❏ discuss the aetiology of overweight and underweight, including an understanding of some eating disorders;
❏ identify appropriate ways of measuring components of body composition and explain the significance of particular results;
❏ suggest ways of increasing or reducing weight by diet and lifestyle changes.

Most people maintain their bodies in a state of energy balance within quite narrow limits, as evidenced by a constant body weight. When changes in energy balance occur, they are rarely sudden or unexplained, but are most likely to occur gradually and over a long period of time. This may make them difficult to correct, since they often go unnoticed until a marked change has occurred.

In Chapter 7, the components of energy balance are described. Energy intake derives from the food we eat and is regulated by a number of different factors, including physiological (such as hunger), psychological (appetite or mood), social and environmental factors, all of which interact in complex ways, and are thus difficult to study and to control. Energy output represents the energy used to maintain physiological and biochemical activities (as basal metabolic rate), to digest and process the food we eat and to fuel all physical activity. Normally, these two aspects are in equilibrium with the energy intake being sufficient to meet the energy output (see Figure 8.1).

$$\text{Energy intake} = \text{Energy output (basal metabolic rate} + \text{thermogenesis} + \text{physical activity)}$$

However, this equilibrium is not necessarily maintained on a day-to-day basis; some days our intake is greater than our output, and on other days the opposite applies. When this happens, some of the surplus energy is stored as fat in the adipose tissue. At other times, these stores have to be drawn on to provide energy needed at a particular moment. Evidence suggests that overall, there is a stability of body weight, and data from a long-term study of the population in Framingham, Massachusetts, shows that, over a period of 18 years, most people were at a body weight within 5 kg of their original weight. This energy imbalance represented less than 0.5 per cent of the total turnover in energy, implying that reasonably efficient regulation was occurring. Subjects whose weight changed the most were also the most likely to suffer from disease.

Figure 8.1 Components of energy balance.

Nevertheless, weight changes do occur; in the UK and most other Western countries, statistics show that incidence of overweight and obesity among the adult population has been increasing rapidly. Trends of increased weight are also now seen in children, often from a very young age. In all of these cases, there is an increase in fat stores. Thus, the energy balance equation above has to be rewritten:

$$\text{Energy intake} = \text{Energy output} \pm \text{energy stores}$$

ADJUSTING THE BALANCE

When the energy balance is disturbed, the body tries to restore it by making various adjustments to the different components of the equation. Some of these may be brought about consciously by our own efforts, others occur at the molecular or cellular level and are outside our direct control. For example, we may deliberately increase or decrease our food intake, or alter our activity level, but the changes that occur to our metabolic rate and the metabolic mixture that the body uses cannot be consciously regulated, but may alter as a consequence of other changes we make. The ways in which its components may be adjusted to achieve energy balance are considered below.

Energy intake

Food is the source of energy entering the body, thus regulation of food intake will control the input side of the balance equation. The factors that are involved in the control of food intake

are considered in Chapter 2. Food intake may change or be adjusted in a number of ways:

- Deliberate reduction or increase of overall intake, with less/more food eaten in general. This may include omitting particular meals, e.g. breakfast.
- Limiting or increasing particular types of food in the diet – such as high-fat foods, or those containing sugar, starch or non-starch polysaccharides (dietary fibre). For example, cakes and confectionery may be excluded, or more fruit and vegetables included in the diet.
- Eating more of particular foods – perhaps low-energy (or 'slimming') foods, or foods that are perceived as causing weight loss. This category may also include foods that are believed to promote development of particular aspects of body composition, such as 'body-building' foods, or those with perceived health properties. Functional foods is a name applied to this category of foods; these are further discussed in Chapter 17.
- Eating more snacks throughout the day, allowing greater flexibility to match appetite and energy needs.
- Changes in appetite, causing rejection of all or some foods, or increasing the desire for foods (general or specific).
- Inability to eat, for medical or psychological reasons, or owing to lack of availability of food. In the case of a person who is unable to eat, nutritional support in the form of modified, possibly liquid feed, may be provided. This needs to be supplied and consumed in an adequate quantity to ensure sufficient energy intake.

In each of the above cases, energy intake is likely to change from the current one to a higher or lower level. This may be the result of a conscious desire to change or can occur as a secondary phenomenon, perhaps in association with illness or disease. There are also likely to be changes to the nutritional composition of the diet in some of the cases.

In addition to changes in food intake, in some cases of disease or in eating disorders, there may be interference with the process of digestion or absorption. Disease of the digestive tract may prevent normal digestion, so that food is either lost by vomiting or passes undigested through the gut. Malabsorption may also affect the transfer of the digestion products into the blood. The presence of stomas (where an opening to the outside of the body has been made from the digestive tract, generally as a result of disease) or a reduced absorptive area following partial removal of the bowel will have similar consequences.

Certain forms of eating disorders also include deliberate interference with digestion and absorption, either with the use of induced vomiting once food has been eaten, or by using laxatives or purgatives to prevent the food being absorbed.

Finally, a drug developed for the management of obesity inhibits the enzyme responsible for the normal digestion of fat, so that malabsorption occurs and undigested fat is lost in the faeces. This has the effect of reducing the energy available from the food eaten.

Energy output

Basal metabolic rate

Changes in basal metabolic rate (BMR) are most likely to occur as a result of changes in body weight or composition. BMR is influenced particularly by lean body mass, so any alteration in this will affect the rate of metabolism. Ageing is accompanied by a reduction in lean body mass and, therefore, there is a gradual fall in BMR. Immobility as a result of illness or ageing will cause a loss of lean tissue and a consequent reduction in metabolic rate.

Conversely, training which involves exercising the whole body or specific blocks of muscles will gradually result in an increase in lean muscle mass (although this can take many weeks) and can result in an elevation of the metabolic rate. It must, however, be remembered that these changes in lean mass may not be immediately apparent by straightforward whole body weighing. The changes may be accompanied by loss of adipose tissue, which may cancel out the overall weight change. More specific measurements of body composition may need to be done to identify changes in these components.

An increase in overall body weight is more commonly associated with an increase in body fat. In this case, there is an increase in BMR because the larger tissue mass requires more energy to sustain it. Furthermore, an increase in the mass of adipose tissue is associated with an increase in the supporting cellular structure, which includes protein-containing cell wall material and water. There are also increases in the heart and skeletal muscle, digestive tract and liver to cope with the increased demands put on them. However, the overall effect on the BMR is smaller as a result of an increase in fat rather than lean tissue, as the latter is more metabolically active. Nevertheless, it is important to remember that a heavier person has a higher BMR than a smaller, thinner individual. This fact is sometimes overlooked by people that are overweight, who claim that their problem is the result of 'slow metabolism'.

When weight is lost, there is a reduction in BMR, consequent on the fall in the mass of metabolically active tissue to be maintained. This is one of the major problems encountered by dieters. As they lose weight, the smaller body actually requires less energy to sustain it and, therefore, the energy deficit becomes smaller. The result is that the rate of weight loss slows down.

Thermogenesis

This comprises the thermic effect of food as well as possible 'adaptive thermogenesis'. The thermic effect of food is equal to approximately 10 per cent of the energy consumed. It follows that any changes in food intake will be accompanied by changes in the amount of heat lost in processing this food. Someone who increases their food intake in a meal from 3.3 MJ (800 Calories) to

5.0 MJ (1200 Calories) will use 17 kJ (40 Calories) more in processing this food. However, these values are not consistent between individuals; some are more efficient in their energy transformations than others. Data suggest that the obese have a smaller thermic response to food than the non-obese, but both will exhibit an increase in thermic effect on overfeeding.

Adaptive thermogenesis is energy expended as heat in response to a number of stimuli, such as cold, infection, injury or cancer cachexia as well as overfeeding. It is particularly important during hibernation in animals, and in the very young mammal is a means of controlling body temperature, before the capacity to shiver has developed. In both cases, it is a particular type of fat cell, known as brown adipose tissue (BAT), which is responsible for the production of heat. The cells of BAT have a rich blood supply and extensive sympathetic innervation, a high concentration of mitochondria in each cell, and the presence of myoglobin for oxygen transport.

The extent of any role for BAT in the control of energy balance in humans has not been agreed. Its role in dissipating the energy from overfeeding was demonstrated initially in rats fed on a range of 'cafeteria foods' typical of some human diets. Some of the rats remained at a normal weight, whereas others gained weight and became obese. Those rats that were able to control their weight were shown to have hypertrophied BAT. It became clear that this had become more active and had dissipated the excess energy as heat, rather than trapping protons in the formation of usable ATP (the energy 'currency unit'). This response of BAT is under the control of the sympathetic nervous system and several key receptors have been identified of which the most important is the β_3-adrenergic receptor. A number of uncoupling proteins (UCP) that are involved in the production of heat in BAT have also been identified in the inner mitochondrial membrane. Recently, markers have been developed that allow this protein to be located; these studies have shown that, contrary to the earlier view that BAT was only present in infants, there is a small amount of BAT in adults. The advances in molecular biology and human gene mapping have allowed many of these features of BAT activity to be identified in humans. A gene associated with reduced β_3-receptor activity has been identified and linked with increased abdominal fat deposition, reduced metabolism and a greater capacity for weight gain. Genes for UCP have also been identified and variants discovered. Nevertheless, the importance of BAT in normal subjects is still unknown; it may possibly account for up to 10 per cent of energy balance. Certainly, the response of individuals to overfeeding does vary, with some gaining more weight than others. Physiologists have believed for many years that there might be a mechanism that allows subjects to 'adapt their energy expenditure to match the intake'. It is possible that BAT is one component of this mechanism that links with other aspects of energy balance regulation.

Physical activity

This is the aspect of our daily energy output that is most variable, both between and within individuals and, therefore, provides the greatest potential to increase energy output.

There has been a major change in the level of activity of people in most Western countries in the last 30–40 years, and particularly in the last decade. The advances in technology have reduced the need for physical effort in work, transport and leisure activities. Few people now have very physically demanding jobs, compared with 30 years ago. Many tasks related to everyday life are now less physically demanding, e.g. shopping with a supermarket trolley and car, compared to carrying shopping from the local high street, and making a bed with sheets and blankets, compared with straightening a duvet. Leisure activities themselves have become more sedentary, with television, video and computer games constituting a substantial proportion of many people's entertainment (see Figure 8.2). In addition, children play outside much less and are generally transported to school much more with the result that the pattern of low activity levels is established at a young age. School sport has also decreased, as pressure on the curriculum for academic subjects, as well as the loss of school playing fields to building and development have their effects.

Figure 8.2 Using energy in everyday life.

There is considerable concern about the steady decline in activity levels and various initiatives exist to raise awareness about the importance of activity. Current advice in the UK is that a minimum of 30 minutes of moderate activity should be undertaken by everyone, with most people aiming for at least 30 minutes moderate activity on 5 days of the week, or 20 minutes intense activity on 3 days a week. Associated with this there is an increasing emphasis on incorporating more 'routine' activity into the lifestyle. This may include using the car less or walking up stairs; the intention is to include activity as part of the normal day, rather than separating it into 'exercise', which tends to become a chore and often stops when the initial enthusiasm wears off. Many schemes exist to encourage physical activity, including 'the walking bus' to take a number of children to school, 'exercise on prescription' (Figure 8.3) to prevent or treat disease and many 'get fit' campaigns promoted in the media and local leisure centres. There are indications that a small increase in moderate to vigorous activity has taken place both in the UK and USA. However, this is seen among the better-educated and better-off groups, rather than in the more deprived areas. In addition, this small increase is insufficient to compensate for the downturn in 'lifestyle' activity that has been occurring.

Many people in Britain are classed as having light occupational activity levels and sedentary leisure activity; an overall physical activity level (PAL) of 1.4 or less is, therefore, estimated.

Figure 8.3 Exercise on prescription.

Studies of free-living populations in Britain confirm these assumptions, with some finding average PAL as low as 1.27. This means that the amount of energy expended during 24 hours is only an additional 27 per cent of the BMR. This represents minimal physical effort. (PAL is discussed in Chapter 7.)

Changing PAL requires periods of activity that involve movement of the body and, therefore, muscle activity, raising cardiac output and respiration for a reasonable period of time to make an impact on the calculation of a 24-hour energy output. It is for this reason that incorporating several smaller increases in activity during a normal day can have more of an impact on total expenditure than one intense bout of activity, which lasts for perhaps only 20 minutes. In fact, after intense exercise, there may be a period of complete inactivity, while the subject recovers from the effort. The overall level of activity may be much less, therefore, than might at first appear.

Spontaneous low-level activity, or fidgeting, is also of interest. It has been noted that subjects in overfeeding studies varied substantially in their levels of fat storage, which was attributed to differences in 'non-exercise activity

Activity 8.1

You will need to refer to information in Chapter 7 to complete this activity.

Three friends have undertaken a study of their activity. They are all male, aged 25 years, with body weights of 60 kg (Tom), 70 kg (Sam) and 80 kg (Harry). The results of their activity diaries are given below

Tom		Sam		Harry	
Activity	Duration (h)	Activity	Duration (h)	Activity	Duration (h)
Work: sedentary	8	Work: mixed standing/sitting	8	Work: mainly moving about	8
Other:		*Other:*		*Other:*	
Personal activities	3	Personal activities	2	Personal activities	2
Watching TV	4	Watching TV	1	Watching TV	2
Drive to work	1	Walk to work	1	Drive to work	1
		Walking dog (brisk)	1	Football	1
		Gardening	2	Swimming	1
		Tidying house	1	Playing computer games	1
Sleeping	8	*Sleeping*	8	*Sleeping*	8
Total hours	24		24		24

Calculate each man's daily energy expenditure, and express the answer as the physical activity level, to allow comparisons to be made between them.

- What similarities and differences are there?
- What impact do their various leisure activities have on the total expenditure?
- How important is the level of work activity?
- What conclusions can you draw about the optimal way of increasing daily energy output?

thermogenesis', or fidgeting. This is also related to sympathetic nervous system activity but the exact involvement of this aspect of activity in total energy output is as yet unclear.

HOW WELL IS ENERGY BALANCE CONTROLLED?

Humans consume different amounts of food each day, with differing proportions of macronutrients, and also expend different amounts of energy in varying activities. The preceding sections have discussed the components of energy balance and shown that changes can occur in each component, consciously or unconsciously, to bring about a restoration of energy balance. The body, therefore, strives to achieve homeostasis by a number of mechanisms. The regulation of energy balance is neither perfect nor rapid and, as a consequence, changes in weight occur, reflecting these fluctuations in energy balance.

By adjusting food intakes in experimental subjects and concurrently measuring energy expenditure, it can be shown that changes in weight and energy expenditure are not matched precisely. Both experimental and long-term observational studies show that the body resists an energy deficit, whether this is induced by diet or exercise, and there is a drive to compensate for this either by increasing energy intake in subsequent days, or reducing energy expenditure. These results confirm that maintaining a weight loss can be difficult. Strong cognitive control, or will power may be needed to resist the physiological drive to restore energy balance, although exercise has been shown to help in the maintenance of weight over the long term. Restoration of energy balance during or following overfeeding is less effective, especially if high-fat diets are consumed. Exercise appears to be an important adjunct to maintaining energy balance on high-fat diets. However, there is a varied response to these disturbances of energy balance between individuals and between genders.

The relative ease of weight gain and difficulty of weight loss associated with physiological mechanisms for homeostasis means that, in some individuals, there is a fluctuation in weight over periods of time, as weight lost is regained. This has been termed 'yo-yo dieting'. Long-term studies of population cohorts have shown that there is an increased morbidity and mortality in people whose weight fluctuates compared with those who have a stable weight. It is not, however, possible to state that weight fluctuation is the cause of the increase health risks, as it may equally be true that poorer health is a cause of weight fluctuation. Nevertheless, it is likely that weight loss followed by weight regain, repeated on many occasions, is detrimental to the psychological well-being of the individual.

When an individual is ill, the achievement of energy balance may be complicated by factors such as the metabolic response to the illness, effects of drugs or other treatments and the accompanying inactivity. Further, feeding or the lack of it will also have an effect on energy utilization. Careful monitoring is required to ensure that energy balance is maintained.

Control mechanisms

For almost 50 years, it has been suspected that body weight is controlled by signals that monitor the quantity of adipose tissue. However, the nature of the signal was not identified until 1994, when a protein produced by adipose tissue was identified and named leptin. The amounts of leptin in the circulation are correlated with measures of adiposity, such as BMI and percentage body fat. Leptin is present in the circulation in both a bound and a free form. Receptors for leptin were found originally in the hypothalamus but many other tissues are now known to

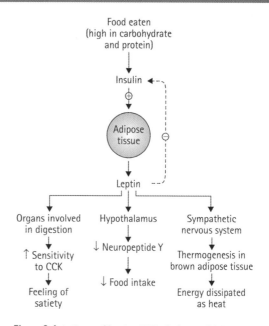

Figure 8.4 Actions of leptin. CCK, cholecystokinin.

contain leptin receptors. These include organs involved in energy storage, metabolism and digestion. Other sites that contain leptin receptors include tissues or organs involved with immunity, blood pressure regulation and reproductive organs; the role of leptin in these functions is still being investigated.

Leptin levels provide information to the brain about the abundance of body fat. Energy balance is regulated by the actions of leptin in the hypothalamus resulting in inhibition of food intake and increase in energy expenditure. Food intake is regulated through the release of neuropeptides, most notably neuropeptide Y, which is associated with increases in food intake. An increase in leptin levels will inhibit neuropeptide Y and, therefore, reduce food intake. The central action of leptin also stimulates the sympathetic nervous system, which in animals has been linked to thermogenesis in brown adipose tissue, allowing dissipation of energy as heat. In subjects with a high fat mass, evidence suggests that a failure of the leptin receptors to respond, results in a breakdown of energy balance, allowing fat deposition to occur (see Figure 8.4).

There are also close links between leptin and insulin. Insulin has similar effects in the hypothalamus, and reduces food intake and increases energy expenditure. It is now clear that insulin is involved in the secretion of leptin from adipose tissue, and also that leptin can inhibit insulin secretion. Therefore, when food is eaten, polypeptides (such as glucose-dependent insulinotropic polypeptide; GIP) released from the intestine, together with absorbed metabolites (glucose, amino acids), stimulate insulin release. Glucose metabolism in adipocytes eventually causes leptin release, which acts in the brain to cause a reduction in food intake. This pathway will be most effective with foods that trigger insulin release, such as carbohydrate- and protein-containing foods, and ineffective with high-fat foods. It, therefore, seems probable that the balance of macronutrients in the diet may influence leptin secretion.

The feedback loop described above identifies the role of leptin in a medium to long term control of energy balance. Leptin is also involved in short-term control of food intake, by increasing the sensitivity of the response to cholecystokinin (CCK). This is one of the gut hormones associated with satiation, released when food enters the duodenum (see Chapter 2). Leptin levels are not constant in an individual, as they exhibit a peak around midnight, which for many people is approximately 4–6 hours after an evening meal. The timing of the peak changes if meal times are altered. Levels are reduced during fasting, and cause increases in hunger even before any change has occurred in body fat levels. This is not helpful for weight reduction, but is a normal physiological response to an energy deficit. A great deal of research effort is currently focused on the potential use of leptin, its analogues or triggers, in order to manipulate energy balance. In addition, investigations into the genetic codes for various leptin receptors and intermediaries in the pathways are ongoing, but research to date has found very few individuals in whom mutations in genes for leptin production or leptin receptors are the cause of overweight. It has recently been noted that pre-term babies who were assigned to receive an enriched formula rather than human milk, had higher leptin levels relative to fat mass, at adolescence. This suggests that the leptin feedback mechanism may already be less sensitive at this age. This finding suggests one possible way in which early feeding may programme the later development of overweight.

BODY WEIGHT AND COMPOSITION

When an individual is in energy balance, the body weight and composition stay constant. Therefore, a growing child or an athlete in training aiming to increase muscle bulk will need to be in positive energy balance to accrue body mass. On the other hand, an individual who is aiming to lose weight will need to be in negative energy balance. Measuring the body mass and its composition is, therefore, important. Most people assume that, in adults, a gain in weight is associated only with an increase in body fat, but some increase in supporting tissues also occurs. Subjects who are physically active and engaging in training schedules may gain weight as a result of an increase in muscle (lean) mass. Similarly, when weight is lost, there can be a loss of lean tissue, particularly if rapid weight loss occurs. This might be the result of a badly planned slimming diet, or perhaps due to illness. It would be more accurate to describe people as overfat rather than overweight, to differentiate between the heavy, but lean individual and the person with a high percentage of fat in the body. Similarly, a light person may still have a relatively high percentage of fat in their body, but this may be not apparent if their lean mass has shrunk. This may be true of an older adult who has perhaps become very sedentary.

Body mass index

The body mass index (BMI) is calculated as the individual's weight (in kilograms) divided by height (in metres) squared: W/H^2, in kg/m^2. Indices can range from less than 20 to above 40. The World Health Organisation (WHO) has recommended that the following categories be used:

BMI	Grade
<18.5	Underweight
18.5–25	Normal weight
>25–29.9	Overweight (Grade 1 obesity)
>30	Obese (Grade 2 obesity)

These data are based on the greater health risks associated with increasing weight, as shown by actuarial life expectancy tables, as well as information about morbidity. In general, risks increase with rising BMI, even within the band categorized as 'normal'. For example, for women the risk of coronary heart disease in an American study was shown to be twice as great at a BMI between 25 and 29 as at a BMI of less than 21. Above a BMI of 29, the risk was almost 3.5 times greater. For diabetes, the prevalence is about three times greater for people with a BMI above 28.5 than for those whose BMI is below 24.4. Thus, the classifications of BMI are rather arbitrary and useful for convenience, rather than being major boundaries between levels of risk. It should be noted also that BMI is not an ideal measurement for everyone, and is mainly focused on those who are overfat, rather than overweight due to other reasons. It takes no account of the components of the body weight and may, therefore, classify as obese a trained athlete who has a high percentage of lean tissue and little body fat. BMI is also useful for classification of degrees of malnutrition in adults, as follows (Ferro-Luzzi et al., 1992):

BMI	Grade of malnutrition
<16	3
16–16.9	2
17–18.4	1

In addition, a chart may be used to check the degree of overweight (see Figure 8.5).

Distribution of body fat

Additional information about the health consequences of increasing weight can be obtained from the waist-to-hip ratio, which compares the girth of the body at these two sites, expressing the result as a single figure. For individuals with a predominance of fat deposition in the trunk, and particularly around the abdomen (central obesity), the ratio is higher than for those whose fat is mainly laid down in the buttocks and hips (peripheral obesity).

In general, women exhibit peripheral obesity (also described as gynoid or 'pear-shaped'), and men tend towards central obesity (android or 'apple-shaped'). Ratios of more than 0.95 in

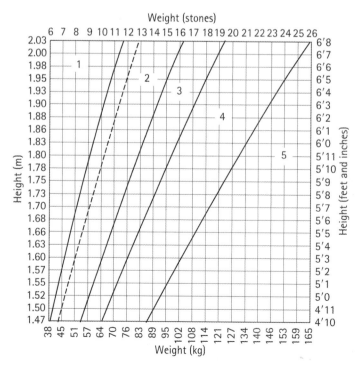

Figure 8.5 Weight assessment chart for adults. Take a straight line across the chart from your height and a straight line up from your weight. Make a note of where the two lines meet. This will indicate if you are within the desirable weight for your size. 1, underweight; 2, desirable weight; 3, overweight; 4, fat; 5, obese.

men and 0.8 in women are taken as indicating increased risk. After the menopause, women become more android in their shape, and this is accompanied by greater risk of obesity-linked disease (see Figure 8.6).

Girth measurements of various parts of the body including abdomen, buttocks, thigh, calf, forearm and upper arm have also been used. Age- and gender-specific equations have been derived and cross-validated with good results. They are useful for ranking individuals within a group according to fatness, and levels of error are in the region of 2.5–4 per cent. The advantage of these measuring techniques is that they require only the simplest of equipment – a tape measure – and can, therefore, be performed almost anywhere. They are particularly useful for monitoring changes in body shape over a period of time. They should, however, be used with caution in people who are very thin, very fat or have undergone periods of physical training.

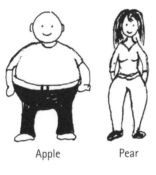

Apple   Pear

Figure 8.6 Central (apple) and peripheral (pear) fat deposition.

Recently, good predictability has been obtained using waist measurement only as an indicator of the need for weight management and this is now being recommended as a very simple public health message. Most people are able to measure their waist circumference or are aware of the measurement for clothes sizing. The measurement should be taken midway between the lowest rib and the iliac crest. Levels for action, based on the cut-off points can be promoted as part of the weight management message. These are shown in Table 8.1.

MEASURING BODY COMPOSITION

Skinfold measurements

Skinfold (or fatfold) measurements are a useful and inexpensive way of obtaining a measurement of body fat content. In the hands of an experienced operator, the specially designed callipers can yield results within 3–5 per cent of those obtained by more complicated and accurate methods, such as hydrostatic weighting (see below). Figure 1.2 illustrates the technique. The results from skinfold measurements can be used simply to quantify the subcutaneous fat at specific sites and monitor this in a particular individual over a period of time. Alternatively, the results can be entered into appropriate equations to calculate the total body fat content. Ideally, measurements should be taken at the four common sites: mid-biceps, mid-triceps, subscapular and supra-iliac, and the total

TABLE 8.1	Action levels for weight management based on waist circumference	
Level of health risk	**Waist circumference – men (cm)**	**Waist circumference – women (cm)**
Healthy/normal	<94	<80
Action level 1		
Increasing risk – no further weight should be gained	94–102	80–88
Action level 2	>102	>88
High risk – medical advice should be sought for weight management		

Adapted from Scottish Intercollegiate Guidelines Network (1996).

skinfold measurement used to calculate the body fat.

A drawback of this technique is that it may not be suitable in individuals who are very fat, elderly (fat is more compressible in older age groups) or highly trained (muscular development makes it difficult to pinch a fatfold). In addition, it should be remembered that, in young adults, about 50 per cent of the body fat is found subcutaneously; with increasing age more is deposited internally. Thus, a similar fat-fold reading will represent a greater total body fat content in an older person than a younger one. Tables of typical skinfold results in population groups are available as standards.

Underwater weighing

This method is based on Archimedes' principle, which states that an object's loss of weight in water is equal to the weight of the volume of water it displaces, because the object in the water is buoyed up by a counterforce, which equals the mass of water it displaces. In applying this to human body composition measurements, the body's volume is determined by the difference between body weight measured in air and measured when submerged in water. The density of the body can, therefore, be calculated using the following equation.

$$\text{Density of the body} = \text{Weight in air} - \text{Weight in water}$$

The body density is composed of fat and fat-free tissue (together with a small correction for gases in the lungs and intestinal tract, which may be added to the calculation). It is assumed that fat has a density of $0.9\,\text{g/cm}^3$ and fat-free tissue a density of $1.1\,\text{g/cm}^3$. Errors may arise from assumptions about bone density and the water content of the body, but these are assumed to be small.

The body density can then be used in the equation derived by Siri, to calculate percentage body fat:

$$\text{Body fat (\%)} = (495/\text{body density}) - 450$$

Clearly, this technique is not suitable for some people, for example, those with a fear of immersion, the sick and elderly people.

Other indirect methods

There are a variety of techniques that can be used to determine the internal composition of the body from external measurements.

Bioelectrical impedance

This is based on the flow of electricity through the body, which is facilitated by the fat-free tissue and extracellular water because of the electrolyte content. The resistance (or impedance) to the flow of current is related directly to the level of body fat. Attaching electrodes to the hand and foot of a subject and passing a localized electrical signal allows impedance to be measured quickly and painlessly. The results obtained will vary with the level of hydration of the subject and with skin temperature. However, when details about age, weight and height are entered, the technique gives a quick readout of percentage body fat, and is widely used.

Ultrasound

This can be used to measure the thickness of the fat layer at various points of the body, as the ultrasound beam is deflected at each interface between different tissues. A similar method is the use of near-infrared interactance, which records the absorption and reflection of an infrared light beam, and computes fat thickness from the readings obtained.

Other techniques

Other techniques that require expensive equipment and are not generally available for routine use include computerized tomography, magnetic resonance imaging and dual-energy X-ray absorptiometry (DEXA). The DEXA technique has been used particularly in the measurement of bone density.

WHAT ARE THE AVERAGE VALUES FOR BODY COMPOSITION?

Various attempts have been made to represent the 'ideal body', not as a goal for individuals to strive for, but to provide a reference against which variations could be compared. Many authors use the terms 'reference man' and 'reference woman' to describe these hypothetical individuals. There are clear gender differences in body composition with a higher lean body mass in males (and consequently higher body water content) than in females. Females have a greater body fat content. These gender differences become apparent at puberty, when girls gain a greater proportion of fat than lean tissue, whereas boys gain predominantly lean tissue, and may actually lose fat during the teenage years.

Average values are as follows:

	Reference man	Reference woman
Weight (kg)	70	60
Lean body mass (kg)	60	48
Body fat (per cent)	15	25–28

Total body fat exists as essential and storage fat. The essential fat is needed for normal physiological functioning, and is believed to represent 3 per cent of total body mass in males, but 10–12 per cent in females. Highly trained athletes of both genders may have fat levels approaching these minimum values. The gender-specific fat in females is related to the reproductive role and hormone activity. At puberty, the growth spurt generally begins at a body weight of 30 kg, and, in addition, a minimal level of body fat must be achieved (13–17 per cent) for menstruation to begin, and a body fat content of up to 22 per cent may be needed to maintain menstrual regularity. If levels fall below these thresholds, menstruation will become erratic or cease. This can happen in girls who diet excessively for psychological or sporting reasons, and is discussed later in the chapter.

POSITIVE ENERGY BALANCE

Throughout Western societies, the end of the twentieth century and the beginning of the twenty-first century have seen a rapid rise in the prevalence of overweight and obesity, that has been described as an 'epidemic'. In the USA, the increase in adult obesity is progressing at 1 per cent per annum, and currently affects 20 per cent of men and 33 per cent of women.

Although the proportions affected are not yet as high, there are signs of increasing prevalence of overweight in some lower-income countries, such as Brazil and India. It is suggested that up to 10 per cent of the adult population worldwide is now obese. The WHO (1998) found that in most countries the prevalence of obesity is higher among women than men, with the exception of Finland and the Netherlands. In the UK in 1980, 6 per cent of men and 8 per cent of women were obese. In the Health Survey for England 1991, the prevalence of obesity was 13.2 per cent of men and 16 per cent of women. The National Audit Office in 2001 reported that 17 per cent of men and 21 per cent of women are obese in England, and a further 46 per cent of men and 32 per cent are overweight. This represents an almost three-fold increase in obesity in 20 years. It is estimated that, at current rates, the average BMI by 2010 in Britain will be 28. There is great concern that obesity is increasingly found in children, with 13 per cent of 8 year olds and 17 per cent of 15 year olds reported as obese in 1996.

What are the reasons?

There is an enormous amount of literature on the complexity of the problem of obesity. Fundamentally, the problem is that at some point the individual has been in positive energy balance, where intake has exceeded output. The reasons for this are considered here.

Dietary intake
Data collected routinely in Britain, for example, by the National Food Survey, show that the average level of energy consumption has fallen. Furthermore, the interest in healthy eating has resulted in a greater awareness about food intake, and many 'low-calorie' or 'low-fat' products are available in shops. Yet the weight of the population is increasing, suggesting that the energy intake is in excess of energy output. Recognition of the extent of underreporting of dietary intakes in survey records, however, suggests that this fall in energy intake may not be quite as large as appears from the published figures.

It has been proposed that one of the main problems with the typical Western diet is its high fat content, which is affecting the control of energy balance. It is clear from diet records over the last 50 years that the percentage of fat in our diet has increased, at the expense of the carbohydrate content.

Over 50 years ago, 53 per cent of dietary energy was derived from carbohydrates and 35 per cent from fats. Thus, for every 1 kJ from carbohydrates, the UK diet provided only 0.6 kJ from fats. By the early 1990s, carbohydrate intakes provided only 44 per cent of energy and 42 per cent came from fats, so that for each 1 kJ from carbohydrates, intakes now provided 0.95 kJ from fat. This represents an increase of 50 per cent in the relative intake of fats. By 2000, the ratio had improved a little to 0.8 kJ of fat for each 1 kJ of carbohydrates. This is the result of a fall in fat intakes. The extra carbohydrates that are being consumed are frequently more refined than those eaten 50 years ago, and lack the accompanying non-starch polysaccharide (NSP) and micronutrients of 'whole' foods that provided additional health benefits.

Studies of dietary intakes and weight in both men and women also indicate that the average BMI, and the proportion of those overweight and obese, decreases as total carbohydrate intake increases, largely as a result of differences in added sugar intake. The BMI increases as the proportion of fat in the diet increases, regardless of the total level of energy intake. Figure 8.7 shows the results of a large Scottish study that demonstrates these relationships clearly. These data suggest that it is, therefore, a high fat intake that is more likely to result in overweight and that the condition is a result of a positive fat balance, rather than positive energy balance. The results of four separate meta-analyses, reviewed by Astrup et al. (2000) consistently show that a reduction in dietary fat without restriction of total energy intake, causes a reduction of energy intake and weight loss in a dose-dependent manner. This can produce a modest but clinically important weight loss in overweight patients, with a typical weight loss of 3–4 kg over 6 months.

Studies on the metabolic fate of dietary macronutrients confirm that there is an oxidative

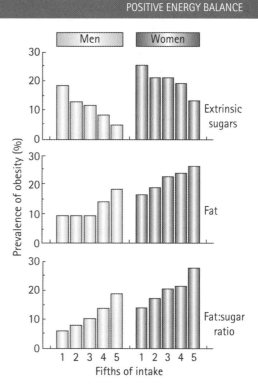

Figure 8.7 The relationships between fat and sugar intakes and body weight. From Bolton-Smith and Woodward (1994). Reproduced with kind permission of Nature Publishing.

hierarchy, with metabolism extremely well matched to intake in the case of alcohol, proteins and carbohydrates, but not for fats. Alcohol must be broken down and eliminated quickly from the body because of its toxic nature and absence of storage site. Therefore, it dominates metabolic pathways and suppresses metabolism of other substrates. Amino acid oxidation matches protein intake effectively. Glycogen levels have to be regulated in the body to maintain blood glucose levels, particularly for the brain and nervous system. Thus, if carbohydrate intake falls, glucose oxidation is reduced to maintain circulating levels and satisfy the obligatory use of glucose. Conversely, a high carbohydrate intake will trigger storage and inhibit fat oxidation. In addition, carbohydrate intake induces satiety through the release of several satiating hormones, including insulin, noradrenaline and gastric-inhibitory polypeptide. There is, therefore, very precise autoregulation of carbohydrate metabolism. These adjustments made to the metabolic mixture being used are reflected in changes in the RQ, which rises as more carbohydrate is used in metabolism.

However, there appears to be almost no autoregulation of fat metabolism to match intake, probably because the capacity for storage of fat is so large. Thus, an increase in fat intake does not trigger an increase in fat oxidation; instead, any fat that is in excess of immediate needs is stored. Thus, fat metabolism 'fills the gap' between the amount of energy available from the other macronutrients and the total required to meet energy output needs.

This is not a problem if the total intake of energy from the macronutrients equals the output. In this situation, the metabolic mixture reflects the proportions of macronutrients in the diet. When intakes are in excess of needs, fat oxidation is inhibited and it is stored in preference to the other metabolic products. In addition, fat is stored very efficiently, with only 4 per cent of its energy content being wasted in the process. If carbohydrate was stored, the initial conversion into fat would waste up to 25 per cent of the potential energy, making this a much less energy-efficient process. Hence, storing fat wastes less energy than storing carbohydrate as fat; this implies that dietary fats are potentially more 'fattening'. In humans, there is effectively no new synthesis of fats (*de novo* lipogenesis) by conversion of other nutrients to fat in the body, although the biochemical capacity to do this exists. Only in circumstances where experimental diets have contained very large quantities of carbohydrates (in excess of 600–800 g/day) for several consecutive days has there been some lipogenesis.

Dietary fat is likely to contribute to overeating. The satiating effect of carbohydrates is greater than that of fats. This, therefore, makes it easier for individuals to overconsume fat-containing diets without reaching satiety. Having consumed excess fat, subsequent food intake is not reduced, so continued overconsumption can occur, almost without the subject being aware of it. In addition, a fat-rich diet has a high energy content per gram and consequently is of a small bulk.

When the fat stores have increased, there is an increase in fat oxidation, which is reflected in a fall in RQ towards 0.7, indicating that fat oxidation is providing the major metabolic fuel. If fat stores are reduced by weight loss, more carbohydrate is used in metabolism and the RQ increases. It is still not clear, however, why some individuals respond in this way to fat intakes, and others apparently do not.

Physical activity

Maintaining adequate levels of physical activity has been shown to help in achieving energy balance. Societies in the West have become increasingly sedentary in the last decades of the twentieth century. A study across Europe by the Institute of European Food Studies (1999) has shown that an average of 32 per cent of adults were having no leisure time physical activity during a typical week. Work-related physical activity was also low, with almost half the population studied spending 2–6 hours sitting down at work and 20 per cent spending 6 or more hours sitting down. Across the age range, physical activity falls sharply after the mid-30s, contributing further to increasing levels of overweight.

Genetic predisposition

Much work has been carried out on identical and non-identical twins, and adoptive and natural parents to quantify the genetic component in weight. It is clear that there is a relationship between parents' weights and those of children, some of which is inherited. The patterns of fat distribution in individuals also show familial characteristics. Nevertheless, it is also evident that obesity is not only the result of a simple genetic defect, but is determined by an interplay between factors that include genetic, environmental, nutritional, psychological and social variables. From the research base, it has been estimated that between 40 and 70 per cent of overweight may be heritable. The contribution of environmental factors may account for a further 30 per cent of the cases of obesity. The importance of the role of the environment has become clearer in the last decades, as prevalence of obesity has increased rapidly, from a constant gene pool in the population. Advances in human genome research will in the future be able to identify candidate genes contributing to human obesity. There are a small number of single gene disorders, such as Prader–Willi syndrome, where obesity is part of the clinical picture. However, these aside, it is likely that overweight and obesity occur as a result of an interplay of factors and that, with suitable targeting and appropriate lifestyle adjustments, even subjects with a genetic predisposition to overweight should be able to maintain their weight within a reasonably normal range.

Age and gender

Scientific evidence proposes several critical periods in obesity development that include pregnancy, early infancy, 5–7 years and adolescence. These are believed to be associated with biological functions and regulated by hormonal action. Fat cell volume and numbers may change at these times. There is debate about the tracking of obesity from childhood into adulthood. Certainly an overweight child has a greater risk of becoming an overweight adult. However, most overweight adults were not overweight as children, and have experienced positive energy balance in adulthood, as a result of factors operating later in life.

Weight gain tends to occur with increasing age in Western societies, with particular increases in fat occurring between the ages of 25 and 45. For example, in England overweight or obesity is reported in 28 per cent of men and 27 per cent of women aged 16–24, 65 per cent (men) and 51 per cent (women) aged 35–44, and 76 per cent (men) and 70 per cent (women) aged 55–64. In women, increases in body weight may follow pregnancy, when weight gained is not lost. Peak prevalence among men is up to the age of 50; in women increases in body weight tend to continue until the mid-sixties. Both genders exhibit weight loss in older ages. It is possible that the trend in weight gain throughout the middle years of life is simply a reflection of reduced activity levels. However, it should also be remembered that basal metabolic rate declines with age and a failure to adjust food intake to compensate for this will contribute to a positive energy balance. In women, the loss of oestrogen activity after the menopause results in an increased central deposition of fat and an increased waist to hip ratio.

Socio-economic status

In Britain, there is an increased prevalence of obesity and overweight with low socio-economic status. In cross-sectional studies, this is seen consistently for women but less strongly for men. However, longitudinal studies demonstrate a consistent relationship between socio-economic status of origin and adult obesity. This finding awaits explanation but suggested reasons include: a poorer intrauterine or early life environment, increased likelihood of bottle feeding rather than breastfeeding and psychological/behavioural factors relating to social norms. These may include poorer self-esteem and attitudes to weight transmitted by parents. In addition, environmental factors such as food availability and selection are important, with evidence consistently showing that low income creates barriers to obtaining a healthy diet. Lifestyle may include low activity levels, where the environment precludes outdoor exercise, and costs prevent the use of leisure centres or gym facilities. Culturally acceptable body size will determine how much an individual may want to change their weight and, therefore, their acceptance of current weight or success in weight loss.

Many of the factors described above apply to people from the ethnic minority groups within British society, who are disproportionately represented among lower income groups. The National Audit Office report (2001) identified women of Black Caribbean and Pakistani origin as groups in whom there is a high rate of obesity. Asian men and women also have a greater prevalence of central adiposity that carries greater health risks.

Psychological factors

It has been suggested that some individuals overeat and become obese for psychological reasons. Both emotional disturbances and personality disorders have been proposed as a cause of obesity, although in both cases there is little good scientific evidence to support the theory. Depression and anxiety may occur among some obese individuals, especially those who binge eat. In addition, emotional distress and low self-esteem appear to be higher among the obese. It is difficult to separate cause and effect in these cases, as there can be improvement on weight loss. Stress has been linked to weight gain, both through a consumption of higher fat foods, but also raised levels of cortisol that is involved in regulation of abdominal fat stores. Those subjects who give up smoking are particularly vulnerable to an increase in weight, and the effects may be both psychological and physical in this case. An addiction to carbohydrate has been proposed, with the addict craving carbohydrates (chocolate, for example) in the way others crave alcohol or drugs. There is little sound scientific evidence to support this.

Overweight may also be the result of abnormal dietary restraint and disordered eating, as is also seen in anorexia or bulimia nervosa. These may be associated with poor or distorted body image, and greater sensitivity to external eating cues. In women, an inability or reluctance to achieve the ideal female stereotypical body shape created by society is believed to play a part in the aetiology of these disorders. It is widely believed that the current media preoccupation with idealized, thin and successful women, in film, fashion or music industries is driving greater body dissatisfaction among young women in the West. This also impacts on the willingness of some young women in particular to engage in physical activity owing to reluctance to expose their bodies in sports settings. This demonstrates an interaction between social and psychological factors resulting in poor control of energy balance.

If psychological factors are contributing to energy imbalance, it must be remembered that they are likely to play a major role in any attempts to normalize weight and should, therefore, be addressed in any weight loss programme.

These contributory factors are summarized in Figure 8.8.

HEALTH RISKS OF OVERWEIGHT AND OBESITY

Many people have the impression that being overweight or obese is only an aesthetic issue, linked simply to the appearance of the individual. As such, then, it is considered to be up to the individual to determine if they are content with their appearance. However, this is not the whole picture – overweight and obesity bring with them major health risks that can become life threatening. Health risk increases with BMI in a J-shaped relationship. Below a BMI of 20, there is increased mortality, linked to diseases that may cause loss of weight, such as cancers and the consequences of smoking. However, as BMI rises above 25 and especially above 30,

Figure 8.8 A summary of factors contributing to positive energy balance.

there is a progressive and accelerating increased risk of mortality. This has been recognized for almost a century when life insurance companies used body weight as a predictor of the 'risk' that a particular client might represent.

In addition to a greater risk of death, overweight and obesity carries increased morbidity, often starting at lower levels of BMI than for mortality. Obesity itself has been classified by the WHO as a disease, but also brings a host of medical consequences. Those that have received particular attention are cardiovascular disease, diabetes and cancers. Cardiovascular disease has received particular attention, as there is striking interaction between obesity and the known risk factors, such as smoking, hypertension and raised blood lipids. In addition, Type 2 diabetes is also a risk factor and is, in turn, strongly associated with obesity. In fact, the risk of Type 2 diabetes is 12.7 times greater in an obese woman and 5.2 times greater in a man than in non-obese individuals. This potentiating effect between risk factors makes it particularly difficult to separate the many aspects of metabolic consequences of obesity.

There are, however, also many other effects, some of which are listed in Table 8.2.

TABLE 8.2	Medical and other consequences of obesity (adapted from Lean 2000)
Type of consequence	**Specific examples**
Metabolic effects	Hyperlipidaemia
	Hypertension
	Cardiovascular disease (coronary heart disease and stroke)
	Type 2 diabetes mellitus
	Abnormality of blood clotting
	Risk of gallstones
Endocrine effects	Oestrogen-dependent cancers (including breast, endometrium and prostate)
	Infertility
	Menstrual dysfunction
	Increased risk in pregnancy
Physical effects	Joint disorders, arthritis, back pain
	Varicose veins
	Oedema
	Breathlessness
	Physical inactivity (possibly linked to bowel cancer)
	Stress incontinence
	Excessive sweating
Psychological effects	Tiredness
	Low self-esteem
	Depression
	Agoraphobia
Social effects	Isolation
	Unemployment
	Family problems/marital stress
	Discrimination
Surgical risk	Poor wound healing
	Chest infections
	Anaesthetic risk
	Venous thrombosis
	Sleep apnoea

Many of the consequences listed above develop slowly and insidiously, and are relatively uncommon in people below the age of 40. However, with the increased prevalence of obesity in younger adults and children, it is likely that the age of first presentation will fall.

The physical consequences of obesity increase with its duration, as organs and systems fail to cope with the increased demand put on them.

The National Audit Office report (2001) attempted to quantify the economic costs of obesity in England. It was estimated that obesity costs £2 billion from the national economy, including at least £0.5 billion in treatment costs to the NHS. Life expectancy is shortened by an average of 9 years, there are 18 million sick days taken each year from work and the overall mortality related to obesity accounts for 6 per cent of all deaths annually. Recent policy documents issued within the UK have included strategies to reduce the burden of ill health associated with obesity, both by helping overweight and obese people to lose weight as well as by preventing weight gain.

TREATMENT OF OBESITY/OVERWEIGHT

Whatever the reasons for weight gain, it is only by reverting to a negative energy balance that excess weight can be lost. Studies performed in carefully controlled metabolic ward environments have shown that even subjects who claim that they cannot lose weight on very small energy intakes when at home will start to lose weight when their food intake is monitored and regulated. Unfortunately, there is a tendency among a large proportion of the population to mislead both themselves and researchers about their food intakes. Some studies have shown that overweight subjects are particularly likely to do this, with some underreporting food intakes by up to 3.3 MJ (800 Calories) per day. There may not be a deliberate intention to deceive; indeed, foods are forgotten about as they are consumed without thought, or considered 'not to count'.

The common objective of these treatments is to reduce the amount of energy taken as food and/or to increase the amount of energy expended by the body. More specifically this should have as its aims:

- to provide a diet that meets all the nutritional requirements to maintain health, with the exception of total energy;
- to satisfy the individual subjects dietary preferences, as well as any financial and lifestyle constraints;
- to have a realistic goal for weight loss, within a specific time scale;
- to aim for a long-term strategy to maintain the target weight through appropriately chosen diet, behaviour and physical activity.

The major factor that will determine success is the motivation of the individual; hence, it is vitally important to assess the expectations as well as the willingness to adopt change. Targets can be modest, as a success in a small weight loss can be more satisfying than a failure in a large one. Even maintaining weight stability after a period of weight gain can be seen as a successful outcome. Dietary intervention needs to be accompanied by practical advice on eating patterns, exercise or other physical activity and long-term planning (see Figure 8.9).

Energy-controlled diets

These may be exactly specified or more flexible, and can be constructed in many different ways. They generally exclude those items in the regular diet that provide mostly energy (such as sugar and alcohol) and are also likely to restrict fat intakes. The most successful will be those that take into account the individual's personal preferences and circumstances. In general, these should be set at up to 2.5 MJ (1000 Calories) less than the subjects habitual intake, depending on the size of the individual. Some very low calorie diets have been developed, which provide even less energy than this. They are attractive to people wishing to achieve rapid weight loss, but are unlikely to lead to better eating habits and maintenance of the lower weight. In addition, as many of these are commercially promoted, their use may be less carefully regulated. Some subjects respond to a variety of energy-restricted diets, changed over time, to limit boredom. A novel approach may also be to eat more frequently,

Figure 8.9 Some possible interventions for weight loss: slimming group, surgical intervention and exercise.

fat storage. Furthermore, a large intake of food, at whatever time of day, induces lethargy so that no physical activity is taken afterwards. Small meals taken at intervals throughout the day allow activity levels to be maintained better. This pattern of eating may suit some individuals, and as with other weight loss advice, needs to be negotiated with the subject.

Pharmacological agents

Two types of drugs are currently used. The first are drugs acting on the digestive tract, of which Orlistat is a major example. This is a pancreatic lipase inhibitor that decreases fat digestion and absorption. The drug, therefore, causes steatorrhoea, with undigested fat appearing in the faeces, often as loose and oily stools. Some initial weight loss needs to have been achieved by normal dieting before the drug is prescribed. Most subjects do achieve some weight loss with the drug, although this may in part be as a result of changes made spontaneously to the diet, to limit some of the unpleasant consequences when fat has been eaten.

A new generation of centrally acting drugs that act to block serotonin and noradrenaline reuptake, and, therefore, promote satiety, has been developed. An example of this class is sibutramine. Earlier examples of centrally acting drugs, such as fenfluramine and dexfenfluramine, have been withdrawn owing to concerns about their safety. It is likely that more drugs will be developed in the near future to act on other aspects of energy balance, such as thermogenesis, or parts of the leptin-controlled pathways. In addition to drugs that have been tested through proper scientific procedures, there are a large number of other weight loss agents on the market that claim to be the 'new answer' to weight loss. These have often not been properly tested and do not come under the auspices of any legal protection as drugs. Unfortunately, people spend money on these, with little chance of obtaining the promised results. If weight loss does occur, it is likely to be as a result of better attention to diet than to the 'therapy' being taken. In some cases, the treatments may actually be harmful. For all pharmacological treatment, there remains the

using carbohydrate-rich snacks and cutting down on fat-rich foods. Eating small amounts frequently allows better matching of intake to needs. It also avoids the 'one large meal a day' pattern of food intake that some people have. This is generally in the evening when there is a higher level of insulin released that may more readily promote challenge to re-educate the subject to better eating habits, for long-term maintenance.

Surgical intervention

Various approaches may be used, all of them designed to assist in a weight loss plan, rather than to be the only means of weight loss. These procedures may attempt to restrict feeding (jaw wiring), mimic satiety (stomach stapling, gastric banding or balloons) or reduce absorption (bypass operations). These surgical procedures are seen as a first step in a long-term weight loss plan for obese patients. Fatty tissue may also be surgically removed, for example, in morbidly obese patients in whom large amounts of fat hang down from the abdomen. This is done to relieve breathing problems, and does not make an important difference to total fat mass. Liposuction is offered as a part of cosmetic surgery, to draw subcutaneous fat deposits, often from the buttocks or thighs. However, the amount of fat removed this way is minimal and makes little difference to overall body fat content.

Behaviour therapy

This may be formal or informal. The use of a psychologist together with a dietitian may help to uncover some of the reasons for the initial eating disorder, and perhaps address the causes. Much informal behaviour therapy occurs in slimming groups, where peer pressure and encouragement from the group leader may achieve better results than those seen in individual dieters. Motivation is a key aspect of group settings and may help the subject to continue with the process rather than relapsing. A group setting also provides the societal support that may be absent in the subject's home environment, and can make them feel more 'normal'.

Exercise

This is often perceived as a useful method of weight loss. However, the energy deficit that can be achieved by exercise alone would not bring about significant loss of weight. For example, jogging for 45–60 minutes, three times a week,

would use up 4.2 MJ (1000 Calories) in a week and it would, therefore, take up to 2 months to lose 1 kg of body fat. This can be contrasted with the possible loss of 1 kg within 1 week by a dietary intake deficit of 6.3 MJ (1500 Calories) per day.

However, exercise can be beneficial in achieving energy balance. It has been reported that exercise enhances fat rather than carbohydrate oxidation and can, therefore, promote greater fat utilization, allowing energy balance to be maintained at higher percentage fat intakes in the diet.

In addition, regular exercise has been shown to increase insulin sensitivity, reduce plasma triglyceride and very low density lipoprotein (VLDL) levels, raise high-density lipoprotein (HDL) levels and lower mildly elevated blood pressure in overweight people. It is also suggested that exercise prior to a meal enhances the thermic effect of eating in overweight people. There are also reports that exercise induces an elevation of the resting energy expenditure, even after the activity itself has stopped. This, however, depends on the severity of the exercise and is most likely to occur in highly trained athletes who incur an 'oxygen debt' during exercise; it may be less effective in people who exercise less vigorously.

Overall, the effect of exercise on changes in total body weight may be small. However, exercise may make it easier to achieve energy balance and, once weight is lost, it may also help in the maintenance of the new weight. There may also be protection of lean tissue during the period of weight loss, if the energy restriction is accompanied by exercise. Finally, exercise produces feelings of well-being, as a result of the release of opiates in the brain. This effect may be particularly beneficial to a subject attempting to lose weight. A restricted food intake may induce feelings of dissatisfaction, possibly even depression, which could be counteracted by the stimulation produced by exercise.

Unsafe methods of weight loss

There are very many dietary regimes that offer rapid weight loss, often linked to the consumption of particular 'wonder remedies'. They may require the dieter to eat more of a particular food (grapefruit is a classic example), or a specific product, which has to be bought from the 'counsellor'. Almost without exception, these are unproven and possibly unsafe, and should be avoided.

At present, there is no 'magic wand' remedy for overweight, but weight loss is possible by reversing the energy balance to a negative balance, and making the body use up some of its stores of energy. The more slowly this weight is lost, the better the chances of maintaining the loss. For most people, weight gain has occurred over a period of months and years; it is reasonable to expect the body to adapt better to a similar gradual reduction, than to a sudden crash diet. However, the best remedy remains to avoid becoming overweight in the first place.

NEGATIVE ENERGY BALANCE

Why does weight loss happen?

Weight loss can occur for a number of reasons.

- It may be deliberate, as in an overweight subject who desires to lose weight to a new target for health or medical reasons. (This has been discussed above.)
- Some sports require a particular body size for competition and demand that participants fall into the appropriate weight category.
- It may begin as being deliberate but become out of control, as in the eating disorders of anorexia and bulimia nervosa.
- It may occur in association with an addiction, perhaps to alcohol or drugs, which replace normal food intake, resulting in weight loss.
- It may be the consequence of ill-health, with the subject unable to eat or absorb adequate amounts of food and becoming malnourished as a result.
- It may occur in cancer, where the substances produced by the tumour may cause alterations in metabolism and severe weight loss (cancer cachexia).

Individuals may also simply have a low body weight, despite an apparent high energy intake. This is likely to be genetically determined.

If weight is maintained at this level, then no intervention is needed; however, if the subject has difficulty maintaining even the low weight further investigation may be necessary.

A negative energy balance may be evidenced by a failure to grow rather than by a loss of weight; this may be particularly true during childhood or adolescent growth spurt, when energy and nutrient needs are high. If these are not satisfied, the growth rate will falter and this can be demonstrated on a growth chart, which will show the deviation from the predicted pattern. This might happen in a young child who becomes ill and consequently has a reduced food intake, or perhaps in an adolescent who is using a great deal of energy in physical activity, for example, training for sport, so that insufficient is left for normal growth.

In all cases, the energy intake does not match the expenditure and, although the homeostatic response of the body is to try to minimize the energy deficit, weight is lost by mobilization of fat stores and lean tissue in an attempt to maintain the energy supplies to the tissues. Eventually, when stores become depleted, the organs themselves may be broken down, resulting in death. The length of time that a person can withstand such negative energy balance depends on the initial size of the stores, and the magnitude of the negative energy balance. Individuals on hunger strike who continue to take liquids may survive for periods up to 100 days. If food is eaten, even in small amounts, then survival can be for much longer. After the first few days, when weight loss can be quite rapid, fasting results in a loss of about 0.5 kg/day in the obese subject and 0.35 kg/day in a non-obese subject. A smaller energy deficit results in slower weight loss; for example, diets providing 5.9–7.9 MJ (1400–1900 Calories) may result in a weight loss up to 0.20 kg/day in obese males and up to 0.12 kg/day in obese females.

Underweight generally is associated with a higher mortality rate, so excessive weight loss is undesirable and should be avoided. Those who have a tendency to gain weight often yearn to be underweight, yet this is also not a healthy state! Subjects who appear to be genetically thin may wish to increase their body weight but may find this difficult. To avoid simply gaining fat, exercise to build lean tissue may need to be included, in association with increased dietary intake. It is also important that healthy eating principles are not ignored, and that adequate intakes of both macronutrients and micronutrients are included in the diet.

Eating disorders

The eating disorders anorexia and bulimia nervosa cause particular concern. Despite considerable research on both of these disorders, no effective way of preventing them has been discovered. The conditions are much more prevalent among females than males, although recent work suggests that 5 per cent of anorexia sufferers may be males. The key element of both disorders is a distorted body image, which perceives the body weight to be greater than it is in reality. Consequently, attempts are made to reduce it. In anorexic patients, these attempts may involve eating very little, with foods chosen carefully to include only those with very low energy content. In addition, the sufferer may exercise frequently and compulsively. There may be mood swings and a denial of the problem, with baggy clothing being worn to disguise thinness. In girls, a diagnostic sign is amenorrhoea and fine hair may grow on the face and body. In the case of bulimia nervosa, body weight may be in the normal range. The pattern of eating involves binges, during which abnormally large amounts of food are consumed. These are then almost immediately followed by deliberately induced vomiting. In both cases, laxatives and diuretics may be used in an attempt to reduce weight.

There are medical consequences of both conditions: anorexic patients may lose so much weight that they die. If weight loss is not quite so drastic, other changes will still be present, which include loss of muscle and bone mass, dry and itchy skin, hair loss, digestive tract irregularities (including constipation or diarrhoea), loss of tooth enamel due to vomiting, fainting and cardiac arrhythmias. Knowledge about both conditions is widespread among young people; websites occur on the World Wide Web that are perceived as encouraging eating disorders, with examples of how to avoid eating, how to prevent feelings of hunger and personal stories. It is unlikely that such a site would cause an eating disorder in a healthy individual but there is potential for someone who is experiencing body dissatisfaction to be influenced by such information.

Treatment requires both clinical and psychiatric intervention, but often takes a long time and may not be successful. There has to be a wish on the part of the sufferer to get better; this is sometimes easier to achieve in the case of bulimic patients than in those with anorexia.

Weight loss due to illness

This requires careful examination and management. The aim is to increase energy intake and, therefore, obstacles to this should be minimized. It may also be useful to assess energy expenditure and thereby obtain an indication of energy needs. A record of food intake for several days should normally be kept to establish where changes could be made. If poor appetite is a problem, it is important to identify foods that are liked. Other possible courses of action include:

- adding energy supplements to these foods if possible;
- reducing low-energy and low-fat foods in the diet and replacing them with high-energy snacks and meals containing some fat (preferably of vegetable origin);
- avoiding drinking with meals, as fluids can induce earlier satiety;
- reducing the amount of dietary fibre (or NSP) in the diet, as this has a satiating effect and will reduce total energy intake;

		Change in fat	
		Increase	Decrease
Change in lean body mass	Increase	Obesity Overfeeding Pregnancy Puberty (in girls)	Exercise Puberty (in boys) Use of androgens
	Decrease	Ageing Bedrest Zero gravity	Underfeeding Anorexia/bulimia nervosa Malnutrition Hibernation

Figure 8.10 The relationship between changes in lean body mass and in fat.

■ reducing physical activity (if appropriate) and perhaps including some muscle building activity, such as work with weights.

Changes in nutrition cause changes in body composition. Generally, these move in the same direction for the major constituents – lean body mass and fat. However, changes in lean body mass and fat can oppose one another, with the result that total body weight shows little overall change (Figure 8.10).

SUMMARY

1 Energy balance can be affected by changes in energy intake, energy output, or both of these.

2 Changes in energy intake may be the result of deliberate manipulation or secondary to changes in appetite perhaps related to disease.

3 Energy output is affected predominantly by basal metabolic rate and physical activity.

4 Changes in body composition occur as a result of alterations in energy balance as the body tries to re-establish homeostasis.

5 There is an increased prevalence of overweight in the UK, which may be linked to a high-fat diet. Low levels of activity may also play a part. Weight loss can only be achieved by measures that cause a negative energy balance.

6 Underweight may also be a problem and may occur by deliberate food restriction, or as a result of illness and disease. There may also be some individuals who are genetically thin.

STUDY QUESTIONS

1 Use your knowledge of the components of energy balance to analyse this case fully. Ann is a reasonably fit 40-year-old woman, weighing 58 kg. She takes regular exercise. This includes swimming for 1 hour three times each week, walking her dog for 1 hour each day and spending about 1 hour each day gardening. Recently, Ann broke her leg in a skiing accident and has been immobile for 6 weeks. She finds that her body weight is now 64 kg, although she has not increased her food intake.
  a Explain what has happened, in terms of the energy balance process.
  b Once her leg has healed and she starts to walk again, what could she do to return to her previous weight as quickly as possible?

2 How has your level of physical activity changed:
  a in the last year;
  b in the previous 5 years?

Can you suggest reasons for any change and possible consequences for your diet?

3 a It is suggested that people in the West should become more physically active. What activities do you consider to be the most appropriate, and likely to be the most effective in the longer term?
  b In some of the developing countries, levels of activity have also decreased. Can you offer an explanation?

4 Design some advertising material to promote physical activity in:
  a children, aged 8–11 years;
  b older teenagers, aged 16–18 years;
  c middle-aged women, aged 45–55; and
  d retired men, aged 65–70 years.

REFERENCES AND FURTHER READING

Astrup, A., Ryan, L., Grunwald, G. et al. 2000: The role of dietary fat in body fatness: evidence from a preliminary meta-analysis of ad libitum low-fat dietary intervention studies. *British Journal of Nutrition* 83(Suppl. 1), S25–32.

Bolton-Smith, C., Woodward, M. 1994: Dietary composition and fat to sugar ratios in relation to obesity. *International Journal of Obesity* 18, 820–8.

Bouchard, C., Perusse, L. 1993: Genetics of obesity. *Annual Review of Nutrition* 13, 337–54.

British Nutrition Foundation 1999: *Obesity. The Report of the British Nutrition Foundation Task Force.* Blackwell Science: London.

Clydesdale, F.M. (ed.) 1995: Nutrition and health aspects of sugars. Proceedings of a workshop. *American Journal of Clinical Nutrition* 62(1S).

Davies, J. 1994: Review of fad diets. *Nutrition and Food Science* 5, 22–4.

DoH (UK Department of Health) 1995: *Obesity: reversing the increasing problem of obesity in England.* A Report from the Nutrition and Physical Activity Task Forces. Wetherby: Department of Health.

Ferro-Luzzi, A., Sette, S., Franklin, M. et al. 1992: A simplified approach of assessing adult chronic energy deficiency. *European Journal of Clinical Nutrition* 46, 173–86.

Fruhbeck, G. 2001: A heliocentric view of leptin. *Proceedings of the Nutrition Society* 60, 301–18.

Havel, P.J. 2000: Role of adipose tissue in body-weight regulation: mechanisms regulating energy production and energy balance. *Proceedings of the Nutrition Society* 59, 359–71.

Hellerstein, M.K. 1999: De novo lipogenesis in humans: metabolic and regulatory aspects. *European Journal of Clinical Nutrition* 53(Suppl.1), 553–65.

Institute of European Food Studies 1999: *A Pan-EU survey on consumer attitudes to physical activity, body weight and health.* IEFS: Dublin.

Jebb, S.A., Elia, M. 1993: Techniques for the measurement of body composition. *International Journal of Obesity* 17(11), 611–21.

Kirk, T.R. 2000: Role of dietary carbohydrate and frequent eating in body weight control. *Proceedings of the Nutrition Society* 59, 349–58.

Lean, M.E.J. 2000: Pathophysiology of obesity. *Proceedings of the Nutrition Society* 59, 331–6.

Lean, M.E.J., Han, T.S., Morrison, C.E. 1995: Waist circumference as a measure for indicating need for weight management. *British Medical Journal* 311, 158–61.

Lissner, L., Heitmann, B.L. 1995: Dietary fat and obesity: evidence from epidemiology. *European Journal of Clinical Nutrition* 49(2), 79–90.

Moloney, M. 2000: Dietary treatment of obesity. *Proceedings of the Nutrition Society* 59, 601–8.

Moore, M.S. 2000: Interactions between physical activity and diet in the regulation of body weight. *Proceedings of the Nutrition Society* 53, 193–8.

Murgatroyd, P.R., Shetty, P.S., Prentice, A.M. 1993: Techniques for the measurement of human energy expenditure. *International Journal of Obesity* 17(10), 549–68.

National Audit Office 2001: *Tackling obesity in England – a report by the Comptroller and Auditor General.* London: The Stationery Office.

Parsons, T., Power, C., Logan, S. et al. 1999: Childhood predictors of adult obesity: a systematic review. *International Journal of Obesity* 23(Suppl. 8), 1–107.

Prentice, A.M., Jebb, S.A. 1995: Obesity in Britain: gluttony or sloth? *British Medical Journal* 311, 437–9.

Scottish Intercollegiate Guidelines Network (SIGN) 1996: *Obesity in Scotland: integrating prevention with weight measurement.* Edinburgh: Royal College of Physicians.

Singhal, A., Farooqi, I.S., O'Rahilly, S. et al. 2002: Early nutrition and leptin concentration in later life. *American Journal of Clinical Nutrition* 75, 993–9.

White, A., Nicolaas, G., Foster, K. et al. 1993: *Health Survey for England 1991.* Office of Population Censuses and Surveys. London: HMSO.

World Health Organisation 1998: *Obesity: Preventing and managing the global epidemic.* Geneva: WHO.

CHAPTER

9

VITAMINS

The aims of this chapter are to:

❏ describe the role of water-soluble and fat-soluble vitamins in the body;
❏ show the importance of the vitamins to health;
❏ demonstrate the interactions between vitamins.

On completing the study of this chapter, you should be able to:

❏ explain the role of vitamins in metabolism;
❏ account for the problems that arise if vitamins are not supplied;
❏ identify the groups in the population who may be at risk of an inadequate intake, and the reasons for this;
❏ discuss when supplements may be needed.

Throughout the body there are catalysts acting on a host of chemical reactions within living cells. Most of these are proteins acting as enzymes; some of these require additional 'cofactors' to complete their function. Some of these cofactors are minerals, such as magnesium, calcium and copper. There are also organic cofactors that must be consumed in the diet because the body (in general) is unable to synthesize them for itself. These are the vitamins.

Vitamins possess a number of specific characteristic features.

■ They are organic and, unlike the minerals, can be readily destroyed.
■ They are essential and, in their absence, particular functions of the body fail and may cease. Ultimately, deficiency of a vitamin can be fatal.
■ They generally work individually in a particular aspect of metabolism. However, some vitamins work in cooperation with one another. They may have similar effects and can thus replace one another (up to a point). They may be involved at different stages of the same pathway and a lack of one member may prevent the others being used.

■ They are present in food in small amounts, usually in both plant and animal foods. They vary in their chemical composition. Vitamins can be synthesized in the laboratory and can be taken as supplements, which will function in a similar way to those found in foods, since they are chemically identical.
■ They are needed by the body in small amounts, measured in milligram or microgram quantities. In some cases, excessive amounts of a vitamin are harmful. The body has varying capacity to store the vitamins; thus, for some, a regular intake is needed.

As vitamins occur in such small quantities in foods, their discovery was a slow process. Traditional cultures had many practices incorporated into their food habits, which ensured that vitamins were adequately supplied, although they would not have been able to offer an explanation. These include the making of drinks from pine-needle infusions to supply vitamin C, and soaking maize in lime water to liberate niacin. Limes were included in the cargo on long sea voyages in the eighteenth century in response to a perceived lack of 'a nutritional factor' in the remaining provisions, which had traditionally resulted in death among sailors.

Identification of the vitamins in the early twentieth century came from studies observing people and animals eating poor or restricted diets. Some of the substances that cured the signs and symptoms were found to be fat soluble, others were water soluble. In the beginning, these vitamines, as they were initially known, were allotted names according to the letters of the alphabet: A, B, C, etc. As the knowledge of the vitamins expanded, and they were chemically isolated and identified, it became more sensible to call them by their proper names. Nevertheless, the alphabetic naming is still used, particularly when there are several members of the group having similar properties, where using individual names would be cumbersome.

There have continued to be new findings about the functions of the vitamins ever since their original discovery. Clearly, our understanding of the vitamins is still incomplete and new findings will continue to be made. In addition, some of the vitamins have been found to have pharmacological properties when present in amounts much greater than those required for their metabolic function, and have, therefore, been used as medication, both therapeutically and prophylactically. Further understanding of this role is also needed.

FAT-SOLUBLE VITAMINS

As a group, these vitamins share several properties.

- They are found in the fat or oily parts of foods, and are, therefore, absent from foods that are devoid of fat.
- Their absorption and transport from the digestive tract requires the secretion of bile and normal fat absorption mechanisms. On the whole, they are absorbed with the digested fats into chylomicrons and transported in the lymph ultimately to reach the blood.
- Their transport in the blood requires carriers that are lipid soluble.
- They are stored in lipid fractions of the body, for example, in the adipose tissue, or in association with lipid components of cells.

- Because of their insolubility in water, they are not excreted in the urine and accumulate in the body, especially in the liver and adipose tissue. Large stored amounts, particularly of vitamin A and D, may be harmful and, therefore, care must be taken to avoid high intake levels.

Vitamin A

The deficiency associated with inadequate levels of vitamin A in the body, night blindness, has been recognized for many centuries. Vitamin A was the first fat-soluble vitamin to be identified; it is now known that there are several related compounds that have vitamin A activity, hence the name vitamin A will be used.

Three forms possess vitamin A activity in the body: retinol, retinal and retinoic acid; collectively they are called the retinoids. There is interconversion between the first two forms, but once the acid has been formed it cannot be reconverted. In addition, there are provitamin A compounds, the carotenoids, which can be converted, with varying degrees of efficiency into retinol (Figure 9.1). The most important of these is beta-carotene.

Vitamin A in foods

Foods derived from animals mostly contain preformed vitamin A, usually in the form of retinyl palmitate, which is easily hydrolysed in the intestine. Good sources are eggs, butter, milk and milk products, liver and fish or fish oils. Margarines contain vitamin A added as a legal requirement to domestic size packs in the UK.

Plant foods contain carotenoids, which are red or yellow pigments found in many fruit and vegetables. In the UK, most of the provitamin is in the form of beta-carotene, although in other parts of the world, alpha- and gamma-carotenes may be important. Red palm oil used in parts of Africa is rich in alpha-carotenes. Rich sources of carotenoids in the West include carrots, dark green leafy vegetables, broccoli, red peppers and tomatoes; in addition, apricots, peaches and mango are good sources.

Ordinary cooking processes do not harm retinol or the carotenoids. Cooking of carrots,

One molecule of beta-carotene

Two molecules of retinal (vitamin A)

Figure 9.1 Conversion of beta-carotene to retinol.

for example, enhances their digestibility and so makes more of the carotene available for absorption.

In order to obtain an estimate of the total amount of vitamin A activity consumed from both preformed retinol and carotenoids, it is necessary to devise a combined unit. This is the retinol equivalent, which represents the amount of retinol consumed + (the amount of beta-carotene ÷ 6). This accounts for losses in both absorption and conversion to the active vitamin.

In the UK mean total retinol intakes have been found (DEFRA, 2001) to be 780 µg retinol equivalents/day, which represents 126 per cent of the mean reference nutrient intake (RNI). Intakes have fallen quite sharply in the last 10 years as a result of lower fat intakes (e.g. from whole milk and spreads) and, in several groups within the population, particularly households with three or more children, the mean intake is less than 100 per cent of the RNI.

The major contributors overall are:

Vegetables (mostly carrots)	29%
Meat (mostly liver)	20%
Fats	22%
Milk and cheese	19%

The contribution of pre-formed vitamin A is approximately 64 per cent of the total intake, the remainder being provided by carotenoids.

In many parts of the world, the carotenoids are the more important source as few animal foods are consumed. Because the conversion of carotenoids to retinol is inefficient and their absorption is low, vitamin A status is poor in many countries. This has implications for health, as discussed later in this section.

Absorption of vitamin A

Both forms of vitamin A in the diet have to be released from complexes for absorption across the intestinal membrane, but the retinol is quickly re-esterified once inside the mucosal cell, and then incorporated into chylomicrons for transport. Carotenes are broken down to yield retinol. Although this conversion should theoretically yield two molecules of retinol from each beta-carotene, only one is thought to be produced normally. Some carotenoids remain unconverted and are absorbed as such. These include some hydroxy-carotenoids, such as lutein, alpha- and beta-cryptoxanthin. Absorption of retinol from pre-formed sources has an overall efficiency of 70–90 per cent if fat intakes are adequate, but only 15–50 per cent of carotenes are absorbed.

Protein deficiency, fat malabsorption, intestinal infections and diarrhoea will all reduce the efficiency of absorption.

Functions of vitamin A in the body

The majority of vitamin A is stored in the liver and the size of the stores can be used to assess vitamin status. It is transported to its target sites attached to a specific retinol-binding protein (RBP), and a pre-albumin in the plasma. This double carrier molecule is too large to be excreted through the kidneys, which protects the body from loss of vitamin A, and is received on target tissues by specific receptors.

Retinol levels in the plasma do not reflect intake and are not a good indicator of vitamin status because of the normal size of liver stores. However, a normal status is indicated when levels are in the range of 20–50 mg/dL. Plasma retinol levels are generally tightly controlled.

Carotenoids also occur in the plasma and tend to reflect dietary intake; lutein comprises 10–40 per cent of plasma carotenoids and may be a useful marker of green vegetable intakes.

The different forms of vitamin A appear to have differing functions in the body.

Vision

The retina is the light-sensitive cellular layer at the back of the eyes. It contains two types of cells: the rods (sensitive to dim light) and cones (sensitive to daylight and colour). In both types, the opsin proteins are associated with 11-*cis*-retinal, derived from retinol. Rhodopsin, found in rods, is much more sensitive to a lack of vitamin A than is the pigment in the cones.

When light strikes rhodopsin, the 11-*cis*-retinal changes to the all-*trans* configuration, triggering a series of complex changes resulting in the initiation and propagation of a nerve impulse, which is detected by the visual cortex. This occurs continuously in daylight so that rhodopsin is constantly being broken down. Most of our daylight vision is the result of changes occurring to the pigment in the cones.

Before it can be useful in dim light, rhodopsin needs to be resynthesized by conversion of the all-*trans* retinal back to the 11-*cis* isomer, for further visual signals to be detected. This can only occur in the dark, and in daylight occurs only when we blink. However, on entering a dark room, rhodopsin resynthesis occurs quickly, provided that there is a supply of retinol/retinal available, and we quickly become 'accustomed to the dark', and can see again. If there is insufficient supply of retinol to restore the rhodopsin, our dim light vision fails, and we suffer from 'night blindness' (see Figure 9.2).

The speed with which we can become accustomed to see in the dark is a measure of our vitamin A status. This is the basis of the dark adaptation test used to assess vitamin A status.

Cellular differentiation

Retinoic acid appears to be the major form of the vitamin involved in gene expression and control of cellular differentiation. In particular, the differentiation of epithelial cells is under the control of vitamin A, which determines their mucus-secreting properties. There are specific binding sites on cellular nuclei, from which retinoic acid interacts with DNA and controls synthesis of proteins and gene expression.

Epithelia constitute most of the body's surfaces and linings, and the ability to secrete mucus and keep these surfaces lubricated and washed is essential in the body's defence. Thus, sites as varied as the conjunctiva of the eye, the trachea and lungs, the digestive tract linings, and the urethra and bladder are all dependent on adequate vitamin A to maintain their integrity and function.

A failure to maintain this epithelial integrity and mucus secretion results in one of the classic signs of vitamin A deficiency: xerophthalmia, or dry eye. In this condition, there is a failure of tear production and the eye lacks lysozyme to keep it clean. It becomes susceptible to bacterial infections, resulting in conjunctivitis and, ultimately, damaged patches develop, known as Bitot's spots. If left untreated, the xerophthalmia progresses to a full breakdown of the eyeball, known as keratomalacia and accompanying loss of sight.

Vitamin A has a key role as an anti-infective vitamin, this is now believed to be closely linked

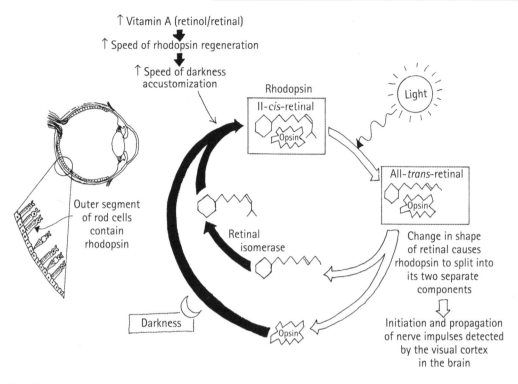

↑ Vitamin A (retinol/retinal)

↑ Speed of rhodopsin regeneration

↑ Speed of darkness
accustomization

Rhodopsin
ll-*cis*-retinal
Opsin

Light

Outer segment
of rod cells
contain
rhodopsin

All-*trans*-retinal
Opsin

Retinal
isomerase

Change in shape
of retinal causes
rhodopsin to split into
its two separate
components

Darkness

Opsin

Initiation and propagation
of nerve impulses detected
by the visual cortex
in the brain

Figure 9.2 Role of vitamin A in vision.

to its role in the maintenance of epithelial integrity. For example, impaired gastrointestinal epithelial integrity may allow the translocation of bacteria across the mucosa. Infection reduces the levels of circulating acute phase proteins that transport vitamin A, further exacerbating the problem of epithelial integrity. Children with vitamin A deficiency are also more susceptible to respiratory infections and measles. Supplementation of sick children with vitamin A has been shown to improve recovery rates.

Growth

Vitamin A is required for normal growth. In addition to the role described above in epithelial differentiation, vitamin A regulates bone remodelling, involving resorption and deposition of bone, required for linear growth. In deficiency there is a thickening of bones resulting from a relative lack of resorbing cells. Thickening of the bones of the skull can cause pressure on the brain and cranial nerves.

Antioxidant role

In recent years, the carotenoids have been found to have an important antioxidant role in quenching free radical reactions, particularly those involving singlet oxygen. This prevents damaging chain reactions, which could result in lipid peroxidation or damage to DNA, both of which have been postulated as being precursors of disease processes, leading to coronary heart disease and cancer, respectively. These properties have been attributed both to beta-carotene and lycopene (found especially in tomatoes). Antioxidant nutrients are discussed further in Chapter 14.

Other functions

A number of other functions have been attributed to vitamin A, although the exact mechanisms are not fully elucidated. The vitamin plays a key role in immunity, especially for T-lymphocyte function and the antibody response to infections. It appears to have a role as an anti-inflammatory agent. In addition, severe infections are associated with loss of the vitamin in urine.

There is a link between vitamin A and red blood cell formation, possibly involving the utilization or transport of iron; anaemia is a frequent finding in vitamin A deficiency, despite apparently adequate iron status.

Vitamin A deficiency

Aspects of vitamin A deficiency have already been referred to. A summary is provided here and is shown in Figure 9.3.

- Vitamin A deficiency is one of the top three major public health problems in the world, with 500 000 new cases each year, of whom 250 000 become blind. It is responsible for 70 per cent of cases of childhood blindness. Prevention with adequate vitamin A supplementation is possible.
- Early signs of deficiency include mild anaemia, impaired dark adaptation, abnormalities of smell, taste and balance, and roughened skin (follicular hyperkeratosis). In children, night blindness may be the first sign.
- Xerophthalmia, with Bitot's spots, may remain as a chronic condition.
- Keratomalacia, with involvement of the whole cornea, is often linked to more acute deficiency, accompanied by an increased risk of infection and mortality.
- In adults, vitamin A deficiency may take many years to develop.

Toxic effects of excess vitamin A

Acute poisoning can be induced by eating polar bear liver, but a more common risk of poisoning occurs when supplements are taken in excessive amounts. In the last 20 years, the levels of retinol in animal livers have increased dramatically and were recently reported to be 19 000 μg/100 g and 25 200 μg/100 g in lamb and calf liver, respectively, as a result of the use of feed supplements. This is of concern, especially for women, in whom high doses of vitamin A may be harmful to the embryo in early pregnancy. Intakes in excess of 3000 mg/day have been associated with birth defects (teratogenic effect). Clearly, a very small amount of liver would exceed this intake level.

Vitamin A derivatives are also used in treatment for acne and as an aid to tanning. Both should be used with care.

Requirement for vitamin A

Report 41 (DoH, 1991) based its reference values on the amounts needed to maintain an adequate pool of the vitamin in the liver at a concentration of 20 μg/g wet weight. On this basis, the RNI for men and women was set at 700 and 600 μg/day, respectively. Upper limits for

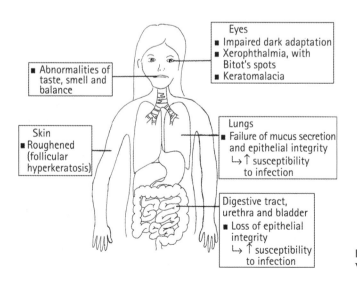

Figure 9.3 Summary of the signs of vitamin A deficiency.

regular intakes are also given, at 9000 µg/day in men and 7500 µg/day in women.

Vitamin D

The principal physiological role of vitamin D is to maintain serum calcium and phosphorus concentrations at a level appropriate for the formation of bone, support of cellular processes, and functioning of nerves and muscles.

Considering vitamin D amongst the vitamins creates a problem. The definition of vitamins states that they are substances that (generally) cannot be synthesized in the body and that a dietary intake is required. However, vitamin D can be made in the skin from a provitamin under the influence of ultraviolet (UV-B) light of wavelength between 290 and 320 nm. There has been considerable debate, therefore, whether vitamin D should continue to be considered as a vitamin. However, there are circumstances when individuals may not be able to synthesize the vitamin, for example, owing to insufficient exposure to UV light and most nutritionists agree that a dietary source is required. In the UK, no synthesis occurs in the skin between October and March because light of the correct wavelength does not reach the earth's surface. Consequently, synthesis that has taken place during the summer months has to provide the body's vitamin D needs during the winter. In addition, those who are housebound or those living in an environment with high levels of air pollution may have to depend on a dietary source all year round.

There are two potential provitamins for vitamin D: 7-dehydrocholesterol (vitamin D_3) and ergosterol (vitamin D_2). The former is present in animal fats, including the skin of humans, having been made in the body from cholesterol. Ergosterol is found in yeast and fungi, and is used as a source of commercial vitamin production.

Vitamin D in the diet

There are few sources of vitamin D that are consumed on a regular basis. Butter, spreading fats (including margarine, low-fat spreads), eggs and milk are the most regularly consumed sources. Levels in the dairy products vary with the seasons and are higher in the summer months. Where vitamin D is added by law as fortification, for example, to margarine, levels are constant throughout the year. In the UK, 7.05–8.82 µg/100 g margarine is the prescribed level added to margarine. Low-fat spreads may be fortified at the manufacturers discretion. Meat has relatively recently found to be a useful source of the vitamin. Other sources include oily fish and liver, although these may occur rarely in the diet. A number of manufactured foods may also be fortified with vitamin D, e.g. breakfast cereals, evaporated milk, bedtime drinks, yoghurts and infant foods. It is important to check on the label to discover which have added vitamin D. Fish oil supplements are a rich source of vitamin D, and may be taken by individuals as a prophylactic treatment for rheumatism and joint pains.

Recorded intake levels of vitamin D are 3.3 µg/day; there is no RNI figure for the majority of the population. The main food groups contributing to dietary vitamin D are reported by DEFRA (2001) to be:

Fats and oils	31%
Meat and meat products	19%
Fish	16%
Fortified breakfast cereals	14%
Milk and cheese	8%

Most people in the UK obtain vitamin D by skin synthesis during the summer months on exposure to UV light from the sun. The day does not have to be sunny nor the skin completely uncovered for synthesis to occur, the light can penetrate thin cloud and light clothing. There is now greater awareness of the dangers of exposure to solar radiation with respect to skin cancer, with recommendations to cover the skin with sun-screening creams or clothing. It is likely that this reduces the potential synthesis of vitamin D. A balance between the harmful (cancer risk) and beneficial outcomes (vitamin D synthesis) is required; it has been suggested that about half an hour per day of exposure to sunlight (avoiding the hottest part of the day) can achieve the beneficial synthesis, without risking harmful consequences.

Absorption of vitamin D

About 50 per cent of the dietary vitamin is found in the chylomicrons leaving the digestive tract in the lymph; most of this vitamin finds its way to the liver with the remnants of the chylomicrons. Vitamin D synthesized in the skin diffuses into the blood and is picked up by a specific vitamin-D-binding protein (DBP), which transports it to the liver, although some may remain free and be deposited in fat and muscle.

Before the vitamin D can perform its functions in the body, two activation stages occur. In the liver, an –OH group is added at position 25 on the side-chain (see Figure 9.4), to form 25 hydroxy-cholecalciferol (25-OH D_3), which is secreted into the blood and circulates attached to the carrier protein. This first activation is controlled by levels of the biologically active product of the second activation in a feedback mechanism.

The next stage occurs in the kidneys, where a second hydroxyl group is added at position 1, to yield 1,25-dihydroxy vitamin D (1,25-$(OH)_2$ D_3, or calcitriol). This is the biologically active form of the vitamin, and its levels are tightly controlled to maintain calcium homeostasis. The activity of the enzyme 1-alpha-hydroxylase, which catalyses this reaction, is determined by parathyroid hormone and low blood calcium levels, which increase its activity. High levels of phosphate inhibit calcitriol production. When the body does not require calcitriol to be produced, the kidneys perform an alternative hydroxylation at position 24, producing 24,25-dihydroxy vitamin D. The role of this metabolite is unclear, but it may be a way of 'switching off' production of the active hormone.

Figure 9.4 The formation of biologically active vitamin D occurs in two stages. First, in the liver, an –OH group is added at position 25. Then, in the kidneys, a second –OH group is added at position 1.

Action of vitamin D

Calcitriol, the biologically active form, has a number of target tissues containing specific receptors for the vitamin, the most notable of which are the intestine, bone and kidney. In each case, the function of the vitamin is to cause an increase in the plasma level of calcium.

- In the intestines, this is achieved by the vitamin-stimulated synthesis of calcium-binding protein, required for absorption of calcium.

- In the bone, calcium can be mobilized by the action of the osteoclasts and also made available for the osteoblasts to resynthesize bone. Thus, calcitriol enables appropriate amounts of calcium (and phosphorus) to be available in the bones for synthesis, while at the same time facilitating their release to maintain plasma levels.

- In the kidneys, calcium reabsorption is promoted by the action of vitamin D.

In summary, when plasma calcium levels fall, parathyroid hormone is released. This causes synthesis of calcitriol in the kidneys. In response, more calcium is absorbed by the gut, some calcium is mobilized by the bone and less calcium is lost at the kidneys. Overall, these changes raise plasma calcium levels, thus cancelling out the original stimulus.

If, however, the kidney is unable to respond to the original stimulus in this way (because there is insufficient 25-OH vitamin D being brought to the kidney, or the kidneys themselves are diseased), more parathyroid hormone will continue to be secreted. This can create a state of hyperparathyroidism, which may be a feature of vitamin D deficiency. Before the role of the kidneys in vitamin D and bone metabolism was fully understood, patients with kidney disease developed unexplained bone diseases. Treatment with active vitamin D can now prevent these problems arising.

In addition, recent work has discovered calcitriol receptors in other tissues, including placenta, gonads, skin and cells of the immune system, suggesting roles that are not directly linked to calcium homeostasis. Potent effects on cell proliferation and cell differentiation both in normal and malignant cells have been described. The vitamin may also be involved in downregulating the immune response, and vitamin D defects may be involved in autoimmune reactions.

Vitamin D deficiency

The lower cut off for adequate vitamin D status is taken as a plasma 25-OH vitamin D level of 10 μg/L (25 nmol/L). Elevated parathyroid hormone levels may be an alternative indicator of poor vitamin D status, but at present accurate limits have not been published. Furthermore, there is a diurnal variation in levels of parathyroid hormone, with a nocturnal rise. Parathyroid hormones tend to rise in the winter months in Britain, reflecting poorer vitamin D status, and this can be reversed with supplementation.

The consequence of deficiency in growing children is a condition known as rickets. The child is miserable and in pain. The bones are poorly mineralized and soft, so that limb bones bend under the body weight, the spine becomes curved and the pelvis and thorax may become deformed. The gait becomes waddling, with bow-legs or knock knees. The cartilage at the ends of the bones continues to grow and enlarge without becoming mineralized. Plasma 25-OH vitamin D concentrations may be below 8 μg/L (20 nmol/L; see Figure 9.5).

Figure 9.5 Vitamin D deficiency in children – rickets.

Curved spine

Thorax and pelvis may be deformed

Bow-legs

Muscular and bone pain

In adults, the comparable condition is called osteomalacia. The clinical picture is of bone gradually becoming demineralized and soft, with unmineralized areas and loss of bone detail, although total amount of bone remains normal. There is likely to be bowing of the spine and difficulty in walking. Depression, neuromuscular changes and generalized pain of uncertain origin may also be present. Plasma 25-OH D_3 levels are likely to be as low as 4 μg/L (10 nmol/L).

In both cases, there is muscular weakness and bone pain; plasma calcium, and phosphorus levels may be low and plasma alkaline phosphatase is raised.

Vitamin D deficiency was prevalent in Europe in the nineteenth century, especially in urban slum areas, where children had little exposure to sunlight. Improved environmental conditions saw the disappearance of rickets as a major problem. There is an increased awareness that rickets may be returning in various parts of the world for a number of reasons. These can be attributed to:

- reduced sunshine exposure, for example, owing to increased pollution, less playing outdoors, increased use of sun creams and highly covering clothing;
- reduced vitamin D intakes, as a result of longer breastfeeding (beyond 6 months), vegan/vegetarian diets, decreased use of milk and replacement with non-vitamin D containing drinks.

In the UK, there are a number of groups who are vulnerable. In particular, this includes:

- Asian immigrants, especially living in the northern regions;
- elderly people who are housebound;
- premature infants;
- individuals with malabsorption conditions;
- those with disease of the parathyroid, liver or kidneys;
- those treated with anticonvulsants.

Vitamin D deficiency had largely been eradicated by the use of fortified infant milks and supplementation with cod liver oil, but reappeared in the UK in the early 1960s amongst the new Asian immigrant communities. A number of factors are believed to interplay in its aetiology in this group.

- The darker skin pigmentation, more concealing clothing and a tendency to spend less time outdoors may limit the amount of skin synthesis (especially among women).
- Calcium intakes are low, as many groups use few dairy products.
- The high incidence of strict vegetarianism, including large amounts of non-starch polysaccharides and phytate, may reduce absorption of calcium, and possibly remove some vitamin D from the digestive tract. Possible intake of vitamin D from meat is excluded.
- Few sources of vitamin D are consumed.

Programmes aimed at increasing supplement use among the Asian population have been successful in reducing rickets among children, although poor vitamin D status continues to be found across all age groups. It has now been recognized that people within a household are likely to exhibit similar plasma levels of vitamin D, suggesting a common, probably dietary aetiology. Diagnosis of deficiency in one member should be followed by investigations of vitamin D status in other members of the household group, and appropriate intervention.

Older adults who are housebound or institutionalized may not be getting sufficient dietary vitamin D to compensate for lack of outdoor exposure. A significant proportion of those experiencing a bone fracture due to osteoporosis may have concurrent osteomalacia. Often plasma vitamin D levels are very low, with reports suggesting that 30–40 per cent of the over-75 age group have levels below 5 μg/L. Even when the individual is not totally housebound, exposure to sunlight may be brief and inadequate to raise plasma vitamin D levels. The efficiency of vitamin D synthesis in skin may decline with age, as the skin becomes thinner and contains less of the vitamin D precursor. Supplementation with 10 μg vitamin D/day seems to be an appropriate prophylactic measure in this group, recommended by the Department of Health.

Vitamin D deficiency in pre-term infants may be linked to inadequate phosphorus supplies in the milk and resultant undermineralization of bone. There are high requirements for vitamin D and feeds should provide 20–25 μg/day.

Various malabsorption conditions interfere with both calcium and vitamin D absorption and may deprive the body of both. This is most likely to occur in coeliac disease, but can also be a consequence of gastrectomy and intestinal bypass surgery. Failure of the various stages in the activation of the vitamin associated with liver or renal disease, or its excessive breakdown may also result in deficiency. Anticonvulsants and alcohol both induce the enzymes that increase the loss of vitamin D in bile and may deplete the body.

Vitamin D toxicity

Excess cholecalciferol can be toxic. This is most likely to occur in children by accidental ingestion of vitamin supplements. It causes a loss of appetite, thirst and increased urine output. The blood calcium may rise and calcium deposits may be laid down in soft tissues.

The margin of safety with vitamin D is not great and raised blood calcium may occur with regular intake of 50 μg/day.

Dietary reference value

This is difficult to establish for vitamin D because, for the majority of the population with a normal lifestyle who are able to synthesize the vitamin in the skin, a dietary source is unnecessary. However, children under the age of 3 years have high needs to sustain rapid growth, which may not be met readily from the diet or by exposure to sunlight and, therefore, an RNI value of 8.5 μg/day up to 6 months and 7 μg/day from 6 months to 3 years is given. Pregnant or lactating women may also benefit from a regular intake of vitamin D to sustain calcium metabolism. Older adults, who may have a reduced ability to synthesize the vitamin, or who are less likely to spend time outside may also benefit from a dietary source of the vitamin. For both of these groups, the RNI is given as 10 μg/day (DoH, 1991). People of Asian origin, for whom vitamin D status may be marginal for cultural or dietary reasons, may also benefit from additional vitamin D, but no RNI has been specifically given. It should be noted that an intake of 10 μg/day is difficult to achieve through dietary means, and a supplement may be needed.

Figure 9.6 Structures of tocopherols and tocotrienols.

Vitamin E

Vitamin E was first identified as an antisterility substance necessary for normal reproductive performance in rats. The rats could be successfully treated with whole wheat. This role has, however, been difficult to identify in humans. In recent years, it has become clear that vitamin E is possibly the most important antioxidant vitamin in the body, playing an essential protective role against free radical damage.

It is now known that vitamin E consists of a group of substances belonging to two closely related families: tocopherols and tocotrienols (Figure 9.6), with each existing in a number of isomeric forms, alpha, beta, gamma and delta, making a total of eight different members of the group. The most important member, with the greatest biological potency and accounting for 90 per cent of the vitamin activity in the tissues, is alpha-tocopherol. It is this form that is often taken as the representative of the whole group.

Vitamin E in food

Animal foods provide only alpha-tocopherol, whereas plant foods may contain the other isomeric forms of tocopherol and the tocotrienols as well. Among plant foods, vegetable oils are the most important sources. The germ of whole cereal grains contains vitamin E (a rich source of tocotrienols). In addition, some is found in green leafy vegetables, and some fruits and nuts. Margarines manufactured from vegetable and seed oils contain some vitamin E, although amounts vary. Breakfast cereals may be fortified with the vitamin, but specific information should be sought on the label.

Animal foods generally are not rich sources of vitamin E, although small amounts occur in poultry, fish and eggs.

In the National Food Survey (DEFRA, 2001), the mean intakes are shown to be 9.9 mg/day. Most important contributors are:

Fats	46%
Cereals and cereal products	14%
Potatoes and potato products	11%
Vegetables	9%

Absorption of vitamin E

Tocopherols generally occur free in foods; tocotrienols are esterified and must be split from these before absorption. In the presence of fats, absorption rates of the vitamin are 20–50 per cent, with lower rates of absorption occurring as dosage increases. Thus, absorption from supplements may be as little as 10 per cent.

In the plasma, the vitamin is transported in the low-density lipoprotein (LDL) fraction and concentrates in the cell membranes. Highest concentrations are found in the adipose tissue; levels increase here with increasing intakes. Other organs and tissues that contain the vitamin include liver, heart, skeletal muscle and adrenal glands. Levels in the plasma and liver are the first to decrease when intakes are inadequate to meet requirements.

Functions of vitamin E

The chemical structure of tocopherols and tocotrienols, with an –OH group on the ring structure, makes them very effective hydrogen donors. Therefore, vitamin E is a potent antioxidant and, as it is fat soluble, this activity is expressed particularly in lipid environments. In donating hydrogen the vitamin E becomes oxidized itself, while preventing the oxidation of something more metabolically important, for example, polyunsaturated fatty acids in cell membranes. This is important when free radicals are present, as these highly reactive substances can attack double bonds, setting up chain reactions, with more free radicals being produced. In the case of damage to fatty acids, lipid peroxides are produced that alter the function of the cell membrane and cause possibly irreversible damage to metabolic pathways.

There is interaction between vitamin E and other nutrients, particularly selenium and vitamin C in the antioxidant role. Vitamin C is involved in the regeneration of vitamin E.

Vitamin E is particularly important in those parts of the body where large amounts of oxygen are present, including the lungs and the red blood cells. In addition, the lungs are also exposed to environmental pollutants, which contain free radicals and, therefore, protection here is essential.

In summary, vitamin E is essential in maintaining cell membranes, contributing to their integrity, stability and function. Cell membrane function is closely related to their structure and, for this reason, vitamin E has been considered an important protective factor in the prevention of degenerative diseases, such as cardiovascular disease and cancer. There is some evidence that vitamin E plays a role in the prevention of cardiovascular disease but the results of intervention trials have not been conclusive. It has also been proposed that vitamin E is essential for the maintenance of vascular integrity in the brain, where low levels may result in impairment of cognitive function and possibly contribute to dementia.

Deficiency of vitamin E

Deficiency of vitamin E may occur in people with fat malabsorption due to liver, pancreatic or biliary disease, cystic fibrosis or coeliac disease, and in individuals with increased or unmet needs, such as:

- premature infants, who have received little vitamin E via the placenta, and whose needs are high because of growth or exposure to high levels of oxygen in incubators;
- adults exposed to a high free radical load, such as smokers or those working in polluted environments; and
- people consuming high levels of polyunsaturated fats in their diet, which require protection by antioxidants.

In all of these cases, deficiency may include the following signs:

- red cells haemolysis;
- oedema owing to increased permeability of membranes; or
- neurological symptoms, including loss of muscle coordination, impaired vision and speech, all of which may progress rapidly, and early treatment is required.

Fortunately, these deficiencies are rare and, as knowledge increases, appropriate preventive treatment can be given.

High intakes of vitamin E

Many claims have been made for potential effects of vitamin E megadoses. These include improved sports performance, slowed ageing processes, cure for muscular dystrophy, improved sexual potency and improving cardiac function. Most of these are based on extrapolation from animals; unfortunately, evidence in humans is lacking. At present, it is believed that an adequate level of vitamin E is important in the diet to compensate for the free radicals in our environment. Research on cancer and heart disease prevalence suggests that fewer cases occur in those with adequate vitamin E status (see Chapter 14). Intakes of vitamin E higher than can be obtained from a normal diet can be achieved by supplementation. At these levels, there is evidence of reduced blood platelet stickiness and improved immunity. In women taking vitamin E supplements, there is evidence of a lower incidence of strokes. Despite this, most nutritionists would recommend that vitamin E is obtained from a balanced diet, rich in grains, fruit and vegetables, rather than from vitamin supplements.

At present, there is no evidence of harm from high doses of vitamin E.

Dietary reference value

The vitamin E requirement depends on the polyunsaturated fatty acid (PUFA) content of the tissues and, in turn, of the diet. On the basis of current levels of intake, it is proposed that intakes of 4 mg and 3 mg/day for men and women, respectively, are adequate. An alternative used in other countries relates the vitamin E intake to the PUFA content of the diet in the ratio of 0.4 mg tocopherol/g of dietary PUFA. In the UK, the average diet provides a ratio of 0.6 mg tocopherol/g PUFA.

Some authors have suggested that intakes should be considerably higher than this, up to 87–100 mg/day, to protect against cardiovascular disease. More work in this area is needed.

Vitamin K

This vitamin was initially isolated as a factor involved in blood clotting, with a haemorrhagic disease observed in its absence. A number of compounds are now recognized as having vitamin K activity, all related by their structure as members of the naphthoquinone family. The most important naturally occurring members are phylloquinone (K_1) (Figure 9.7) and menaquinone (K_2); there is also a synthetic compound, menadione (K_3), which is water soluble and therefore has advantages in absorption.

Sources of vitamin K

The menaquinones are synthesized by bacteria, including those which inhabit the human terminal ileum and colon. It is, therefore, possible to obtain some of the vitamin requirement from synthesis in the gastrointestinal tract. Very little is known about the site or mechanisms of absorption of this potentially large pool of vitamin K. It is unlikely that this can meet all the needs, therefore a dietary source is also required. If the colonic bacteria are eliminated, for example, by antibiotic use, the individual is totally dependent on dietary supplies. Phylloquinones are obtained from plant foods, with rich sources being the green leafy vegetables (such as broccoli, cabbage, spinach, Brussels sprouts) and peas. Green vegetables supply about 50 per cent of the total dietary intake of vitamin K_1. Vegetable oils and margarines together with foods that contain these, such as biscuits and cakes, provide a further 20–25 per cent of the intake. Menaquinones occur in animal foods, especially liver; meat and dairy products contain smaller amounts. Generally, vitamin K is widely distributed in foods and a dietary deficiency is rare. Tea also contains a useful amount of vitamin K.

Intakes in the UK were found to be 72 µg/day and 64 µg/day in men and women, respectively, averaged over the year. In a study of people aged over 65 years in the UK, the mean intake was 65 µg/day. This was calculated to be below the current guideline (DoH, 1991) of 1 µg/kg body weight, in 59 per cent of the subjects. The major dietary source in this group was vegetables, which contributed 60 per cent of the total intake.

Absorption of vitamin K

Between 40 and 80 per cent of the ingested vitamin appears in the chylomicrons entering the lymph. When fat absorption is impaired, as little as 20 per cent may be absorbed. The water-soluble synthetic form is absorbed directly into the hepatic portal vein and carried to the liver, where it is activated and then released along with the naturally occurring forms of vitamin K. These are carried in the LDL to target sites.

Figure 9.7 Phylloquinone (vitamin K_1) is derived from plants and is lipid soluble.

Turnover of vitamin K is rapid and stores are small.

Function of vitamin K

The major role of vitamin K is to take part in the gamma-carboxylation of glutamic acid residues. This is part of a cycle in which the vitamin changes from an oxidized form (quinone) to the reduced form (quinol). On completion of the carboxylation, the vitamin is converted back to the quinone form, and can be reused. The vitamin-K-dependent proteins (or gla-proteins) that are produced participate in many reactions in the body. The most important of these is the blood clotting cascade, in which four of the factors needed contain gamma-carboxyglutamate, namely prothrombin and Factors VII, IX and X. It is thus clear why a vitamin K deficiency has serious effects on blood clotting. Anticoagulants such as warfarin interfere with the regeneration of the reduced vitamin K, thus breaking the cycle.

Another gla-protein is osteocalcin, found in bone, which is needed for the normal binding of calcium in bone matrix. It is now recognized that vitamin K supplementation may increase bone density in osteoporosis. Further evidence suggests that vitamin K may also inhibit bone resorption by causing osteoclasts to undergo apoptosis.

Vitamin K appears in the brain as menaquinone 4 where its role may be associated with the formation of a class of brain lipids. Other gla-proteins occur in many other organs in the body, although at present their roles are unclear.

Deficiency of vitamin K

Primary deficiency of vitamin K due to a dietary lack is almost never seen, except in newborn infants. These are at risk because of low levels of vitamin K in milk (especially human milk) and because the sterile gut of a young infant is incapable of contributing bacterial vitamin K. It has been common practice to give an intramuscular injection of vitamin K to young infants to prevent possible deficiency. However, some concern has been expressed in the last few years that this practice may contribute to an increased risk of leukaemia in childhood, although the evidence is controversial. Some neonatal units now give the vitamin by mouth, although it is believed to be less effective via this route. Infants who become deficient are at risk of a haemorrhagic disease of the newborn, with spontaneous bleeding, which can occur in the brain, resulting in brain damage and death. This typically occurs in totally breastfed infants between 3 and 8 weeks of life.

In adults, deficiency is most likely due to malabsorption of fat, resulting from liver, biliary or pancreatic disease. Chronic use of mineral oil laxatives and a poor intake may also contribute to deficiency; this may occur in anorexia nervosa. Long-term use of antibiotics may reduce intestinal synthesis; this may be a risk after intestinal surgery, when coupled with a low dietary intake. In all cases, there is an increased tendency to bleed.

Dietary reference value

This is difficult to set because of an indeterminate amount of bacterial synthesis in the colon. The Department of Health (DoH, 1991) uses normal blood clotting factor concentrations as an indicator of adequate status. This can be achieved with an intake of $1\,\mu g/kg$ per day in adults. It has been suggested that a higher level of vitamin K than this may be needed for optimal bone function, but evidence to propose a new level is lacking. Prophylactic vitamin K is recommended in all infants.

WATER-SOLUBLE VITAMINS

With the exception of vitamin C, the water-soluble vitamins belong to the B-complex group. Many of the B vitamins share similar functions and often work together; they can be broadly described as cofactors in metabolism. They facilitate the use of energy and are involved in the interconversion between different groups of metabolites. Folate and vitamin B_{12} are involved in cell division.

Owing to their chemical nature, the water-soluble vitamins have different characteristics from the fat-soluble vitamins.

- They are absorbed into the portal blood after digestion.
- When present in excess they are excreted in the urine.

■ The body has limited storage capacity for these vitamins (with the exception of vitamin B_{12}); most reserves in the body are found in association with enzymes where the vitamin plays a cofactor role.

■ They are more readily lost during food preparation processes, since they are soluble in water (in particular, this occurs on heating, especially in water and also on exposure to light and air).

Thiamin

The deficiency disease associated with thiamin, beriberi, has been known for 4000 years, although the name was first used in the seventeenth century. The nutritional links were first recognized at the beginning of the twentieth century in Japan. The water-soluble agent was eventually isolated in 1911, and named vitamin B to differentiate it from the first fat-soluble vitamin – A.

The structure of thiamin is unusual in that it contains a sulphur group in the thiazole ring (Figure 9.8).

Sources of thiamine

The most important sources of thiamin in the British diet are cereals, which provide 45 per cent of the intake. The whole cereal grain is rich in the vitamin but losses on milling are high, as most is concentrated in the outer layers; thus white flour and polished rice are low in thiamin. However, thiamin is added to white flour at the rate of 2.4 mg/kg, which restores the level. Many breakfast cereals are also enriched with thiamin and, therefore, provide a useful source. Beans, seeds and nuts are also rich in thiamin, and may provide an important amount in the diet, especially in vegetarian populations. In rice-eating countries, they are one of the main sources of thiamin.

Figure 9.8 Structure of thiamin.

Meat is generally not rich in the vitamin, with the exception of pork and liver, and meat and meat products provide only 15 per cent of dietary thiamin. Milk and related products provide 8 per cent of total intake and potatoes provide 9 per cent. Both of these have low concentrations but, as they are consumed frequently, their contribution can be useful.

Mean daily intake in the UK is 1.44 mg, which represents 171 per cent of the RNI (DEFRA, 2001).

Thiamin is one of the more unstable vitamins, especially in alkaline conditions, and at temperatures above 100°C. Estimates suggest an average of 20 per cent is lost in domestic food preparation. The presence of sulphur dioxide as a preservative accelerates destruction of thiamin.

Absorption and metabolism of thiamine

Thiamin is readily absorbed from the diet by both active and passive mechanisms. At high levels of intake, most absorption is passive. Absorption may be inhibited by alcohol and by the presence of thiaminases, which are found in some fish. However, because these are destroyed on cooking, the problem exists only where raw fish is eaten regularly, as in Japan and Scandinavia.

On absorption, thiamin is phosphorylated to thiamin pyrophosphate (TPP) (also called thiamine diphosphate), especially in the liver. The major tissues that contain thiamin are the skeletal muscle (about 50 per cent of all thiamin), heart, liver, kidneys and brain.

The major role of TPP is as a cofactor in a number of metabolic reactions, especially involved with carbohydrate utilisation. The most important of these is as a coenzyme for pyruvate dehydrogenase in the production of acetyl coenzyme A from pyruvate at the start of the Krebs cycle, through which 90 per cent of the energy from glucose is released as ATP. Acetyl coenzyme A is also needed for the synthesis of lipids and acetylcholine (a neurotransmitter), and this demonstrates how thiamin is linked to nervous system function.

TPP is also required to complete the metabolism of branched-chain amino acids (large doses of thiamin may help in maple-syrup urine disease, which is caused by a genetic defect in this pathway). Interconversions between sugars of different carbon chain length also require TPP, acting as a cofactor for the enzyme trans-ketolase.

Recently, thiamin triphosphate has been found to control a chloride ion channel in nerves and may be a further link to neurological functions of thiamin.

Thiamin status can be assessed by measuring the activity in the red blood cell of the enzyme transketolase, which is TPP dependent.

Thiamin deficiency

It is not surprising that thiamin deficiency affects the nervous system, as this requires carbohydrate almost exclusively as its source of energy. Lack of thiamin prevents pyruvic acid metabolism, and this accumulates in the blood, with some being converted to lactate. The onset of the deficiency is slow, since most diets will contain a trace of the vitamin. However, on a totally thiamin-free diet, symptoms may begin within 10 days, reflecting the absence of stores.

Two separate clinical pictures may exist, and these have been termed 'dry' and 'wet' beriberi. In the 'dry' form, there is excessive fatigue, heaviness and stiffness in leg muscles, inability to walk far and abnormal breathlessness on exercise. Sufferers may also complain of mental and mood changes, and later of sensory loss and abnormal sensations from the skin. The paralysis may become so severe that the patient is unable to stand and walk, and may become bedridden. This picture is more commonly seen in older adults who have consumed an inadequate diet for many years. There may be anaemia and the heart rate is abnormally fast on exercise. In 'wet' beriberi, excessive fluid collects in the legs indicating cardiac involvement. Respiration may be compromised because of oedema in the lungs. In addition, there may be serious damage to the brain, which can cause neurological changes affecting the cerebellum, and eventually a confusional state leading to psychosis; this is the Wernicke–Korsakoff syndrome.

Classically, thiamin deficiency occurred in poor, rice-eating communities. It can still be found in undernourished communities in Asia.

In the West it is associated particularly with alcoholism, which results in a poor dietary intake and interference by the alcohol with thiamin absorption and metabolism. The clinical picture in chronic alcoholics often presents as Wernicke–Korsakoff syndrome. People with low thiamin intakes, perhaps exacerbated by vomiting, and those with malabsorption, for example, with biliary or inflammatory bowel disease, are at risk. Increased needs, such as in pregnancy, lactation, strenuous exercise and in cancer, also create a risk.

Consumption of a diet rich in carbohydrate increases the demand for thiamin; this may not be met if the foods consumed are highly refined. It has been proposed that there may be a genetic variant of transketolase that may predispose to Wernicke–Korsakoff syndrome. Thiamin deficiency has also been proposed as a factor in Alzheimer's disease, although this may be a consequence of the condition rather than an aetiological factor.

Thiamin has also been proposed as an ergogenic (i.e. energy releasing) factor in sports performance, to enhance aerobic capacity and limit lactic acid production, but results of trials have not supported a beneficial effect.

Dietary reference value

Thiamin requirements are related to energy metabolism and, therefore, to energy intake. Deficiency occurs when intakes fall below 0.2 mg/1000 Calories. The dietary reference value report (DoH, 1991), therefore, based its RNI at 0.4 mg/1000 Calories to allow for variance and provide a margin of safety.

Excessive intakes above 3 g/day are reported to be toxic and should be avoided.

Riboflavin (vitamin B₂)

Riboflavin (Figure 9.9) was originally identified as a growth-promoting substance, rather than a factor to cure a specific deficiency disease. It was isolated from a number of food substances, including milk, eggs and yeast, and for a time was known as 'vitamin G'. One of its most characteristic features is that the crystalline substance has a yellow–orange colour.

Figure 9.9 Structure of riboflavin.

Riboflavin in foods

The diet contains both free riboflavin as well as its two phosphorylated forms, flavin adenine dinucleotide (FAD) and flavin mononucleotide (FMN). Foods rich in riboflavin include milk and milk products, meat (especially liver) and eggs. The major sources in the British diet derive from milk and dairy products (43 per cent of total intake), cereal products that contain milk and eggs (27 per cent of total) and meat (14 per cent of total). Cereals alone are not a good source of the vitamin, unless enriched. A small amount of riboflavin is supplied by tea. Fruits and most vegetables are not important sources of the vitamin, although the dark green leafy vegetables may be important contributors, if eaten regularly.

Mean intakes of riboflavin in Britain are 1.75 mg/day; this represents 154 per cent of RNI.

Riboflavin is more stable to heat and less soluble than many of the B vitamins, but may be lost in cooking water. It is also destroyed by exposure to sunlight. Leaving milk exposed to sunlight in glass bottles will result in the loss of 10 per cent of the vitamin per hour. Paper and plastic cartons are better for protecting the vitamin content of milk.

Absorption and metabolism of riboflavin

Absorption occurs readily from the small intestine as riboflavin. It is believed that absorption is better from animal than plant sources. In the plasma it is carried in association with albumin, which carries both the free vitamin and coenzyme forms. In the tissues, riboflavin is converted into the coenzymes FMN and FAD, which constitute the active groups in a number of flavoproteins. Greatest concentrations are found in the liver, kidney and heart.

Both FMN and FAD act as electron and hydrogen donors and acceptors, which allows them to play a critical role in many oxidation–reduction reactions of metabolic pathways, passing electrons to the electron transport chain. Examples include the following.

- FAD is used in the Krebs cycle and in beta-oxidation of fatty acids, forming $FADH_2$.
- FAD also functions in conjunction with a number of oxidase and dehydrogenase enzymes, including xanthine oxidase (used in purine catabolism), aldehyde oxidase (needed in the metabolism of pyridoxine and vitamin A), glutathione reductase (selenium-requiring enzyme, used to quench free radicals), monoamine oxidase (for neurotransmitter metabolism) and mixed function oxidases (used in drug metabolism).
- FADH2 is needed in folate metabolism.

The examples listed above show not only the crucial role that riboflavin has in macronutrient metabolism and energy release, but also the interrelationships that exist with other nutrients in the body.

Assessment of riboflavin status is most accurately performed using the activation of glutathione reductase (a riboflavin-dependent enzyme) in red blood cells.

Deficiency of riboflavin

Mild cases of riboflavin deficiency occur around the world, often seen in conjunction with other B vitamin deficiencies. This is in part due to the coexistence of many of the B vitamins in similar foods, as well as the interaction between them at the metabolic level. Signs of deficiency are generally non-specific, but may involve the following.

- The mouth – with cracks and inflammation at the corners of the mouth (angular stomatitis), sore, burning lips, which may become ulcerated (cheilosis), and a purple–red (or magenta) coloured tongue, with flattened papillae and a pebbled appearance (glossitis).
- The eyes – with burning and itching, sensitivity to light, loss of visual acuity and a gritty sensation under the eyelids. Capillary blood vessels may also invade the cornea, and there may be a sticky secretion, which makes the eyelids stick together.

- The skin – with an oily dermatitis, particularly affecting the nose, cheeks and forehead. Occasionally, the reproductive organs may also be affected.
- Anaemia – may be seen in long-standing riboflavin deficiency.

Some of these signs are also found in deficiencies of niacin and vitamin B_6, which may coexist.

Deficiency, which includes inadequate riboflavin status, may arise from an inadequate intake, particularly when this is associated with increased needs for growth. Cases have been reported in adolescents consuming no milk or dairy products. Poor intakes may also be found in the elderly and in alcoholics. There has been a reported association between ocular lens opacity in the elderly and riboflavin status, but more research is needed.

Pathological states, which include negative nitrogen balance, such as cancers, trauma and burns, may increase the turnover and thus increase requirements. Increased excretion in the urine has been reported in diabetics.

Dietary reference value

Intakes of 0.55 mg/day over a period of 4 months have been reported to result in riboflavin deficiency. Earlier recommendations had been based on levels producing tissue saturation. The upper range of glutathione reductase activity is now considered a more sensitive indicator of saturation. Surveys have shown that intakes in the UK achieve this level. The RNI was set at 1.3 mg/day for men and 1.1 mg/day for women.

Excessive intakes of riboflavin are poorly absorbed and, therefore, no evidence exists of potential harmful effects.

Nicotinic acid (niacin)

The deficiency disease associated with niacin is pellagra, named from the Italian for 'rough skin'. The disease was recognized as endemic among maize-eating populations, and its occurrence spread with the introduction of maize throughout Europe and into Africa. In the early twentieth century, it reached epidemic proportions in the southern states of America. A dietary cause

Figure 9.10 Structures of nicotinic acid and nicotinamide, collectively known as niacin.

was suspected in the 1920s, and a protein-free extract of meat or yeast was found to prevent the deficiency. The association with maize was not explained for a further 20 years. The pellagra-preventing factor in yeast and meat extract, nicotinic acid, can be made in the human body from the amino acid tryptophan. The conversion is very inefficient, with only 1 mg of vitamin produced from 60 mg of tryptophan. However, tryptophan is the limiting amino acid in maize protein, so none is available for vitamin synthesis. In addition, the nicotinic acid in maize is present in a bound and unabsorbable form. These two factors make a deficiency of the vitamin likely when the diet is poor and mainly composed of maize.

Nicotinic acid and its amide nicotinamide (Figure 9.10) are nutritionally important, and are collectively termed niacin.

Sources of niacin

In addition to niacin provided as pre-formed vitamin, the body makes a certain amount of niacin by conversion from tryptophan. In the West, the large amount of protein in the diet probably supplies enough tryptophan to meet the whole of the need for niacin and a dietary intake of pre-formed niacin may not be needed. However, if protein intakes are low, insufficient tryptophan may be available to meet the need for niacin.

Food composition tables provide an estimate of the amount of niacin supplied from tryptophan, given as 'nicotinic acid equivalents'. (This is calculated as 1/60th of the tryptophan content.) Adequate amounts of vitamin B_6 and riboflavin are required for this conversion. An overall figure for total niacin equivalents can then be obtained by adding preformed niacin + nicotinic acid (or niacin) equivalents from tryptophan.

Rich sources of niacin equivalents are meat (especially liver), fish, peanuts and cereals (especially if fortified). In the British diet, meat is the main source (38 per cent of total intake), followed by cereals (25 per cent of total), milk and dairy products (13 per cent of total) and vegetables (including potatoes) (11 per cent of total). It is also worth noting that coffee and cocoa provide some niacin. The total amount of niacin equivalents in the UK diet is reported as 27.8 mg (DEFRA, 2001), which represents 200 per cent of the RNI.

In some foods, niacin is bound to complex carbohydrates or peptides, which makes it largely unavailable. This is particularly a problem with maize, but to a lesser extent applies to other cereal grains. However, soaking of maize in lime water releases the bound niacin, making it available. This is a traditional practice in Mexico and, consequently, although maize is the staple food in this country, pellagra does not occur.

Since most of the niacin in the diet is in the form of its coenzymes, it is relatively stable to light, heat and air, and losses on cooking occur only by leaching into water.

Absorption and metabolism of niacin

There is rapid absorption of dietary niacin, both by active and passive mechanisms. The main role of niacin in the body is in the formation of nicotinamide adenine dinucleotide (NAD) and NAD phosphate (NADP), which can be made in all cells. Once the niacin has been converted to NAD or NADP, it is trapped within cells and cannot diffuse out.

Excess free niacin may be methylated and excreted in the urine. A low level of this metabolite in the urine (<3 mg/day) is indicative of a deficiency state, and may be used as an assay method.

NAD and NADP act as hydrogen acceptors in oxidative reactions, forming NADH and NADPH. These, in turn, can act as hydrogen donors. On the whole, NAD is used in energy-yielding reactions, for example, glycolysis, the Krebs cycle and the oxidation of alcohol. The hydrogen they accept is eventually passed through the electron transfer chain, to yield water. NADPH is mostly used in energy-requiring, biosynthetic reactions, most importantly, for fatty acid synthesis. Overall, NAD and NADP play a part in the metabolism of carbohydrates, fats and proteins and are, therefore, central to cellular processes. In addition, they are involved in vitamin C and folate metabolism, and are required by glutathione reductase.

Niacin has been described as a component of the glucose tolerance factor, which also contains chromium and which facilitates the action of insulin. This role is separate from its function in NAD.

Niacin deficiency

Pellagra has been described as having three main features: dermatitis, diarrhoea and dementia.

Dermatitis affects particularly those parts of the body exposed to sunlight, and may have the appearance of sunburn. In chronic cases, it becomes worse in sunny weather, and improves in the winter months, forming patches of thickened rough skin. The dermatitis is almost always symmetrical. The skin may become cracked and infected in more acute cases. The inside of the mouth is also affected, resulting in a 'raw beef' tongue, which is sore and swollen. (There may also be concurrent riboflavin deficiency contributing to this sign.) The mouth may be so painful that even taking liquids is impossible.

The whole lining of the gastrointestinal tract may be affected by mucosal inflammation, resulting in heartburn, indigestion, abdominal pain, diarrhoea and soreness of the rectum.

Dementia tends to occur only in advanced pellagra, and may range from headache, vertigo and disturbed sleep, through anxiety and depression to hallucinations, confusion and severe dementia with convulsions. If untreated, the condition results in death.

Niacin deficiency is still found in parts of the world where the diet is poor and based on maize, such as among poor communities in South Africa. In India, millet diets, which are high in lysine and inhibit the use of tryptophan for niacin formation, may lead to pellagra. In the West, low intake, as in alcoholics, or increased needs due to cancer, may result in deficiency.

In addition, altered metabolism caused by isoniazid (an antituberculosis drug) or Hartnup disease (inability to absorb tryptophan) may also result in pellagra, if the problem is not anticipated.

Dietary reference value

The level of niacin needed to prevent or cure deficiency is 5.5 mg/1000 Calories. On this basis, the RNI has been set at 6.6 mg/1000 Calories for adult men and women. High doses of nicotinic acid (in excess of 200 mg/day) may cause vaso-dilatation, flushing and a fall in blood pressure.

Large doses (1 g/day) have been used in the treatment of hypercholesterolaemia; however, side-effects, which include flushing, gastrointestinal discomfort and possible damage to the liver, mean that this is not a treatment of choice. At other times, niacin has been used as a treatment for chilblains and schizophrenia, although the benefits are uncertain.

Vitamin B₆

This vitamin was isolated as a cure for a scaly dermatitis seen in rats fed on purified diets. It is now clear that there are three closely related compounds that have biological activity. These are pyridoxine (found predominantly in plant foods), pyridoxal and pyridoxamine (both of which are present in animal foods, generally in the phosphorylated form) (Figure 9.11).

Sources of vitamin B₆

Vitamin B₆ is widely distributed in small quantities in all animal and plant tissues. Rich sources are liver, whole cereals, meat (including poultry), peanuts, walnuts, bananas and salmon. Moderate

R = CH₂.OH   Pyridoxine (pyridoxol)
R = CHO   Pyridoxal
R = CH₂.NH₂   Pyridoxamine

Figure 9.11 Structures of the three closely related compounds known as vitamin B₆: pyridoxine, pyridoxal and pyridoxamine.

amounts are found in vegetables, such as broccoli, spinach and potatoes. The availability from animal sources of the vitamin may be greater than that from plant sources, because of binding to glucoside.

Vitamin B₆ is also susceptible to processing losses in heating, canning and freezing. It is estimated that between 10 and 50 per cent may be lost in this way.

Mean daily intakes in the UK are 2.0 mg (DEFRA, 2001). Main contributors in the total diet are vegetables (32 per cent of total), meat (30 per cent of total) and cereals (25 per cent of total). In men, beer may make a useful contribution to the total intake of the vitamin.

Absorption and metabolism of vitamin B₆

The vitamin has to be released from its phosphorylated forms prior to absorption; once in its free form, absorption is rapid. The liver and muscles are the main sites for pyridoxal phosphate in the body; once it is phosphorylated, the vitamin is trapped in the cell.

Pyridoxal phosphate is involved in many biological reactions, particularly those associated with amino acid metabolism. Some examples are:

- decarboxylation, e.g. production of histamine from histidine, production of dopamine and serotonin (important neurotransmitters);
- transamination – for the synthesis of non-essential amino acids; synthesis of porphyrin (for haem), nicotinic acid from tryptophan and cysteine from methionine.

The formation of cysteine from methionine has homocysteine as an intermediate product, and there has been a great deal of interest in the possible role of vitamin B₆ as a factor for reducing homocysteine levels. At present, the evidence on its usefulness as a protective factor against hyperhomocysteinaemia is equivocal.

Vitamin B₆ also plays a role in:

- fat metabolism in the conversion of linoleic acid to arachidonic acid, and in synthesis of sphingolipids in the nervous system;
- glycogen metabolism, particularly in muscle.

Some recent work has shown that vitamin B₆ may also have a role in modulating the action of steroid and other hormones at the cell nucleus.

Deficiency of vitamin B_6

There is no clear clinical deficiency syndrome, as a lack of this vitamin often coexists with inadequate intakes of some of the other water-soluble vitamins. Signs of deficiency may include:

- anaemia (due to reduced synthesis of haem);
- smooth tongue, cracks at corners of mouth (may be linked to riboflavin deficiency);
- dermatitis (as above, and niacin deficiency);
- nervous/muscular system signs – irritability, headaches, fatigue, muscle twitching, numbness, difficulty walking, convulsions (especially in infants).

Deficiency may occur because of reduced availability of the vitamin. This may be the result of a poor dietary intake (due to ageing, alcoholism or abnormal eating patterns), in which case the deficiency is likely to involve several vitamins and be multifactorial in origin. Alternatively, it may be caused by increased demand, for example, during periods of growth (especially in young infants born with low levels of the vitamin), during pregnancy and in women taking the contraceptive pill.

Abnormal vitamin B_6 metabolism leading to deficiency may occur as a result of some drugs, particularly isoniazid (used in tuberculosis), anticonvulsants and steroids, or due to liver disease, which sometimes reduces activation of the vitamin. Dialysis for renal disease causes increased losses of vitamin B_6.

Vitamin B_6 therapy has been recommended for the relief of symptoms associated with the pre-menstrual syndrome. Although there is no evidence of a deficiency, supplementation may be of benefit to some women.

Dietary reference value

Depletion studies have shown that deficiency develops faster on high protein intakes. The RNI has been set in relation to protein intake at $15\,\mu g/g$ protein for both men and women. The elderly may have poorer rates of absorption and metabolism, but currently there is insufficient evidence to set a higher RNI.

Care should be taken with supplement use, as some cases of sensory neuropathy have been reported with chronic intakes of $100–200\,mg/day$.

Folate

This vitamin was originally identified as a factor present in yeast extract, which could cure a type of anaemia that had been described in pregnant women. This anaemia was similar to pernicious anaemia, with large macrocytic cells, but the lesions of the central nervous system were absent. The active agent was found in crude liver extract and in spinach, and was thus named folate (from foliage).

Folate is now used as the generic name for the group of substances with related vitamin activity; this includes the synthetic form of the vitamin folic acid (or pteroyl glutamic acid) (Figure 9.12) and various polyglutamate forms (containing several glutamic acid residues) that are commonly present in foods, including the 5-methyl- and 10-methyltetrahydrofolates, which are the coenzyme forms of the vitamin.

Folate in foods

Food is analysed for folate content using a microbiological growth assay with *Lactobacillus rhamnosus* (formerly *Lactobacillus casei*). This

Figure 9.12 Structure of folic acid.

may not always give an accurate measurement of the amount of folate obtainable by humans on ingestion of the food. New methods continue to be developed, for example, high-performance liquid chromatography and antibody-based techniques. Reference standards have also been developed, which should contribute to more reliable assays. However, at present there is still uncertainty about the validity of figures for folate contents. The majority of food sources contain polyglutamates, with probably less than 25 per cent being present as monoglutamate. Folic acid itself does not occur in nature, and is used only in supplements and fortification.

Richest dietary sources are green leafy vegetables (spinach, Brussels sprouts) and liver, with lower but useful amounts in broccoli, cabbage, cauliflower, parsnips, fortified cereals and bread, oranges and whole wheat. Folate intakes are, in general, correlated with income; families on a high income may have substantially more folate in their diet than those on a low income. Folate intake also correlates with vitamin C intakes, as many of the sources provide both of these vitamins. The main foods contributing to total intakes include cereals and cereal products, mainly as a result of fortification (34 per cent of total intake) and vegetables, including potatoes (31 per cent of total). Milk and fruit both provide small amounts. Beer intake can contribute important amounts of folate, as a result of its yeast content. Mean intakes in studies in the UK were found to be 248 µg/day (DEFRA, 2001). Levels have increased since the mid-1980s with the gradual introduction of fortified products, especially breakfast cereals, and the increased consumption of fruit juices. The mean intake achieves 132 per cent of the mean RNI, but there are groups identified by the National Food Survey, in whom the mean intake is just 100 per cent of RNI. These are particularly found in large households and those with three or more children.

Folate in foods is susceptible to cooking losses; it is less soluble in water than many of the B vitamins, but is sensitive to heat and, therefore, most cooking procedures will cause a loss of some of the vitamin. Keeping food hot for periods of time or reheating are particularly damaging, and can destroy all of the folate originally present. The extent of loss will depend on the particular form of the folate in food. Folic acid itself is more stable chemically than natural folates in foods.

Absorption and metabolism of folate

Most folate in the diet is in the bound form and, for optimal absorption, glutamates have to be removed to produce the monoglutamate, 5-methyl tetrahydrofolate (5-methyl THF); this is achieved with conjugase enzymes found in the brush border and lysosomes of the duodenum and jejunum. These enzymes are zinc dependent and can also be inhibited by alcohol. There may also be conjugase inhibitors in some foods, such as beans, which prevent the freeing of folate. Overall, 50 per cent of dietary folate is believed to be absorbed. The absorption of folic acid is more efficient, with up to 85 per cent of intake being bioavailable (i.e. well absorbed or assimilated). In the USA, a Dietary Folate Equivalent has been introduced to allow an overall folate provision to be estimated from a variety of sources with varying bioavailabilities.

Most folate is stored in the liver, which is, therefore, also a good dietary source of folate. Once taken up by target cells, folates are conjugated to produce polyglutamates. Intracellular folate, as tetrahydrofolate (THF) is used to carry one-carbon units from one molecule to another. Thus, it can accept such single-carbon groups from donors in degradative reactions and then act as the donor of such a unit in a subsequent synthetic reaction. Such transfers are important in a number of steps during amino acid metabolism, for example:

- synthesis of serine from glycine (and vice versa);
- synthesis of homocysteine from methionine (and vice versa);
- conversion of histidine to glutamic acid; and
- synthesis of purine and pyrimidine bases, for DNA and RNA synthesis. This explains the crucial role of folate in cell division.

The removal of the methyl group from 5-methyl THF is a particularly important step, which is catalysed by the vitamin B_{12}-dependent enzyme methionine synthase. Without the

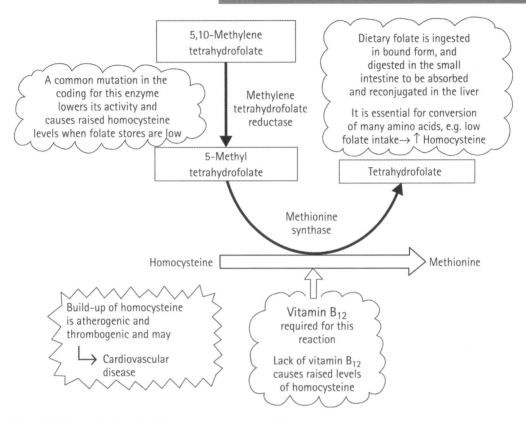

Figure 9.13 The metabolic role of folate homocysteine metabolism.

presence of vitamin B_{12}, the THF is 'trapped' in its methyl form and can no longer carry single-carbon units. This reaction is an essential link between the two vitamins and explains some of the common features of their deficiency states (see Figure 9.13).

Furthermore, the methyl group removed during this reaction is used to generate methionine from homocysteine. Evidence suggests that elevated homocysteine levels may be associated with an increased risk of some diseases, and thus metabolic pathways that serve to reduce homocysteine levels have been extensively studied. The 5-methyl THF needed for methionine synthesis is formed from 5,10-methylene tetrahydrofolate, by the action of methylene tetrahydrofolate reductase (MTHFR). A recessive genetic mutation in the coding for this enzyme has been found, with 5–18 per cent of individuals estimated to be homozygous for this mutation. This results in a lower level of enzyme activity and, consequently, higher homocysteine levels

when folate status is low. These findings may offer some explanation for the benefits of folate supplementation in certain circumstances, for example, the prevention of neural tube defects. Other roles for folate supplementation are discussed below.

Folate deficiency

Deficiency of folate will affect rapidly dividing cells, which have a high requirement for purine and pyrimidine bases. The cells particularly affected are those making blood cells (in the bone marrow) and those lining the gastrointestinal tract.

The effect on red cell formation results in a megaloblastic anaemia, in which the cells are immature, larger than normal and released into the blood as macrocytes. These cells are fewer in number, affecting the oxygen-carrying capacity of the blood and producing the signs and symptoms of anaemia. There may also be loss of appetite, nausea and diarrhoea or constipation;

the mouth may be sore with a smooth red tongue. White blood cell division is also affected and there may be depression of the immune system.

Folate deficiency is most likely to occur in pregnancy in Britain. This is because the needs for folate are increased and the mother's stores may be inadequate to supply the extra amount needed. In general 20–25 per cent of pregnant women in Britain may exhibit signs of mega-loblastic changes in their bone marrow.

Alcoholics are also at risk, in part because of a reduced intake, as well as due to the negative effects that alcohol exerts on the absorption of folate. Folate deficiency may be an indication of an alcohol problem.

Folate deficiency may arise for a number of other reasons, such as inadequate intake, ineffi-cient absorption or altered metabolism.

Inadequate intake may be linked to poverty, poor food choices, careless cooking techniques or a small appetite. Particularly vulnerable are the elderly, in whom low red blood cell folate levels have been reported. Infants have rela-tively high needs for folate; premature babies may have low blood levels, and this may hinder their growth and development. Heating of milk may lower its folate content. Infants who are fed on goats' milk are also at risk, as this has a very low content of folate.

Inefficient digestion and absorption may occur in a number of malabsorption conditions, for example, in inflammatory bowel disease, coeliac disease or tropical sprue and in protein–energy malnutrition. Folate deficiency itself also affects the gut's absorptive capacity.

Altered metabolism may be largely due to interactions with drugs, such as anticonvulsants. Some commonly used drugs, such as aspirin, indigestion remedies and the contraceptive pill, may interfere with folate metabolism; smokers may also need more folate. In addition, some drugs used in chemotherapy for cancer are specific folate antagonists, and will cause a deficiency during treatment.

Folate supplements

In general, low dietary intakes of folate lead to raised plasma homocysteine levels and these can be reduced by giving folic acid, with the greatest effects seen in those with the highest initial levels of homocysteine.

Folate has been shown to be a particularly important nutrient at the time of conception. A number of UK and international studies have shown that supplementing women who have previously given birth to a child with a neural tube defect (affecting either the brain or spinal cord) can reduce the risk of a further such affected pregnancy by almost 75 per cent. There is no indication that the mothers had been defi-cient in folate, although recent work has shown that plasma levels of folate and B_{12} were signif-icantly lower (but still within the 'normal' range) than in control subjects. Evidence now suggests that a genetic mutation increases the need for folate in some women. However, as it is not feasible to screen all women to identify those at risk, many countries now advise all women who are planning to or may become pregnant to ensure they have adequate folate intakes. Some foods, such as breads and most breakfast cere-als, are now fortified with folate to facilitate this. Bioavailability of folate from foods is relatively poor, and thus a folate supplement of 0.4 mg/day is recommended to ensure an adequate folate status. This should be taken ideally from at least 12 weeks before conception and continued until the 12th week of pregnancy. Health promotion campaigns have been used to increase aware-ness of the need for folate supplementation in this group.

Elevated plasma homocysteine levels may have both atherogenic and thrombogenic actions, and these have been implicated in cardiovascu-lar disease. Homocysteine is reported to promote oxidation of LDL cholesterol, to stimulate pro-liferation of vascular smooth muscle cells and to reduce the endothelial production of nitric oxide, an important vasodilator. Across popula-tions from Europe, Japan and Israel, a positive relationship has been shown between total plasma homocysteine level and cardiovascular mortality. Although increasing the intake of folate has been shown to reduce homocysteine levels, at present, there is no strong evidence that there is a parallel reduction in cardiovas-cular disease and further work in this exciting area is required. Nevertheless, folate supplements may in future be shown to be of benefit in cardiovascular disease prevention.

Low folate status has been reported in both psychiatric and psychogeriatric patients. In many cases this may be due to poor dietary intake. Response to drug treatment is enhanced if folate status is improved. Dementia states have been linked to elevated homocysteine levels in some patients and supplementation with folate may be a preventive measure in the future.

In view of potential benefits of an adequate intake of folate, there has been debate in a number of countries, including the US and UK, about the introduction of fortification with folic acid of a staple foodstuff. The debate resulted in the introduction of fortification in the USA from January 1999, where folic acid is added at a level of $140\,\mu g/100\,g$ of grain. This aims to achieve an additional mean intake between 100 and $1000\,\mu g/day$. A recent review (Honein et al., 2001) in the USA found that the incidence of neural tube defects had fallen by almost 20 per cent since the introduction of folate fortification. In the UK, the debate continues, despite a recommendation by the Committee on Medical Aspects of Food Policy (DoH, 2000) that universal fortification of flour at $240\,\mu g/100\,g$ should be introduced. Concerns related to fortification with folic acid are that increased intakes may mask vitamin B_{12} deficiency, and result in development of neuropathy in vulnerable individuals. Some drugs, especially those used in epilepsy, may also be less effective with a higher folate intake. Further consideration is required of this issue (see Gibson, 2002).

Dietary reference values

On the basis of surveys of habitual intakes of folate, liver and blood levels of folate and amounts that prevent deficiency, the RNI (DoH, 1991) is $200\,\mu g/day$ for both men and women. A folate supplement of $400\,\mu g$ is now recommended prior to and for the first 12 weeks of pregnancy.

Vitamin B_{12}

The existence of vitamin B_{12} had been accepted since the 1920s, when it was found that a protein- and iron-free extract of liver given by injection could cure pernicious anaemia. However, the biologically active agent was not isolated and identified until 1948. An additional finding was the requirement for a factor in gastric juice, which would enable the vitamin B_{12} to be absorbed when it was given by mouth. For this reason, dietary treatment with liver previously had to use very large amounts (of raw liver) on a daily basis to provide any improvement. Even at this stage, there was some confusion with folate, as some of the signs of deficiency are similar for both the vitamins. It is now recognized that vitamin B_{12} is needed to release folate from its methyl form so that it can function as a carrier of single-carbon units. However, not all of the functions of vitamin B_{12} are associated with folate.

Vitamin B_{12} is the name given to a group of compounds called the corrinoids; their characteristic feature is the presence of an atom of cobalt in the centre of four reduced pyrrole rings. Four important forms are recognized:

- hydroxycobalamin;
- cyanocobalamin (synthetic form found in supplements and fortified foods);
- adenosylcobalamin – active coenzyme;
- methylcobalamin – active coenzyme.

Vitamin B_{12} in foods

For humans, the only dietary sources of vitamin B_{12} are animal foods; none is obtained from plant foods. Ruminant animals, such as cows and sheep, synthesize the vitamin in the stomach by the actions of the bacterial flora found there. Humans benefit from this by consuming the products from these animals.

Trace amounts of the vitamin may occur in a plant-only diet, resulting from contaminating yeasts, bacteria or faecal contamination of water sources. Richest sources are animal livers, where the vitamin is stored in life. Meat, eggs, milk and dairy products contain smaller concentrations.

Mean intakes in the UK are $5.8\,\mu g/day$. This is predominantly derived from meat and fish (38 per cent of total intake) and milk and cheese (45 per cent of intake).

It is essential that vegans, who exclude all animal foods from their diet, should have an alternative source of vitamin B_{12}. Most vegans are aware of this, and supplement their diet either with a specific vitamin supplement or vitamin-enriched products.

Excess amounts of vitamin C can interfere with vitamin B_{12} availability, converting it to an inactive form; care needs to be taken with high levels of intake.

Absorption and metabolism of vitamin B_{12}

Ingested vitamin B_{12} has to be combined with intrinsic factor produced by the stomach before it can be absorbed. The binding occurs in the duodenum where the pH is less acid than in the stomach. The vitamin–intrinsic factor complex is then carried down to the terminal ileum (the last part of the small intestine), from where the vitamin is absorbed, leaving the intrinsic factor behind. The process is slow, although at low levels of intake, 80 per cent of dietary vitamin may be absorbed. Absorption rates fall as intake increases. In the absence of intrinsic factor, there is only minimal absorption of the vitamin by passive diffusion and eventually a deficiency state will develop. Although some of the vitamin may be synthesized by bacteria in the bowel, it is not absorbed from here and does not form a useful source.

The metabolic role of vitamin B_{12} is associated with two enzyme systems, one involved in the availability of THF and the other in the metabolism of some fatty acids.

Vitamin B_{12} acts as a cofactor for methyltransferase, the enzyme needed to remove a methyl group from methyltetrahydrofolate, making THF available. Therefore, if vitamin B_{12} levels are low, this effectively also causes folate deficiency. A further consequence is that an inadequate amount of methionine is produced. It is believed that this eventually results in damage to the myelin coating of nerve fibres.

Vitamin B_{12} is needed for the metabolism of fatty acids with an odd number of carbons in their chains.

Vitamin B_{12} deficiency

This deficiency takes many years to develop, unless the inadequate intake starts in infancy. Most people have adequate reserves of the vitamin, and with the body's careful conservation of the vitamin, these can be made to last for up to 30 years. However, if the reserves were never accumulated, a deficiency can develop within 3–4 years.

There are two aspects to a vitamin B_{12} deficiency.

- There is a failure of cell division, which is similar to that described for folate deficiency, as the ultimate cause is the same, i.e. a failure to provide sufficient purines and pyrimidines for DNA and RNA synthesis. The main sign of this deficiency is megaloblastic anaemia. Treatment with folate can reverse the signs of this aspect of the deficiency. However, this is potentially dangerous, as the underlying deficiency of vitamin B_{12} will still lead to the second, neurological manifestation.

- There is a neurological element, which involves progressive damage to the myelin sheaths of the nerve fibres, with loss of conduction velocity and gradual loss of sensory and motor function in the periphery. If this has been masked by folate treatment, progression may have occurred beyond a reversible stage.

Although masking of B_{12} deficiency by folate is unlikely to happen at normal levels of folate intake, there is a theoretical risk that supplementation at high doses with folate ($>1000\,\mu g/day$) or high levels of fortification may lead to this problem, particularly among the older population.

It should also be noted that even a modest reduction in vitamin B_{12} status will cause an elevation of plasma homocysteine levels. There is growing evidence that this may be a risk factor in coronary heart disease and dementia.

Deficiency of vitamin B_{12} arises most commonly due to a failure of intrinsic factor production, resulting in an inability to absorb the vitamin. This form of the deficiency is known as pernicious anaemia, and occurs most commonly in middle-aged or elderly individuals. It is believed that the body destroys the cells producing its own intrinsic factor, possibly as part of an autoimmune response. The production of hydrochloric acid in the stomach is also affected. This is needed to release vitamin B_{12} from bound sources in food. In addition, the recycling of the body's store of the vitamin travelling through the enterohepatic circulation is also affected. The consequence is that deficiency develops relatively quickly. Injections of vitamin B_{12} are given to restore levels of the vitamin in the body; oral intakes would not be absorbed.

Deficiency may sometimes develop for other reasons, such as:

- inadequate intake over many years (occasionally occurs in strict vegetarians) and may lead to raised homocysteine levels;
- failure to absorb the vitamin due to malabsorption conditions following removal of the ileum, excessive bacterial flora in the gut consuming the vitamin, or interference from drugs (including alcohol, potassium supplements, biguanides);
- repeated exposure to nitrous oxide anaesthetics, which may inactivate the vitamin in the body and lead to signs of deficiency.

Overall, it can be seen that dietary lack of vitamin B_{12} is not a common cause of deficiency, largely because, if the diet contains any animal products, then the very small requirement for the vitamin will be met.

Dietary reference value

Turnover of the vitamin is very slow and conservation very efficient, thus it is difficult to induce deficiency. Evidence for the level of requirement is based on habitual intakes and responses to treatment in pernicious anaemia. The RNI has, therefore, been set at 1.5 mg/day for adult men and women; this is believed to be sufficient to produce stores that would allow the subject to withstand a period of low intake.

Pantothenic acid

The name for this member of the B group of vitamins derives from the Greek word for everywhere, suggesting that it is widespread. Biochemically, it is part of the coenzyme A molecule, which plays a role in the metabolic pathways for all the macronutrients. It is, therefore, central to energy transformations in the cell.

Deficiency has only been studied when induced experimentally. It includes a diverse and unspecific number of symptoms. An abnormal sensation in the feet and lower legs, termed 'burning foot syndrome', has been attributed to pantothenic acid deficiency in malnourished patients, as it responded to treatment with the vitamin. In rats, pantothenic acid deficiency was associated with loss of colour from the fur, and the vitamin is still included in some shampoos as an anti-grey hair factor, although there is no evidence that it has this role in humans.

No dietary reference value has been set, although it has been noted that mean intakes in the UK are 5.4 mg/day. Main sources are meat, cereals and vegetables.

Biotin

Deficiency of biotin (a member of the B group of vitamins) can be induced experimentally by the feeding of raw egg white. This contains avidin, which has a high binding affinity for biotin and makes it unavailable for absorption. The clinical signs include loss of hair and a fine scaly dermatitis. Biotin is needed as a cofactor for several carboxylase enzymes, which carry carbon dioxide units in metabolic pathways. Carboxylases occur in the metabolism of all the major macronutrients and hence biotin has a widespread role.

Biotin occurs in many foods: richest sources are egg yolks, liver, grains and legumes. There is also significant synthesis of biotin by the bacterial flora in the colon, although whether this is available or not is unclear.

Occasional cases of biotin deficiency have been reported in subjects with unusual dietary practices, unbalanced total parenteral nutrition or in severe malabsorption consequent on bowel disease or alcoholism. Deficiency has also been reported in epileptics treated with some of the common anticonvulsant drugs.

Intakes of biotin in Britain average 26–39 mg/day; in the absence of deficiency, these appear to be adequate. Main contributors to the diet are cereals, eggs, meat and milk (together with beer, usually greater in men).

Vitamin C

As early as 1601 it was known that oranges and lemons or fresh green vegetables could protect a person against scurvy, a disease that broke out after several months of a diet devoid of fresh vegetables or fruit. The disease was a particular problem for sailors in the sixteenth to eighteenth centuries, when long sea voyages of discovery were being made. Classical experiments by James Lind in 1747 compared the curative properties of cider, hydrochloric acid, vinegar, seawater and oranges and lemons in sailors suffering from scurvy. Only those eating the citrus fruits recovered, within 1 week. However, the inclusion of citrus fruits and attention to adequate fresh vegetables was by no means routine thereafter in expeditions, and even Scott's expedition to the South Pole at the beginning of the twentieth century came to a tragic end because of scurvy. Populations in Europe throughout the Middle Ages suffered scurvy during the winter months, and it was probably the introduction and rapid rise in popularity of the potato in the sixteenth century that contributed most to the decline of this disease.

It is important to remember, however, that scurvy is still with us: it occurs among refugees around the world, in relief camps where the diet does not provide adequate vitamin C. It has also been reported among teenagers eating highly refined diets, and among the homeless of Britain.

Two forms of the vitamin have biological activity: these are ascorbic acid (Figure 9.14) and its oxidized derivative, dehydroascorbic acid. The two forms are interconvertible, and are collectively termed vitamin C. If further oxidation takes place, the vitamin loses its potency.

Vitamin C is unique among the vitamins in that it is essential as a vitamin for only a few animal species; most members of the animal kingdom can synthesize vitamin C from glucose and have no dietary requirement for it. The exceptions are the primates, including humans, and the guinea pig, together with a fruit-eating bat and a rare bird. It has been calculated that primates originally had the gene to perform this synthesis, but the ability was lost some 70 million years ago.

Sources of vitamin C

Most dietary vitamin C is supplied by fruit and vegetables (see Figure 9.15). Only very small amounts come from animal sources, mostly from milk, although levels here may be reduced by pasteurization and other processing.

Among the fruits, the richest sources are blackcurrants and rosehips, but for the general population, oranges (and orange juice) probably provide the most vitamin. Other sources are mangoes, papayas and strawberries. Vegetable sources include green peppers, broccoli, cauliflower and Brussels sprouts. Potatoes have a varying content of vitamin C: new potatoes are rich in the vitamin, but content declines as the storage time increases. Traditionally, potatoes have been a very important source of the vitamin in UK diets. However, potato consumption has fallen markedly in Britain, and other sources of vitamin C, notably fruit juice, have become more common, resulting in a changing profile of vitamin C intake. The National Food Survey (DEFRA, 2001) found the mean vitamin C intake to be 59 mg/day, which represents 152 per cent of the mean RNI. Intakes were lowest in Scotland, Northern Ireland and North West England, and also in lower income households.

Figure 9.14 Structure of ascorbic acid.

Figure 9.15 Some dietary sources of vitamin C.

Contributors to vitamin C intake were:

Fruit 52% (half of this from fruit juice)
Vegetables 34% (includes 9% from potatoes)
Milk 7%

Vitamin C is readily lost on cooking and processing. It is probably the least stable of all the vitamins, and its destruction is accelerated by exposure to light, alkali, air as well as heat. Therefore, most parts of the food preparation process may cause some loss of the vitamin. Anyone who is involved in preparing fruit and vegetables should consider the following ways of conserving vitamin C:

- handle food with care, with minimum bruising when cutting, to prevent release of oxidizing enzymes;
- immerse vegetables directly into boiling water to destroy the enzymes and thus protect the vitamin; this is also true of immersion into hot fat (e.g. in the cooking of potato chips);
- cover the saucepan with a lid to reduce exposure to air;
- use a small volume of water, or preferably steam to minimize the leaching of vitamin into water; if the cooking water can subsequently be used, then the vitamin C may still be included in the meal;
- avoid adding sodium bicarbonate, which enhances the green colour of some vegetables but destroys much of the vitamin C;
- avoid keeping vegetables hot after cooking, as this continues the destruction of the vitamin, so that almost none may remain after 1 hour. This is a particular problem when food is cooked in bulk and kept hot on serving counters during a service period which may span 1–2 hours.

Vitamin C in fruit is subject to much less destruction, as the lower pH in acidic fruits protects the vitamin. However, fruit juice loses its vitamin content if left to stand in the refrigerator after squeezing or after opening of a carton. The best way to maximize intake of vitamin C from fruit and vegetables is to consume as many as possible in their raw form.

Absorption and metabolism of vitamin C
Both forms of the vitamin are readily absorbed by active transport and passive diffusion mechanisms, although dehydroascorbic acid is believed to be absorbed better than ascorbic acid itself. The percentage of the ingested dose absorbed falls as the amount consumed increases. Overall, at levels of vitamin C usually consumed, absorption rates are 80–95 per cent. In the plasma, vitamin C occurs principally as free ascorbate; plasma levels are a reflection of the size of the dietary intake and continue to increase until they reach a plateau at 1.4 mg/dL (100 μmol/L) at intakes of 70–100 mg/day.

The adrenal gland, pituitary and the lens of the eye have high concentrations of vitamin C. Among other tissues that have a significant content of the vitamin are the liver, lungs and white blood cells. The content of vitamin C in the white blood cells is used as an indicator of tissue levels of the vitamin.

The total content of vitamin C in the body is known as the body pool. Normal values for this are 2–3 g in the adult; when this falls to less than 300 mg, clinical signs of scurvy may appear. Vitamin C status, in other words the amount of vitamin C within body tissues and fluids, is dependent on many factors (see Figure 9.16). These include the following.

- Intake: this depends on the composition of the food, its length of storage, processing and cooking methods.
- Absorption: this is affected by the total dose of vitamin ingested, the speed of travel through the digestive tract and the presence of other factors in the tract, such as glucose levels, trace elements and nitrosamines.
- Metabolism: rates of usage will vary with metabolic demand and the ability to recycle the vitamin; demand may be higher in smokers, pregnancy, exercise, inflammation, diabetes and in polluted environments. Plasma levels are lower with increasing age.
- Excretion in urine: this depends on the levels in the plasma, glomerular filtration rate and the renal threshold.

Roles of vitamin C
Most of the roles of vitamin C in the body are related to its being a reducing agent, as the ascorbate is readily oxidized to dehydroascorbate. In this way, vitamin C can act as a

In

Intake

Dependent on:
- Composition of food
- Length of food storage
- Processing and cooking methods

Absorption

Dependent on:
- Total dose of vitamin ingested
- Speed of travel through digestive tract
- Presence of other factors in tract,
  e.g. glucose levels
    trace elements
    nitrosamines

Vitamin C status

Out

Metabolic usage

Dependent on:
- Demand – higher in
  smokers
  pregnancy
  exercise
  inflammation
  diabetes
  polluted environments
- Ability to recycle vitamin
- Age → ↓ plasma levels

Excretion in urine

Dependent on:
- Levels in plasma
- Glomerular filtration rate
- Renal threshold

Figure 9.16 Summary of factors influencing vitamin C status.

hydrogen donor to reverse oxidation and, therefore, may be termed an antioxidant. As an antioxidant, vitamin C can react with free radicals and inactivate them before they cause damage to proteins or lipids. Once vitamin C has acted in this way, it must be regenerated. This is achieved by a number of reductase enzymes, which restore the ascorbate from dehydroascorbate, making it available for further reactions. Reductases that are used in this way include reduced glutathione and NADH and NADPH.

The other major role of vitamin C is as a cofactor for a number of hydroxylation reactions. This too may be an antioxidant role, whereby the vitamin is protecting metal ions, which act as prosthetic groups for these enzymes. Examples of hydroxylation reactions requiring vitamin C include:

- formation of hydroxyproline and hydroxylysine, for collagen synthesis;
- synthesis of carnitine, needed for release of energy from fatty acids, especially in muscle;
- synthesis of noradrenaline;
- synthesis of brain peptides, including a number of hormone-releasing factors found in the brain.

Vitamin C is closely linked to iron metabolism. It enhances iron absorption from food by reducing ferric iron to ferrous iron to facilitate absorption. It may also be involved in the incorporation of iron into ferritin. This may become a problem in individuals with excessive amounts of iron in the body. As always, caution should be exercised if large amounts of any single nutrient are taken.

Other roles have been proposed for vitamin C, including detoxification of foreign substances in the liver and the promotion of immune function. The latter has received a great deal of publicity and many people believe that consumption of large amounts (often several grams) of vitamin C will help to prevent the occurrence of the common cold. Evidence has been reviewed and has failed to show a consistent effect on prevention of the cold. However, moderate doses (up to 250 mg/day) may reduce the severity of the symptoms of a cold. It should also be remembered that very high intakes of the vitamin are poorly absorbed (absorption may be 10 per cent or less), may cause intestinal irritation and diarrhoea, and chronic ingestion may result in kidney stones.

Overall, there is a great deal of evidence from many studies that a higher intake of vitamin C is associated with a lower disease risk.

Vitamin C deficiency
General features of scurvy include progressive weakness and fatigue, muscular and bone pains,

oedema and depression. As the deficiency progresses, there may be delayed wound healing and subcutaneous bleeding, appearing as bruising and bleeding gums. Enlargement of the hair follicles causes roughness of the skin. There may be anaemia and possible pathological bone fractures due to failure of normal bone formation. Death results from pneumonia and cardiac failure.

Many of the signs of scurvy can be linked to the known functions of vitamin C, as described above. Thus, the failure of collagen synthesis may account for the bleeding from capillaries, failure of wounds to heal and bone fractures. Lack of carnitine synthesis may contribute to the feelings of tiredness. Depression may be linked to poor neurotransmitter synthesis.

Although scurvy is relatively rare in the West at the present time, sporadic cases are still reported. Generally, these arise from an inadequate intake of the vitamin, associated either with poor food choices or insufficient income. There is a positive association between income and vitamin C intake. Disease states that affect the appetite, such as anorexia or cancers, may also reduce intakes to deficiency levels.

Subclinical scurvy with low blood levels of vitamin C and possible biochemical changes is found in some elderly people and alcoholics. Elderly residents of institutions may be particularly vulnerable if large-scale catering practices are wasteful of vitamin C. On the whole, elderly women tend to have better vitamin C status than men. Recent findings suggest that vitamin C may protect blood vessel integrity, and in the elderly may prevent cognitive impairment and possibly stroke. There is also a possible role in the prevention of cataract formation by normalizing metabolism in the lens of the eye.

Smokers also have poorer vitamin C status. The explanation for this is not clear, but may include a lower intake, poorer absorption and increased turnover in combating the free radicals generated by the smoking.

There is growing interest in optimizing vitamin C status to promote health. Chronic disease, such as coronary heart disease, cancer and cataracts have been reported to be associated with low intake or plasma concentration of vitamin C. Supplementation with vitamin C is reported to decrease blood pressure and blood lipids, improve glucose metabolism, endothelial function and prevent free radical damage of lipids. It is, however, very difficult to attribute all of these effects solely to vitamin C intakes, as these often vary in line with other nutrients in a healthy diet.

Dietary reference value

The requirement for vitamin C may be defined in terms of the amount needed to prevent scurvy: the majority of studies agree that an intake of 10 mg/day will be preventive. Further increases in intake do not increase plasma levels until the intake reaches 40 mg/day, when measurable amounts start to appear in the plasma. This level of intake has, therefore, been set as the RNI by the Department of Health (DoH, 1991), as indicative of sufficient supply of the vitamin to distribute to the tissues.

There is a recommendation that smokers should consume up to 80 mg/day more than the RNI, to allow for the increased needs. In terms of optimal intakes, 200 mg/day has been suggested, which will achieve a saturation level of the vitamin in the plasma. More work is needed to support this proposal.

SUMMARY

1 The fat-soluble vitamins perform diverse functions, acting as regulators of metabolic reactions (vitamin D and K), protective agents (vitamin E), or constituents of essential chemicals in the body (vitamin A).

2 New roles are emerging for these vitamins as metabolic regulators at the nuclear level, perhaps involved in gene expression.

3 Adequate levels of these vitamins are required, although excessive amounts are stored in the body and may be toxic.

4 The water-soluble vitamins perform many key functions in the body; without them there is a considerable risk of failure of specific metabolic functions. Several of the vitamins act cooperatively, for example, folate and vitamin B_{12}, riboflavin and niacin, and vitamin B_6 and niacin.

5 The deficiency syndromes associated with some of these vitamins sometimes overlap, with similar pictures, particularly involving the skin, mouth and tongue, occurring with several vitamins, for example, niacin, riboflavin and vitamin B_6. This is also the case with folate and vitamin B_{12}, with a similar blood picture.

6 Many of the water-soluble vitamins are sensitive to cooking procedures and may be lost in substantial amounts. Care should be exercised when preparing foods that are important sources of these vitamins.

7 Several of the vitamins occur in similar foods:
   - meats provide thiamin, niacin, riboflavin and vitamin B_{12};
   - milk and dairy products are important sources of riboflavin and vitamin B_{12}
   - cereals provide thiamin, niacin and folate and vitamin E
   - fruits and vegetables are important sources of vitamin C and folate, as well as carotenes and vitamin K.
   Thus, omitting one of these groups of foods can have implications for more than one nutrient. A balanced diet, prepared with care, will ensure that all of these vitamins are supplied.

8 Care should be taken not to consume too much of any of the vitamins. Some harmful effects have been recorded with excessive intakes of niacin, vitamin C and vitamin B_6. Even though these vitamins are water soluble and, therefore, any excess is excreted in the urine, large concentrations in the body obtained from megadoses of supplements should be avoided.

9 Supplementation with some vitamins, for example, folate or vitamin E may have positive health benefits and more research is ongoing in this area.

STUDY QUESTIONS

1 A 25-year-old mother with three young children, aged 2, 4 and 6 years, is concerned that she is not giving them a balanced diet, as most of what they eat is made up of simple convenience foods. She herself tends to eat with the children and often finishes their leftovers. She feels tired and depressed. She asks if the whole family should take supplements of vitamins and/or minerals. What do you think?

2 a Why might an individual who has had a substantial part of their intestines removed (for medical reasons) be at risk of vitamin deficiencies?
   b Explain which vitamins in particular may be at risk.

3 Consider the various reasons why the following may not meet their vitamin requirements:
   a a college student, living in self-catering accommodation;
   b a middle-aged man, working long hours and living alone;
   c a recently bereaved, elderly woman.

4 Construct tables to compare common features (e.g. functions, sources, signs of deficiency) of the following pairs of vitamins:
   a riboflavin and niacin;
   b vitamin B_{12} and folate;
   c vitamins C and E.

5 Can you identify any other vitamins that might share features in common with any of the pairs in Q.4, above?

REFERENCES AND FURTHER READING

Abrams, S.A. 2002: Nutritional rickets: an old disease returns. *Nutrition Reviews* 60(4), 11–115.

Bates, C.J. 1995: Vitamin A. *Lancet* 345, 31–5.

Bender, D.A. 1994: Novel functions of vitamin B6. *Proceedings of the Nutrition Society* 53, 625–30.

Boushey, C.J. 1995: A quantitative assessment of plasma homocysteine as a risk factor for vascular disease: probable benefits of increasing folic acid intakes. *Journal of the American Medical Association* 274, 1049–57.

Bower, C., Wald, N.J. 1995: Vitamin B12 deficiency and the fortification of food with folic acid. *European Journal of Clinical Nutrition* 49(11), 787–93.

Buttriss, J., Bundy, R., Hughes, J. 2000: An update on vitamin K: contribution of MAFF-funded research. *British Nutrition Foundation Nutrition Bulletin* 25, 125–34.

DEFRA 2001: *National Food Survey 2000 Annual Report on food expenditure, consumption and nutrient intakes.* London: The Stationery Office.

DoH (UK Department of Health) 1991: *Dietary reference values for food energy and nutrients for the United Kingdom.* Report on Health and Social Subjects No. 41. Report on the Panel on Dietary Reference Values of the Committee on Medical Aspects of Food Policy. London: HMSO.

DoH (Department of Health) 2000: *Folic acid and the prevention of disease.* Report on Health and Social Subjects 50. London: The Stationery Office.

Fraser, J.D. 1995: Vitamin D. *Lancet* 345, 104–7.

Gale, C.R., Martyn, C.N., Winter, P.D. et al. 1995: Vitamin C and risk of death from stroke and coronary heart disease in cohort of elderly people. *British Medical Journal* 310, 1563–6.

Gibson, S. 2002: Report from the folic acid public stakeholder meeting. *British Nutrition Foundation Nutrition Bulletin* 27, 107–15.

Honein, M.A., Paulozzi, L.J., Mathews, T.J. et al. 2001: Impact of folic acid fortification of the US food supply on the occurrence of neural tube defects. *Journal of the American Medical Association* 285, 2981–6.

Iqbal, S.J., Garrick, D.P., Howl, A. 1994: Evidence of continuing 'deprivational' vitamin D deficiency in Asians in the UK. *Journal of Human Nutrition and Dietetics* 7, 47–52.

Khaw, K.T., Woodhouse, P. 1995: Interrelation of vitamin C, infection, haemostatic factors, and cardiovascular disease. *British Medical Journal* 310, 1559–63.

MAFF (Ministry of Agriculture, Fisheries and Food) 1994: *Dietary and nutritional survey of British adults: further analysis.* London: HMSO.

Maxwell, J.D. 1994: Seasonal variation in vitamin D. *Proceedings of the Nutrition Society* 53, 533–43.

Meydani, M. 1995: Vitamin E. *Lancet* 345, 170–5.

Morrissey, P.A., Quinn, P.B., Sheehy, P.J.A. 1994: Newer aspects of micronutrients in chronic disease: vitamin E. *Proceedings of the Nutrition Society* 53, 571–82.

Scott, J.M. 1999: Folate and vitamin B12. *Proceedings of the Nutrition Society* 58, 441–8.

Thane, C.W., Paul, A.A., Bates, C.J. et al. 2002: Intake and sources of phylloquinone (vitamin K1): variation with socio-demographic and lifestyle factors in a national sample of British elderly people. *British Journal of Nutrition* 87, 605–13.

Vermeer, C., Jie, K-S.G., Knapen, M.H.J. 1995: Role of vitamin K in bone metabolism. *Annual Review of Nutrition* 15, 1–22.

Wald, N.J. 1994: Folic acid and neural tube defects: the current evidence and implications for prevention. *CIBA Foundation Symposium* 181, 192–211.

10

MINERALS, ELECTROLYTES AND FLUID

The aims of this chapter are to:

❑ identify the major elements found in the human body;
❑ describe the functions of each element;
❑ consider the interactions between certain elements;
❑ review the role of the different elements in the maintenance of health;
❑ examine the importance of fluids.

On completing the study of this chapter, you should be able to:

❑ discuss the importance of the inorganic elements to health;
❑ recognize the consequence for health of an inadequate or excessive intake of particular minerals;
❑ identify food sources of particular minerals;
❑ discuss the causes of an inadequate intake of specific minerals in certain groups of the population;
❑ describe the rationale for the levels of inorganic minerals given as reference values;
❑ discuss the body's need for fluid and how this can be met.

This chapter considers those substances that appear in food analyses as ash. These are the substances that are left behind when the carbon, hydrogen and nitrogen have all been burnt away in the presence of oxygen as, for example, in a bomb calorimeter. Commonly called minerals, these substances occur in nature in water, the soil and in rocks, and are taken up by the roots of plants and thereby find their way into animals. Humans, therefore, consume minerals both from plant and animal sources, although foods of animal origin generally have a higher content as the minerals have been concentrated in the tissues.

The body contains about 22 known minerals, of which the majority are believed to be essential to life. Those that are considered to be nutritionally important are shown in Table 10.1. Their amounts in the human body and in food have an extraordinarily wide range, from over 1 kg of calcium in an adult to 5–10 mg of chromium. Altogether they account for 4 per cent of the weight of the body.

TABLE 10.1	Average amounts of minerals found in the adult human body
Minerals	**Total body content**
Major minerals	
Calcium	1200 g
Phosphorus	780 g
Potassium	110–137 g
Sulphur	175 g
Sodium	92 g
Chloride	84 g
Magnesium	25 g
Trace minerals	
Iron	4.0 g
Zinc	2.0 g
Manganese	12–20 mg
Copper	80 mg
Iodide	15–20 mg
Chromium	<2.0 mg
Cobalt	1.5 mg
Selenium	3–30 mg

Some of the minerals are present in the body as contaminants from the environment and, as far as is known at present, have no essential function in the body. These include vanadium, arsenic, mercury, silicon, tin, nickel, boron, lithium, cadmium and lead.

The major minerals are those present in amounts greater than 5 g; this applies to calcium and phosphorus. Also of great importance, although present in rather smaller quantities, are the electrolytes, namely sodium, potassium and chlorine (as chloride ion). Although sulphur is listed, it does not occur freely in the body but is an essential component of the sulphur-containing amino acids.

In addition, there are the trace minerals that together amount to approximately 15 g. Although present in small amounts, these trace substances are vital for particular functions in the body.

The minerals have several features in common.

- They exist in the body in one of two forms:
  - as biological components – in the skeleton, in haemoglobin, in thyroid hormones and many enzymes;
  - in their ionized state in the body fluids, where they serve to maintain homeostasis. Whichever of these forms occurs, the minerals retain their chemical identity.
- Once in the body, it is sometimes difficult for the mineral to be excreted. Those that dissolve in water can be lost in the urine; others are lost in the faeces, either by being secreted into the digestive tract (usually in bile), or by being lost when cells are shed from the intestinal lining. Toxic minerals are harmful in the body because they may be difficult to excrete without the use of special drugs to chelate and remove them. In addition, those that are similar in size and properties to the essential minerals may displace them. This is what happens when strontium and caesium find their way into bones and milk in place of calcium.
- Minerals are generally resistant to heat, air and acid, which is why they remain when a food has been burned in a bomb calorimeter. This also means that they are rarely lost during food preparation procedures, although the ones that are water soluble can be lost into cooking water.
- A problem with some minerals is that they are found in food as large complexes attached to a number of different compounds. Probably the most prevalent is inositol hexaphosphate (phytate), which is found in cereals, legumes and nuts, and which binds calcium, iron and zinc. This interferes with their absorption in the digestive tract, reducing their bioavailability. A similar problem can occur where minerals are present in foods containing large amounts of dietary fibre (non-starch polysaccharides; NSPs).
- Some minerals interfere with the absorption of other minerals, competing for the same carrier mechanism in the digestive tract. For example, large amounts of calcium may interfere with the absorption of iron and magnesium, and zinc can reduce absorption of iron and copper. For these reasons, taking supplements of one mineral may cause an imbalance of other minerals in the body.

MAJOR MINERALS

Calcium

Calcium is the most abundant mineral present in the body, amounting to almost 40 per cent of the total mineral mass. The majority is present in bone where, together with phosphorus (as hydroxyapatite $Ca_{10}(PO_4)_6(OH)_2$), it plays an essential part in hardening the skeleton and teeth. In addition, this calcium is a reserve of the mineral for its role in body fluids as ionic calcium, which is essential for nerve impulse transmission, muscle contraction and blood clotting.

Sources of calcium

The main dietary sources of calcium are milk and dairy products. For vegetarians who do not use dairy products, tofu set with calcium salts or calcium-enriched soya milk may be important sources of calcium. In addition, cereals and cereal products may supply a reasonable amount of calcium, although this may be less well absorbed from wholegrain cereals owing to the presence of NSP and phytate. All wheatflour in the UK, with the exception of wholemeal has, since 1943, been fortified with calcium carbonate by law, and provides the equivalent of 94–156 mg calcium/100 g of flour. Although a number of expert reports have in recent years considered this addition to be no longer necessary, it currently remains in force. Green leafy vegetables, such as spinach, broccoli and kale, contain good amounts of calcium, but its absorption may be inhibited by the presence of oxalates.

Other sources of calcium may include small fish, such as sardines, whose bones (when eaten) supply calcium, dried figs, nuts (e.g. almonds, brazil nuts), parsley, watercress and black treacle. Unless these foods form a major part of the diet, their contribution to the total dietary intake will be small.

In parts of the world where the water is hard (i.e. contains many dissolved salts), it can supply a significant amount of calcium to the day's intake.

Daily intakes in the UK, reported by the 2000 National Food Survey (DEFRA, 2001), are 863 mg. This represents 125 per cent of the mean reference nutrient intake (RNI); in households with three or more children, the mean intake only just exceeds the RNI, suggesting that there are groups that do not meet this figure. The main contribution comes from milk and cheese (54 per cent), and cereals (30 per cent).

Absorption of calcium

Calcium salts are generally not highly soluble, which makes their absorption from the diet problematic. Several factors can enhance or inhibit the absorption of calcium.

Enhancing factors

The most important of these is vitamin D, which causes the synthesis of a calcium-binding protein in the intestinal cells that transports calcium into the plasma. The ability to synthesize this protein and the amounts made are regulated by homeostatic mechanisms involving parathyroid hormone and active vitamin D, in response to changes in circulating levels of plasma calcium. In this way, calcium absorption

can be increased to meet increased needs in the body.

Lactose (present in milk) also enhances calcium absorption by keeping it in a soluble form. The presence of lactose and the large amounts of calcium found in milk make this an excellent source of the mineral. Other sugars and protein also enhance calcium absorption. The acidic environment of the upper digestive tract also facilitates the solubility of calcium. Therefore, taking large amounts of 'indigestion preparations' that lower acidity may compromise calcium absorption.

Inhibitory factors

Calcium absorption is reduced by phytic acid present in whole cereals, owing to the formation of insoluble calcium phytate. However, yeast fermentation probably breaks some of this down in the making of bread. It is also believed that people who regularly eat foods containing phytate develop a phytate-splitting enzyme, allowing them to make greater use of the calcium.

Oxalates (present in spinach, rhubarb, beetroot, chocolate, tea infusions, wheat bran, peanuts and strawberries) may also inhibit calcium absorption owing to the insoluble nature of the calcium oxalate salt. Non-starch polysaccharides may trap some calcium making it unabsorbable in the small intestine. However, fermentation of the soluble NSP in the large intestine may release the calcium for absorption here.

Unabsorbed fats will combine with calcium to form soaps, removing the calcium from the body. This is a particular problem in steatorrhoea, in which loss of vitamin D, a fat-soluble vitamin, may aggravate the problem of calcium absorption. However, more recently, it has been suggested that a high calcium intake, with large amounts lost in the faeces, may help to remove some fats from the body and be of benefit in preventing raised blood lipid levels. This is discussed further in Chapter 14.

There has been some doubt about the role of the calcium:phosphorus ratio in determining the bioavailability of calcium. At normal 1:1 ratios of the two minerals, there is no adverse effect of phosphorus on calcium absorption.

If phosphorus intakes are very high (ratio of 1:3 with calcium), calcium metabolism may be altered, with hypocalcaemia and oversecretion of parathyroid hormone, but there is little evidence that absorption of calcium is affected.

Overall absorption of calcium in adults averages about 30 per cent at a low-moderate intake (up to 500 mg); as intakes increase, the percentage absorption falls. Generally, as the need for calcium increases, for example, during growth and in pregnancy and lactation, the efficiency of absorption improves. A summary of factors involved in calcium balance is shown in Figure 10.1.

Role of calcium in the body
In bones
Calcium is principally located in bones, where it is found both in the dense cortical bone and in the less dense trabecular bone. The skeleton is an active reservoir of calcium. The mineral is continually being laid down (by osteoblasts) and resorbed (by osteoclasts) as bone growth (in childhood and adolescence), and maintenance (in adults) take place.

During growth in childhood and adolescence there is a net gain of bone and, therefore, of calcium. In the early adult decades, the amount of bone remains relatively constant in health, although it is in a state of constant flux with a balance between the activities of osteoclasts and osteoblasts. However, if there is a period of immobility or changes in levels of some hormones, such as cortisol or oestrogens, then bone loss will occur. The amount of bone gradually declines with age. This happens earlier and more rapidly in women at the time of the menopause, particularly in the first 2–3 years. The gradual

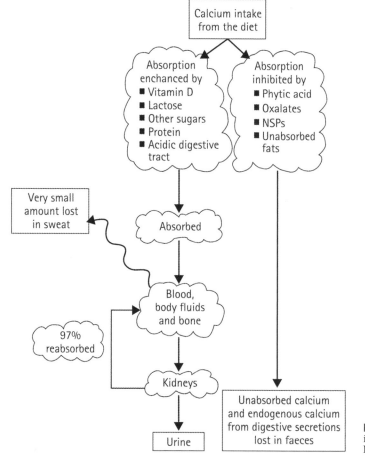

Figure 10.1 A summary of factors involved in calcium balance. NSPs, non-starch polysaccharides.

decline then continues as the rates of bone breakdown exceed bone repair. This may result in the bone becoming so fragile that it is easily broken; this condition is called osteoporosis and is discussed later in this section.

In blood and body fluids

The calcium present in body fluids is crucial to the normal homeostasis of the body and the levels are tightly regulated to remain within narrow limits of 2.2–2.6 mmol/L. This is achieved by the regulatory hormones, namely, parathyroid hormone, active vitamin D (1,25-dihydroxycholecalciferol) and calcitonin, acting on the gut, bones and kidneys in response to changes in circulating calcium levels (see Figure 10.2).

Overall, when plasma calcium levels are low (or phosphate levels are high) parathyroid hormone is secreted. This increases calcium levels by promoting synthesis of active vitamin D and, thus, increasing calcium absorption from the gut, reducing calcium excretion at the kidney and stimulating calcium release from the bone. Conversely, high calcium levels cause the release of calcitonin from the thyroid gland. This inhibits bone mobilization and promotes calcium uptake into bone.

Why does plasma calcium need to be closely regulated?

Calcium is essential for blood clotting; it is part of the clotting cascade by which insoluble prothrombin is converted into the thrombin of a blood clot by the action of fibrin and several other clotting factors. If calcium levels are insufficient, blood will not clot. Muscle contraction and nerve impulse transmission at nerve endings both involve the movement of calcium across the cell membrane, increasing intracellular levels and triggering contraction or depolarization.

Calcium excretion

Calcium is lost from the body via the faeces and urine, with very small amounts lost in sweat. Loss in the faeces represents the calcium unabsorbed from the diet, together with endogenous calcium from digestive secretions, especially bile and cells shed into the digestive tract, amounting to approximately 100 mg/day. Total losses in the faeces, therefore, depend on the amount consumed. Urinary calcium represents the final adjustment of plasma calcium levels, with the majority (up to 97 per cent) of the calcium filtered being reabsorbed by the renal tubules.

Levels of urinary calcium are increased:
- on a high calcium intake;
- by a high protein diet;
- by high sodium intake;
- in women at the menopause.

Levels of urinary calcium are decreased:
- in old age;
- by a high potassium intake;
- by a high magnesium intake;
- by a high phosphorus intake.

Figure 10.2 The regulation of plasma calcium.

Health aspects of calcium

Bone health and osteoporosis

As the numbers of older adults increase in most Western societies, as a result of a number of demographic changes and longer life expectancy, there is growing public health concern about the rising incidence of osteoporosis among this ageing population. Bone loss is a normal component of ageing and in many people the progressive bone loss causes no clinical problems, whereas in others the bone is sufficiently weak to fracture even under a minor impact. Osteoporosis is thus the loss of bone mass and micro-architecture with age resulting in fragile bones, which are susceptible to fractures. The most vulnerable sites for fracture are the radius at the wrist, the vertebrae of the spine and the neck of the femur in the pelvis. All of these fractures cause pain and disability, and represent a significant cause of morbidity and mortality, resulting in immense costs to the health services. In the UK alone, in 2000, there were a reported 90 000 fractures associated with this condition; other Western countries are experiencing a similar 'epidemic'.

The problem is much more common, but not exclusive to, older women, in whom it is estimated that one in three may suffer from the condition. This is because of the accelerated loss of bone at the time of the menopause, linked to the withdrawal of the female hormones. In men, the loss is much slower and more consistent.

Adult bone health is determined by the 'peak bone mass' (PBM) achieved at the end of bone accretion, and the later rate of bone loss. Current evidence suggests that the most desirable method of prevention is to achieve a high peak bone mass by the age of 20–25, so that the critical point for fracture is not reached when bone is lost in later life. Figure 10.3 shows the average rate of bone accretion up to peak bone mass, and the decline in bone mass with ageing. Bone mineral is lost from about the age of 35–40, at the rate of 0.3–0.4 per cent of the bone mass per year. Bone accretion is most efficient and rapid during the teenage years, with 90 per cent of peak bone mass achieved by a mean age of 16.9 years, and 95 per cent by 19.8 years. Both endogenous and exogenous factors play a part in determining bone mass. It has been estimated that genetic

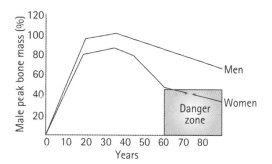

Figure 10.3 Changes in bone mass with age. (From British Nutrition Foundation, 1991. Reproduced with kind permission of the British Nutrition Foundation.)

components may account for 75 per cent of the variation in mass. However, exogenous factors have an important role to play. It is evident that several factors needed for optimal bone formation should be in place at this critical time. The raw materials for bone formation must be supplied in sufficient amounts. This includes principally calcium, but also other minerals and vitamins. Rates of calcium deposition have been reported to peak during puberty, reaching levels up to 1960 mg/day. In comparison, daily turnover in an adult is between 300 and 600 mg/day. It has been proposed that intakes as high as 1300 mg/day may be needed for maximum calcium retention. Calcium sources need to feature at all meals during the day for teenagers to ensure this level of intake. Unfortunately, data about calcium intakes in teenagers show that these are often below the reference levels of 800 mg for females and 1000 mg for males.

Other factors that may help in the development of a high peak bone mass in young adults are the following.

- Exercise. Weight-bearing exercise in particular promotes bone metabolism. In addition, exercise promotes food intake, ensuring higher intakes of calcium as well as helping to maintain a normal body weight.
- Body weight. Excessively thin females (with a body mass index (BMI) below 20) may be amenorrhoeic. The absence of normal menstrual cycles and lack of oestrogen will prevent normal bone accretion. This may be a problem both in girls suffering from eating disorders, and those who train excessively and

try to reduce their body weight. Body size is generally a good indicator of bone mass. Increased muscular development requires stronger bones to support movement, thus promoting greater bone density. The larger frame of the male is also associated with a greater bone mass than the smaller female.

- Alcohol and smoking. These both reduce bone accretion and are, therefore, detrimental to bone health.
- Vitamin D. Adequate exposure to sunlight for the synthesis of vitamin D is important, because of the critical need for vitamin D in calcium absorption.
- Vitamin K. Osteocalcin and matrix gla-protein are both vitamin K-dependent factors involved in bone mineralization. An adequate intake of this vitamin is, therefore, important to facilitate bone development.
- Vitamin C. This is an essential factor for the synthesis of collagen that forms part of the structural framework for bones.
- Other dietary factors. Inclusion of phytate, non-starch polysaccharides, high protein, sodium or phosphorus intakes in the diet may play a part. They may hinder calcium absorption or promote increased urinary excretion.

Once peak bone mass has been achieved, weight-bearing exercise and a healthy dietary intake are required to maintain it. Any period of immobilization will have a detrimental effect on the bones. All of the factors listed above continue to be important for bone health. The bones are a major source of alkaline buffering capacity in the body, consequent on their content of citrate, carbonate and sodium ions. In general, the Western diet is rich in foods that produce acid residues on metabolism, which, therefore, need to be buffered, drawing ions out of the bones. Such foods include protein sources (both animal and plant) and cereals. Osteoclasts are stimulated by a more acidic pH and thus resorb more calcium from the bones. This is excreted in greater amounts in an acidic urine, perhaps contributing to osteoporosis.

Some foods, such as milk, produce a relatively neutral residue, whereas fruit and vegetables produce an alkaline residue. Evidence to support the beneficial effects of milk, fruit and vegetables on bone was provided by the DASH (Dietary Approaches to Stopping Hypertension) study (Sacks et al., 2001), in which an increase in the number of servings of fruit and vegetables resulted in a substantial reduction in urinary calcium excretion.

Vegetarianism and high-fluoride intakes have been linked to lower incidence of osteoporosis, although the mechanisms are not clear.

At the menopause, the use of hormone replacement therapy for a period of about 5 years is recognized as an important means of preventing bone loss. Women who are overweight at this time of life appear to have a lower risk of the condition; it is believed that naturally occurring oestrogens produced by metabolism in the adipose tissue offer some protection to the bones. Smoking accelerates the normal rate of bone loss after the menopause. Male smokers also have an increased risk of bone loss. Exercise can promote bone health even in the elderly, and can minimize the progressive reduction in bone mass. Exercise is also important in helping to maintain mobility and balance, and reduce the risk of falls that could result in a fracture. Supplementation with calcium and vitamin D after the menopause has been shown to delay bone loss and reduce the risk of fractures in some studies, but there is still debate about the general application of this measure and the doses needed. Soy protein isoflavones have also been shown to reduce the loss of bone density around the time of the menopause, although more research is needed. These factors are summarized in Figure 10.4.

General screening for osteoporosis is not currently a public health recommendation in the UK, although those at high risk would benefit from early diagnosis. Risk of osteoporosis is greater in people with coeliac disease, inflammatory bowel disease and on prolonged steroid therapy. Individuals with a family history of (maternal) osteoporotic fracture may be at greater risk. Dual x-ray adsorptiometry (DEXA) is the most widely used method, although new techniques include biochemical markers of bone resorption, such as urinary pyridinium crosslink excretion and quantitative ultrasound (QUS). Overall, there are many unanswered questions on the subject of osteoporosis. It seems clear,

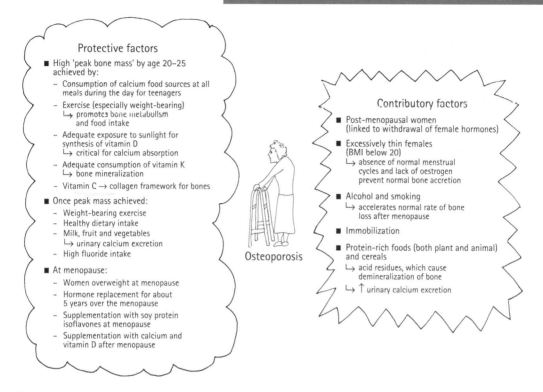

Figure 10.4 Factors influencing bone health.

however, that achieving a high peak bone mass in early adulthood is probably one of the best ways of preventing the development of the condition.

Colon cancer

There is some evidence that calcium may reduce the incidence of colon cancer. It has been suggested that bile acids and fatty acids are bound to unabsorbed calcium, and are thus removed from the colon. This reduces the potential for harmful effects if they were to linger in the colon.

Blood pressure

Individuals who have higher intakes of calcium, especially from dairy products, have been shown in several studies to have lower blood pressure. In addition, calcium supplementation can lower blood pressure.

Dietary reference values

These are difficult to determine, as there is no single satisfactory approach. The figures recommended in Report 41 (DoH, 1991) are, therefore,

based on the factorial approach, taking into account needs for growth and maintenance. The average absorption is assumed to be 30 per cent; the reference nutrient intake for adults is 700 mg/day. There are no specific recommendations made to take into account possible health implications.

Phosphorus

Phosphorus is often considered together with calcium, as both are present in bone. In blood, they have a reciprocal relationship and are controlled by similar mechanisms. Phosphorus is widely available in both animal and plant foods including meat, poultry, fish, eggs and dairy products, and in cereals, nuts and legumes. Small amounts occur in tea and coffee. It is widely present as a food additive in bakery goods, processed meats and soft drinks.

Absorption and metabolism

The body absorbs phosphorus more efficiently than calcium, at rates of 60–90 per cent, depending on body needs. An inadequate intake is, therefore, unlikely.

Dietary phosphorus can be either organic or inorganic in origin, most absorption taking place in the inorganic form. Phosphorus found in cereals and legumes as phytate is only partly liberated during digestion, with approximately 50 per cent being absorbed. Absorption from the digestive tract is reduced by the presence of magnesium and aluminium, both of which may be found in indigestion preparations. This is unlikely to lead to phosphate deficiency, unless there is also a metabolic problem involving the kidneys or parathyroid gland that regulate phosphate levels. Calcium also reduces phosphorus absorption.

Together with calcium, phosphorus is the major mineral constituent of bone where it occurs as hydroxyapatite, and 85 per cent of the body's phosphorus is found here. The remaining 15 per cent is distributed within the soft tissues, as phospholipids in red blood cells and plasma lipoproteins, in DNA and RNA, and a small amount as inorganic phosphate. The inorganic phosphate compartment is, however, critical, as it receives phosphate from the diet and from bone resorption, and loses phosphate to urine and bone mineralization. It is also the primary source for all of the biochemical reactions that require phosphates as the currency for energy transformations. It is, therefore, central to the functioning of the metabolic machinery. Phosphates are also critical as buffers to maintain normal pH in the body. Cells have limited storage capacity for phosphate and, therefore, draw on the inorganic phosphate pool for their needs.

Phosphorus levels in the body are regulated mainly by renal excretion under the influence of parathyroid hormone, which causes increased urinary loss. (This allows plasma calcium levels to rise – a major function of the hormone.) Abnormal levels of phosphate in the blood are generally the result of renal or parathyroid dysfunction, rather than dietary excess or deficiency, since there is extensive recycling of the mineral. However, intakes may be low in premature infants, vegans, alcoholics and people who use aluminium-containing antacids regularly. Deficiency of phosphorus can cause bone loss, and result in rickets and osteomalacia.

A low level of extracellular inorganic phosphate (hypophosphataemia) will result in cellular dysfunction. Signs and symptoms may include anorexia, anaemia, muscle weakness, bone pain, parasthesia (pins and needles) and, if acute, confusion and death.

Intakes of phosphorus in the UK average 1.2–1.3 g/day; a minimum intake of 400 mg/day had been proposed to maintain adequate plasma phosphate levels. The RNI (DoH, 1991) is given as 550 mg/day for adults, based on an equimolar ratio with calcium intakes.

Magnesium

The human body contains approximately 25 g of magnesium, of which 60 per cent is found in the bones, the remainder in the soft tissues and 1 per cent in the extracellular fluid. It is the most abundant divalent intracellular ion.

Food sources of magnesium include whole grain cereal, nuts, legumes, seafoods, coffee, tea, cocoa and chocolate. Chlorophyll found in green leafy vegetables contains magnesium. Intakes in the UK are reported to be around 227 mg/day.

Absorption and metabolism

Absorption of magnesium occurs in the small intestine and appears to be more efficient when intakes are low. Absorption is improved by vitamin D, and reduced by the presence of fatty acids and phytate. Plasma magnesium levels are kept constant by precise regulation of excretion via the kidney to match amounts absorbed. The magnesium found in bones is thought to act as a reservoir to sustain plasma levels. The remaining magnesium is largely found in muscle and other soft tissues. It occurs as part of cell membranes but is also an essential activator of over 300 enzyme systems. Most notably it is involved in all enzyme systems utilizing ATP. In addition, magnesium is involved in protein synthesis, energy production, muscle contraction and nerve impulse transmission.

There are many situations in which magnesium competes with or interferes with the action of calcium in the body. For example, magnesium inhibits the blood clotting process, it may also inhibit smooth muscle contraction by blocking the calcium binding sites. However, the actions of vitamin D and parathyroid hormones, which regulate calcium, both require the presence of magnesium.

Magnesium deficiency

In humans this is most likely to be secondary to other disturbances in the body. These may include:

- inadequate intakes in protein–energy malnutrition;
- prolonged intravenous feeding;
- in alcoholics, excessive gastrointestinal tract losses as in vomiting, diarrhoea or malabsorption;
- excessive excretion as in the use of certain diuretics, or in uncontrolled diabetes involving tissue catabolism.

Studies of patients in intensive care units have shown that hypomagnesaemia may occur in up to 65 per cent of cases, often in association with low potassium levels.

Hypocalcaemia is a major sign in magnesium deficiency and may contribute to the clinical picture. Low levels of magnesium result in gradually progressive muscle weakness, neuromuscular dysfunction, irregular heartbeat and ultimately coma and death.

Health aspects of magnesium

Epidemiological evidence suggests that coronary heart disease is more common where magnesium levels in the water supply are low; however, evidence on this is conflicting. It has been proposed that adequate magnesium protects the cardiac muscle against ischaemic injury. Furthermore, magnesium has been advocated as therapy in acute myocardial infarction to strengthen cardiac muscle contraction and possibly reduce mortality. Magnesium supplementation has also been proposed as a treatment for osteoporosis but more work is needed. Magnesium has been used successfully as a treatment in pre-eclampsia of pregnancy, to reduce the risk to both mother and infant.

Because of the absence of a clear-cut deficiency in healthy adults, a reference value is difficult to define. The Department of Health (DoH, 1991) suggests that an intake of 3.4 mg/kg per day, equal to 270 mg in women and 300 mg in men, is an adequate intake.

Sulphur

Sulphur enters the body as the sulphur-containing amino acids methionine and cysteine. The sulphur-containing side-chains in these amino acids can link to each other forming disulphide bridges, which give great strength to the peptide produced. These bonds are found in proteins that form the hard parts of the body, such as skin, nails and hair. Sulphur is also present in the vitamins thiamin and biotin.

These amino acids are required for the synthesis of proteins and connective tissue constituents, such as chondroitin sulphate. Sulphur also has an important role in the detoxifying pathways used by the liver for removal of waste products and participates in acid–base balance.

A mixed diet is unlikely to be short of sulphur as most proteins contain over 1 per cent sulphur. Egg and milk proteins are particularly rich in methionine, which is especially important in tissue growth and regeneration after illness and injury.

MICROMINERALS OR TRACE ELEMENTS

Iron

Iron is part of the haemoglobin molecule in blood and, as such, accounts for two-thirds of the body's iron content. In this role, combined with the protein globin, it is the carrier of oxygen from the lungs to the tissues and, therefore, plays a vital role in survival. In addition, some is found in myoglobin, which is the pigment found in muscles that has a high affinity for oxygen.

The remainder is used in enzymes (especially cytochromes, which are essential in oxidation-reduction reactions), stored in the body or is found in the blood, being carried between sites in the body.

The total amount of iron present in the body varies with the body weight, gender and long-term nutrition. It is also affected by the state of health, growth and pregnancy. On average, the body iron content averages 50 mg/kg of body mass in men and 38 mg/kg in women.

Sources of iron

Iron occurs in the diet in two forms: as haem iron mainly in foods of animal origin, and non-haem, or inorganic iron, predominantly from plant foods. The richest sources of haem iron are meat and fish (liver is one of the richest sources of iron, although many people never eat it). Cereals contain inorganic iron, which may also be bound to insoluble compounds such as phytate. However, fortification of white bread flour with iron does ensure that some additional iron is available without competition from phytate, which is removed in the milling process. Legumes and green vegetables also provide iron, although the availability of this is much less than from the animal sources. Other sources of iron include nuts and dried fruits. Milk and dairy products are very low in iron, and intakes of large amounts of milk may be linked to poor iron status.

Iron supplements are widely available. They contain a variety of iron salts – sulphate, succinate, gluconate and fumarate – and have varying levels of bioavailability. It is stated that in those taking supplements, these contribute 7.5 mg/day of iron.

Average intakes of iron in the UK are 10.1 mg/day, which represents 97 per cent of the average RNI (DEFRA, 2001). Most of the groups studied in the National Food Survey had mean intakes that fell below 100 per cent of the RNI. Only households with no children achieved intakes of 100 per cent or more of the RNI. In the *Health survey for England 1994* (Colhoun and Prescott-Clarke, 1996), low iron stores were reported for 4 per cent of men and 26 per cent of women. Main contributors in the UK to iron intakes are cereal products (53 per cent), meat (13 per cent) and vegetables (16 per cent).

Absorption of iron

The two forms of iron in the diet are absorbed with different efficiency. Organic (haem) iron must be hydrolysed from any protein to which it is attached and is then absorbed relatively easily, albeit slowly; the overall absorption of iron

from meat may be 20–25 per cent. The absorption takes place most effectively in the duodenum, and is inversely related to the level of iron stores.

Non-haem, inorganic iron must first be solubilized and hydrolysed before absorption can occur. Hydrochloric acid in the stomach performs this function and also converts any ferric (Fe^{3+}) iron in food to its (absorbable) ferrous (Fe^{2+}) state. This reaction is also facilitated by ascorbic acid (vitamin C), which can dramatically improve inorganic iron absorption. Other factors that can enhance the absorption of inorganic iron include citric acid, lactic acid, fructose and peptides derived from meat; all of these form ligands with the ferrous iron, maintaining its solubility and thus facilitating absorption. Alcohol is also believed to enhance iron absorption.

There are, in addition, a number of factors that reduce absorption of inorganic iron. These generally bind with the iron, making it unavailable for absorption. Most notable are:

- phytate (in whole cereal grains);
- polyphenols (in tea, coffee and nuts);
- oxalic acid (in tea, chocolate, spinach);
- phosphates (in egg yolks);
- calcium and zinc.

These interactions make it extremely difficult to predict how much iron will be absorbed from a particular meal. For example, iron absorption from plant foods can be as little as 2–5 per cent, but can be enhanced tenfold by the presence of vitamin C. Tea will reduce iron absorption by as much as 60 per cent. Overall, iron absorption from the diverse UK diet is estimated to be 15 per cent. Under certain circumstances, for example, in pregnancy, absorption may be 90 per cent. However, if the diet contains little or no meat, and substantial amounts of phytate-rich foods, absorption is likely to be less than 10 per cent. Factors influencing iron absorption are summarized in Figure 10.5.

Advice to people who have marginal intakes of iron should, therefore, include simple guidelines about food combinations that may be beneficial. However, it is clear that there is often little relationship between dietary iron intake and iron status, and mechanisms exist in the body that regulate uptake in response to physiological

Figure 10.5 Influences on iron absorption.

circumstances in as yet incompletely understood ways.

Control of absorption

Once iron has been absorbed into the body, there is no means of eliminating a surplus, which can be toxic in excess, other than by loss of blood. In severe iron overload, the patient may be bled to remove iron, or is prescribed a chelating drug, which binds to the iron and allows it to be excreted. It is clearly preferable to have a mechanism that can prevent the entry of iron into the body when it is not needed. In a healthy individual a 'mucosal block' operates, which regulates the amount of iron allowed into the circulation according to the level of stores present in the body. Thus, more is absorbed when the body stores are low or the needs are increased, for example, in pregnancy.

As it passes through the mucosal cell, the iron is oxidized back to the ferric state and attached to the transport protein transferrin for circulation around the body. Iron not required by the body is trapped within the mucosal cell and is lost in the faeces when the lining cells of the gut are shed at the end of their life cycle.

Iron in the body

The main endogenous source of iron is the breakdown of red blood cells by the reticuloendothelial system. This is added to the iron from the diet (exogenous iron) for use and storage.

Iron is carried in the body fluids attached to the protein transferrin, which takes it from sites of absorption or release to sites of iron utilization or storage. A substantial amount of iron is transported around the body each day; normal concentrations of transferrin are 2.2–3.5 g/L, which at any time are carrying 3 mg of iron. During the course of a day, 25–30 mg of iron are transported around the body in a very efficient 'recycling' mechanism.

Red blood cells have an average lifespan of 120 days, which means that, each day, 1/120th of the total red cell count is broken down and has to be replaced. The bone marrow requires 24 mg of iron per day to make red blood cells. This daily need for iron demonstrates how important it is that recycling of iron occurs in the body: it would be impossible to take in these quantities of iron on a daily basis. With an absorption rate of 10 per cent, the diet would have to contain 240 mg of iron simply to meet the needs for red cell synthesis.

Iron is used:

- predominantly by the bone marrow, for red blood cell synthesis (between 70 and 90 per cent is used here);
- by muscle cells for myoglobin synthesis;
- in metabolically active cells for the production of cytochromes in mitochondria;
- in synthesis of hormones and neurotransmitters; and
- in immune function.

Losses of iron

Small amounts of iron are lost daily from the digestive tract lining, skin cells, in bile, urine and any small blood losses. Overall, this 'obligatory' loss of iron amounts to approximately 0.9 mg/day in men. In women, there is a monthly loss of iron in menstrual flow, estimated to be equivalent to an additional 0.7 mg/day on average. However, up to 10 per cent of women may have heavy menstrual losses, which may equate to an additional daily iron loss of up to 1.4 mg. Additional iron loss is generally associated with pathological changes in the digestive tract, such as ulcers or cancer causing bleeding. Some drugs such as aspirin, taken regularly, may also cause small blood loss into the gut, which, over time, can amount to a significant loss of iron.

Ideally, the obligatory losses are compensated by iron absorbed from the diet, which should be sufficient to restore iron balance. However, if insufficient iron is ingested there will be a gradual depletion of iron stores, eventually resulting in iron deficiency.

Stored iron

Iron in excess of immediate needs is taken to storage sites in the liver, bone marrow and spleen, where it is stored in association with a protein called ferritin. Ferritin can accommodate over 4000 atoms of iron in its interior and thus prevent any toxic effects. It has been suggested that even a moderate level of iron storage may be a risk factor for cardiovascular disease and cancer. Stored iron, acting as a pro-oxidant, has the potential to cause oxidative stress through the production of free radicals and thus dysregulate antioxidant–oxidant balance. Small amounts of ferritin are present in the circulation, and this can be measured to reflect the size of the iron stores. Plasma ferritin levels of 12 mg/L or less are suggestive of depleted iron stores. If the iron stores become very large, ferritin molecules can clump together to form haemosiderin, which allows safe storage of more iron. However, in excess, this too can be toxic and is associated with a serious condition called siderosis, in which liver function deteriorates.

Iron deficiency

When iron stores become depleted, the amount of ferritin in the blood will fall. This will be the first sign of iron deficiency. The daily physiological need for iron will still be met with recycled iron, but as this gradually becomes depleted, and the saturation of transferrin becomes less, the supply of iron for the synthesis of new red blood cells will become inadequate and the cells produced will contain less haemoglobin and be smaller and fewer in number. This is the typical blood picture of iron-deficiency anaemia. Markers of iron status can, however, be misleading. For example, both ferritin and transferrin are affected by the acute phase response associated with infection, and levels fall. Thus, measurement of these indicators can give misleading results during periods of infection and may lead to inappropriate treatment with iron.

When the number of red cells becomes so low that the oxygen-carrying capacity to the tissues is affected, the individual will suffer the symptoms of anaemia, including fatigue, apathy, loss of appetite and poor temperature regulation. There may also be changes to the mouth and digestive tract symptoms, linked to reduced cell replication. The nails may become brittle.

In addition, it is now recognized that low iron status also affects other physiological parameters. Capacity for physical work is affected owing to inadequate oxidative mechanisms.

Deficiency of iron that occurs in the first 2 years of life can significantly impair mental and motor development. This may result in poor memory and learning, and a low attention span. There is still ongoing debate concerning the reversibility of this effect on treatment with iron, with some studies indicating a permanent reduction in mental test scores. Equally, there are conflicting results in studies of older children, with some aspects of learning, such as language scores, affected more than maths scores.

Immune status is also depressed, related to a reduced bactericidal capacity of phagocytes owing to a lack of oxidative enzymes. However, iron is also needed for bacterial growth, and an iron deficiency in malnourished children may actually protect them from bacterial infection. As treatment starts, the increased availability of iron for the bacteria without an associated improvement in immune function can result in rapid and fatal infections. Adequate vitamin A status is also needed for normal recovery to take place.

Iron deficiency is a major health problem worldwide, with anaemia affecting up to 10 per cent of the world population. Evidence from surveys indicates that in Western countries between 20 and 30 per cent of women of child-bearing age have negligible iron stores. Iron-deficiency anaemia probably only occurs in between 2 and 8 per cent of these populations.

There are certain subgroups who are at much greater risk of deficiency and anaemia for a number of reasons. These include people with:

- inadequate intake due to low income, poor food choice or vegetarian diets;
- low absorption rates due to interference from other dietary components, low stomach acidity or parasites;
- increased needs or losses owing to growth, pregnancy, heavy menstrual losses or bleeding from other causes.

These factors tend to occur in infants, children, teenagers and women of child-bearing age, and these constitute the main vulnerable groups.

Diagnosis of poor iron stores can be made on the basis of low ferritin levels in plasma, and a reduction in the saturation of transferrin. Low levels of haemoglobin signify advanced iron deficiency. Anaemia is diagnosed when the blood haemoglobin levels falls below 13 g/L in men and 12 g/L in women. Patients often fail to recognize the early symptoms of iron deficiency, as these develop over a long period of time.

Prevention of iron deficiency is important. It can be achieved by:

- including more sources of iron in the diet;
- using more bioavailable iron;
- reducing foods that compromise iron absorption;
- using iron-fortified foods, especially in infants and young children; and
- taking iron supplements when iron losses are high (e.g. in menstruation).

Dietary reference values

Report 41 (DoH, 1991) takes into account the obligatory losses of iron and estimates of the average absorption rates for iron. Assuming this to be 15 per cent from mixed diets, the RNI for adult men is 8.7 mg and for women is 14.8 mg. However, it is accepted that there will be some 10 per cent of the female population whose needs will be greater than this, and who may need supplements. After the menopause, the RNI for women falls to the same level as that of men.

No additional increment is proposed for pregnancy, although it is recognized that there are increased iron requirements amounting to 680 mg over the whole pregnancy. It is assumed that women will have adequate stores of iron on which to draw and there is also a saving on daily iron balance from the cessation of the menses. Some women with inadequate stores may, however, require additional iron. Levels of haemoglobin that fall below 10 g/L in pregnancy have been shown to be associated with progressively increasing risk to the baby, pre-term delivery and associated complications. Iron absorption may increase between five- and nine-fold during pregnancy as needs increase. It is, therefore, difficult to make predictions of the exact dietary needs at this time, and serum ferritin or haemoglobin levels should be monitored.

Zinc

Human zinc deficiency was first reported in the 1960s in the Middle East in teenage boys found to have poor growth and delayed sexual maturation (hypogonadal dwarfism). It was subsequently reported among children and among hospitalized patients on intravenous nutrition in the USA. It is now recognized that zinc is essential for the activities of many enzymes and regulatory proteins, and plays a part in numerous, diverse functions of the body.

Sources of zinc

Dietary intake of zinc is correlated with the protein content of the diet because zinc occurs complexed with proteins and their derivatives. Particularly good sources are lean meat (especially offal), seafoods and dairy products. Pulses and whole grains are a moderate source, but are of importance in vegetarian diets. Low levels of zinc occur in leafy vegetables, fruit, fats, alcohol and refined cereals. As with other divalent minerals, bioavailability is a determinant of the usefulness of particular dietary sources. Animal sources of zinc are generally more readily available than plant sources.

The average daily intake in the UK is 8.0 mg (DEFRA, 2001). Main contributors of zinc in the British diet are meat and meat products (30 per cent), cereal products (27 per cent) and dairy products (23 per cent). In many groups, especially in households with three or more children, the average intake fell below 100 per cent of the RNI, indicating some groups at risk of low intakes.

Absorption of zinc

Both ingested zinc as well as that secreted in various digestive juices, such as bile and pancreatic juice, are available for absorption. Zinc is released from bound sources and attaches to amino acids, which facilitate its absorption. The amount absorbed is regulated to match the needs of the body, although the mechanisms are unclear. There is competition for the absorption mechanism from other divalent ions, such as calcium and iron, which may reduce zinc uptake. Stress has been shown to increase zinc uptake.

Inhibitors of zinc uptake include phytate (especially in the presence of calcium), oxalic acid, polyphenols and folic acid. Zinc taken into the mucosal cells may be bound to metallothionein and then lost from the body when the cells are shed. This is thought to provide an important mechanism for regulating body levels of zinc. Overall, rates of zinc absorption average 30 per cent, although considerable variation may occur with different dietary combinations.

Zinc in the body

Zinc is involved in:

- the metabolism of all the macronutrients;
- the production of energy;
- nucleic acid synthesis (and therefore cell division);
- oxygen and carbon dioxide transport (in carbonic anhydrase) antioxidant mechanisms (through superoxide dismutase);
- the immune system;

- protein synthesis, and is especially important in wound healing and growth:
- the storage and release of insulin;
- nuclear transcription and activation of proteins that regulate gene expression.

With so many roles, it is not surprising that zinc is widely distributed throughout the body. Major sites are the muscle (60 per cent), bone (30 per cent), skin (4–6 per cent), with the remainder found in liver, kidney and plasma. There is no readily identified store of zinc, although in catabolic states, zinc is released from muscle and made available to the plasma. The liver provides 'fine tuning' of plasma zinc levels, which are tightly controlled, by releasing zinc from metallothionein–zinc complexes in its cells. In infection, zinc is taken up by the liver metallothionein and plasma levels fall. Levels of zinc in other tissues, such as bone, brain, lung and heart, remain relatively stable in the event of low zinc intakes.

Excretion of zinc occurs mostly via the faeces through secretion into the digestive tract. Small amounts are lost in the urine and in skin cells.

Zinc deficiency

Zinc status is difficult to measure because plasma zinc levels can be affected by a number of situations unrelated to status. Measures that have been used but are believed to be insufficiently reliable include white blood cell zinc levels, urinary excretion and hair zinc.

Signs of mild deficiency may include depressed appetite, poor taste acuity, delayed wound healing, immunosuppression, poor growth, skeletal abnormalities and delayed sexual maturation in children (see Figure 10.6). People in Western societies are increasingly eating foods in which the zinc content has been reduced by processing. It is likely that poor zinc status may be an increasing problem. Reports from both the USA and Europe have found that the amounts of zinc provided by typical diets are below the recommended allowances for children, adolescent girls, women of reproductive age and elderly men and women. There is concern that individuals have insufficient zinc reserve to cope with increased demand, e.g. growth and

Figure 10.6 Signs of zinc deficiency.

tissue repair. In developing countries, the opposite problem exists: there may be sufficient zinc in the diet, but the absorption is inhibited by other factors.

Marginal zinc deficiency may be a problem in children and in elderly subjects who have poor appetite and who consume little meat. It has been suggested that poor zinc status in pregnancy, especially in the first trimester, may be linked to intrauterine growth retardation, although the evidence is conflicting. Other situations in which zinc deficiency may occur include protein–energy malnutrition and prolonged intravenous nutrition. Alcoholics, patients with malabsorption and diabetics may also exhibit abnormal zinc status.

Severe zinc deficiency is associated with an inborn error of zinc metabolism, known as acrodermatitis enteropathica, which affects the intestinal uptake of zinc. This produces a severe rash, which is prone to secondary infections, growth failure and behavioural abnormalities. Maintenance on large doses of supplemental zinc is necessary.

It has been suggested that zinc deficiency may be a component in anorexia nervosa and treatment with zinc sulphate has been reported to help in restoring normal eating patterns. However, although zinc status may be poor in sufferers, it is unlikely to explain the whole syndrome.

Dietary reference value

Figures for the daily turnover of zinc are used as the basis for setting dietary reference values. In adults, systemic needs appear to be 2–3 mg/day, and these can be converted into RNI, using an estimate of 30 per cent for absorption of dietary zinc. Thus, RNIs for adult men and women are 9.5 mg/day and 7.0 mg/day, respectively. No additional increment is recommended in pregnancy, since it is assumed that metabolic adjustment takes place to provide the extra zinc.

Excessive intakes of zinc may cause nausea and vomiting, and at 50 mg/day may interfere with immune responses, and the metabolism of iron and copper. Caution should, therefore, be exercised in taking zinc-containing supplements.

Copper

There are approximately 100 mg of copper in the adult human body and the amount decreases with age. Deficiency of copper is well known in animals, and results in anaemia and failure to mature. In humans, deficiency has been recognized for many years, but the diagnosis and significance of any suboptimal status in populations is still uncertain.

Sources of copper

The content of copper in plant foods varies with soil conditions and food processing techniques. However liver, shellfish, nuts, seeds (including cocoa) and legumes together with the outer parts of cereals are reported to be the richest sources (0.3–2.0 mg/100 g). Bananas, potatoes, tomatoes and mushrooms have intermediate levels (0.05–0.3 mg/100 g). Low levels are found in milk, bread and breakfast cereals. Drinking water can be an important source, where copper piping is used, and can provide up to 6 mg/day.

Estimated daily intakes of copper in the UK were 1.8 mg/day, the range for developed countries being 0.6–1.6 mg/day. Intakes among vegetarian populations have been reported to range from 2.1 to 3.9 mg/day. Analysed values are reported to be higher than those calculated from food composition tables, reflecting the variability in foods. Meat and meat products (27 per cent), together with cereal products (27 per cent) are the main contributors of copper in the UK diet.

Absorption of copper

Copper is absorbed mainly in the duodenum and jejunum, at rates of 35–70 per cent. The efficiency of absorption appears to vary inversely with intake. The transfer of copper across the baso-lateral membrane of the enterocyte is energy dependent and carrier mediated, and there is competition for the pathway from other minerals, most notably zinc and iron. Other inhibitors include an alkaline pH, molybdenum, calcium and phosphorus, and possibly the presence of phytates and sulphides. Absorption is enhanced by the presence of animal protein, human milk and fructose. On absorption, copper is bound to plasma albumin, but becomes rapidly bound to caeruloplasmin in the liver, which then forms the major circulating source of copper. Copper is also secreted into the digestive tract, especially in bile, and this forms the main excretory route and is believed to be an important mechanism for maintaining a constant body pool of copper.

Copper in the body

Copper is found tightly bound to proteins, termed metalloproteins, some of which are cuproenzymes and take part in a variety of intracellular and extracellular reactions.

Of the total amount of copper in the body, 40 per cent is found in muscle; the remainder is in the liver, brain and blood (in red cells and as caeruloplasmin in plasma). Essential for iron metabolism, caeruloplasmin converts ferrous iron into its ferric state. The ferric iron then binds to transferrin and enters cells. An absence of caeruloplasmin, therefore, results in accumulation of iron in liver and brain. Caeruloplasmin is also involved in the response to infection as one of the acute-phase proteins. Copper occurs as a component of several enzyme systems, including cytochrome oxidase, superoxide dismutase and various amine oxidases. Cytochrome oxidase is the essential final link of the electron transport chain for the production of energy as ATP. Copper is a component of the free-radical-quenching enzyme superoxide dismutase, which also has an important role in protecting the body from damage by products of the response to infection. Amine oxidase is used in cross-linkage formation in the connective tissue proteins collagen and elastin. Copper-containing enzymes are also involved in melanin production, formation of myelin, and for neurotransmitter synthesis (such as catecholamines, dopamine and encephalins). A summary of the roles of copper in the body is in Figure 10.7.

Deficiency of copper

Copper deficiency has been reported in small premature infants, malnourished infants and in adults fed intravenously for long periods.

Premature infants lack the copper normally transferred from the mother in the later stages

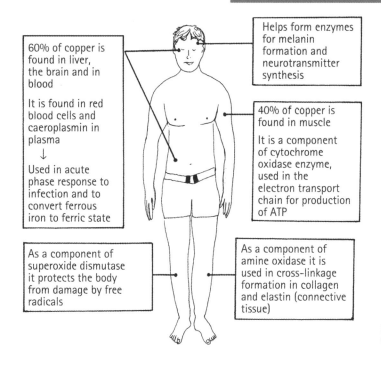

60% of copper is found in liver, the brain and in blood

It is found in red blood cells and caeroplasmin in plasma
↓
Used in acute phase response to infection and to convert ferrous iron to ferric state

Helps form enzymes for melanin formation and neurotransmitter synthesis

40% of copper is found in muscle

It is a component of cytochrome oxidase enzyme, used in the electron transport chain for production of ATP

As a component of superoxide dismutase it protects the body from damage by free radicals

As a component of amine oxidase it is used in cross-linkage formation in collagen and elastin (connective tissue)

Figure 10.7 The role of copper in the body.

of pregnancy. As milk is also low in copper, these infants are particularly vulnerable to inadequate copper status. They may suffer anaemia, neutropenia, skeletal fragility and a susceptibility to infections. Similar signs may be seen in infants being rehabilitated from malnutrition.

In animals, studies have shown increased cholesterol levels and vascular weakness in copper deficiency, which may lead to cardiovascular disease. *In vitro*, copper has been shown to be a pro-oxidant, causing oxidative damage to lipoproteins, thus implying a possible contributory role in atherosclerosis. However, in the body, it is mainly bound to caeruloplasmin, which prevents this damage occurring, and may, therefore, act as an antioxidant. Studies in which subjects were supplemented with additional copper, at 6 mg/day, found no increase in susceptibility of lipoproteins to oxidation.

A rare genetic defect, Menkes' disease has now been shown to be caused by a defect in a copper-transporting ATPase. In this disease, the transport of copper across the placenta, the gastrointestinal tract and the blood–brain barrier is defective, and the individual suffers from acute copper deficiency, with growth failure, mental retardation, bone lesions and anaemia.

Copper toxicity

Copper accumulates in the body in Wilson's disease, a rare genetic disorder, now also found to be due to a defective copper-transporting ATPase. In this case, transport into bile for excretion is affected, so that copper accumulates in the body, and becomes deposited in soft tissues; the condition used to be fatal. Treatment involves chelating agents, which allow the excess copper to be excreted.

Accidental ingestion of excess copper causes vomiting and diarrhoea, which may eliminate the mineral from the body. Chronic poisoning has been reported in patients on haemodialysis, where copper pipes were used, and in vineyard workers using copper fungicide sprays. A maximum safe range for adults has been set at 12 mg copper/day by the World Health Organisation (WHO).

Copper balance is reported to be achieved with intakes of 1.62 mg/day, and a minimum daily requirement has been given as 0.4–0.8 mg/day, by trials on healthy young men. Report 41

(DoH, 1991) proposes an RNI of 1.2 mg/day for adults.

Selenium

The amount of selenium present in the body varies with the local environment, as its content in soil is variable. Levels are low where soils are acid, and rainfall heavy. In some countries, for example, Finland, fertilizers contain added selenium to enhance the content in the soil. In recent years, there has been a reduction in the dietary intake of selenium in some parts of the world, including Britain, and epidemiological evidence suggests a possible link between selenium and certain diseases. As a result, more attention has been paid to this trace element.

The selenium content of foods is related to the protein level, since it is found as selenocysteine (in animal products) or selenomethionine (in cereals). However, it should be remembered that the actual content within a particular sample of food will depend on the level in the soil or in the diet of the animal, and variation may be up to 100-fold. In addition, many Western diets contain foods from different parts of the world. This makes it very difficult to calculate selenium intakes accurately using food tables. Only where there is dependence on local produce can a more accurate prediction of selenium intake be made.

In the UK, brazil nuts are the richest dietary source, with fish (especially shellfish), and offal (kidney and liver) providing a moderate source. Meat and eggs also provide moderate amounts of the element. Cereals and cereal products can provide a useful source, depending on their origin. In the UK, bread was an important source in the past, when flour was imported from North America. Presently, European flour is used, and the selenium levels in bread have fallen considerably. It is believed that this has had a major effect on average selenium intakes in the British diet, which have fallen from an average of 62 μg/day in the late 1980s to 39 μg/day. Fruit and vegetables are generally low in selenium. In the UK, selenium intakes derive mostly from meat and eggs (39 per cent), cereals (22 per cent), dairy products (15 per cent) and fish

Figure 10.8 Sources of selenium in the diet.

(13 per cent). Intakes in vegetarians have been found to be lower than the average in the UK. Selenium is also consumed in the form of supplements (see Figure 10.8 for some sources of selenium).

Absorption and metabolism

Absorption of selenium, especially as selenomethionine, appears to be efficient and may be as high as 80 per cent. Inorganic forms are less well absorbed. In the body, selenium is incorporated into proteins (known as selenoproteins) and found particularly in the liver, kidneys, muscle, red blood cells and plasma. The red blood cell levels remain fairly constant and can be used to assess long-term intake, whereas the plasma level tends to reflect recent intake. Selenium levels in toenail clippings are also used as an indicator of long-term intake. Activity of glutathione peroxidase in red cells is a useful indicator of selenium status; however, it reaches a plateau with high exposure levels.

Urinary excretion is the main means of regulating selenium levels in the body; after high intakes, some selenium may be lost in the breath.

Glutathione peroxidases are the major selenium-containing enzymes in the body. The enzymes occur in several variants, in different locations to provide protection against damage by reactive oxygen species. They occur both intracellularly and in plasma, within cell membranes, and have recently been found in sperm and in the gastrointestinal tract. Their role is to act as a catalyst for the reactions that remove hydrogen peroxide and other hydroperoxides to produce water or other harmless products. Glutathione peroxidase works in conjunction with other cellular enzymes, such as catalase and superoxide dismutase, as well as other dietary antioxidants such as vitamin E and C (see Chapter 14 for more information on antioxidants). Selenium is also involved with iodine metabolism in the conversion of thyroxine (T4) to its active form triiodothyronine (T3), in the thyroid gland.

Selenium has recently been shown to play a role in the normal functioning of the immune system. Defence against infection involves the production of reactive oxygen species, which must be removed by antioxidants to protect immune system cells from damage. It is suggested that selenium plays a key part in this, by protecting cells of the immune system in the lymph nodes, spleen and liver from damage.

The presence of a glutathione peroxidase in sperm has led to research on links between male subfertility and selenium status, with some positive results indicating improvements in sperm motility following supplementation with selenium in men with low status of this mineral.

Deficiency of selenium

Selenium deficiency is closely related to that of vitamin E and adequate amounts of one of the nutrients can in part compensate for a lack of the other. Two conditions found in China – Keshan disease and Kashin–Beck disease – have been linked to low selenium status.

Keshan disease, named after the region where it was originally found, is an endemic cardiomyopathy, characterized by multiple necrosis throughout the heart muscle, which becomes replaced with fibrous tissue. It affects mainly children under 15 years and women of childbearing age living in rural areas, where selenium content of the soil is low. It has a seasonal presentation, and other factors apart from selenium, such as a viral infection, may also be involved. Since the recognition of the involvement of selenium, public health measures, including a more varied diet, have largely eliminated this disease.

Kashin–Beck disease involves degeneration of the joints and cartilage in young people up to the age of 20, leading to painful swelling of joints. Selenium deficiency appears to be a causative factor, but low iodine intake and toxins or contaminants in food, coupled with a poor and unvaried diet probably contribute to this disease. Neither disease is seen in other parts of the world, although selenium intakes may be equally low.

Patients fed intravenously are at risk of deficiency, if attention is not paid to selenium levels. Semi-purified synthetic diets may also be devoid of selenium.

Public health roles of selenium have been studied particularly in relation to cancer and coronary heart disease. Epidemiological evidence points to a possible inverse relationship between selenium status and cancer mortality, especially for prostate, colon and rectal cancers. Prospective studies and supplementation trials provide further evidence that, in populations with low selenium status, there is a possible increased risk of cancer and that supplementation may reduce this risk. However, other evidence suggests that high levels of selenium may stimulate tumour development, so at present a cautious approach is needed. Damage by oxygen reactive species is believed to contribute to the development of atherosclerosis, so the role of selenium within the antioxidant defences is an important aspect of coronary heart disease prevention. At present, data on the specific role of selenium in cardiovascular disease is equivocal.

The effect of supplementation with selenium has also been studied in the context of immune function, which is shown to be impaired in selenium deficiency. Although some benefits have been noted following supplementation with selenium, for example, in infectious disease in the elderly and respiratory tract infection in children, it is too early to assume that this effect would be replicated in everyone, regardless of prior nutritional status. Selenium status declines early in HIV infection, and administration of selenium at this time may slow replication of the virus and progression of the disease.

On the basis of the evidence from China, Report 41 (DoH, 1991) gives the lower reference nutrient intake (LRNI) for selenium as 40 μg/day. The basis of the RNI is the level of intake that will sustain a blood selenium level at which glutathione peroxidase levels reach a plateau in the red blood cell. The values are 75 μg/day for men and 60 μg/day for women. These values are higher than current (2000) recommendations in the USA (55 μg/day for men and women) and figures provided by WHO (1996) of 40 and 30 μg/day for men and women, respectively. Concern has been expressed that the use of selenium supplements may pose a health risk from toxic levels. Maximum upper safe levels have been proposed in a number of countries, ranging from 200 to 450 μg/day.

Iodine

Iodine exists in the body as iodide, which is far less toxic than the iodine from which it derives. Any iodine ingested in food is rapidly converted to iodide in the gut. Iodide is necessary for the production of the thyroid hormones, which maintain the metabolic pattern of most cells in the living organism. In addition, the hormones play a key role in early growth and development of organs, especially that of the brain. In humans, this occurs in fetal and early post-natal life. Therefore, iodine deficiency at this time of life, if it is severe enough to affect thyroid function, will cause hypothyroidism and brain damage, and mental retardation. In the adult, an absence of iodide results in an enlargement of the thyroid gland, but has major consequences when it occurs in pregnant women.

Sources of iodide
Most of the iodine in the world is in the oceans, since the land masses have had the iodine leached from them by glaciation, rain and floods. Thus, soils that are mountainous, land-locked or subject to frequent flooding, together with the crops grown on them are most likely to be devoid of iodine. This is true of many of the central regions of large continental landmasses. In Europe, most countries are still characterized by mild to moderate iodine deficiency, although iodine is added to salt in many of these. However, low urinary excretion of iodine is still found in Belgium, Italy, Czech Republic, Hungary and Romania.

In the UK, iodine status is considered adequate. Milk is the major source of iodide, as a result of increased use of cattle-feed supplements containing iodine as well as iodine in medications and disinfectants used in animal husbandry. In addition, seafoods are a rich source, particularly haddock, whiting and herring. Plaice and tuna have a lower iodine content. Seaweed and products made from it may be rich in iodine, although not all have a high content. Vegans who rely on these sources should ensure that the intake is adequate. In the USA, bread contains iodine from improvers used in the baking industry. Iodized salt is an important source of iodine in areas where food sources are low in the mineral.

Mean intakes of iodine in adults in the UK are 180–250 μg/day.

Absorption and metabolism
Iodide absorption is efficient and the free iodide is concentrated by the thyroid gland, which takes it up actively against a concentration gradient. The gland contains 70–80 per cent of the body's iodide and uses it in the synthesis of thyroid hormones, combining it with the amino acid tyrosine in a stepwise process. The completed hormones contain three or four atoms of iodine. These are stored attached to a protein colloid until required. Release is regulated by the thyroid-stimulating hormone (TSH) produced by the anterior pituitary gland. Any iodine that is not used in the final hormones is recycled. Most organ systems in the body are under the influence of thyroid hormones, which control metabolism.

If the intake of iodine is insufficient, thyroid hormone levels fall and the pituitary responds by increasing secretion of TSH to accelerate uptake of iodine by the gland. Normally, the resulting hormone shuts off the release of TSH. However, in the absence of iodine, insufficient hormone is produced to cause this and TSH secretion continues. This results in enlargement of the cells of the gland as they attempt to trap iodide from the circulation. In addition, unfinished thyroid hormones may accumulate in the gland, contributing to the swelling. The overall size of the gland increases and it may become prominent as a swelling in the neck. This is known as a goitre. Gross enlargement of the thyroid may compress other structures in the neck, leading to difficulties in breathing and swallowing.

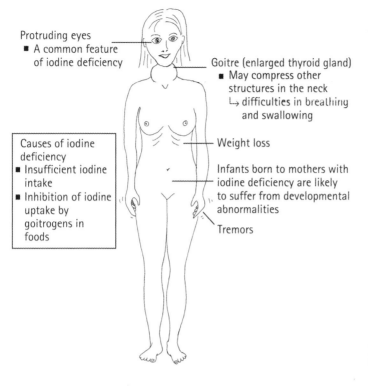

Protruding eyes
■ A common feature
  of iodine deficiency

Goitre (enlarged thyroid gland)
■ May compress other
  structures in the neck
  ↳ difficulties in breathing
    and swallowing

Weight loss

Infants born to mothers with
iodine deficiency are likely
to suffer from developmental
abnormalities

Tremors

Causes of iodine
deficiency
■ Insufficient iodine
  intake
■ Inhibition of iodine
  uptake by
  goitrogens in
  foods

Figure 10.9 Causes and effects of iodine deficiency.

Goitres most commonly become apparent in puberty and during pregnancy, as the needs for iodine increase. The extent of damage to the infant depends on the severity of iodine deficiency but is associated with the failure of hormone transfer across the placenta to function in fetal brain development. Figure 10.9 shows some of the causes and effects of iodine deficiency.

In mild iodine deficiency (intakes of 50–99 μg/day), there is likely to be thyroid enlargement in pregnancy, but no measurable effect on development of the neonate or child. With moderate iodine deficiency (intakes of 20–49 μg/day), there is likely to be congenital hypothyroidism in the infant, and abnormalities of psychoneuromotor and intellectual development in children and adults. In populations with severe iodine deficiency (intakes below 20 μg/day), goitre occurs in 90 per cent of females of child-bearing age. Infants born to these mothers are likely to suffer endemic cretinism, a syndrome of mental retardation, several neurological signs including deaf mutism, spasticity and motor rigidity as well as dwarfism. Up to 15 per cent of children in these areas may be affected.

It has been estimated that this intellectual impairment results in the loss of 10–15 IQ points at a population level, and can severely limit national development.

This is a preventable disorder, since iodide supplements can be given to women in vulnerable areas, either in the form of salt, iodized oil or by injection. Up to 1 billion people live in areas of the world where iodine levels are inadequate, and the use of supplements is a major public health priority to prevent such disability.

There are some interactions between selenium and iodine, whereby selenium deficiency together with iodine deficiency may reduce neurological damage.

Goitre may also arise because of inhibition of iodide uptake by the gland by substances known as goitrogens. These include goitrins, which originate in the cabbage family, and thioglycosides, which are found in cassava, maize, bamboo shoots, sweet potato and lima beans. They are largely destroyed by cooking, but may contribute to 4 per cent of cases of goitre in the world.

Excessive intakes of iodine can also cause thyroid enlargement; this may occur when people consume large amounts of seaweed.

Report 41 (DoH, 1991) states that an intake of 70 μg/day appears to protect populations against the occurrence of goitre; with a margin for safety, the RNI is stated to be 140 μg/day for adults. A European figure for recommended intake is 150 μg/day for adults, with an increase to 200 μg/day in pregnancy.

Chromium

Chromium can exist in either trivalent or hexavalent form, with the former being more biologically active. Both forms appear to exist in tissues and may interconvert.

The richest sources of chromium are spices, brewer's yeast, meats (especially beef), whole grains, legumes and nuts. However, doubts have been expressed about the accuracy of some of the analytical methods used to assay chromium in foods, and values may need to be revised when better techniques are developed. Refining of foods causes a significant reduction in levels of chromium, and consuming a refined diet results in a very low intake of chromium. It has also been suggested that sugars may stimulate loss of chromium in the urine.

Absorption of chromium may be very poor, with less than 2 per cent of inorganic chromium and 10–25 per cent of organic chromium being absorbed in animal studies.

It is postulated that chromium potentiates the action of insulin by combining with nicotinic acid and amino acids to form glucose tolerance factor (GTF). The effectiveness of insulin is, therefore, greater with chromium than in its absence. In addition, chromium may have roles in lipid metabolism, specifically by affecting lipoprotein lipase activity, and in nucleic acid metabolism, by affecting the integrity of nuclear strands.

Chromium is excreted mainly in the urine, at levels of 1 μg/day. Chromium deficiency is not clearly defined, with many people apparently consuming less than the requirement for chromium. Glucose tolerance is improved by chromium supplementation at levels of 150 μg/day of chromium. In general, levels of chromium in Western populations decline with age. There are a very small number of reported cases of chromium deficiency in patients maintained on intravenous nutrition for long periods. Symptoms included impaired glucose tolerance or hyperglycaemia. Chromium is available as a supplement, and suggested roles include amelioration of diabetes and gestational diabetes, lipid abnormalities and insulin resistance. Doses of trivalent chromium up to 1000 μg/day appear to be safe.

Report 41 (DoH, 1991) suggests a 'safe intake' for chromium of more than 25 μg/day, for adults.

Fluoride

Fluoride is essential for the production of hard, caries-resistant enamel in the teeth but, when present in water supplies in amounts greater than 2–3 mg/L, it causes mottling of the dental enamel. Even though these teeth are discoloured, they are still resistant to caries.

Fluoride intake is largely determined by the level in the water supply, as few foods contain significant amounts. Tea and seafoods are the major dietary sources. Where naturally occurring levels are low, fluoride has been added to the water supply of parts of the world for over 50 years as part of the effort to reduce the incidence of dental caries. In addition, fluoride toothpastes are widely available in many countries. These can provide an additional source of fluoride, especially for children, who may swallow significant amounts from the toothpaste.

Fluoride in solution is very readily absorbed from the digestive tract; absorption of food sources ranges from 50 to 80 per cent. After absorption, fluoride is taken up, particularly by the bones and teeth, where it becomes incorporated into the calcium phosphate crystal structure apatite, replacing the (–OH) group, and forming fluoroapatite. This is a harder material, and more resistant to decay than apatite. The presence of fluoride also accelerates the remineralization process when teeth have started to demineralize in the presence of low oral pH. Finally, the presence of fluoride in saliva alters the bacterial flora in the mouth and reduces acid production. Thus, the pH fall after sugar consumption is less in the presence of fluoride. All of these mechanisms help to protect teeth.

In communities where fluoride is present in the water supply at recommended levels of 1 mg/L, there is at least a 50 per cent reduction in tooth decay when compared with areas that have no fluoride. There has been considerable controversy about the desirability of adding fluoride to water supplies, and human rights cases have been heard by the courts. The safety of the procedure has been thoroughly investigated and, at present, there are no scientific data to support the claim that fluoridation is harmful to health. The widespread availability and use of fluoride toothpaste has made a significant difference to caries incidence in most European countries. For individuals who regularly use this, there are few additional advantages from fluoridated water. However, in every society, there are sectors for whom tooth cleaning and the use of toothpaste is not a habit; in these cases, fluoridated water can make an important contribution to dental health. Dental health is discussed further in Chapter 6.

There appear to be no other requirements for fluoride apart from this role in dental health promotion.

Sodium and chloride

These two minerals are considered together, because they occur together in foods and in the body, as well as in seawater and the earth's crust. Salt has been held in very high regard by people throughout history, and there are many expressions in common speech that use the word salt to indicate worth or value. The word 'salary' is derived from salt, indicating the use of salt as a means of payment, or payment as a means of getting salt!

Together with potassium, sodium and chloride contribute in large measure to the osmolality of the body fluids, which, in turn, determines their distribution and balance. Changes in osmolality may involve changes in the content of minerals or of water. Restoration of a normal balance activates mechanisms that regulate mineral excretion or water loss via the kidney, by means of hormonal control, through aldosterone, rennin–angiotensin or antidiuretic hormone, as appropriate.

Sodium is the major cation of extracellular fluid, comprising over 90 per cent of the cations in the blood. Some 40 per cent of the body's sodium is present in bone as an integral part of the mineral lattice, but it is not clear how readily this can be mobilized to maintain sodium levels in extracellular fluids.

Sodium plays a crucial role in:
- maintaining osmolality of body fluids;
- maintaining the extracellular fluid, and hence the blood volume;
- acid–base balance;
- maintaining the electrochemical gradients across cell membranes.

The electrochemical gradients are especially important in nerve and muscle cells, where they are vital for the propagation of nerve impulses and for muscle contraction. They are also important in the absorption of substances across cell membranes against concentration gradients, for example, in the digestive tract and kidneys. The maintenance of electrochemical gradients at all times in the body consumes the greatest part of the daily energy requirement for life, as the ATP pumps move the ions across cellular membranes.

Since sodium is essential to homeostasis, it is clear that the levels of sodium in the body must be carefully regulated, regardless of levels of intake. Further, there is no functional store of sodium, so the daily needs must be met by control of excretion when intake is variable.

Chloride occurs generally in association with sodium as the major anion in extracellular fluid, but it is not found in bone. It can also associate with potassium in intracellular fluids, and can readily cross the cell membrane. In addition to its role in electrolyte balance associated with sodium, it is also essential for the transport of carbon dioxide in red blood cells, and in the formation of hydrochloric acid secreted by the stomach. Chloride is the major secretory electrolyte of the whole digestive tract. Losses of digestive juices, especially in vomiting, can deplete the levels of chloride in the body.

Sodium and chloride in foods

Most foods naturally contain a low level of sodium: plant foods contain very little sodium, while animal foods contain low to moderate levels. The majority of sodium in the diet comes from foods that have undergone some processing or manufacture and to which salt has been added. In addition, salt may be added during home cooking or at the table. In general, the greater the consumption of processed foods, the higher will be the sodium intake. Not surprisingly, sodium intakes are very variable, both within a population, and between people in different countries.

In the UK, average daily sodium intakes are 2.6 g, although the range usually quoted is from 2 to 10 g. Main food sources quoted by DEFRA (2001) contributing to the total intake in the UK are meat products (21 per cent), bread (13 per cent) and other cereal products (24 per cent). If no salt is added to foods, the sodium intake from natural sources would be between 0.5 and 1 g/day. Thus, it is evident that the greater part of our intake originates from added salt.

Sodium comprises 39 per cent by weight of sodium chloride, which represents the major source of sodium in the diet. Total daily intakes of sodium chloride (salt) in the UK average 7.7 g in women and 10.1 g in men, with a range of 3–14 g and 4–18 g, respectively.

Sodium (usually as chloride) is used in food processing and manufacture because of its properties as a:

- preservative (e.g. in meats, dairy products, preserved vegetables);
- flavouring agent (e.g. in breakfast cereals, crisps, packet soups, bread); and
- texture enhancer (e.g. in cheese, preserved meats).

Other sodium salts are used as raising agents (see Figure 10.10).

It is not easy to measure sodium intakes, as there is so much variability between individuals and a proportion of that used in cooking may be discarded before consumption, e.g. in cooking water. A more reliable approach is to measure 24-hour urinary sodium excretion, which closely mirrors the intake. Lithium can be used as a marker of cooking or table salt and measured in the urine.

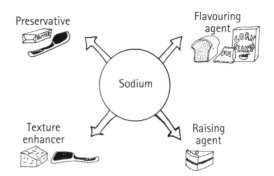

Figure 10.10 Sources of sodium.

Absorption of sodium and chloride

Both sodium and chloride are readily absorbed. Sodium has been shown to be absorbed by a series of pathways that can function in both the small intestine and the colon.

In the West, intakes of sodium are generally much greater than the requirements and, thus, the sodium taken into the body must be regulated by excretion.

Chloride is absorbed passively, generally following electrochemical gradients established by the absorption of cations. It is also extensively secreted into the digestive tract, although most of this is subsequently reabsorbed.

The concentration of sodium in extracellular fluids is maintained at 3.1–3.3 g/L (135–145 mmol/L). If levels increase above this, water is retained to maintain osmolality and the extracellular fluid volume increases. This is subsequently lost by increased sodium and water excretion over 1–2 days. Conversely, a fall in sodium levels will result in conservation by the kidneys of both electrolytes and water. These mechanisms result from the interplay of a number of hormonal and nervous system factors; a full explanation will be found in physiology textbooks.

Sodium excretion occurs principally via the kidneys, which filter and then reabsorb large amounts of sodium in the course of a day. This provides a great deal of flexibility to adjust the plasma levels precisely. Significant losses may also occur in sweat, when physical work is performed in hot conditions. Acclimatization results in a lowering of the sodium losses in sweat; in the short term, exposure to conditions causing excessive sweating may necessitate an increased salt intake.

Excretion of chloride is primarily through the kidneys, where it accompanies sodium loss.

Sodium and health

It is estimated that approximately 30 per cent of the variance in blood pressure is attributable to genetic predisposition and 50 per cent to environmental influences. Genetic variants may affect the functions of the kidney, but also interact with hormonal and metabolic alterations. Salt is one of the environmental influences, and intakes of sodium have been shown to correlate positively with blood pressure, with high intakes considered to be risk factors for stroke and cardiovascular disease. The relationship with blood pressure has been shown in cross-cultural studies and in a meta-analysis of data from a large number of separate studies. The relationship is, however, complicated by the influence of alcohol and BMI, which also influence blood pressure. Nevertheless, when these are taken into consideration, there is a predictable increment of blood pressure with increasing sodium intakes. This increment also increases with age, so that a small increase in salt intake has a greater impact on blood pressure at age 65 than at age 25. Conversely, reducing salt intake can lower the blood pressure, although this effect may take up to 5 weeks to become apparent. Reductions in salt intake have also been shown to potentiate the effects of blood pressure lowering medication. The effects of salt reduction are greater in those individuals with a higher blood pressure and there is still debate as to the effectiveness of salt reduction in normotensive individuals. The amount of potassium in the diet will also modify the response.

In terms of public health measures, the INTERSALT study showed that deaths from stroke were highly correlated with urinary sodium excretion levels in various communities. Community intervention studies, such as in Portugal and North Karelia (Finland), have demonstrated that reducing salt intakes can have substantial effects on the average blood pressure in the community. In North Karelia, the mean reduction in blood pressure was >10 mmHg in adults. In the Netherlands, reducing the salt content of infant formulae resulted in lower blood pressures in the children at follow up, aged 15 years, with no further measures in the intervening period. Results from the DASH-Sodium trial (Sacks et al., 2001) in the USA have indicated that a highly significant reduction of blood pressure can be achieved in normotensive subjects with salt intakes of 3.8 g/day. Modest reductions were obtained at levels of 6.5 g/day. This confirms earlier results found in the original DASH trial in hypertensive subjects. It is important to note that the DASH diet includes a combination of interventions, i.e. the diet is rich in low-fat dairy products, wholegrain cereal, vegetables and fruit as well as low salt intake.

The UK Department of Health (DoH, 1992) in its report on the nutrition of elderly people has recommended that intakes of salt should not exceed 6 g/day; this implies a reduction in average salt intakes in the UK by 3 g/day.

Many people find it difficult to reduce salt intake as they have become accustomed to the taste of their food at a particular level of salt addition. Practical advice needs to be given to help people achieve a reduction; most importantly, this should be attempted over a period of time to allow the taste buds to adapt to lower levels. Depending on the original level of intake, reduction can be achieved by:

- using less or no salt at table;
- reducing amounts of salt used in cooking;
- using alternative flavouring agents, such as herbs and spices; and
- reducing the amounts of processed and manufactured foods in the diet, perhaps by selecting 'lower salt' varieties.

Dietary reference value

The RNI for sodium is 1.6 g/day for adults, with an LRNI of 575 mg/day. The majority of people in the UK consume levels in excess of the RNI. There appears to be no physiological advantage to this, and in the light of evidence of the relationship with blood pressure, it is suggested that current intakes are needlessly high and should not rise further. A reduction in the salt content of manufactured foods would make a significant contribution to reducing salt intakes in the population.

Activity 10.1

If you have previously kept a record of your daily food intake, you can return to this for the activity. If not, first make a list of all the things you have eaten in the last 24 hours.

- Identify the main sources of salt/sodium in this intake (you may need to check food labels to do this accurately).
- What sort of foods are contributing to this salt intake? Are there lower salt alternatives available?
- Plan a modified diet that contains less salt.
- What problems would you have in achieving this? Are there some foods you could avoid straight away?

Special care should be taken with sodium intakes in young infants, as their ability to regulate sodium levels in the body is not well-developed in the first weeks of life. In addition, if there is vomiting and diarrhoea, serious depletion can result.

Potassium

Potassium is the major intracellular cation of the body, with almost all of the body's content found within the cells, the majority of it bound to phosphate and protein. Like sodium, potassium is essential for cellular integrity and the maintenance of fluid, electrolyte and acid–base balance. It is also involved in the propagation of the nerve impulse and muscle contraction. Potassium that leaks out into the extracellular fluids is quickly pumped back to maintain the differential between the composition of the fluids outside and inside cells, on which much of the cellular function depends.

Potassium in foods

Daily intakes of potassium in the UK are reported as 2.7 g. Thus, the levels are similar to those of sodium. Main contributors of potassium in the British diet (DEFRA, 2001) are vegetables and potatoes (29 per cent) and moderate levels are obtained from cereals (15 per cent), dairy products (18 per cent), meat (13 per cent) and fruit (11 per cent). Foods that are rich in potassium include dried fruit and nuts, chocolate, treacle, meat and raw vegetables.

Potassium absorption

This occurs readily in the upper small intestine and colon with 90 per cent of ingested potassium absorbed, although the mechanisms are not fully understood. Potassium levels in the body are carefully regulated to maintain low levels in the plasma (3.5–5.5 mmol/L) and much higher levels (150 mmol/L) in the intracellular fluid. The total amount of potassium in the body is related to the lean body mass.

Regulation occurs by means of hormonally controlled secretion into the glomerular filtrate in the kidneys. The kidneys are very efficient at removing surplus potassium from the body, but less precise at preventing loss when body levels are low. Small amounts of potassium may be lost in the faeces and sweat.

Potassium deficiency is unlikely to occur for dietary reasons because of the widespread occurrence of the mineral in foods. However, low blood potassium may result from excessive losses of gastrointestinal fluids, for example, in vomiting, diarrhoea, purgative or laxative abuse. Certain diuretic drugs may also remove excessive amounts of potassium from the body. These result in mental confusion and muscular weakness. The muscular effects may affect the heart, causing sudden death, or the smooth muscle of the intestinal tract, resulting in paralytic ileus and abdominal distension. This may be a first sign of low plasma potassium in children.

High levels of blood potassium are generally associated with tissue breakdown, in catabolic states and starvation. More potassium is lost in the urine and the body gradually becomes depleted of potassium with shrinkage of the intracellular fluid volume. In uncontrolled diabetes mellitus, accelerated tissue breakdown will cause increased urinary loss of potassium. Treatment with insulin can cause plasma levels to fall dramatically, resulting in cardiac arrhythmias, and care must be taken to avoid this.

Potassium and health

Studies on the relationship between blood pressure and diet have indicated that a high

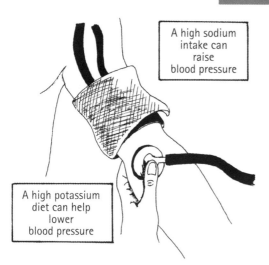

A high sodium intake can raise blood pressure

A high potassium diet can help lower blood pressure

Figure 10.11 Roles of sodium and potassium in blood pressure.

potassium intake is beneficial in reducing blood pressure (see Figure 10.11). In many primitive communities, potassium intakes are much higher than those of sodium. Consequently, these societies tend to have low levels of blood pressure, possibly because of the beneficial ratio of the two minerals. In Western societies, the consumption of fruit and vegetables has tended to decrease, as the intake of processed and manufactured foods has increased, thereby reversing the Na:K ratio. Studies indicate that a higher level of potassium intake (3.5 g/day) facilitates the body's ability to deal with sodium excess. Further, potassium intakes between 2.5 and 3.9 g/day have been shown to reduce blood pressure in both normotensive and hypertensive subjects.

Potassium intakes may need to be restricted in renal disease, when the kidney is not regulating plasma levels effectively. The roles of sodium and potassium in blood pressure regulation are summarized in Figure 10.11.

Dietary reference value

The RNI for adults has been set at 3.5 g/day, although it is recognized that intakes may be much higher than this. Toxicity is unlikely, however, at normal dietary levels. Intakes in excess of 17.6 g/day may cause harmful effects, but these are only likely to occur with supplement use.

FLUIDS – KEEPING THE BODY HYDRATED

Humans can survive for long periods of time without food; several weeks' survival has been reported. However, if fluids are withheld, there is a rapid deterioration and death may result within 10 days.

This is not surprising when we recognize that water is the single largest component of body composition, comprising 50–60 per cent of the total body weight in an average adult. Water content is somewhat higher in males than in females, as the higher percentage body fat in females is associated with less water than is muscle.

Water is an essential component of the body because:

- the process of ingestion, digestion and absorption is facilitated by the presence of water, including the various secretions along the digestive tract containing digestive enzymes;
- elimination of unabsorbed material via the colon requires water to facilitate its passage;
- metabolic reactions occur in an aqueous environment;
- nutrients and metabolites are transported in solution within extracellular or intracellular fluids;
- mucous membranes must be kept moist for normal functioning, including the exchange of gases during respiration in the lungs;
- the excretion of waste products via the kidney occurs in water;
- regulation of body temperature by transfer of heat within the circulation and the production of sweat.

Fluid intake is, therefore, essential for our survival and we require a regular intake. Yet, despite these key roles, there is no recommendation made on the intake of water in the Dietary Reference Values Report in the UK (DoH, 1991).

Fluid balances

There is a daily turnover of body water equivalent to approximately 5 per cent of our body weight. The actual amount depends on a variety of circumstances. The average values for a

TABLE 10.2	Average values for daily turnover of body water in a temperate climate		
Input (mL)		**Output (mL)**	
Food	1000	Urine	1300
Drinks	1200	Faeces	100
Metabolism	350	Skin	750
		Lungs	400
Totals	2550		2550

healthy individual who is sedentary and lives in a temperate climate are given in Table 10.2.

Water loss

It can be seen from the above that water is lost from the body in a variety of ways.

Urine

The amount of urine produced is under hormonal control and is adjusted to achieve fluid balance in the body. Therefore, the volume and concentration of urine will reflect the state of hydration of the individual. Following large intakes of fluid, the urine will be dilute and pale and straw-like in colour. Pale urine is an indicator of a good level of hydration in the body. As fluid intake decreases, or other losses of fluid increase, the colour of the urine becomes darker. Thus, dark yellow or even brownish urine is a sign of severe dehydration. This is a very simple guide that anyone can follow to monitor his or her state of hydration.

The volume of urine is affected by certain dietary items. Protein and sodium contents of the diet can both increase the volume of urine that needs to be excreted (known as obligatory loss). This is associated with the need to eliminate waste products (urea from protein metabolism, and sodium) and maintain homeostasis. Thus, both a high-protein or a high-salt diet will increase obligatory urine losses. In these cases, it is important to increase fluid intakes to ensure adequate levels to meet excretory needs.

Alcohol is a diuretic and, therefore, increases the loss of urine from the body. Whether this will have a dehydrating effect depends on the volume of fluid ingested with the alcohol. It is estimated that a 10 mL diuresis occurs for each gram of alcohol ingested. In practice, therefore, an 8 g intake of alcohol (equal to 1 unit), would cause 80 mL of diuresis. If this was taken as a half pint of beer, then more fluid would have been taken in than was being lost, and dehydration would not result. However, with stronger drinks, taken in a smaller volume, such as wine and spirits, alcohol ingestion will lead to diuresis, causing dehydration.

Caffeine-containing drinks, such as coffee, tea, chocolate and colas, together with some of the 'energy drinks' on the market also have the potential to act as diuretics. This also applies to related compounds, such as theophylline and theobromine, that are found in tea and chocolate. There has been considerable debate about this matter, and widely repeated advice that all of these drinks are of no value for hydration because of their diuretic effects.

However, it has now been established that there is no evidence in the scientific literature to show that at normal intakes of caffeine, that is, less than 300 mg/day, there is any diuretic effect and the beverage can contribute fully to the hydration of the body. In the UK, the daily caffeine intake from tea and coffee has been found to be 239 mg/day, well within the limit stated above. Studies that have indicated a diuretic effect of caffeine have used higher doses than this (300–700 mg), in caffeine-depleted well-hydrated individuals. In this case, caffeine does have a diuretic action.

Although hot beverages, such as coffee and tea, vary in their actual caffeine content, dependent on the method of preparation, average values for these drinks are shown in Table 10.3. It is, therefore, recommended that all of these drinks can be used to hydrate the body without causing a diuretic action.

Faeces

The fluid loss here is generally small. However, amounts can increase if there is diarrhoea when up to 2 L may be lost via this route each day. Diarrhoeal disease associated with contaminated water is a major cause of death in children in developing countries, and emphasizes the importance of aiming to maintain hydration in this situation.

TABLE 10.3	Average caffeine (in milligrams per average serving) for some beverages
Beverage	**Caffeine content (range)**
Tea	40 (30–55)
Instant coffee	58 (42–68)
Filter coffee	90 (60–120)
Decaffeinated coffee	2 (1–4)
Hot chocolate	5 (1–8)
Cola	23 (11–70)
'Energy drinks'	48 (1–70)

Skin

Losses through the skin occur continuously and are an essential part of the body's temperature control mechanism. They will, therefore, vary with the environmental temperature and the amount of physical activity. In a hot environment, the body loses heat by evaporation of large amounts of sweat, and the fluid balance may become disturbed. Amounts of sweat may increase to 2–3 L as a result. Physical activity compounds these losses. Any increase in physical activity generates body heat, which must be lost through sweating. Moderate exercise may increase sweat losses to 1 L/hour. If this occurs also in a warm environment, sweat losses may be as high as 2–3 L/hour. Individuals working in hot environments, such as steel workers, miners and catering workers also have high sweat losses that need regular replacement.

Children exposed to heat may lose proportionately more sweat because of a greater surface area to volume, and will have a more critical need for water to replace this. Thirst mechanisms may not be very sensitive, so encouragement to drink may be needed.

In a person who has a raised body temperature, it is estimated that skin losses of water as part of thermoregulation are increased by 500 mL for each 1°C above normal.

Lungs

Losses occur here continuously, as gaseous exchange in the lungs takes place in a moist environment. Losses increase when there is low humidity, for example, in dry climates or air-conditioned offices, as well as in aircraft and at high altitude. Increased respiratory rates during exercise also increase the hourly rate of water loss from the lungs. Water loss also increases via this route in patients who are attached to ventilators.

Water gain

Water is produced in the body during metabolic reactions and this contributes a small amount to the body's water economy. This is a continuous source of water for cellular needs.

Water is also obtained from the food consumed. Almost all food contains some associated water. Semi-liquid foods, such as soups, yogurts and ice cream, are obvious examples; fruit and vegetables contain a high percentage of water. Even foods that appear to be relatively 'solid', such as bread, cereal foods, cakes, meats and dairy products, contain some water. Some examples are shown in Table 10.4.

It follows that a person who has a small appetite, or is unwell and, therefore, eating very little will gain small amounts of water by this route, and will need to make up for this by increasing their fluid intake. A normal mixed diet, however, will provide up to 1 L of water from the food consumed.

Consumption of liquids is governed by thirst and habit, both of which can be overridden. When fluid volumes fall in the body, there is normally a rise in osmolality of body fluids, and an increase in sodium concentrations. These trigger the thirst mechanism. It can be seen that thirst does not prevent the fall in fluid volume, but follows on from it, by which time there is already some dehydration. Furthermore, the thirst mechanism is not a very sensitive trigger for fluid intake. Other triggers might include a dry mouth and reduced saliva production. Overall, it is much better to be in the habit of taking fluids regularly, without waiting to be thirsty. In people with a high fluid turnover, such as athletes, anticipating the need for fluid and keeping hydrated is a sensible precaution against dehydration. In unusual circumstances, if large amounts of salt have been lost through profuse sweating, an intake of a large volume of water may reduce plasma osmolality further and cause continued

TABLE 10.4	The water content of some foods (as a percentage)
Food	**Water**
White flour	14
White bread	37
Semi-sweet biscuits	2.5
Doughnut	27
Ice cream	62
Lentil soup	78
Baked white fish	76
Peas	78
Boiled potatoes	80
Lettuce	95
Banana	75
Orange	86
Boiled rice	68
Cornflakes	3
Sponge cake	15
Cheddar-type cheese	36
Fruit yogurt	77
Cooked meat	60
Grilled oily fish	65
Carrots	90
Potato chips	52
Tomato	93
Apple	85
Grape	82

urine loss. This situation is potentially dangerous and requires an intake of salt with water to restore normal electrolyte balance. In the majority of circumstances, adequate salt is obtained from normal dietary intakes to prevent this happening.

Large intakes of fluid can also be taken voluntarily, for example, on social occasions. In this situation, there is rarely any thirst for the drinks, but the normal controlling mechanisms are overridden by conscious control.

Similarly, thirst sensations may be weak or can be ignored. The sense of thirst decreases with age, so the risk of dehydration is greater in older adults. Children may also not respond adequately to the sensation of thirst and become vulnerable to dehydration, especially if undertaking physical activity in which they become very involved. The urge to drink may also be ignored if it is inconvenient or difficult to empty the bladder. This may be for social reasons, or because of a lack of facilities, or incontinence or impaired mobility. All of these situations may present a risk of dehydration.

Dehydration

Although there is no doubt about the essential nature of water in the body, the signs and symptoms of dehydration are less well described.

Mild dehydration (a deficit of 500 mL–1 L, or 1–2 per cent of body weight) will cause thirst to be triggered. There is no clear evidence whether this level of dehydration has a detrimental effect on cognitive function. Mild to moderate dehydration (a deficit of 1–3.5 L or 2–5 per cent of body weight) will lead to headaches, early fatigue, loss of precision in tasks, inability to concentrate, irritability and nausea. Progressively greater dehydration will cause an elevation of body temperature, increased heart rate and respiration, dizziness, weakness and raised blood pressure. Ultimately, renal function will be impaired and the person may become comatose. Death can follow if fluid balance is not restored.

The prevalence of mild dehydration is not known, although it is likely that a substantial proportion of the population of all ages have inadequate fluid intake. Concern has been voiced about the need to ensure that schoolchildren have access to fluids during the day to prevent loss of concentration owing to dehydration. Among older persons who are admitted to hospital, dehydration and confusion are common findings.

Some long-term studies have indicated that chronic hypohydration may be associated with higher incidence of colon and breast cancer, although further research in these areas is needed.

How much to drink?

From the above discussion it is clear that fluid intake is important, and the optimal way of avoiding dehydration is to develop a habit of regular fluid intakes without waiting for thirst to intervene. The quantities needed will depend on the factors discussed above that affect fluid losses and will vary between individuals. As a general rule, however, most sedentary adults, in a temperate environment require to drink between 1.2 and 1.5 L each day. This assumes that a further 1 L of fluid is obtained from the food consumed. In this way, a fluid intake of 35 mL/kg body weight per day would be achieved.

What to drink?

Some guidelines suggest 6–8 glasses of water per day, although it is not necessary to consume only water.

As has been discussed above, it is only alcohol that, in practice, has a diuretic effect and may not contribute to hydration. However, low alcohol beers can be used to help towards hydration. Most other commonly consumed beverages can be counted towards the fluid intake allowance. However, it is important to consider some of the other attributes of common drinks when selecting what to consume.

Water
This is often the easiest and cheapest fluid to drink. Consumption of water has increased in recent years, with the popularity of bottled waters. The habit of carrying a bottle of water during the day has become widespread and is a useful reminder to drink.

Soft drinks
These include carbonated drinks, dilutables (squash/cordial) and fruit juice drinks. These are of varying nutritional quality. Some may be 'low calorie' but others may provide up to four teaspoons of sugar per portion. Levels of phosphoric acid are often high in the carbonated drinks and this has cariogenic potential. Some fruit juice drinks have added nutrients, such as vitamin C, but may also be high in sugar.

Fruit juices
These are useful as they provide both vitamin C and possibly phytochemicals that may have additional health benefits.

Milk
This is less popular than in the past, but there is a growing market in flavoured milks and probiotic products based on milk. These may, however, contain added sugar. Milk provides a useful range of nutrients, especially calcium and riboflavin. In addition, it is a useful source of vitamin B_{12}, vitamin A, iodine, magnesium, phosphorus, potassium and zinc. It is a nutrient-dense food, in relation to its energy intake, especially if a reduced-fat milk is drunk.

Tea and coffee
Both of these are popular beverages. They can make a useful contribution to hydration. If drunk with milk, additional nutritional value may be gained.

Overall, it is sensible to consume a range of drinks, according to taste. Care should be taken that drinks do not cause damage to teeth or provide unnecessary additional energy, if there is concern about weight management. Most importantly, fluid intake should be frequent and adequate to maintain hydration.

SUMMARY

1   The minerals constitute a diverse group. Their roles may be structural, protective or regulatory.
2   Levels of the minerals are generally closely regulated, either by control of absorption or by control of excretion, to prevent excessive amounts accumulating in the body.
3   Some of the minerals, especially calcium, zinc, copper and iron, may compete with one another for absorption.
4   Many of the minerals function as cofactors for enzymes involved in metabolic processes. These range from energy transformation to synthesis of essential biological materials in the body.
5   Intakes of the minerals in the UK are generally adequate, with the exception of iron and zinc, where there is evidence of inadequate intake, and absence of stores in a significant proportion of the population.
6   Deficiency states for some of the minerals are more clearly defined than for others. However, in many cases, deficiency is more likely to develop as a secondary consequence, rather than due to primary dietary lack.
7   Fluid intakes may be marginal in some people and represent a significant risk of dehydration. Developing a habit to drink regular amounts of fluids is important.

STUDY QUESTIONS

1 List those groups in the population who are at risk of poor iron status and provide a discussion of the causes for each group.

2 Construct a table to identify some common and contrasting features of iron, calcium and zinc. You could consider the following in your comparison: dietary sources, influences on absorption, functional role and how reference values are set.

3 a Explain why healthy eating advice recommends a reduction in sodium intakes.

   b Which foods might need to be restricted in this case?

4 A number of minerals have a regulatory role in the body. These include iodine and chromium (a role in the function of hormones in the body) and selenium (involved in antioxidant function).

   a Explain these roles.

   b What are the consequences of deficiencies?

5 Develop a table to distinguish those minerals in which a deficiency is most likely to be of primary (dietary) origin from those where a secondary cause is more likely.

REFERENCES AND FURTHER READING

Appel, L.J., Moore, T.J., Obarzanek, E. 1997: A clinical trial of the effects of dietary patterns on blood pressure. *New England Journal of Medicine* **336**, 1117–24.

British Nutrition Foundation 1991: *Calcium.* Briefing Paper No. 24. London: British Nutrition Foundation.

British Nutrition Foundation 1995: *Iron nutrition and physiological significance.* The Report of the British Nutrition Foundation Task Force. London: Chapman & Hall.

British Nutrition Foundation 2001: *Selenium and health.* Briefing Paper. London: British Nutrition Foundation.

Colhoun, H., Prescott-Clarke, P. (eds) 1996: *Health survey for England 1994.* London: HMSO.

DEFRA 2001: *National food survey 2000.* Annual Report on food expenditure, consumption and nutrient intakes. London: The Stationery Office.

Delange, F. 2000: The role of iodine in brain development. *Proceedings of the Nutrition Society* **59**, 75–9.

DoH (UK Department of Health) 1991: *Dietary reference values for food energy and nutrients for the United Kingdom.* Report on Health and Social Subjects No. 41. Report of the Panel on Dietary Reference Values of the Committee on Medical Aspects of Food Policy. London: HMSO.

DoH (UK Department of Health) 1992: *The nutrition of elderly people.* Report on Health and Social Subjects No. 43. London: HMSO.

EURODIET Working Party: Final report. 2001: European diet and public health: the continuing challenge. *Public Health Nutrition* **4**(2A), 275–92.

Hamet, P. 1995: The evaluation of the scientific evidence for a relationship between calcium and hypertension. Report of the Life Science Research Office, Federation of American Societies in Experimental Biology. *Journal of Nutrition* **125**, 311–400.

Heaney, R.P. 2000: Calcium, dairy products and osteoporosis. *Journal of the American College of Nutrition* **19**(2), 83S–99S.

Jeejeebhoy, K.N. 1999: The role of chromium in nutrition and therapeutics and as a potential toxin. *Nutrition Reviews* **57**(11), 329–35.

Maughan, R., Shirreffs, S. 2002: Keeping the body hydrated: why it's necessary and how to achieve it. *Nutrition in Practice* **3**(1), 1–4.

National Osteoporosis Society 1999. *Diet and bone health.* London: National Osteoporosis Society.

New, S.A, 2001: Exercise, bone and nutrition. *Proceedings of the Nutrition Society* 60, 265–74.

Nutrition Society Symposium 1994: Newer aspects of micronutrients. *Proceedings of the Nutrition Society* 53(3), 557–636.

Rayman, M.P. 2002: The argument for increasing selenium intake. *Proceedings of the Nutrition Society* 61, 203–15.

Sacks, F.M., Svetkey, L.P., Vollmer, W.M. et al. 2001: Effects on blood pressure of reduced dietary sodium and the Dietary Approaches to Stop Hypertension (DASH) diet. DASH-Sodium Collaborative Research group. *New England Journal of Medicine* 344, 3–10.

Sojka, J.E. 1995: Magnesium supplementation and osteoporosis. *Nutrition Reviews* 53(3), 71–80.

Strain, J.J. 1995: Micronutrients interactions (symposium). *Proceedings of the Nutrition Society* 54(2), 465–517.

WHO, Food and Agriculture Organisation, International Atomic Energy Expert Group 1996: *Trace elements in human nutrition and health*. Geneva: WHO.

PART THREE

THE APPLICATION OF NUTRITIONAL KNOWLEDGE

11

PREGNANCY AND LACTATION

The aims of this chapter are to:

❏ establish the importance of nutrition in preparation for and throughout pregnancy;
❏ discuss the nutritional needs during pregnancy;
❏ identify specific groups in the population who may be at particular risk in pregnancy;
❏ describe the possible links between pregnancy outcome and long-term health;
❏ discuss the nutritional needs in lactation;
❏ identify some of the influences on the mother in choice of feeding method.

On completing the study of this chapter, you should be able to:

❏ explain the importance of good nutritional status at conception;
❏ discuss some of the metabolic changes that occur in pregnancy in the mother and how these influence her nutritional needs;
❏ explain why certain dietary patterns may be associated with increased vulnerability in pregnancy;
❏ devise general dietary advice for optimal pregnancy outcome.

Based on studies of well-fed pregnant women in the 1950s in the UK, the physiological norm for weight gain in a 40-week pregnancy was set at 12.5 kg. This appeared to be associated with optimal outcome of pregnancy and has been used as a reference since then. The 12.5 kg comprises:

Fetus	3.5 kg
Increased maternal tissues (including uterus, mammary glands and blood volume)	5.0 kg
Stored fat	4.0 kg

These increases were also believed to prepare the mother's body for lactation, in the form of stored energy for milk production.

On the basis of such figures, it would seem reasonable to conclude that the mother needs to consume a significantly greater amount of food during the pregnancy in order to provide sufficient nutrients and energy to build these extra tissues. The corollary of this is that pregnancy outcome, both in terms of the mother's health and the well-being of the baby, would be adversely affected if her nutritional intake were not increased.

In recent years, a better understanding has emerged of the relationship between nutrition of the mother and pregnancy outcome. This has shown it to be very much more complex than stated here, as well as far from fully understood.

This chapter considers the importance of nutritional status before pregnancy, at the time of conception, and in the presence of major physiological changes, which occur during pregnancy. The indicator of outcome of pregnancy that is widely used is the birthweight of the baby. A favourable outcome is the delivery of a healthy full-term infant, weighing between 3.5 and 4 kg (in the UK; some countries use 4.5 kg as the upper end of the range). This is associated with the lowest risk of infant and perinatal morbidity and mortality. Above this birthweight there is an increased likelihood of obstetric complications as well as neonatal mortality and morbidity. Babies born weighing less than 2.5 kg (termed 'low birthweight') have a 40-fold greater risk of neonatal mortality than those born at optimal weight, and the survivors have an increased risk of neurological disorders and handicap, as well as infection. Work by Barker (1998) and others indicates that infants who experience growth restriction in the womb or in early life may be more susceptible to later degenerative disease. It is, therefore, important to minimize these risks wherever possible. It is, however, also important that the mother herself arrives at the end of pregnancy in a healthy state and well enough to be able to care for her newly born infant.

NUTRITION BEFORE PREGNANCY

The nutritional status of a woman at the time of conception reflects her diet and lifestyle over a number of years, even perhaps going back to her own infancy and childhood. These are dependent on many environmental and social factors, which must be taken into account.

Several features of the pre-pregnancy diet may affect the chances of conception or the success of pregnancy. For example:

- vitamin D deficiency in adolescence may have resulted in rickets with pelvic malformations, making a normal delivery impossible;
- a dietary deficiency of vitamin B_{12} may cause infertility; and
- a history of dieting, or in its extreme form anorexia nervosa, can result in poor nutritional status, with low reserves of many nutrients.

Research on underweight women has found that low body fat stores are associated with amenorrhoea and infertility. Evidence of this association comes from records obtained in wartime from places where food supplies were critical, such as Holland and Leningrad, as well as from more recent studies in infertility clinics and on women with anorexia. These indicate that a body mass index (BMI) of 20.8 appears to be a threshold for normal pregnancy, and that there is a minimum ratio of fat:lean body mass needed to support pregnancy.

Women who are obese (BMI above 30) may also experience infertility, as the associated changes in insulin activity and sex hormones may reduce the viability of the ovum.

It would, therefore, appear to be desirable that a woman planning to become pregnant should aim to achieve a BMI within the range of 20–26. If this is achieved by adopting healthy nutritional practices, then the reserves of micronutrients will also be maximized.

Research on primates and human volunteers suggests that the most crucial phase is the 14 days prior to conception, when the follicle in the ovary is growing rapidly before it extrudes the ovum at ovulation. The environment for the developing ovum in the ovary requires appropriate hormone levels. These are crucially dependent on the maternal state of nutrition both in terms of protein as well as other nutrients. These may include iodine to ensure normal thyroid hormone function, magnesium and zinc for the binding of hormones at their receptor sites, and folic acid for the normal growth of the follicle.

It is clear that nutrition prior to pregnancy has long-term implications and that, for an optimum outcome, diets should be adequate and well-balanced before conception.

NUTRITION AT THE TIME OF CONCEPTION

The embryo at conception and in the first weeks afterwards is extremely vulnerable. The majority of the organs and systems develop in the first 8 weeks after conception. The essential energy and nutrients for this are derived from the mother's circulation and from the lining of the womb. It is, therefore, critical that these can provide the necessary nutrients in appropriate amounts. At this stage in the pregnancy, the placenta has not yet formed, so there is no mechanism to protect the embryo from deficiencies in the maternal circulation. It is, therefore, not surprising that nutritional status and nutritional reserves at this time are vital. Studies from the Dutch hunger winter (1944–45) showed that, among the women who did bear children, it was the ones who had experienced the full duration of hunger (8 months) prior to conception who had the most severely affected infants with respect to malformations.

Trials on the prevention of neural tube defects (NTDs) have shown that supplementing the diet of 'at risk' women with folic acid (4 mg/day) for 3 months before conception and up to the 12th week of pregnancy significantly reduced the risk of NTD in the fetus. Since folate is needed for cell division, it is suggested that these levels override a metabolic abnormality linked to neural tube closure. In the majority of cases, it is impossible to predict which women might be at risk and only those who have already had one affected fetus can be identified as requiring particular supplementation. As a result of these studies, women who might become pregnant are now advised in the UK by the Department of Health (HEA, 1996) to increase their intake of folate by at least 400 μg daily. This is more than the typical diet provides and, therefore, foods fortified with folic acid, or folic acid supplements, are needed. The Folic Acid Campaign is further discussed in Chapter 18.

Foods that are a good source of folate are listed in Figure 11.1.

Retinol has also received particular attention in recent years. Reports have suggested that extreme intakes of retinol (doses from 8000 to 10 000 μg/day) are teratogenic (i.e. cause fetal malformations). Such a level of intake is likely to be taken regularly only in the form of supplements. The main dietary source of retinol that might contain these levels is liver. A 100 g serving of liver might contain up to 10 000 μg of retinol; it is unlikely, however, that this would be eaten on a daily basis. Nevertheless, women who may be trying to become pregnant are advised to avoid liver and liver products, as well as supplements that contain megadoses of retinol, as there is a very small risk of harm. No cases of fetal damage attributable to liver intakes have been reported in Britain.

Alcohol is also a potential teratogenic agent, particularly if taken in large amounts, for example, in binge drinking. Women who are

Figure 11.1 Sources of dietary folate.

considering becoming pregnant should, therefore, avoid consuming large amounts of alcohol. This is important in view of the likelihood that damage may be done in the first weeks after conception, before the woman realizes she is pregnant. Later in pregnancy, alcohol taken in moderate to large amounts may result in growth retardation, or more seriously in fetal alcohol syndrome. This includes a series of characteristic malformations and defects affecting the face, heart, brain and nervous system, and is generally associated with reduced mental capacity. For this reason, general advice in the UK is to limit alcohol intake in pregnancy to no more than one standard drink per day and, in any case, to avoid consuming more than 15 units per week. In men who drink heavily, there is likely to be a reduced sperm count, which may be a contributory factor in reproductive failure in a couple.

The weight of the woman and, in particular, her body fat content at the time of conception is also an important determinant of the metabolic changes that occur during pregnancy. Research suggests that a low fat content at conception is a signal to the body to conserve energy so that the metabolism during the pregnancy becomes very efficient and the total energy costs of the pregnancy are low. This is mediated by altered leptin levels. Conversely, in women with high fat stores at conception, there is little energy conservation and the cost of pregnancy is high. Nevertheless, even with this adaptability, mothers with low fat stores give birth to lower birthweight babies than do those with higher fat stores.

Research also suggests that there are nutrients that may be protective at this stage of pregnancy, having an antimutagenic effect. These include riboflavin, vitamins C and E, and mono-unsaturated and polyunsaturated fats. Foods that are particularly rich in antimutagens are fruit and vegetables, although their activity is likely to be destroyed by cooking.

NUTRITION DURING PREGNANCY

Considerable changes occur in the mother's body during pregnancy. In addition to the developing fetus, there are changes in her own tissues, with an expansion of the plasma volume and red cell mass, increase in the size of the uterus and mammary glands and deposition of fat.

In the 1970s, incremental calculations of the amount of extra protein and fat laid down during pregnancy were performed, which gave an estimate of the energy and protein needs of these 'capital gains'. In addition, an allowance was added for the extra 'running costs' of the heavier maternal body. Such calculations produced a figure for the total additional energy cost of pregnancy of about 335 MJ (80 000 Calories). These figures were used in many countries as the basis for setting recommended intake levels for pregnant women.

Recent findings have shown that energy metabolism exhibits considerable variation, with pregnancy being maintained successfully at an additional energy cost of 523 MJ (125 000 Calories) in well-nourished women in Sweden, and with an energy deficit of 30 MJ (7150 Calories) in women in the Gambia not receiving nutritional supplementation. A woman's adaptive mechanisms to pregnancy can include:

- an increase in food intake to meet energy needs;
- laying down of fat stores/mobilizing fat stores;
- an increase or reduction in the basal metabolic rate (including the costs of synthesis and maintenance of new tissues);
- a reduction in physical activity costs (see Figure 11.2).

Activity 11.1

Think about what you have just read, and answer the following question.

How would the following cases cope with the metabolic demands of pregnancy?

- A rural peasant woman in a food-deficient, poor country.
- A normal-weight woman living in an industrialized Western country.
- An overweight woman, living in a Western country.
- A 14-year-old girl, living in a Western country.

In this way, the energy costs of supporting a developing fetus can be maintained at very different levels of energy intake.

In addition to metabolic adaptations in terms of energy, the body also undergoes other physiological changes to increase the efficiency of nutrient utilization and to optimize the supply to the fetus. Many of these changes commence in the early weeks of pregnancy while the fetus is still very small and its nutritional demands low. At this time, the mother may conserve nutrients in her tissues. Evidence suggests that this applies to protein in particular, with reduced amino acid oxidation occurring in the liver. In the later stages of pregnancy, as the fetus enters a rapid growth phase, this protein can be made available from the mother's tissues to supplement that consumed in the diet. In this way, the needs can

be met without a major increase in intake being necessary.

The mother also makes greater use of lipids as a source of energy for her own needs, thus sparing glucose for the needs of the fetus. This change is brought about by alterations in hormone levels, particularly insulin. There are adaptations also in the muscular activity of the intestines, so that food spends a longer time being digested and absorbed. This increases the efficiency of absorption, particularly for minerals such as calcium and iron. In addition, both of these may be better absorbed in response to the physiological regulation, which occurs as a result of the increased need for the minerals.

The slowed activity of the intestines may cause heartburn and constipation. Heartburn arises because the muscles at the top of the

- Increase in food intake to meet energy needs

- Reduction in physical activity costs

- An increase or reduction in the basal metabolic rate (including the cost of synthesis and maintenance of new tissues)

- Laying down of fat stores/ mobilizing fat stores

Figure 11.2 Adaptive mechanisms in pregnancy to conserve energy.

stomach are more relaxed, which allows reflux of the acidic stomach contents into the lower part of the oesophagus, causing irritation and pain. Some practical suggestions for relieving heartburn include:

- eating small, frequent meals;
- taking liquids separately from meals;
- avoiding spicy or fatty foods;
- sitting upright while eating;
- waiting 1 hour after eating before lying down;
- not exercising for at least 2 hours after eating.

Constipation occurs because of the longer time available for absorption of water from the digestive tract. Increasing both fluid and non-starch polysaccharide (NSP) intakes can help to relieve this problem, as will maintaining a moderate level of activity.

WHAT ARE THE DIETARY GOALS IN PREGNANCY?

Generally, pregnant women do not eat a diet substantially different from that eaten by the rest of the female population. Studies around the world of pregnant women in different cultures and at different levels of income show that pregnancy can occur successfully at varying levels of nutritional intake, although there are limits to the protection afforded the fetus at low intake levels. Whether the baby that is born is as healthy as possible may not necessarily be apparent in the first instance, since current research suggests that the intrauterine environment is crucial to long-term health (this is discussed later in the chapter).

Birthweights are lower in babies born to women who have lower energy and nutrient intakes, with particularly strong relationships seen with intakes of the minerals magnesium, iron, phosphorus, zinc and potassium, and the vitamins thiamin, niacin, pantothenic acid, riboflavin, folic acid, pyridoxine and biotin. Increasing the food intake does not result in progressively larger and larger infants. Studies by Doyle and colleagues (1990) show that there is a threshold birthweight (of 3.27 kg) above which extra food intake makes little difference, but below which there is a progressively lower birthweight as intakes are reduced.

TABLE 11.1	Guidelines on weight gain in pregnancy
Pre-pregnancy BMI (w/h^2)	Recommended weight gain (kg)
<19.8	12.5–18
19.8–26.0	11.5–16
26–29.0	7–11.5
>29.0	6 (minimum)

Institute of Medicine 1990. *Part I, Weight gain*. Committee on nutritional status and weight gain during pregnancy. Food and Nutrition Board. Washington DC: National Academy Press. Reproduced with permission.

For optimal outcome measured in terms of lowest perinatal mortality, women who are underweight before pregnancy need to increase their food intake more and gain more weight than those of normal weight. The converse is true of overweight women. Various guidelines are now available for the recommended weight to be gained in relation to pre-pregnancy BMI (see Table 11.1 for figures recommended in the USA).

THE DIET IN PREGNANCY

From what has already been said, it is clear that a pregnant woman does not need to 'eat for two'. The mother's appetite should be a good guide to her overall needs for energy.

In the first three months of pregnancy, up to 70 per cent of women suffer from nausea and vomiting. Although this is commonly termed 'morning sickness', probably only 10–15 per cent of women experience sickness in the morning. In the remainder, it can actually occur at any time of day or night – and in some women occurs continuously. Nausea and vomiting of pregnancy (NVP) is a better name for this syndrome. It may range from a mild nausea to quite severe, frequent vomiting. The condition appears to be more prevalent in societies that consume animal products and it has been suggested that NVP is a protective mechanism against potential parasites and pathogens that may be ingested at a critical time in early pregnancy and threaten the embryo. Paradoxically, NVP appears to be associated with a favourable outcome of pregnancy, including higher birthweight and longer gestation. It has

Diet tips for pregnancy...

To relieve heartburn:
* eat small, frequent meals
* take liquids separately from meals
* avoid spicy or fatty foods
* sit upright while eating
* wait 1 hour after eating before lying down

To avoid constipation:
* increase fluid & NSP intakes (fruit, veg, cereals)
* maintain moderate level of exercise

To avoid nausea & vomiting:
* Eat frequent nutritious meals or snacks
* High carbohydrate foods best tolerated

To avoid dehydration:
* Eat salty foods to trigger thirst

To provide extra nutrients necessary for fetus in last 3 months of pregnancy:
* Increase total food intake
* Eat a variety of different foods
* Increase fruit & vegetable intake to provide vitamins A & C, riboflavin, folate & vitamin D.
* Take extra milk or dairy products for protein, calcium & riboflavin

If pregnant through the winter:
* may need to take vitamin D supplements.

Figure 11.3 Some general diet tips for pregnancy.

been proposed that this may be the result of the adaptation of the placenta to a reduced food intake in the first trimester, which then favours fetal growth once NVP resolves. Frequent meals or snacks are recommended, even if the woman has little appetite for them. It is important that the food eaten is as nutritious as possible and often it is high carbohydrate foods that are best tolerated. Dehydration is also a risk and salty foods that trigger thirst mechanisms may also be useful. An improved quality of the diet may be important to compensate for the period when food intake is low (see Figure 11.3 for general diet tips in pregnancy).

Appetite is usually good in the middle part of pregnancy, so that food intake is at or a little above normal pre-pregnant levels. This ensures an adequate provision of energy and nutrients to form a reserve for the greater needs of the last months.

In the last 3 months, the needs of the fetus are high and the mother's appetite may increase. She is limited in her capacity for food, however, because of the pressure of the enlarged womb on her stomach. The diet chosen should contain a variety of foods to supply the necessary nutrients. Report 41 (DoH, 1991) recommends a small increase in energy intake of 0.8 MJ (200 Calories) per day during the last trimester of pregnancy. This should be provided by increasing total food intake. Together with the adaptations to absorption efficiency and the metabolic changes already mentioned, this will ensure that the additional needs for many other nutrients will be covered.

Particular attention should be paid to certain nutrients for which the increase recommended is greater than can be achieved from a diet designed to just meet the energy requirement. These nutrients are vitamins A and C, riboflavin, folate and vitamin D. Increasing fruit and vegetable intake should provide extra amounts of folate, vitamins A and C. Taking extra milk or dairy products, which can contribute to the extra energy intake and also supplies protein and calcium, will also contribute to meeting the riboflavin needs. Vitamin D requirements may be a problem, especially in women who are pregnant through the winter and are, therefore, unable to synthesize skin vitamin D. If stores have not been accumulated during the previous summer, a supplement of vitamin D is advisable to ensure adequate calcium metabolism. A particular problem may arise in strictly vegetarian women of Asian origin, whose vitamin D status may be precarious, and in whom supplementation with vitamin D has been shown to be of positive benefit for the birthweight and subsequent growth of the baby.

The NSP content of the diet is important in pregnancy because of the tendency for constipation. Including fruit and vegetables and cereal fibre in bread or breakfast cereals can provide sufficient NSP to relieve problems of constipation.

A summary of the dietary reference values for pregnancy is given in Table 11.2.

It should be noted that many of the recommendations made by the UK Department of Health (DoH, 1991) assume an adequate pre-pregnancy diet, resulting in good nutritional status and stores at the outset of pregnancy.

Where these are not present, extra intakes will be necessary during pregnancy.

This is a particular problem with iron because it is recognized that a substantial proportion of women have a chronically low intake resulting in poor stores. An early check on haemoglobin and circulating ferritin will confirm if iron status is adequate or whether supplementation is required.

Moreover, where there is a short interval between pregnancies, levels of some nutrients, such as calcium, iron and folate, may be insufficiently restored. It may take 2 years to return levels to their original values. Attention to a nutrient-rich diet is, therefore, important in this situation.

Teenage girls who become pregnant are also particularly at risk, as their own growth needs are high and stores may be insufficient.

Other advice on dietary intake includes food safety issues. The presence of *Listeria monocytogenes* can cause a series of symptoms from mild to severe, but can also result in premature birth or miscarriage and meningitis in a newborn baby. This is a relatively rare condition (estimates are 1 in 30 000 in the UK), but pregnant women are advised to avoid potentially

TABLE 11.2 Summary of dietary reference values for pregnancy	
Nutrient	**Recommendation**
Energy	Increase by 200 kcal (0.8 MJ)/day in last trimester only
Protein	Extra 6 g/day; total recommended 51 g/day
Thiamin	Increase in line with energy: extra 0.1 mg/day; total recommended 0.9 mg/day
Riboflavin	Needed for tissue growth: extra 0.3 mg/day; total recommended 1.4 mg/day
Nicotinic acid	Metabolism becomes more efficient: no increase needed
Pyridoxine	No evidence that increase needed
Vitamin B_{12}	Little information available about needs: no increase
Folate	Increased usage in pregnancy, maintain plasma levels with extra 100 µg/day; total recommended 300 µg/day
Vitamin C	Drain on maternal stores in late pregnancy: extra 10 mg/day; total recommended 50 mg/day
Vitamin D	Seasonal variation in plasma levels of vitamin; 10 µg/day as supplement
Calcium	Maternal store drawn upon in early pregnancy and enhanced absorption: no increase
Iron	Iron stores, cessation of menstruation and increased absorption should cover needs: no increase
Magnesium, zinc and copper	Increased needs, but assumed to be met from increased absorption

From DoH, 1991. Crown copyright is reproduced with the permission of Her Majesty's Stationery Office.

contaminated foods. These include certain cheeses, such as Brie, Camembert and blue-veined cheeses, and meat-based pate. Cooked chilled meats and ready to eat poultry may also be a source of contamination. Other microbiological contaminants include *Salmonella* and toxoplasmosis (mainly from cat litter).

However, there is little evidence to show that education of pregnant women to improve their diet has significant effects. Targeted interventions may make some impact in specific groups and these are considered below. In general, encouragement of healthy eating and increase in nutritional knowledge for the future benefit of the family are useful targets.

SHOULD SUPPLEMENTS BE GIVEN?

There have been many studies of the effects of various supplements on pregnancy outcome. In general, the effects of supplementation during pregnancy are small.

The provision of a balanced energy and protein supplement to undernourished women results in birthweight increases of less than 100 g. High-protein supplements may actually result in reductions in birthweight, possibly associated with development of a larger placenta rather than increasing the size of the fetus. A better understanding of the metabolic adaptations that occur in pregnant women suggests that the result of supplementation is a decrease in the efficiency of energy saving by the mother, with a resulting higher cost of the pregnancy. It is also unclear how much of the supplement the women consume; it may be used to replace intakes rather than add to existing nutrient levels.

Evidence suggests that the greatest effects of supplementation occur when this is given either in the first 3 months of pregnancy or, preferably, before conception. In the latter case, identifying mothers who have already given birth to a low-weight baby and providing supplements in the inter-pregnancy period has proved to be effective in avoiding a subsequent low weight birth. The Women, Infants and Children Program in the USA, which provides food or voucher support to women in low-income groups has demonstrated a consistent benefit in terms of better health of the baby, and reduced need for health and welfare support in the future. This is a cost-effective scheme with greater savings than costs.

In London, supplementation with multivitamins and minerals, of women who had borne a low birthweight infant and who were found to have a poor diet (not meeting the majority of dietary reference values), resulted in a favourable improvement in folate and iron levels up to 9 months after delivery. However, control subjects who did not receive the supplements continued to have low blood levels of these nutrients. This would be an unfavourable start for a subsequent pregnancy and indicates how poor nutrient intakes can be insufficient to restore blood levels of nutrients in the inter-pregnancy period.

Similarly, supplementation with specific nutrients, such as folate or iron, may be most effective if given pre-conceptionally, or in the very early weeks of pregnancy. Although it occurs routinely in much obstetric care, there is controversy about the desirability of supplementation with iron during pregnancy. Some evidence suggests that pregnancy outcome is optimal at haemoglobin concentrations between 96 and 105 g/L, indicating that this level may be the most desirable. Haemoglobin levels above this value can be achieved by supplementation, but this may be counterproductive.

It could be argued that a low iron status is merely a marker of a generally inadequate diet, which may be low in other, less frequently measured nutrients. It would, therefore, appear to be preferable to improve the whole diet, rather than to focus on specific nutrients, which might result in an unbalanced intake.

The need to supplement with long-chain fatty acids has also been debated, particularly for women whose diet is low in dietary sources. Infant growth and development, especially of the brain and retina, is dependent on an adequate supply of docosahexaenoic acid. Poor status in the mother will mean low levels in the infant. Supplementation of the mother in late pregnancy with fish oil has been shown to increase levels of *n*-3 fatty acids in cord blood of the newborn infant. Supplementation can also increase concentrations of *n*-3 acids in breast milk.

Supplementation with calcium has been used effectively to reduce blood pressure in women at risk of hypertension in pregnancy. The greatest benefits have been seen in women with low dietary calcium levels. The amount used is at least 1 g of calcium per day. Longer term studies of the offspring from these pregnancies have shown lower blood pressures in the children.

WHO IS MOST AT RISK IN PREGNANCY?

A number of groups in the population are particularly vulnerable to poor pregnancy outcome.

Teenage girls

The nutritional status at conception may be poor for a number of reasons. Adolescents are less likely to be eating a well-balanced diet. This applies particularly to girls, who may be chronic dieters as a result of the current fashion for slimness. Low intakes of vitamins A and C, folic acid, calcium, iron and zinc have been reported.

Furthermore, if the girl is still growing, her own nutritional needs may be high and, if she continues to grow during the pregnancy, the baby's development will be compromised. A teenage mother may have social problems, including eating very little to conceal the pregnancy, having little money, perhaps smoking and living in poor-quality housing. All of these factors will contribute to a poorer pregnancy outcome with a higher incidence of low birthweight, perinatal mortality, premature delivery and maternal problems of difficult labour, anaemia and hypertension being reported.

Low income

Women comprise the majority of those existing on low income. The cost of a diet appropriate to meet the needs of a pregnant woman has been calculated to be between 40 and 65 per cent of the state benefits payable in the UK. For most women in this situation, it is unrealistic to spend this amount on food for themselves, and a nutritionally inferior diet is eaten, containing insufficient amounts of nutrients to meet the needs. This leads to a high incidence of low birthweight. Of particular concern is the fatty acid profile of the diet, which may include few long-chain polyunsaturated fatty acids (such as arachidonic and docosahexaenoic acids) that are crucial for development of the neural and vascular systems, and are particularly important in the last 3 months of pregnancy when brain growth is at its most rapid. These essential fatty acids are found in vegetable oils, green vegetables and oily fish, which occur less frequently in the diets of the poor. This deficit may have long-term consequences for the growth and development of their children.

Underweight and overweight women

The importance of adequate but not excessive weight gain has already been discussed. Infants born to underweight women may exhibit inadequate patterns of growth at 12 months, suggesting delays in development. Overweight women also have increased pregnancy risks, both for themselves and the outcome for the baby. In overweight women, dieting during pregnancy is never recommended; a low energy intake during pregnancy may result in ketosis and pose a threat for the developing fetus. However, maintaining a reasonable level of activity during pregnancy is desirable to avoid excessive weight gain and benefit the mother's physiological fitness. Aerobic exercise may be particularly beneficial for women with a predisposition to gestational diabetes, as it enhances insulin sensitivity.

Other situations

Other at-risk situations that may occur are summarized in Table 11.3.

LONG-TERM CONSEQUENCES OF INTRAUTERINE EVENTS

Studies on animals have over many years shown that the tissues and organs of the fetus go through critical periods in their development, at specific times in uterine life. It has also been clear that a positive or negative stimulus occurring during a critical period can have permanent,

TABLE 11.3	Possible indicators of nutritional vulnerability in pregnancy
Indicator	**Possible causes**
Low nutrient stores at conception	Adolescent growth spurt
	Closely spaced pregnancies
	Low BMI
	Intake affected by poverty
	History of dieting/disordered eating
Poor intake during pregnancy (evidenced by poor weight gain)	Poor-quality diet due to: poverty; lack of interest in food; smoking; use of drugs or alcohol
	Previous low-weight birth
	Illness/sickness of pregnancy
	Negative attitude to pregnancy
	Cultural taboos on diet in pregnancy
Pre-existing or gestational disease/condition	Requires special diet/monitoring of food and drug balance during pregnancy
	Weight gain/weight loss

lifelong consequences, even after that stimulus has been removed or cancelled. This phenomenon is known as 'programming', and in evolutionary terms is probably an adaptation to improve the chances of short-term survival, while having longer term consequences that may be detrimental. These are less important from the evolutionary perspective, if the consequence is delayed until post-reproductive life. The relevance of programming to humans has only been recognized from the mid-1980s, and since then an enormous amount of research has been published that shows the fundamental impact of events in fetal life on subsequent health of individuals.

Early clues to the need for this research came from observations that the distribution of coronary heart disease in the 1970s in the UK mirrored patterns of infant mortality at the start of the twentieth century. This suggested that events in early life that caused a high rate of infant deaths might in some way contribute to a higher risk of coronary heart disease in survivors. Following improvements in living standards in the middle of the twentieth century, coronary heart disease rates began to show a decrease in the later decades of the century. This fall could not be

attributed to any major changes in adult lifestyle factors. Furthermore, as developing countries are becoming more Westernized, so prevalence of coronary heart disease and other Western diseases is rising there, in much the same way as they did in the UK in the middle of the twentieth century.

Evidence in support of a link came initially from data contained in birth and development records of babies born in the early decades of the twentieth century, together with mortality records of those who have since died and measurements made on the survivors. A strong negative correlation between weight at birth and the incidence of coronary heart disease later in life was found (Barker, 1998). This did not apply only to babies that could be classified as 'low birthweight', but was true across the whole range of normal birthweights at full term. This negative association between weight at birth and coronary heart disease has since been demonstrated in several different study cohorts, in the USA, India and Norway.

Furthermore, relationships have been demonstrated between weight at birth and the presence of some of the accepted risk factors for coronary heart disease. The evidence suggests that restricted growth during uterine life programmes the fetus in a way that increases subsequent risk of coronary heart disease and other degenerative diseases. As the mechanisms underlying these findings are explored, it has become clear that birthweight alone is a crude indicator of changes that have occurred during uterine life. Changes in body proportions, including thinness, length, head and abdominal circumference are able to give more information about possible organs that may have been advantaged or disadvantaged in utero. The ratio of the placental to birthweight has also shown to be a useful indicator. At either extreme, an imbalance between these suggests that either the placenta was too small to provide adequate nutrients for the fetus, or it was excessively large and, therefore, took a greater share of nutrients for its own development.

At the cellular level, it is understood that programming may:

- alter gene expression, for example, resulting in different levels of enzyme activity;
- affect cell division, resulting in fewer cell numbers within a particular organ;
- influence levels of hormone secretion, or sensitivity of receptor sites to hormones.

Examples of these changes have been demonstrated in animal studies, but application of modern experimental techniques will allow more to be studied in humans to further the understanding of processes that happened in the womb.

Lower birthweight has been associated with the following conditions.

Higher blood pressure

A systematic review of 34 studies by Law and Shiell (1996) has shown a consistent decrease in blood pressure for each 1 kg increment in birthweight. The relationship is less clear during adolescence but is consistent at other ages. The relationship with blood pressure is also found when the ratio of placental to birthweight is considered. A disproportion between these weights, in either direction from the normal ratio of 1:6, is associated with a higher blood pressure. A number of mechanisms have been postulated to explain these findings. Poor nutrient supply may compromise renal development, with reduced numbers of nephrons that become more susceptible to raised glomerular pressure, leading to hypertension. The involvement of the hypothalamus, pituitary and adrenals is considered as a probable mechanism. The model proposes that the fetus is exposed to higher levels of cortisol. These may originate from the mother, as a result of physiological stress, and are insufficiently blocked by low activity of 11-beta-hydroxysteroid dehydrogenase in the placenta and thus reach the fetus. Downregulation of this enzyme has been demonstrated in the placenta in the animal model. Alternatively, the fetus itself experiences stress and generates high levels of cortisol. The raised cortisol levels have multiple effects on the development and sensitivity of blood vessels as well as the response of the hypothalamus to signals from blood pressure receptors.

Insulin resistance and diabetes mellitus

Many studies have confirmed the relationship between low weight or thinness at birth with a greater risk of impaired glucose tolerance, insulin resistance or Type 2 diabetes in the adult. Raised plasma insulin concentrations and slower glucose clearance after challenge with glucose have both been demonstrated in children who were thin at birth. In adults who were thin at birth, lower rates of energy production from glucose in skeletal muscle during exercise have been shown. These findings have led to the hypothesis that the fetal metabolism responds to a reduced nutrient supply by reducing its utilization of glucose. This is achieved by a reduction in levels of insulin and insulin-like growth factor I and increased cortisol levels. Skeletal muscle growth and glucose uptake are both reduced, and amino acids and lactate are used for energy. Thus, there is reduced muscle bulk, resulting in a thinner baby, and a relatively lower glucose utilization accompanied by less responsiveness to insulin. If this metabolic pattern persists into adulthood, it predisposes to the insulin resistance syndrome and Type 2 diabetes.

A further consequence of programming that may determine glucose metabolism affects the size and function of the pancreatic cells that secrete insulin. Animal studies have shown that rats fed protein deficient diets produced offspring with fewer pancreatic islet cells and a reduced ability to regulate glucose. Such a situation will result in insulin deficiency in adult life.

Cholesterol metabolism and blood clotting

Animal studies have demonstrated that impaired nutrient supply to the fetus in the latter stages of gestation results in diversion of more oxygenated blood flow to the cranial region to protect development there. As a result, the trunk and particularly the liver becomes relatively deprived of nutrients, with the potential for permanent changes to be programmed at this stage. Studies on rats fed low-protein diets have identified changes in levels of enzymes associated with lipid metabolism and blood clotting in the liver. Studies in humans have indicated that infants born with a relatively larger head and either a shorter trunk or smaller abdominal circumference, have raised levels of factors produced by the liver. These include blood-clotting factors, such as fibrinogen, and cholesterol fractions. Both of these may contribute to a higher risk of coronary heart disease in later life.

Other conditions

Other possible conditions that may have fetal origins have been investigated. For many, there is still only emerging evidence and more research is needed. These include associations of fetal development with: various cancers, intelligence, obesity, atopy and food allergies, immune status, polycystic ovary syndrome and osteoporosis. In addition, ageing processes appear to be associated with growth and nutrition in early life; lower weight at 1 year has been found to be associated with increased lens opacity, thinner skin, poorer hearing and reduced muscle strength in old age. Figure 11.4 summarizes the fetal influences on later health.

It should be stressed here that not every small baby is destined to have a lifetime of ill-health. The effects of programming are inevitably modified by lifestyle factors. However, it is clear from the research to date that the greatest risk of developing degenerative diseases occurs in those who had been small at birth, or small at 1 year of age and who are then exposed to adverse conditions in adult life (such as weight gain, smoking, a high saturated fat diet, lack of exercise).

The largest babies, or the ones who had grown well in the first year of life, were found to have the lowest risk of developing these degenerative diseases.

These correlations are strong and show up to three-fold differences in risk between those with the highest and lowest birthweights, for example, in the development of impaired glucose tolerance and diabetes. If adult BMI is taken into account, the risk increases to almost seven-fold in those who also become overweight.

The most tantalizing aspect of this research is to discover what aspects of maternal diet are the keys that determine fetal nutrition and development. There is strong evidence that the uterine environment is a major determinant of the size of the fetus. Research from embryo implantation studies shows that the recipient mother has a much stronger influence on the size of the baby than the donor mother, even though the baby has the donor's genes.

A fetus whose rate of growth is rapid is much more susceptible than one growing more slowly to a change in the nutrient supply. The latter appears to be better adapted to withstand a faltering nutrient supply. A key question, therefore, is what determines the setting of the growth trajectory. It is suggested, although human evidence is lacking, that the nutrient availability around the time of conception is critical in determining the partitioning of embryonic cells between fetus and placenta, and sets the rates of growth for both. The availability of nutrients within the mother's womb may itself be determined by her own development as a fetus, when her ovary and uterus were developing. Thus, there is a strong possibility of cross-generational effects that determine the growth of a fetus. There is some evidence to support this proposal, both from studies on rats, where effects of deficiency may take up to three generations to be normalized, as well as from human studies following periods of famine in wartime, where effects have been observed in the following generation.

Many populations have lived for generations in an environment where food supply was poor and the workload heavy; these have been associated with slow fetal growth and small babies. Degenerative disease was relatively rare in these

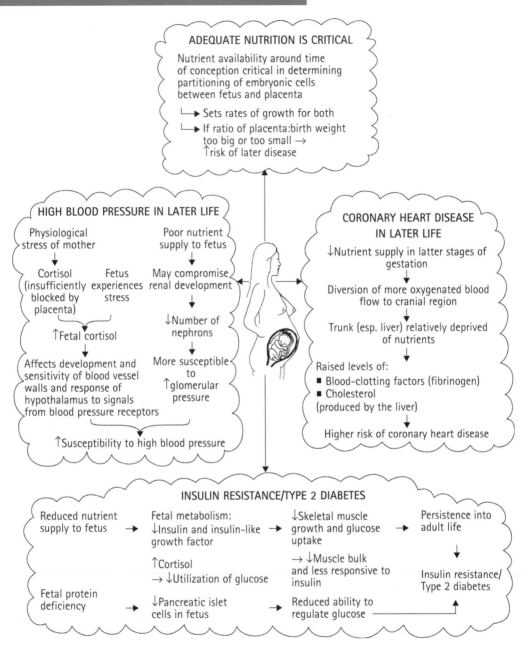

Figure 11.4 Summary of fetal influences on later health.

populations. As Western lifestyles and food habits spread across the world, there is likely to be a transition phase, where maternal capacity to nourish a fetus may still be hampered by a poor uterine environment. Babies will continue to be born small, until the effects of better nutrition improve the overall health of mothers. Thus, there is likely to be an increase in degenerative disease, as small babies become overweight adults, poorly adapted to the plentiful food supplies and lower workloads. This transition phase occurred in the West in the middle of the twentieth century, with a high prevalence of degenerative diseases, but may now be nearing its end, with a decline in some of these diseases. However, developing countries may still be facing the upsurge of diseases, such as coronary heart disease, as they enter the transition phase, especially in urban areas.

Translating this research into practical advice for pregnant women, or those intending to become pregnant is still very difficult. There is insufficient evidence to pinpoint dietary changes that should be made, but overall advice to prepare nutritionally for pregnancy and to maintain healthy eating throughout must remain as the guiding principle. The practice of supplementing the diet during pregnancy may not be beneficial, as the determinants of growth are set very early, before the pregnancy is confirmed. Small babies need to be monitored and the importance of healthy weight and lifestyle stressed in this group, as they have greater vulnerability to disease than those whose weight at birth was higher. The next decade may bring more detailed information about this fascinating area of study.

THE NURSING OR LACTATING MOTHER

Breastfeeding a newborn infant is the natural sequel to pregnancy. The process of lactation (or milk production) does not occur in isolation since the mother's breasts become prepared for lactation throughout pregnancy. By no means all mothers choose to breastfeed their babies. In the UK, prevalence of breastfeeding at birth is around 64 per cent, although there are great differences between middle-class mothers, of whom over 80 per cent may start breastfeeding, and lower social class mothers, where the prevalence is in the order of 25 per cent. For mothers who choose to breastfeed, it is usually a special and enjoyable experience. Those mothers who decide not to breastfeed can provide adequate nutrition for their babies using the many formula feeds available. However, certain aspects of human milk will not be present in the formula. These are discussed further in Chapter 12.

If a woman decides not to breastfeed her child, the breasts return to their normal pre-pregnant size within a fairly short period of time.

THE PROCESS OF LACTATION

There are two stages involved in lactation: milk production and milk ejection (see Figure 11.5).

Milk production or lactogenesis

Milk is made in the mammary glands of the breast, which contain cells arranged in lobules. The synthesis of milk is stimulated by the hormone prolactin released from the anterior pituitary gland, which in turn is stimulated by the process of suckling by the infant at the breast. Thus, the more the infant suckles, the more milk is synthesized and milk production parallels demand.

Some proteins found in milk, such as the immune factors, enter from the maternal circulation, but the majority of the protein content is synthesized by the mammary glands. The fats that contain short-chain fatty acids are synthesized in the breast, but the long-chain fats are derived from the maternal diet. A mother who consumes a high level of long-chain fats will, therefore, have higher levels of them in her milk. The galactose part of the lactose molecule is synthesized in the breast, the glucose part is derived from the maternal circulation.

Milk ejection or let-down

The milk that is formed is not released from the breast until the baby suckles. This initiates a reflex in the mother, involving signals to the hypothalamus, which in turn cause the release of the hormone oxytocin from the posterior pituitary gland. It is this hormone that causes the specialized cells in the mammary gland to contract and eject the milk into the mouth of the infant. The reflex can be inhibited by the mother's mental state: if she is apprehensive, tense or tired, the reflex can fail and milk is not released. An understanding of the nature of the reflex, which allows sufficient relaxation and preparation for feeding, can prevent a great deal of frustration. After about 2 weeks of breastfeeding, the reflex becomes automatic and can be triggered simply by hearing the baby crying.

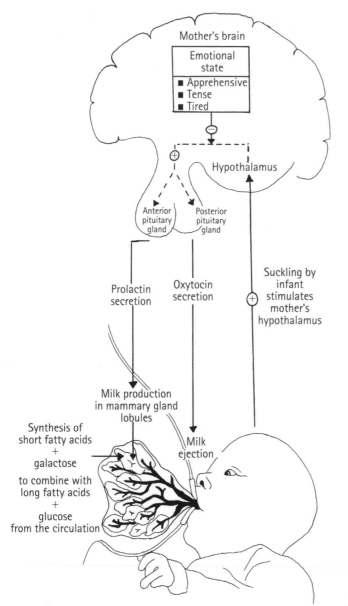

Figure 11.5 The process of lactation.

DIET IN LACTATION

As with pregnancy, no special diet is needed in lactation. It must be remembered, however, that the food eaten by the mother in the first 4–6 months of breastfeeding (before weaning takes place) has to meet all of her own needs as well as those of the baby, which are considerably greater than its needs while in the womb. These increased requirements are reflected in the higher dietary reference values published by the UK Department of Health (DoH, 1991) and summarized in Table 11.4.

Energy

The average daily volume of milk produced varies from mother to mother. Data from the UK and Sweden indicate that the average volume of milk produced in the first 3 months of lactation ranges from 680 to 820 mL/day. The energy cost

TABLE 11.4	Dietary reference values for lactation
Nutrient	**Recommended level**
Energy	Additional 450–570 kcal (1.9–2.4 MJ)/day at 1–3 months
	Additional 480 kcal (2.0 MJ)/day between 3 and 6 months
Protein	To cover protein content of milk, increase by 11 g/day; total recommended 56 q/day
Vitamin A	To cover content in milk, increase by 350 μg/day; total recommended 950 μg/day
Thiamin	Increase only in line with increased energy requirement
Riboflavin	To cover extra content in milk, and its secretion, increase by 0.5 mg/day; total recommended 1.6 mg/day
Niacin	To cover extra content in milk, increase by 2.3 mg/day; total recommended 8.9 mg/day
Pyridoxine	No evidence exists of a need to increase intake
Vitamin B_{12}	To cover the content in milk, increase by 0.5 mg/day; total recommended 2.0 mg/day
Folate	To cover the content in milk, and absorption and utilization by the mother, increase by 60 μg/day; total recommended 260 μg/day
Vitamin C	To cover content in milk and maintain maternal stores, increase by 30 mg/day; total recommended 70 mg/day
Vitamin D	To maintain plasma vitamin D levels: recommend a supplement of 10 μg/day
Calcium	To cover content in milk and allow for efficiency of absorption by mother, increase by 550 mg/day; total recommended 1250 mg/day
Magnesium	To cover content in milk, and allow for absorption, increase by 50 mg/day; total recommended 320 mg/day
Iron	Extra content in milk can be met by lactational amenorrhoea; thus, no extra increment
Zinc	To cover zinc content of milk; no information about enhanced absorption is available; thus increase by 6 mg/day; total recommended 13 mg/day

From DoH, 1991. Crown copyright is reproduced with the permission of Her Majesty's Stationery Office.

of producing this milk, assuming an 80 per cent efficiency of energy conversion, has been calculated as 2.38–2.87 MJ (570–690 Calories) per day in the first 3 months. After 3 months, and assuming that weaning begins at around 4 months, the output of milk falls to 700 mL/day, with an energy cost to the mother of 2.45 MJ (590 Calories) per day.

Some of this extra energy can be met from fat stores laid down in pregnancy, although the extent to which this is mobilized appears to vary between women. It is assumed that, on average, 0.5 kg of stored fat is used per month, although women have been recorded as losing between 0.6 and 0.8 kg/month during the first 4–6 months after delivery. In overweight women, a loss of 2 kg/month may be possible, but feeding on demand should continue to ensure that adequate milk production is maintained. Undertaking intense exercise to speed up weight loss can raise lactic acid levels in the blood, which will pass into the milk and affect the taste.

However, moderate exercise is beneficial and should be encouraged, as long as energy needs continue to be met.

Dietary energy restriction may affect milk output, particularly in the first weeks before lactation is fully established. However, it is also possible that milk output is only compromised when body fat stores are below a particular threshold level. It is also important to recognize that restricting energy intake to a low level will have consequences for the quality of the diet, and may result in other nutrient requirements not being met. There is a concern that toxic chemical residues, which may be present in maternal body fat, will be mobilized and secreted in the milk, if fat stores are used as a source of energy. There is little evidence, however, on which a judgement can be based.

In women who are chronically undernourished and, therefore, have very low body fat reserves, lactation can still occur satisfactorily even in these apparently adverse circumstances.

Studies suggest that the greater efficiency of metabolism seen in pregnancy carries through into lactation, so that costs of maintaining the mother's body remain low, thus providing extra energy for milk production. However, the nutritional content of the milk probably starts to fall from the third or fourth month of lactation.

Protein

The protein content of milk supplies the amino acids necessary for the growth of the baby, and the additional amount should be provided in the mother's diet. If the diet contains sufficient extra energy to satisfy those needs, then the protein content will also be adequate. On a poor diet, where the total food supply is inadequate, it is not possible to provide additional protein, but protein levels in the milk are maintained for several months even under these circumstances.

GENERAL CONSIDERATIONS

It can be seen from Table 11.4 that nutritional needs in lactation are greater than those in pregnancy. However, if a mother satisfies her need for additional energy, then the increased needs for all the other nutrients should be met, assuming the extra food eaten is well-balanced.

Nutrients that warrant special attention are calcium, and vitamins A and D. If it is not possible to increase food intake, then the nutritional quality of the milk may suffer. The water-soluble vitamins, B complex and C, will be present in smaller amounts. The other constituents, namely fats, lactose, protein and fat-soluble vitamins, may remain at an adequate level for 3–4 months, but will then decline. The weight gain of the baby may slow down or stop at this point, and alternative sources of food will be needed for the baby.

THE DECISION TO BREASTFEED

Human milk is ideally suited to the needs of the human infant. Nevertheless, a significant number of mothers do not take advantage of the process of lactation for a number of reasons. The arguments for and against breastfeeding from the mother's perspective are briefly reviewed and summarized in Figure 11.6. An additional

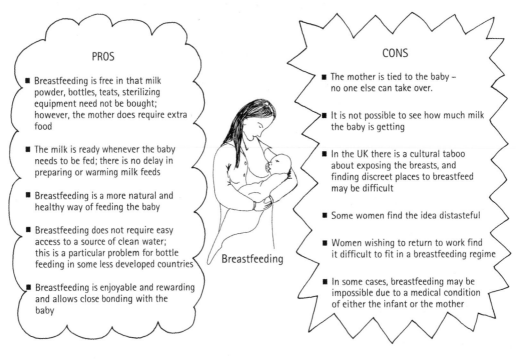

PROS

- Breastfeeding is free in that milk powder, bottles, teats, sterilizing equipment need not be bought; however, the mother does require extra food

- The milk is ready whenever the baby needs to be fed; there is no delay in preparing or warming milk feeds

- Breastfeeding is a more natural and healthy way of feeding the baby

- Breastfeeding does not require easy access to a source of clean water; this is a particular problem for bottle feeding in some less developed countries

- Breastfeeding is enjoyable and rewarding and allows close bonding with the baby

Breastfeeding

CONS

- The mother is tied to the baby – no one else can take over.

- It is not possible to see how much milk the baby is getting

- In the UK there is a cultural taboo about exposing the breasts, and finding discreet places to breastfeed may be difficult

- Some women find the idea distasteful

- Women wishing to return to work find it difficult to fit in a breastfeeding regime

- In some cases, breastfeeding may be impossible due to a medical condition of either the infant or the mother

Figure 11.6 Arguments for and against breastfeeding.

advantage of breastfeeding is that it has been shown to protect women against breast cancer; this may explain the higher rates of breast cancer in developed than in the less developed countries.

The benefits of breastfeeding are discussed further with respect to the infant in Chapter 12.

Because the decision to breastfeed or not is based on so many deeply held beliefs, it should be respected, and mothers who choose not to breastfeed should not be made to feel that they are failing their baby in any way. What matters for the mother and infant is that the mother is confident with what she is doing and can provide all of the nutritional needs that her child requires. She can achieve this with formula milk or by ensuring that her own nutrition is adequate to provide good-quality milk for as long as she wishes to feed her infant.

Activity 11.2

1 Carry out a small survey among your colleagues. Ask whether they have opinions about breastfeeding and try to relate these to their own experience of breastfeeding. This may include seeing siblings breastfed, having breastfed an infant themselves or having seen friends breastfeeding.
   - Is there a gender difference in opinion?
   - Is there an age difference?
   - Do the opinions you collect match those given in Figure 11.6?
   - Can you add others to the list?

2 In what ways do you think health promotion could persuade people to breastfeed their children?

SUMMARY

1 The outcome of pregnancy for both the mother and infant depends on nutritional status of the mother.
2 Nutritional status prior to pregnancy may determine fertility and the early development of the embryo.
3 During pregnancy, the first 3 months are the most critical from the nutritional perspective, as the placenta is not fully developed and the fetus depends entirely on the concentrations of nutrients in the mother's circulation.
4 The needs for some nutrients increase more than others. All nutritional needs can be met from a balanced diet, eaten in sufficient amounts. Many adaptations occur in the mother's body to ensure adequate nutrient supplies.
5 The nutrient supply to the fetus may not only determine the birthweight but also set up the programme for potential health in future years.
6 Lactation is a sequel to pregnancy and also requires adequate nutrition.
7 The quality of the milk is largely protected from shortcomings in the mother's diet for the first 3 months of lactation by increased efficiency in maternal metabolism.

STUDY QUESTIONS

1 Why is it important for a woman to be nutritionally fit at the time of conception?

2 Metabolic adjustments occur in a woman during pregnancy. In the following cases, state what the adjustments are and their consequences for nutritional intake or needs:
   a appetite
   b digestive tract function
   c metabolic rate.

3 Design a poster or leaflet giving practical dietary advice for pregnancy.

4 Why might the following be particularly nutritionally vulnerable while pregnant:
   a vegetarians
   b women on a low income
   c young adolescent girls (aged 13–15)?

5 Identify five reasons commonly cited by women against breastfeeding and consider how you might offer a positive view to counter each reason.

REFERENCES AND FURTHER READING

Allen, L.H. (ed.) 1994: Recent developments in maternal nutrition and their implications for practitioners. *American Journal of Clinical Nutrition* 59(2) (suppl.), 439–541.

Anderson, A.S. 2001: Pregnancy as a time for dietary change? *Proceedings of the Nutrition Society* 60, 497–504.

Barker, D.J.P. 1998: *Mothers, babies and health in later life.* Edinburgh: Churchill Livingstone.

Czeizel, A.E. 1993: Prevention of congenital abnormalities by periconceptional multivitamin supplementation. *British Medical Journal* 306, 1645–8.

DoH (UK Department of Health) 1991: *Dietary reference values for food energy and nutrients for the United Kingdom.* Report on Health and Social Subjects No. 41. Report of the Panel on Dietary Reference Values of the Committee on Medical Aspects of Food Policy. London: HMSO.

Doyle, W., Crawford, M.A., Wynn, A.H.A. et al. 1990: The association between maternal diet and birth dimensions. *Journal of Nutritional Medicine* 1, 9–17.

Food Standards Agency 2002a: *Food portion sizes*, 3rd edn. London: The Stationery Office.

Food Standards Agency 2002b: *McCance and Widdowson's The composition of foods*, 6th summary edn. Cambridge: The Royal Society of Chemistry.

Frisch, R.E. 1994: The right weight: body fat, menarche and fertility. *Proceedings of the Nutrition Society* 53, 113–29.

Godfrey, K.M., Barker, D.J.P. 2001: Fetal programming and adult health. *Public Health Nutrition* 4 (2B), 611–24.

Goldberg, G. 1994: Human pregnancy and lactation: physiological metabolic and behavioural strategies to maintain energy balance. *British Nutrition Foundation Nutrition Bulletin* 19(Suppl.), 37–52.

Goldberg, G., Prentice, A.M. 1994: Maternal and fetal determinants of adult diseases. *Nutrition Reviews* 52(6), 191–200.

HEA (Health Education Authority) 1996: *Folic acid – what all women should know* (leaflet). London: HEA.

Jackson, A.A., Robinson, S.M. 2000: Dietary guidelines for pregnancy: a review of current evidence. *Public Health Nutrition* 4(2B), 625–30.

Langley-Evans, S.C. 2001: Fetal programming of cardiovascular function through exposure to maternal undernutrition. *Proceedings of the Nutrition Society* 60, 505–13.

Law, C.M., Shiell, A.W. 1996: Is blood pressure inversely related to birth weight? The strength of evidence from a systematic review of the literature. *Journal of Hypertension* 14, 935–41.

Livingstone, V. 1995: Breastfeeding kinetics: a problem-solving approach to breastfeeding difficulties. *World Review of Nutrition and Dietetics* 78, 28–54.

Marabou Symposium 1996: Early nutrition and lifelong health. *Nutrition Reviews* 54(2), 1–73.

Rasmussen, K.M. 1992: The influence of maternal nutrition on lactation. *Annual Review of Nutrition* 12, 103–17.

Sayer, A.A., Cooper, C. 2002: Early diet and growth: impact on ageing. *Proceedings of the Nutrition Society* 61, 79–85.

Yajnik, C. 2000: Interactions of perturbations in intrauterine growth and growth during childhood on the risk of adult-onset disease. *Proceedings of the Nutrition Society* 59, 257–65.

The aims of this chapter are to:

❏ describe the nutritional needs of the normal infant and how these are met by human and formula milks;
❏ discuss the process and objectives of weaning and consider the problems that might arise;
❏ consider the diets of pre-school children and the key nutritional principles to be addressed in this group;
❏ discuss the diets of school-age children, including adolescents;
❏ consider the special nutritional dilemmas encountered by teenagers.

On completing the study of this chapter, you should be able to:

❏ explain the relative merits of human and formula milks in feeding normal infants and how these may need to be modified for infants with particular needs;
❏ relate nutritional needs and intakes to the development of the child;
❏ explain some of the reasons why intakes may not be nutritionally sound in school age children;
❏ suggest ways in which nutritional intakes in adolescents could be improved.

Adequate dietary intake and nutritional status among children are important for their own growth and development and function. However, there is now also evidence that childhood nutrition influences adult health. Research has shown that intrauterine nutrition influences adult morbidity and mortality, but childhood diet and nutritional status can modify the consequences of being born small. Diet in all the stages of childhood needs to be taken seriously because of its potential for producing normally developed children as well as determining their lifelong health and thus having an impact on a nation's health. With many diets in transition owing to changing social, economic and environmental conditions, consideration of the impact of these changes on the diets of children is important. Particular issues of concern include the establishment of good dietary habits, together with adequate physical activity to prevent the development of overweight, adequate intakes of calcium to promote bone health, and sufficient intakes of minerals and vitamins in the face of a culture often centred on fast food. There are many gaps in our current understanding of children's food habits and influences on these. It is difficult to obtain good-quality information about these and, therefore, health promotion inputs may be missing their target.

INFANTS

Infants are totally dependent on other people for their food supply. During the first year of life, there is very rapid growth, so for its age and size the infant has very high nutritional needs. Neither of these situations normally occur again in a healthy individual. The main aim of infant feeding is to satisfy nutritional needs in the best possible way, and to achieve a healthy infant who is growing at the appropriate rate and developing normally. Although the main emphasis here is on the principles of feeding normal infants, it must be remembered that infants who are premature, ill, disabled or with any other special needs can also be fed successfully, often by only minor adjustment of the normal practice.

Growth

Babies grow faster in their early months and more slowly in the latter part of the first year. An infant's birthweight is doubled within 4–6 months and trebles within the first year.

Growth is slower thereafter, and the weight at 5 years is on average twice that of the weight at 1 year. Standard growth curves (see Figure 12.1) are used to monitor a child's development in terms of height and weight. They are based on percentiles, which represent the range of expected normal results in a group of children. The position of any one child represents their rank if 100 children had been measured. Monitoring weight and height at intervals allows a child's progress to be followed. Deviations over time from the child's usual curve may indicate faulty nutrition, perhaps as a result of concurrent illness. This may be seen frequently in children in developing countries, who may experience periods of infection, possibly often in addition to chronic poor nutrition, resulting in slowed growth.

As in uterine life, post-natal growth may be slowed owing to insufficient cell multiplication or cell growth. The timing of poor nutrition will determine which aspect of growth is affected more. If fewer cells are made, then it is impossible for this to be remedied later by better nutrition. However, failure of cells to grow may be compensated by 'catch up' growth, if nutrition improves. Key periods of cell multiplication occur at different times for different organs. Brain development, for example, occurs very rapidly in the first months after birth and cell multiplication stops by the age of 12–15 months. Although growth continues, the brain is almost at adult size by the age of 5 years. Thus, infancy and childhood are critical periods for nutrient supply to the brain. There has been considerable debate about critical periods for fat cell formation and some evidence suggests that overfeeding in infancy may encourage multiplication of fat cells. These may be associated with higher leptin levels and possible leptin resistance in later life. However, this requires further study.

Growth may also be affected by emotional factors and stress. Where possible, the cause should be investigated and rectified as quickly as possible to prevent long-term consequences.

Nutrition and development

An infant born at full term is able to suck, but is not able to bite or chew pieces of food, so that its diet of necessity is a liquid one. The liquid designed by nature as food for the newborn is milk produced by its mother. This provides not only nourishment, but also immune protection and developmental stimuli.

Alternative milks have been developed; these are highly modified to make them suitable for infants. In Britain, two types of milks derived from cows' milk are available: whey-dominant types based on the dialysed whey protein, and casein-dominant types based on the entire protein fraction. Modern milks are as similar in composition to human milk as is possible, however, they lack the immunological and hormonal factors. Modified soya milks and other hydrolysed protein formulas have also been developed to meet the needs of children with diagnoses of allergy.

From about the end of the third month of life, the baby can cope with a rusk or cereal mixed with milk, by sucking it or swallowing it with saliva. The ability to bite and chew lumps of food begins at 5–6 months, and it is at this stage that an increasing variety of tastes and textures can begin to be introduced into the baby's diet. An ability to chew lumpy food by 6–7 months is an important developmental step and chewing is best learned at this age. If it is delayed, the child may have difficulty in learning to chew later. The ability to chew is also related to early speech development. Early feeding is thus an important preparation for verbal communication.

By the age of 1 year, the infant has progressed from a newborn only able to suck liquids from a nipple or teat, to increasing independence of eating, and attempting to feed itself. By this age, a child may have up to eight teeth, which help in the biting and tearing of food. Molar teeth for proper grinding of food develop late in the second year, when chewing ability becomes more fully developed.

Figure 12.1 Example of a standard growth curve used to monitor child development. (©Child Growth Foundation. Copies of the chart may be purchased from Harlow Printing, Maxwell Street, South Shields NE33 4PU, UK.)

TABLE 12.1 Reference nutrient intakes for selected nutrients for infants				
Nutrient	0–3 months	4–6 months	7–9 months	10–12 months
Protein (g/day)	12.5	12.7	13.7	14.9
Thiamin (mg/day)	0.2	0.2	0.2	0.3
Riboflavin (mg/day)	0.4	0.4	0.4	0.4
Niacin (nicotinic acid equivalents) (mg/day)	3	3	4	5
Folate (μg/day)	50	50	50	50
Vitamin C (mg/day)	25	25	25	25
Vitamin A (μg/day)	350	350	350	350
Vitamin D (μg/day)	8.5	8.5	7	7
Calcium (mg/day)	525	525	525	525
Iron (mg/day)	1.7	4.3	7.8	7.8
Zinc (mg/day)	4.0	4.0	5.0	5.0

From DoH, 1991. Crown copyright is reproduced with the permission of the Controller of Her Majesty's Stationery Office.

Development of the digestive tract

In the young infant, digestive enzymes are not fully developed and certain dietary components may not be readily digested. Only small amounts of lipase are produced by the pancreas during the first 3 months, and pancreatic amylase increases only after 6 months. Breastfeeding is believed to promote the release of gastrin and cholecystokinin in the infant, and may promote both the digestive process and the development of the gut. A young infant has the ability to absorb some undigested protein. This is particularly important for the absorption of antibodies present in maternal milk or colostrum during the first days of breastfeeding. However, it may also result in the absorption of proteins, such as egg albumen or lactoglobulin from cows' milk, if these are consumed in the early part of infancy. These proteins will generate antibodies within the infant and may lay the foundations of future allergic reactions. There is concern about early exposure of infants and children to peanuts in some weaning foods. A rapid increase in the incidence of peanut allergy, which can be life threatening, is believed to be linked to this early sensitization.

Nutritional needs

It must be assumed that the nutritional needs of the infant are ideally met by breast milk, when this is produced in sufficient quantity by a fully breastfeeding mother. For this reason, the UK Department of Health (DoH, 1991) took the view that no dietary reference values were required for breastfed infants. Values were, therefore, set for formula-fed infants, which are based on the nutritional composition of breast milk and the average amounts consumed. In addition, some allowance is made in certain cases for poorer efficiency of digestion and absorption of the nutrients in formula milks.

Dietary reference values for infants are shown in Table 12.1.

Energy

Energy needs are determined primarily by body size and composition, physical activity and rate of growth. Infants have a high basal metabolic rate owing to the large proportion of metabolically active tissue and the large loss of body heat over a relatively great surface area. In the second half of the first year, the growth rate slows, but the level of activity increases as the child starts to crawl and then learns to walk around the age of 1 year. Total energy expenditure in infants has recently been measured using the doubly labelled water technique, which has produced lower results than had been previously reported. Results from studies of energy intakes confirm these results.

Age (months)	Average weight (kg)		Requirement/kg body weight (kJ (Cal))	EAR (kJ (Cal))	
	Boys	Girls		Boys	Girls
1	4.15	4.00	480 (115)	1990 (480)	1920 (460)
3	6.12	5.70	420 (100)	2570 (610)	2390 (570)
6	8.00	7.44	400 (95)	3200 (760)	2980 (710)
9	9.20	8.55	400 (95)	3680 (880)	3420 (820)
12	10.04	9.50	400 (95)	4020 (960)	3800 (910)

TABLE 12.2 The estimated average requirement (EAR) for energy for children up to the age of 12 months

From DoH, 1991. Crown copyright is reproduced with the permission of the Controller of Her Majesty's Stationery Office.

Activity 12.1

Using the information in Table 7.6, calculate the equivalent energy needs per kilogram body weight for adults. Assume that the average adult male weighs 75 kg and the adult female 60 kg.

■ Compare your figures for adults with those for infants, shown in Table 12.2.

■ What is your own energy need per kilogram of body weight?

■ Calculate the protein need per kilogram for both infants and adults (use the information in Table 4.5).

Table 12.2 shows the gradual reduction in the energy requirement per kilogram of body weight as growth rates slow down; however, as body size increases, the total energy needs become greater. The energy requirement for children is up to four times greater than that of the adult, when expressed per unit of body weight. This emphasizes the special need for adequate energy and explains why a shortfall of energy may have such serious consequences for growth.

Protein

In infants, the role of protein is almost entirely to support growth. The infant requires more protein per unit weight than the adult, and has a particular requirement for the essential amino acids histidine and taurine. Human milk provides a relative excess of some of the amino acids (glutamine, leucine and isoleucine) needed for tissue synthesis, and relatively lower levels of others (arginine, alanine and glycine). This means that the neonate has to be very efficient in transforming some amino acids into others to fulfil needs for tissue synthesis. Adequate amounts of feed should be provided to allow the protein to be used for growth, rather than to meet the energy needs. Excessive amounts of protein are undesirable and may be harmful to the infant, as they increase the amounts of waste material to be excreted in the urine, and might result in dehydration. In addition, immature kidneys cannot adequately filter high molecular weight proteins.

Fats

Fat should comprise 30–50 per cent of an infant's energy intake and, above this level, it may be digested poorly. In breast milk, fats supply 50 per cent of the energy. Fats are an important part of an infant's diet because of their energy density, that is, they provide a substantial amount of energy in a relatively small volume. The essential fatty acids found in milk, and particularly the long-chain n-3 acids, are important for development of the brain, vascular systems and retina in early months of life. In particular, docosahexaenoic acid may not be synthesized in sufficient amounts by the infant from precursors in the diet to meet the needs of tissue development.

Carbohydrates

Carbohydrate, predominantly in the form of lactose, supplies 40 per cent of the energy in an infant's diet. Lactose yields glucose and galactose on digestion; the latter is essential in the development of the brain and nervous system. Undigested lactose is fermented in the digestive tract to lactic acid and lowers the pH. This is beneficial as many of the pathogenic organisms that can cause gastroenteritis do not thrive in an acidic environment. Infants can also digest and utilize sucrose, although this sugar is sweeter tasting than lactose and can induce a preference for sweet foods in the infant. The ability to digest starch is limited.

Fluid

Because of their relatively small total body water content, babies have a vital need for fluids. Their small body weight/surface area ratio makes them susceptible to dehydration, for example, in hot weather and illness. As an absolute minimum, the normal infant requires daily between 75 and 100 mL of fluid per kilogram body weight, and should be provided with 150 mL/kg, to ensure that all needs are met. Under normal circumstances, this amount of fluid is provided by the milk feed and no additional water is required.

The infant loses water through the skin and respiratory tract, through sweating in warm environments and through the urine and faeces. The volume of urine produced is dependent on the fluid intake and on the amount of solutes to be excreted. An adult kidney is able to concentrate solutes and reduce water loss, if fluid intake is low, but a baby's kidneys initially lack this ability. Thus, feeding a diet with a high 'solute load', in particular with high protein and sodium contents, results in increased water loss via the kidney. Under normal circumstances, fluid intake should be sufficient to cope with this. However, difficulties may arise if:

- a baby is given an overconcentrated feed (unmodified cows' milk is inappropriate for this reason);
- amounts of feed are very small (due to illness);
- there is fluid loss via other routes (vomiting, diarrhoea, sweating);
- solids are given at a very young age (below 2 months).

In each of these cases, additional water should be given to avoid dehydration.

Minerals

Babies require a wide range of minerals in their diet. These include calcium, phosphorus and magnesium for bone development, iron and copper for red blood cell formation, zinc for cell division and growth, together with other trace elements. The iron content present at birth has usually been used in red blood cell formation by 4–6 months, and an additional source of iron is needed at this stage. Calcium and phosphorus are present in equimolar quantities in human milk, which matches the ratio in the body. An excessive intake of phosphorus can dangerously lower calcium levels. This is a particular problem in premature infants and those fed on unmodified formula. The minerals in human milk are associated with the protein or fat fractions of the milk, which probably facilitates their availability.

Vitamins

The vitamin content of milk is generally adequate, with the exception of vitamins D and K. Human milk is low in vitamin D and the UK Department of Health (DoH, 1991) recommends that breastfeeding mothers should take a vitamin D supplement of 10 μg/day to ensure adequate levels in their milk, especially in the winter months. Formula-fed infants receive adequate levels of the vitamin.

Breastfed infants are also at risk of low vitamin K intakes. It has been routine practice to give newborn infants a dose of the vitamin in the first days of life by intramuscular injection. Although the evidence is not clear-cut, there has been concern that this may increase the risk of childhood cancer and oral administration of the vitamin is now recommended until the issue has been clarified.

Meeting nutritional needs

A baby's nutritional needs are generally met either by the use of human milk from the breast or formula derived from cows' milk, modified to a composition resembling that of human milk. The continued development of formula milks ensures that they come closer to the content of human milk than ever before. In Western societies, mothers are free to make the choice between breastfeeding and bottle-feeding, without fear that their baby will be disadvantaged in any way as a result of their decision. The professional consensus is that breastfeeding is better for the baby, and possibly confers benefits to the mother. In many poor areas of the world, the use of infant formula may increase health problems rather than solving them. Where standards of hygiene are poor, with inadequate water supplies and non-existent or poor sanitary facilities, it is almost impossible to prepare artificial feeds with the degree of cleanliness necessary to prevent infection. In addition, poverty may tempt the mother to prepare excessively dilute feeds in an attempt to extend the supply of the milk powder. This can and does lead to serious malnutrition in the infant. In such a situation, the only safe choice for infant feeding is with human milk from the breast. The spread of formula milk throughout poor regions of the world has resulted not only in greatly increased deaths from infection in infants, but has also removed the birth-spacing benefits of breastfeeding.

BREASTFEEDING OR BOTTLE-FEEDING?

Across the world there are programmes and activities to promote breastfeeding, since it is recognized as nutritionally the best way of feeding the newborn infant. The World Health Organisation (WHO) and the United Nations Childrens Fund (UNICEF) jointly promote the Babyfriendly Hospital Initiative (BFHI), which encourages hospitals to put in place a number of measures that will facilitate the initiation and continuation of breastfeeding. Some 15 000 hospitals have been certified as Babyfriendly around the world, with around 260 in industrialized countries.

A series of studies on behalf of the Department of Health in the UK has taken place since 1975 to provide national statistics on the incidence, prevalence and duration of breastfeeding and other feeding practices adopted in the early weeks and months after birth. The most recently reported of these was carried out in 2000 (Hamlyn et al., 2002). The survey identified the reasons given by mothers for the choice of infant feeding method. Most women decide before the birth how they will feed the baby. The decision is based on the mother's own attitude to the idea of breastfeeding, but is also influenced by the views of her mother, friends and partner. Previous experience of feeding is also a strong influence.

Breastfeeding is more likely in mothers from social class 1, compared with social class 5. However, there have been marked increases in prevalence among women in social class 5 since the earlier surveys. There is also a higher prevalence among older mothers, ranging from 46 per cent in teenage to 78 per cent in mothers over 30 years. Improvements have also been noted in prevalence among mothers educated to age 16 (to 54 per cent), where the rates had been lowest, compared with rates in those educated beyond the age of 19 years (88 per cent prevalence reported).

Reasons cited for choosing breastfeeding are generally very positive, including that it is the best and most natural way of feeding the baby (79 per cent of respondents said this) and that it is convenient (37 per cent said this). Other reasons mentioned included that it develops a closer bond with the baby, is cheaper and more natural. Those who choose to bottle-feed have more negative views about breastfeeding, considering that they would be tied to the baby and wanted others to be able to feed it (25 per cent), worrying about how much milk the baby receives and generally finding the idea distasteful (19 per cent).

The attitude of society in general is important in helping women make the choice, and in supporting and helping breastfeeding mothers. Unfortunately, many people have negative attitudes to breastfeeding, considering it inappropriate and even shameful behaviour, especially if carried out, however discreetly, in public; this can affect the new mother. The ambivalent view of society about the function of breasts can make it difficult for some women to consider feeding their baby themselves.

There has been an increase since 1990 in the number of women attempting to breastfeed their baby, with 71 per cent starting to breastfeed in England and Wales (and 63 per cent in Scotland, 54 per cent in Northern Ireland). The overall figure for the UK is 69 per cent. However, the numbers who continue to breastfeed decrease quite rapidly, falling to 52 per cent by 2 weeks, 42 per cent by 6 weeks and 28 per cent by 4 months. However, 13 per cent of mothers were still breastfeeding at 9 months. These rates are lower than in most other north European countries.

The most common reasons for stopping in the early weeks were given as rejection of the breast by the baby and painful nipples. However, when feeding continued for more than a week, but had stopped by 4 months, insufficient milk was the most commonly cited reason for stopping. In reality, this should rarely be a reason for failure to breastfeed, and probably represents inadequate support and information being made available in the first days of breastfeeding while the process is becoming established. More help for new breastfeeding mothers could increase success rates. An additional reason for stopping breastfeeding between 4 and 6 months was that the mother was returning to work (mentioned by 39 per cent of respondents).

Overall, this survey shows an encouraging improvement in incidence and prevalence of breastfeeding. In particular, improvements have occurred in those groups where previous levels of breastfeeding had been lowest.

Formula milk and breast milk compared

The composition of formula milks available in Britain is governed by a directive from the European Commission (EEC, 1991), and Statutory Instrument 77 (MAFF, 1995). Derived from cows' milk, they are classified as 'casein-dominant', based on the entire protein fraction, or 'whey-dominant', containing the dialysed whey protein. Modifications include the addition of lactose, maltodextrins, vegetable oils, various vitamins and trace elements, and reductions in the level of protein, electrolytes and some minerals, such as calcium.

Bottle-feeding, if carried out correctly, with due attention to hygiene, appropriate concentrations and closeness during the feeding, can provide most of what the infant needs. However, the unique composition of human milk, with over 200 constituents and with a varying content, will probably never be matched by a manufactured formula feed. The composition of breast milk is not constant between women and within the same woman for different lactations and even during the day. The milk secreted towards the end of a feed (hind milk) is richer in fat and, therefore, higher in energy value than the fore milk, at the start of the feed. This may play a part in appetite control, with the richer hind milk providing a feeling of satiety. Obviously, this cannot happen with a formula feed.

Proteins in milk

The proteins in human milk are predominantly whey proteins, including alpha-lactalbumin, lactoferrin and various immunoglobulins; casein forms only 30–40 per cent of the total protein. Although the lactalbumin is a major source of amino acids, the other whey proteins have a non-nutritional role, in particular, as protective agents (see below for their role in immunity).

In cows' milk, casein comprises 80 per cent of total protein, which can form tough, leathery curds in the stomach and be more difficult to digest. In the formula milks based on whey, the casein content is reduced (from 27 g/L in cows' milk, to 6.0 g/L). Beta-lactoglobulin, which is normally found in cows' milk and is a potential allergen, is also absent from these formula milks.

Human milk also contains non-protein nitrogen compounds, including taurine, urea, and a number of hormones and growth factors. Their functions are still uncertain but may well help with the normal development of the infant. Until their function is clearly defined, it is unlikely that these substances will be included in formula milks.

Carbohydrates in milk

Lactose concentrations in human milk are greater than in cows' milk, although levels in formula are similar. Formula milks may also contain maltodextrin as a source of carbohydrate. Lactose enhances the absorption of calcium as a result of the lower pH resulting from fermentation to lactic acid, which makes the calcium more soluble.

Fats in milk

Although the total fat contents of human and cows' milks are similar, the fatty acid compositions are quite different. Modified milks contain added oils to increase the unsaturated fatty acid content towards that of human milk. Nevertheless, there remains a much greater diversity of lipids in human milk, which contains cholesterol, phospholipids and essential fatty acids. Digestion and absorption of fat from human milk is aided by the presence of lipase within the milk secretion, which starts the process of digestion before the small intestine is reached. Some milks have been reformulated to include more essential and long-chain fatty acids.

Vitamins

The levels of the water-soluble vitamins in milk reflect the maternal levels, and thus rely on a sufficient intake by the mother. In the West, it is rare for vitamin levels to be deficient in milk due to maternal undernutrition. Human milk also contains binding factors for folate and vitamin B_{12}, which facilitate their absorption. Most formula milks contain levels of the vitamins greater than those found in human milk. However, apart from vitamins D and K, for which intake may be too low from human milk, there appears to be no advantage in this.

Minerals

Levels of many minerals are modified in the manufacture of formula from cows' milk. This is because their concentrations would generally be too high for the human infant to cope with. In particular, this applies to calcium, phosphorus and the electrolytes. Many of the minerals are associated either with proteins or fat globules, and this appears to facilitate their absorption. Specific binding factors have been identified for iron and zinc, which make the absorption of these minerals from human milk much greater than that from formula.

Immunological factors

Apart from the nutrients and water, human milk contains a number of other constituents. Most importantly, it contains a range of substances that enhance the immune system of the baby.

Among these are:

- white blood cells – T and B lymphocytes, neutrophils and macrophages;
- immunoglobulins, which are the circulating antibodies;
- lysozyme, which has specific antibacterial action;
- lactoferrin, which binds iron to prevent its uptake by bacteria that need it for growth and replication, and also promotes growth of *Lactobacillus* sp.;
- bifidus factor, which promotes growth of *Bifidobacteria* that prevent the growth of potentially pathogenic bacteria;
- cytokines and growth factors.

The overall effect of these constituents is to promote the development of the baby's own immune system and reduce the risk of infection, while it is still immature. Immune factors specific to the environment are produced by the mother's gastrointestinal and respiratory tracts, which then stimulate the mammary glands to synthesize similar compounds. Thus, the immunity provided is 'tailor made'. Evidence from around the world, including both industrialized and developing countries, indicates that there are lower infection rates in breastfed compared with bottle-fed infants.

Other factors

Human milk may also contain substances passed through the mother, such as drugs, alcohol, nicotine and pollutants. This causes some concern to mothers and, where possible, such agents should be avoided when feeding the baby. However, environmental pollutants may be stored in maternal body fat and be released during the lactation process. At present, there is insufficient evidence to decide the risk from these.

HIV infection may be transmitted through breastfeeding. However, whether a woman who is infected chooses to breastfeed is largely dependent on the alternatives available to her and her baby. If these are safe, it is probably better to feed with formula; if not, then the recommendation of the WHO is that breastfeeding is the better option. The advantages of breastfeeding in these situations still outweigh the risk of infection from HIV.

Other milks available

Alternative milks are available for infants who are allergic to cows' milk or lactose. The most widely available are those based on modified soya protein. These milks contain glucose and carry a possible risk to teeth. Their use should be carefully monitored. Hydrolysed protein formulas are available for highly allergic children and these should be used under supervision.

Special milks for babies born pre-term are also available, although their use is still controversial. It has been recognized that mothers giving birth to pre-term infants, produce milk that has a higher content of fat, protein and sodium, and less carbohydrate. This would appear to be necessary to sustain the rapid growth of the baby and to compensate for the lack of reserves with which it is born. A combination of breast milk and pre-term formula is considered the best compromise for these infants.

Future health

It has been claimed that breastfeeding confers advantages in terms of the later health of the baby. Some studies have shown more advanced development during childhood in those children who received breast milk, even for a short period in infancy. A meta-analysis by Anderson et al. (1999) showed that breastfeeding conferred an advantage of 3.2 point increments in cognitive function by adolescence. A study of adults aged 53 (from the British 1946 birth cohort) confirmed that breastfeeding was significantly and positively associated with educational attainment, but this was largely accounted for by the cognitive effect at 15 years.

Other possible advantages that have been proposed include less allergic disease, lower cholesterol levels, less obesity, heart disease and multiple sclerosis. Breastfed infants have higher levels of low-density lipoprotein (LDL) and very low density lipoprotein (VLDL) as infants; this may be linked to lower cholesterol levels in later life, through adaptation of enzyme levels.

Some of these advantages are difficult to show and require long-term studies. However, using records from the early years of the twentieth century, Barker (1994) has shown that men who were breastfed beyond the age of 1 year actually experienced higher mortality rates. It is suggested that this is a reflection of inadequate nutrition and possibly restricted growth, since breast milk is not a complete food beyond about 5–6 months. On the other hand, other work by Barker shows that infants who gained weight well and had highest weights at the age of 1 year had the lowest incidence of impaired glucose tolerance and cardiovascular disease. Clearly, nutrition in the first year of life has to be good enough to promote growth and development for long-term health. However, more information is needed.

WEANING

The process of weaning an infant literally means 'to accustom' the baby to new foods, and in so doing to diversify the diet from milk to one containing solid foods. The age at which this occurs and the foods used vary between different cultures and communities, and may be as early as 2 months or as late as 12 months. Neither of these extremes is nutritionally ideal. The optimal age of weaning is between 4 and 6 months.

In the UK, the Infant Feeding Survey 2000 (Hamlyn et al., 2002) has shown that there had been a move to slightly later introduction of solids. Although 24 per cent of mothers had introduced solids by the age of 3 months, this was less than half the number recorded in 1995. By the age of 4 months, 85 per cent had introduced solids and almost all the babies in the survey were receiving some solids by the age of 6 months.

Early weaning is more common in social classes 4 and 5, in the north of England and Scotland, among bottle-fed babies and by mothers who smoke.

Why should a baby be weaned?

Developmental advantages ensuing from weaning have already been mentioned. Further, from the age of 4 months onwards the physiological development of the baby allows more varied foods to be ingested and digested, and their waste products to be excreted. Early weaning tends to result in faster weight gain but, by the age of 1 year, differences between infants weaned before 8 weeks and those weaned after 12 weeks have disappeared. In addition, there is a small tendency for infants weaned early to experience more respiratory illnesses and cough in the first year of life. Early weaning may precipitate an allergic response, and in infants who are at high risk of developing allergies, weaning as late as possible is advised.

Weaning has important developmental advantages. The ability to manipulate a bolus of food in the mouth and swallow it, to coordinate a utensil and bring food to the mouth and to drink from a cup all help in the development of muscles in the face. These are important in the acquisition of speech.

From the nutritional point of view, weaning is required to provide certain nutrients that can no longer be supplied in sufficient amounts by breast or formula milk. In particular, this applies to energy, protein, iron, zinc, vitamins A and D.

There is particular concern about iron status in infants, with low stores and the possibility of anaemia in 12 per cent of young children. The low iron status may result in delayed psycho-motor development and defects in cellular immunity.

An infant's stomach capacity is considerably smaller than an adult's, which makes it very important to ensure that the foods offered contain enough energy in a compact form. Commonly, the first food introduced to the infant is the local staple cereal. In the West, this may be specially formulated, designed for weaning and enriched with a number of nutrients. Rice (or other non-wheat cereals) is preferred to wheat,

which may cause gluten allergy to develop. In developing countries, the local staple is used, prepared as a gruel or porridge.

Other purées may then be introduced, for example, potato, vegetable, pulse or fruit purées, dairy products such as custard or yoghurt. These are all smooth with a relatively bland taste, with which the infant can gradually become familiar. As the child becomes accustomed to the novelty of solid foods, minced meat, fish and other sources of protein, such as sieved soft cheese can be included, together with vegetables and fruit that have been minced or mashed to retain more texture.

As chewing ability develops, the pieces of food offered become more distinct, allowing chewing to be practised. 'Finger foods' held in the hand allow the child some independence and help to develop coordination, as well as providing some nutritional value. These can include rusks, fingers of toast or pieces of hard cheese.

The diet should aim to provide a variety of different food groups, to ensure that a range of nutrients is consumed (Table 12.3). Particular attention may need to be paid to iron and vitamin D sources; vitamin C will help the absorption of iron and should also be provided. Some examples of suitable foods to provide these nutrients are shown in Table 12.4.

Milk should remain the cornerstone of the infant's diet, as it contains important amounts of protein, calcium and vitamins, as well as providing energy. Amounts of milk offered should be 600 mL at 4 months when weaning starts, but still 350 mL in the 1-year-old. The type of milk offered to the infant is also important. The UK Department

TABLE 12.3 Suggested food groups to be included in the diet at 6–9 months and 12 months

Food group	Number of servings/day	
	6–9 months	12 months
Bread, cereals, potatoes	2–3	At least 4
Fruit and vegetables	2	At least 4
Milk and dairy products	500–600 mL milk	2–3 servings + 350 mL milk
Meat, fish and alternatives	1	1–2
Fatty and sugary foods	Avoid	Limit

TABLE 12.4 Sources of iron, vitamin C and vitamin D suitable for weaning

Sources of iron	Sources of vitamin C	Sources of vitamin D
Red meat (beef, lamb), pork poultry	Unsweetened fruit juice: diluted	Oily fish, e.g. sardines
Liver, liver sausage	Citrus fruits, e.g. oranges, satsumas	Eggs and egg dishes
Oily fish, e.g. sardines	Summer fruits: strawberries, peaches, nectarines	Fortified margarine
Eggs and egg dishes	Green leafy vegetables	Breakfast cereals fortified with vitamin D
Beans and lentils	Tomatoes, green pepper, peas	Baby cereals fortified with vitamin D
Baby foods fortified with iron	Potatoes	Evaporated milk
Breakfast cereals with added iron		Some yogurts
Green leafy vegetables		
Dried fruits, e.g. apricots, prunes		
Fish fingers		

of Health (DoH, 1994) recommends that infants should continue to receive breast milk, formula or a 'follow-on' milk up to the age of 1 year. 'Follow-on' milks have been introduced in recent years, as suitable for infants from 6 months of age. They are less modified than infant formula, but still contain added nutrients to provide a valuable source of nutrition. Drinks should be offered in a cup, and the practice of leaving a child with a bottle or 'trainer' cup (one with a feeding spout) for periods of time is discouraged as it can lead to pooling of drink in the mouth. This can cause decay of newly erupted milk teeth.

Pasteurized cows' milk should not become the major milk drink until after the age of 1 year. This is because it contains low levels of iron and vitamin D, and may contribute to deficient intakes if taken as the main milk in the diet. However, cows' milk may be used to make dishes containing milk, such as custards and sauces. Infants should not be given low-fat milks, such as skimmed milk or semi-skimmed milk, as these contain insufficient fat and, therefore, have a low energy density.

Throughout the weaning process, it is recommended that:

- the child is always supervised during mealtimes;
- sugar and salt are not added to the infant's food;
- foods should not be heavily spiced;
- nuts should not be included in the diet;

- soft-boiled eggs should be avoided because of possible contamination with *Salmonella*; hard-boiled eggs are safe;
- pâté and mould-ripened soft cheeses (such as Brie) should be avoided because of the risk of *Listeria* contamination;
- drinks other than milk should be offered from a cup from the age of 6 months; they should be dilute and unsweetened.

Special 'infant drinks' may contain large amounts of sugar and should be avoided or only used rarely and with care. Infants should never be left with a sugary drink in a feeding bottle, as newly erupting teeth may be damaged.

Commercial weaning products are of value. They are often fortified with additional nutrients, which is especially useful when the child has a very small intake, when home-prepared foods may provide very few nutrients.

Infants cannot cope with large amounts of foods rich in non-starch polysaccharides (NSPs), such as whole grain cereals and pulses, and these should not be an important part of the weaning diet. However, small amounts can be included, and quantities increased when appetite is bigger.

By the age of 1 year, the infant should be eating solids several times per day, and be included in family meals. The complete process of weaning may take longer than this, however, and full chewing ability will not be attained until the molar teeth have erupted towards the end of the second year.

Tips for weaning

★ First try porridge (avoiding wheat which may cause gluten allergy), purées of vegetables, pulses or fruit, custard or yoghurt

★ Next: minced meat, fish, soft cheese, minced fruit & vegetables.

★ To develop chewing & coordination use finger foods: rusks, fingers of toast, hard cheese

★ Continue to breastfeed or use formula or follow-on milk up to 1 yr

★ Don't use pasteurised cow's milk as a separate drink but use full fat milk to mix custards, porridge etc.

★ Avoid sugary drinks and especially never in a feeding bottle

★ Make it a pleasurable learning experience for the infant.

Figure 12.2 Summary of how to wean a baby.

Supplements of vitamins A, C and D are available; these are recommended for all infants from the age of 1 to 5 years, and for breastfed infants from the age of 6 months. The daily dose of supplement provides $200\,\mu g$ of vitamin A, $20\,mg$ of vitamin C and $7\,\mu g$ vitamin D.

It should be remembered throughout that the infant is undergoing a process of learning about food and, to develop a child with a broad appetite for foods, many different tastes should be offered. Variety in the diet helps to ensure an adequate nutritional intake. Nutrients that need attention remain iron, zinc and vitamin D. Refusal of a specific food need not eliminate it completely from the diet. It can be reintroduced later. Important foundations are being laid down at this time and it is essential that the caregiver makes this a pleasurable learning experience for the infant. Sometimes the weaning process falters and a child that has been gaining weight may stop doing so. This has been called 'failure to thrive' and is of multifactorial origin. There is no evidence that it is associated with deprivation and neglect. There appears to be an underlying lack of interest in food in the child, slower eating and diminished appetite. Delayed progression on to solids and a limited variety of foods eaten have also been described. Intervention with dietary advice and practical management of mealtimes can result in rapid improvement, if there is no underlying organic cause. The process of weaning is summarized in Figure 12.2.

THE CHILD FROM 1 TO 5 YEARS OF AGE

These years provide a time to move from the milk-centred diet of the first year of life to the typical diet of the family. In nutritional terms, this represents a change from a diet which contains approximately 50 per cent fat, no NSP and simple sugars rather than starches (as seen in the milk-fed infant), to one meeting or approaching the dietary guidelines, with 35 per cent fat, 11 per cent non-milk extrinsic sugars and plenty of starch and NSPs. Clearly, there needs to be a gradual transition from one to the other.

The food habits developed at this time will be the foundation for the approach to diet and nutrition for the rest of the individual's life. During this period, the child will also develop some independence in relation to food, and this may lead to conflict with the parents. Infants more readily accept new foods and tastes. During early childhood there may be an increasing reluctance to try new foods. This served a protective function in the past, as a young child began to wander off and might have been tempted to try a hazardous food. Exposing children to new foods is, however, important. Perseverance, which may necessitate up to five or ten exposures to the food can pay off. Modelling on others who are eating the food is a helpful way of persuading a young child to accept it. Finally, presenting a novel food together with a familiar taste can be useful, for example, as part of a liked dish. Parents have an important role in determining what food is available for the child in the home. The attitude of parents to food is central, and conscious or subconscious preferences for foods, or attributes attached to a food will be passed on to the child. Foods used as a positive reward ('have some chocolate for being a good boy'), or a hurdle to be overcome to achieve something pleasurable ('eat your vegetables and then you can go out to play') can foster attitudes to these foods that were not necessarily intended. Children need guidance and family food rules are beneficial to provide a framework in which their own food habits can develop. Ideally, these should focus on healthy foods and eating patterns.

Growth is slower than in the first year of life but tends to occur in spurts, often accompanied by surges of appetite. Activity also increases markedly during the second year, as the child becomes increasingly mobile. Full dentition by about the age of 2 also increases the dietary repertoire. Because capacity remains relatively small, between-meal snacks are likely to be needed in addition to the three main meals of the day. It is important to maintain healthy eating

guidelines in mind when selecting snack foods, since these should be contributing to total nutritional intake, rather than being additional to it. Unfortunately, poorly selected snacks, often comprising little more than sugar, in drink or solid form, can seriously compromise nutritional intake, as they dull the appetite at mealtimes. Snacks can include:

- fresh or dried fruit (although the latter may stick to the teeth and be cariogenic);
- wholemeal sandwiches with nutritious fillings;
- raw vegetables as 'finger food' to chew;
- dry breakfast cereal;
- low-sugar or savoury biscuits;
- yoghurt or milk;
- popcorn (plain, rather than sugar coated);
- scones or similar plain cakes.

Meals should consist of nutrient-dense foods, with at least 250 mL of milk daily, and cereal and bread used to fill up to appetite. Appetite remains the best guide to overall food needs at this age.

Food refusal can be a major problem, and can cause a great deal of stress to parents. The child needs a consistent and firm response from the parent, so that the association of eating with mealtimes is learned. If the child does not eat at table and is then allowed to snack between meals, disorganized eating habits may develop for the rest of their life. Experimentation with food within limits is important. Given a wide range of foods to experience, we all develop as individuals in our choice of foods with specific likes and dislikes. Ideally, our children should develop with few dislikes, if we give them the appropriate guidance and personal example.

A national study (Gregory et al., 1995) of children aged 1.5–4.5 years, as part of the National Diet and Nutrition Survey in Britain, found that, on the whole, children were eating large amounts of salt and sugar, and insufficient fruit and vegetables. Although the mean intake of energy was found to be lower than the estimated average requirements, the children appeared to be growing well. As a result, it has been suggested that energy requirements may need to be decreased by 10–12 per cent from their current levels. Other findings included the following.

- Those who had the highest energy intakes also consumed the most NSP.
- Total sugar intakes represented 29 per cent of total energy and starches 22 per cent; the intake of non-milk extrinsic sugars comprised 19 per cent of total energy.
- There was a reciprocal relationship between fat and sugar intakes.
- Fat intakes were generally between 34 and 36 per cent of total energy and, therefore, in line with Department of Health recommendations (DoH, 1991). It should be remembered that young children should not be rigorously put on low-fat diets, as this can compromise their total energy intake. Other studies show that low-fat/high-fibre diets are being given to this age group, reflecting confusion about healthy eating guidelines.
- Iron intakes were low in a proportion of children: 24 per cent of those aged 1.5–2.5 years, and 16 per cent of those under 4 years had intakes below the lower reference nutrient intake (LRNI), with low ferritin levels indicative of low stores of iron, and low haemoglobin levels resulting in anaemia in 1 in 12 of the sample. Apart from help with iron-rich foods, parents may need advice about promoters and inhibitors of iron absorption.
- Dental caries was found in 17 per cent of this age group.

In a secondary analysis of these data, it was found that only 1 per cent of children met the reference nutrient intake (RNI) recommendations for iron, zinc, vitamins A and C, and guidelines on non-milk extrinsic sugars (NMES). Two or fewer of the targets were met by 76 per cent of the children. Compliance with the recommended levels of intake was related to socio-economic status, with more children from lower social groups, with a head of household in a manual category and mothers with fewer educational qualifications meeting the least number of RNIs/recommendations.

Overall, it can be concluded that the quantity of the diet of this age group in the UK is currently adequate, although certain aspects of its quality probably need attention. In particular, there needs to be:

- more attention given to iron-containing foods;
- a reduction in both the amount and frequency of consumption of sugars, especially in the form of soft drinks; these could be replaced by milk or water;
- a reduction in the consumption of savoury snacks that are high in salt;
- an increase in the consumption of fruit and vegetables;
- more attention to the impact of socio-economic factors on food choice in families.

SCHOOL-AGE CHILDREN

Influences on nutritional intakes

When children start school, their eating patterns begin to be increasingly influenced by factors other than the home environment. However, it should be remembered that parents remain the 'gatekeepers' of what is consumed at home and can still have a considerable influence by determining what is provided at mealtimes, and what snack foods are available for children to help themselves. They also continue to serve as important role models.

Autonomy

A study of 9-year-old children in the UK reported that this group felt that parents had a great deal of control over their food choices. However, the greatest number (90 per cent) reported control over the content of breakfast, with 2/3 reporting control over snacks and only 1/3 reporting control over the amount of food eaten (Robinson, 2000). This appears to leave children with a reasonable amount of autonomy in various aspects of their diet.

Adolescence itself is a time of transition, associated with progress towards autonomy. This is reflected in all aspects of the teenager's life, but inevitably impacts on food choice and nutritional intake.

Rejection of food selected or prepared by parents is a normal aspect of this developing autonomy. Foods chosen as alternatives may be less healthy, as a gesture of independence and perhaps peer solidarity. There is also likely to be experimentation with foods and adoption of novel dietary practices. At other times, the adolescent may still want to be part of the family and eat what is provided in the home.

Growth

Growth rates are relatively slow during the pre-adolescent years, but growth still occurs non-linearly with surges accompanied by increases of appetite. Periods of slow growth may be accompanied by a relatively small appetite and, at such times, particular attention must be paid to the nutrient density of the diet. In adolescence, periods of rapid growth take place that have profound effects on appetite.

School may also be emotionally taxing for children, which may affect their food intake. In addition, beginning school is often accompanied by exposure to many childhood infections and periods of (often minor) illness. These can have an impact on food intake and, if numerous, may affect growth.

Activity

Apart from growth, activity is the other main influence on appetite in this age group. Starting school may significantly alter a child's activity pattern, the direction of the change depending on how active the child was during pre-school years. Children of primary school age tend to be relatively more active in their play and levels of activity have been shown to decline in a large proportion of adolescents, especially girls. Following the *Health of the nation* report (DoH, 1992), physical activity in children has become a focus of policy in the UK, with recommendations made for an increase in activity in this age group. There is concern that many hours are being spent watching television, playing computer games and staying in the house, rather than being involved in physical activity or even just walking. Estimates from studies in Scotland suggest that teenagers may now expend between 2 and 3 MJ (500–700 Calories) per day less than their peers did 60 years ago. Average time spent watching television has been shown to be positively associated with increased body weight,

skinfold, fat mass and prevalence of overweight in pre-pubertal children. The reasons for this association are complex.

Societal pressures

Pressures from friends will increasingly influence food intakes as a child goes through school, and this becomes most notable in adolescence. In addition, societal pressures linked to body image have a major impact on the food intake of some individuals, especially girls at this age. Adolescence is the peak age for dissatisfaction with body image and attempts at dieting are prevalent, more so in girls than boys at this age. Changing food trends are particular influences. In recent years, there has been a major shift from traditional meals, and many children and teenagers consume a series of snacks during the day rather than eating 'normal' meals. The choice of foods available in fast-food outlets can be a limiting factor for making healthy selections.

There is also widespread concern about the impact of advertising on food choices in this group. Food advertising is the single largest category of advertisement shown during children's television programmes. The majority of these are for products that are high in sugar and fat and low in fibre, and include confectionery, snack foods and breakfast cereals. This trend is also seen in other countries, such as the US and Australia. The advertisements for these foods are often humorous, animated and easy to follow, so that they are memorable to children. In contrast, there are no advertisements for foods that should form a substantial part of a healthy diet, such as fruit and vegetables. Although advertisements by themselves do not change food habits, there is concern that the balance of those shown is in conflict with health promotion messages.

Nutritional needs

Steady growth during childhood up to adolescence, increasing per year by 10 cm in height and 2.5 kg in weight, is reflected by a gradual increase in the need for nutrients. There is a certain amount of accumulation of stores during this time, most notably of body fat, which then becomes available to contribute to the fuel required for the pubertal growth spurt. Calcium is also laid down and provides some of the needs for bone growth.

At adolescence, growth rates are greater than at any other time of life, except early infancy. In most girls, the growth spurt begins between the age of 10 and 13, in boys between 12 and 15 years. In both cases, rapid growth takes place over a period of 3 years. Girls gain lean tissue and fat, and increase by 20 cm in height and 20 kg in weight. In boys, there is a loss of fat and a gain in lean tissue, with increases of 30 cm in height and 30 kg in weight. These increases account for approximately 40 per cent of adult weight. It is to be expected, therefore, that the nutritional requirements at this time will reflect this growth.

The timing of the need for additional nutrients varies with the individual, and depends on the onset of growth. In the West, peak appetite occurs around the age of 12 in girls and 14 in boys, apparently corresponding to the most rapid growth period. The demand for new tissue synthesis results in increased nutrient requirements for:

■ calcium, phosphorus, magnesium and vitamin D for bone;

■ protein, zinc and iron for muscle;
■ iron, folate, vitamin B$_{12}$ and copper for the synthesis of extra blood cells to supply it with oxygen;
■ adequate energy to sustain this synthesis, and the B vitamins to release it.

If energy needs are not met, the growth spurt may be delayed or reduced. However, energy needs for growth probably do not exceed 10 per cent of total energy requirements at this time.

Once the growth spurt is over, nutrient requirements settle down to adult levels.

Selected dietary reference values are shown in Table 12.5 for the age groups from 4 to 18 years. In addition to these specific guidelines, children's diets should approach the general recommendations on fat and carbohydrates (shown in Table 12.6).

No distinction is made between genders for the majority of nutrient requirements for children up to the age of 10 years. After this age, with the onset of the pubertal growth spurt, different figures are set for male and female adolescents. In part, these reflect the different body weights at these ages. However, special needs for menstrual losses are incorporated in the iron requirement calculations.

TABLE 12.5 Dietary reference values for children from 4 to 18 years								
Nutrient	Age 4–6		Age 7–10		Age 11–14		Age 15–18	
	M	F	M	F	M	F	M	F
Energy								
(MJ/day)	7.16	6.46	8.24	7.28	9.27	7.92	11.51	8.83
(Cals/day)	1715	1545	1970	1740	2220	1845	2755	2110
Protein (g/day)	19.7	19.7	28.3	28.3	42.1	41.2	55.2	45.0
Thiamin (mg/day)	0.7	0.7	0.7	0.7	0.9	0.7	1.1	0.8
Riboflavin (mg/day)	0.8	0.8	1.0	1.0	1.2	1.1	1.3	1.1
Niacin (nicotinic acid equiv.) (mg/day)	11	11	12	12	15	12	18	14
Folate (μg/day)	100	100	150	150	200	200	200	200
Vitamin C (mg/day)	30	30	30	30	35	35	40	40
Vitamin A (μg/day)	500	500	500	500	600	600	700	600
Calcium (mg/day)	450	450	550	550	1000	800	1000	800
Iron (mg/day)	6.1	6.1	8.7	8.7	11.3	14.8	11.3	14.8
Zinc (mg/day)	6.5	6.5	7.0	7.0	9.0	9.0	9.5	7.0

From DoH, 1991. Crown copyright is reproduced with the permission of the Controller of Her Majesty's Stationery Office.

There are no dietary reference values (DRVs) given for vitamin D, as it is assumed that sufficient will be synthesized in the skin during everyday activity. However, some children of Asian origin may require a dietary supplement.

These dietary guidelines should be met in the same way as for adults, by eating a diet in line with the Balance of Good Health, which provides an appropriate balance between the five main groups shown. Thus, the diet should provide mainly starchy carbohydrate sources, fruit and vegetables (five servings per day of each of the two groups). In addition, there should be three servings of milk and dairy produce, and two servings of meat and alternatives. Intakes of fatty and sugary foods should be limited; they may be included in the diet when the needs for the other four groups have been met.

TABLE 12.6	General recommendations on fat and carbohydrates
Total fat	35% of food energy
Saturated fatty acids	11%
Polyunsaturated fatty acids	6.5%
Total carbohydrate	50% of food energy
Non-milk extrinsic sugars	11%
Intrinsic and milk sugars + starch	39%
Non-starch polysaccharides	18 g/day

Activity 12.2

Return to Activity 12.1 and perform a similar exercise for children and adolescents for the following body weights:

Age (years)	Male weight (kg)	Female weight (kg)
5	18	17.75
10	31	31.5
14	49	48
18	65	55.5

It is helpful if meals are planned to include items from each of the food groups wherever possible.

WHAT DO CHILDREN AND ADOLESCENTS EAT?

Studies of children's attitudes to healthy eating in recent years have shown that in general children understand the concept of a balanced diet as described in the 'Balance of Good Health' model. They are also aware of the relationship between diet and health, both present and for the future. Children also demonstrate an awareness of the potential risk for heart health of excessive fat intakes, and the desirability of a normal body weight. The health implications of being too thin and the dangers of eating disorders are also recognized. For this age group, however, social pressures are important, and knowledge does not necessarily translate into behaviour.

A number of studies took place during the 1980s and early 1990s on groups of children from 5 to 17 years of age. In general, these studies showed that the health of schoolchildren in Britain is good. There was no widespread evidence of dietary deficiency, and no biochemical or functional improvements were seen with the use of supplementation. However, a European study has reported that the diet of UK children is amongst the worst in Europe, being high in fat and sugar, low in fibre, iron and calcium and possibly folate.

A new survey of young people aged 4 to 18, which is part of the ongoing National Diet and Nutrition Survey programme in the UK was published in 2000 (Gregory et al., 2000). This was a comprehensive study, including 7-day dietary records, anthropometric measurements, biochemical and clinical assessments, and lifestyle and socio-economic characteristics. Over 1700 children responded to the survey and the data provide a valuable picture of this group.

Some of the main findings are summarized here.

Health-related aspects

■ The young people in the survey confirmed the secular trend, being both taller and heavier than the cohort studied in 1982–83.

- Blood pressure increased with age; it was significantly higher in those children who used salt at table, for boys who smoked and boys in the oldest group who drank alcohol.
- Physical activity levels were recorded as fairly active in the 4–6-year-old children. After this age, activity decreased with increasing age and girls were less active than boys.

Dietary patterns

- Foods eaten by over 80 per cent of the respondents included: white bread, biscuits, chips, potatoes, savoury snacks and chocolate confectionery.
- Meat consumed most commonly was chicken and turkey (65–79 per cent of respondents); beef and veal were consumed by 43–63 per cent of males and 43–52 per cent of females. Ten per cent of the oldest girls reported that they were vegetarian or vegan.
- Raw and salad vegetables were eaten more by girls than boys (37–53 per cent of boys, 49–66 per cent of girls), but consumption of green leafy vegetables was similar, at around 40 per cent of the groups.
- Apples and pears were the fruit consumed most often, but consumption declined sharply with age (from 70 to 39 per cent in youngest and oldest boys and from 66 to 44 per cent in girls). Bananas were the next most popular fruit (average consumption

40 per cent), and citrus fruits the least popular (average 25 per cent).
- Whole milk was consumed most by the youngest group (75 per cent) and declined sharply with age. Conversely, the consumption of semi-skimmed milk increased with age to approximately 60 per cent in the oldest group.
- The most popular beverages were carbonated soft drinks, consumed by up to 85 per cent of boys and 73 per cent of oldest girls. Low-calorie versions were consumed by more girls than boys. Tea was a more common choice of beverage than coffee.

Nutritional intakes

The survey results were affected by underreporting, as is commonly found.

- Total energy intakes were below the estimated average requirements (EAR) for all age groups. In particular the oldest age group of girls and boys reported intakes of only 77 and 83 per cent of their EAR. As body weight and height show no evidence of inadequate energy intakes, it is assumed that these results are underreported. Cereals and cereal foods provided the main source of energy, as found also in the National Food Surveys.
- The contributions to the total food energy intake of the main macronutrient groups are shown in Table 12.7.

TABLE 12.7	Contributions of the main macronutrient groups to total energy intake for young people aged 4 to 18	
Macronutrient	**Contribution to food energy**	**Main contributing food groups**
Protein	13.1%	Meat and meat products
		Cereals and cereal products
Carbohydrate	51.6% (boys)	Cereals and cereal products
	51.1% (girls)	Sugar and preserves
Fat	35.4% (boys)	Cereals and cereal products
	35.9% (girls)	(biscuits, buns, cakes and pastries)
		Meat and meat products
Non-starch polysaccharides	11.2 g (boys)	Vegetables, potatoes and savoury snacks
	9.7 g (girls)	Cereals and cereal products

■ Intakes of non-milk extrinsic sugars provided an average of 16.5 per cent of energy, mainly from carbonated soft drinks and chocolate confectionery.

Micronutrient intakes were generally above the RNI for most nutrients, for most age groups. However, some intakes were below the LRNI, and the prevalence of this increased with increasing age and was more likely in girls than boys.

■ Among the vitamin intakes, vitamin A and riboflavin were most likely to fall below the LRNI. Further, in the oldest age group of girls, there were some intakes below the LRNI for all vitamins studied.

■ For mineral intakes, levels below the LRNI were found in the youngest age groups mostly for zinc. With increasing age, a greater range of mineral intakes fell below the LRNI. These included iron, calcium, magnesium, potassium, zinc and iodine. In the case of iron, 50 per cent of the oldest group of girls (aged 15–18 years) had intakes that fell below the LRNI. Among the oldest boys, magnesium intakes (18 per cent) and potassium (15 per cent) were the most common minerals to fall below the LRNI.

■ Those respondents who took dietary supplements generally had higher intakes from food sources than non-users of supplements. Supplements affected mean intakes for vitamin A and C, iron and zinc, but did not affect the intakes below the LRNI.

■ Poor nutritional status identified in blood analyses was shown in some individuals for vitamin D, vitamin C, folate, riboflavin and thiamin. In addition, serum ferritin levels were below the normal range for adults in 13 per cent of boys and 14 per cent of girls. This finding was more common in younger boys (18 per cent affected), but older girls (27 per cent affected).

Other smaller studies confirm these findings. In general, the transition from primary to secondary school is associated with the beginning of greater independence in food choice and is accompanied by an increased consumption of less desirable foods and a reduction in desirable foods, most notably fruit and vegetables.

In addition, socio-economic status results in differences in the nutritional quality of children's diets, with lower intakes of total energy and lower intakes of nutrients when energy intakes had been taken into account. This trend corresponds to that reported in adults.

School meals

A meal in the middle of the school day is important nutritionally, socially and educationally. In terms of academic performance, it is important that children eat in the middle of the day to maximize their learning opportunities.

Nutritional guidelines for school meals that had existed since the 1944 Education Act were abolished in the UK in 1980. Prior to this date, the meal offered at school had to provide one-third of a child's daily requirements of protein, energy and some minerals and vitamins. From 1980, the only obligation that remained was to provide a meal for those who were entitled to free school meals, by reason of low income. Since this date, considerable concern has been expressed about the nutritional adequacy of the diets of schoolchildren.

Following a period of consultation, Minimum Nutritional Standards have been established, taking effect from April 2001. There is once more a duty to provide a paid meals service in schools, and guidance documents have been produced by the Department for Education and Skills. Schools have more autonomy than in the past and at secondary level hold budgets for the provision of meals. This means that many schools are able to adopt whole-school policies on food and nutrition. The School Nutrition Action Group (SNAG) initiative has provided a framework for the formation of school-based alliances between teachers, pupils and caterers together with help from appropriate health professionals. Many of these are in place and they allow the consumers to be involved in the decision-making process and thereby increase their sense of ownership of the school meal provision. School management also needs to be involved to ensure there is an adequate provision for a lunch break in the timetable and that a suitable environment exists to enable meals to be taken in comfortable surroundings.

When aspects of healthy eating are part of the school curriculum, the food service can provide the practical illustration in a positive way as well as contributing to the pastoral welfare of the children.

Some issues about the provision of meals in school remain to be resolved. These include the following.

■ Ensuring that cultural diversity is recognized in the meals provided.

■ Improving the uptake of free school meals – reports suggest that to achieve this a number of factors, for example, insensitive administration that results in an associated stigma, the quality of the food, eating environment and service, all need to be addressed. Some Local Education Authorities have introduced swipe cards for all children, so that there is no distinction made at the point of purchase between the children receiving free lunches and those who are paying.

■ Provision of drinking water to accompany the meals.

■ Monitoring of the provision of the meals and maintenance of standards. This is a role for the appropriate government agency.

Minimum nutritional standards

The national nutrition standards are based on the food groups in the Balance of Good Health (see Table 12.8). In terms of defining a healthy diet, they incorporate the following principles:

■ a balanced diet with plenty of variety, and enough energy for growth and development;

■ plenty of fibre-rich starchy foods, such as bread, rice, pasta, potatoes and yams;

■ plenty of fruit and vegetables;

■ not eating too many foods containing a lot of fat, especially saturated fat;

■ moderate amounts of dairy products;

■ moderate amounts of meat, fish or alternatives;

■ not having sugary foods and drinks too often.

In addition to these general principles, specific nutrients have been identified as important for children of school age. These are:

■ calcium – important for bone health;

■ iron – important for preventing anaemia;

■ folate – important for adolescent girls and young women, but establishing a good intake in early years forms a sound base;

■ zinc – for normal growth and development.

Slightly different nutritional standards have been established for children in primary and secondary schools. In addition, there are separate standards for children of nursery school age.

TABLE 12.8 Minimum nutritional standards for school meals (DfES, 2001)

Food groups	Primary school	Secondary school
Starchy foods such as bread, potatoes, rice and pasta	Provide at least **one** from this group daily. Items cooked in oil or fat should not be served more than **three** times a week	Provide at least **two** from this group daily. At least **one** of these should not be cooked in oil or fat
Fruit and a vegetable	One item of **both** must be available every day. Fruit-based desserts must be available **twice** a week	**Two** items of **both** should be available daily
Milk and dairy foods	Provide at least **one** from this group daily	Provide at least **two** from this group daily
Meat, fish and alternative sources of protein (cheese may be provided as an alternative for primary school children **only**)	Provide at least **one** from this group daily. Red meat to be served **twice** a week; fish to be served **once** a week	Provide at least **two** from this group daily. Red meat must be served at least **three** times a a week; fish to be served at least **twice** a week

TABLE 12.9	Summary of Caroline Walker Trust Nutritional Guidelines for School Meals
Nutrient	**Guideline**
Energy	30% of the estimated average requirement
Fat	Not more than 35% of food energy
Saturated fatty acids	Not more than 11% of food energy
Carbohydrate	Not less than 50% of food energy
Non-milk extrinsic sugars	Not more than 11% of food energy
NSP (fibre)	Not less than 30% of the calculated reference value
Protein	Not less than 30% of the RNI
Iron	Not less than 40% of the RNI
Calcium	Not less than 35% of the RNI
Vitamin A	Not less than 30% of the RNI
Folate	Not less than 40% of the RNI
Vitamin C	Not less than 35% of the RNI
Sodium	Should be reduced in catering practice

NSP, non-starch polysaccharide; RNI, reference nutrient intake. From Sharp, 1993 with permission.

These standards apply to all lunches (hot or cold) provided during term time. There are additional recommendations for the provision of water, free of charge. Milk to drink should also be available every day. It is recommended that some hot food be offered daily, especially in the winter months.

Caterers are also given guidance on good practice, which includes the following key points:
- reflect the likes and dislikes of children;
- work with the school to check that healthy eating principles are being reinforced by both the curriculum and the lunch service;
- actively encourage children to have a balanced diet;
- aim to offer a selection of foods, which, over the week, reflects the proportions in the Balance of Good Health, and make changes gradually;
- offer a variety of foods;
- use a variety of cooking methods that lead to minimum destruction of nutrients.

In addition to the above, guidance is provided on various foods within each food group, portion sizes, special dietary requirements and monitoring of the nutritional standards. Even though the new minimum standards have been expressed in terms of food groups, and servings from these, caterers are encouraged to use the Caroline Walker Trust Guidelines on School Meals to check the nutritional value of the meal provided. These are shown in Table 12.9. This is particularly important where children have a free choice in a cash-cafeteria selection. Throughout, caterers are encouraged to promote healthy eating and encourage children in a variety of ways to eat the food provided.

Where children can leave school at lunchtime, caterers have to compete effectively with local food outlets. Attractive packaging, advertising and promotions can all help keep children in school for lunch.

Alternatives to school lunch

Packed lunches brought in to school may be of variable nutritional content (see Figure 12.3). Confectionery and soft drinks may also be available in school, often as a fund-raising activity, and may tempt the children to eat these items rather than more nutritious foods. In some schools, children can go out of school at lunch time, and foods purchased away from school may include pizzas, chips, burgers or cakes and soft drinks. The UK Department of Health survey (DoH, 1989) found that foods eaten out of school were generally of lower nutrient density, especially among the older school-children. In particular, these meals contained less protein, iron, calcium, retinol, thiamin, riboflavin and vitamin D. A small section of the

Figure 12.3 Example of a healthy packed lunch.

teenage population have no lunch, with 11 per cent of girls and 5 per cent of boys aged 14–16 reporting this.

Overall, a well-balanced lunch can provide between 30 and 40 per cent of the nutrients required in the day. If no food is taken or a very poor-quality snack is eaten, then the likelihood of daily nutritional needs not being met increases because it becomes more difficult to achieve adequate intakes from the remaining meals. Eating is a social activity and having lunch with one's peers can provide an important socialization activity, teaching the individual about food habits and learning from others. A proportion of children come to school without having eaten breakfast, or a snack on the way to school. In some schools, Breakfast Clubs have been established that provide food before the school day begins. The School Fruit Initiative aims to provide all primary school children with a piece of fruit in school each day. This is still being developed, but pilot schemes report a fair measure of success. School milk is also being reintroduced into some primary schools, to try to address some of the potential nutritional problems in this age group.

However, it must be recognized that providing healthier choices for children in school does not necessarily lead to changes in behaviour. One study reports the outcomes of a 2-year programme in secondary schools (Parker and Fox, 2001). This had a number of dietary targets,

including increasing intakes of high-fibre bread, fruit and vegetables, non-fried potatoes and non-cream cakes. After 2 years, there was some change in consumption of high-fibre bread, but other changes were not sustained. This study demonstrates the challenge of improving dietary intakes of children in school.

SOME POTENTIAL NUTRITIONAL PROBLEMS

As part of the development of increasing independence, children, and particularly teenagers, may encounter difficulties with their diet, which might result in nutritional problems. These are summarized in Figure 12.4.

Vegetarianism

An increasingly common finding among children and teenagers in the UK is the rejection of the omnivorous diet in favour of a vegetarian (non-meat) diet. In addition to the reasons for choosing to be vegetarian that are discussed in Chapter 16, this age group may be subject to peer pressure or initially make the decision as a bid for independence from parental control.

Unfortunately, many young vegetarians may have an inadequate understanding of the principles of nutrition, so that the traditional 'meat and vegetables' becomes just 'vegetables', or cheese omelette, or baked beans on toast. There may be little attempt to introduce other dietary items, such as pulses, cereals or grains, into the diet to replace the animal foods being avoided. In this way iron, zinc and niacin may become inadequate, as well as calcium, if dairy products are omitted. It has already been mentioned that iron intakes are low in teenagers, particularly girls. A small study in London found that anaemia was three times more common among vegetarian 12–14-years olds, with an incidence of 25 per cent, compared to 9 per cent in omnivores.

There is also concern about low calcium intakes and future health. The majority of bone mass is accrued during the teenage years, with high assimilation rates of dietary calcium. Dietary reference values are high to allow for this. If calcium intakes are low, it is likely that less bone will be made. This may have

Figure 12.4 A summary of potential nutritional problems encountered by children and teenagers.

repercussions in later life, with an increased risk of osteoporosis.

Many vegetarian meal replacements are now available, based on soya or quorn, which are acceptable and which can help to maintain an adequate nutritional intake, although they can be expensive as an everyday item. It should be remembered that a well-planned vegetarian diet can be nutritionally adequate and may be advantageous in terms of long-term health benefits.

Teenage athletes

Teenage athletes are particularly vulnerable, if they spend a lot of time training and participating in their chosen sport. This is because the energy needs for their physical activity must be met in addition to their needs for growth. Most schoolchildren participate in some sport, which involves no more than 2–3 hours per week; playing in school teams may occupy a further 3–4 hours a week. This amount of extra physical activity increases nutritional needs slightly, but probably not beyond the limits of the usual recommended levels for nutrients with the exception of energy.

As with adult athletes, there is a particular need for carbohydrate, preferably in its starchy form, to sustain muscle glycogen levels. School sports teachers should be aware of this.

Where a teenager aspires to be of national class standard, training may take up much more time, often from a very young age. This imposes considerable nutritional needs both for energy and associated nutrients in line with the increase in energy. Energy needs may be 50 per cent greater than those for an average teenager. Meeting these necessitates eating an enormous amount of extra food, which can be quite daunting for a teenager. There may be reluctance to do this for fear of becoming overweight, or appearing greedy. However, full athletic potential and normal growth cannot be achieved without the appropriate nutritional input.

Pregnant teenagers

Pregnancy is associated with changing nutritional requirements. When these are additional to the high needs of adolescence, there is a risk that the intake may not be adequate to meet both. Approximately 1 per cent of all conceptions in England and Wales are in girls under 16; this represents 9400 pregnancies.

In addition to the nutritional needs, there may be social and emotional factors that compound the nutritional difficulties. Dietary habits of pregnant teenagers have been shown to be more erratic than those of pregnant adults and low levels of vitamins A and C, folate, calcium, iron and zinc have been recorded. If the pregnancy is unwanted, as is often the case, the girl may try to limit weight gain or even diet to lose weight. There may be parental rejection and she may leave home, which can reduce her opportunities to obtain a healthy diet.

Attendance at antenatal clinics may be erratic or non-existent, so monitoring of the pregnancy to anticipate problems and obtain advice about diet may be missed. Unsurprisingly, there is an increased risk to both mother and fetus in teenage pregnancies. Maternal mortality may be 2.5 times greater at the age of 15 than between 20 and 24; the infant is likely to be of low birthweight, and is at higher risk of morbidity and mortality from a number of causes.

A teenager who becomes pregnant needs to increase her nutrient intakes and gain sufficient weight to allow the normal development of her baby. She requires foods with high nutrient density and cannot afford to include low nutrient density foods in her diet. She may also require supplements.

Dieting

Dissatisfaction with body image is a prevalent phenomenon in Western societies, affecting more females than males. This is transmitted to children from their parents and inevitably influences attitudes and behaviours in children. The preference for slimness is strongly related to the child's current body weight, but a desire to be thinner is found among those with a normal body weight and also those that are underweight. The desire for a thinner body has increasingly been reported in pre-adolescent children. Over half of teenage girls questioned reported feeling fat and wanting to be thinner; the figure for boys in this study was approximately 20 per cent.

Dieting is a natural corollary to this dissatisfaction, with over 40 per cent of teenage girls reporting past attempts at dieting, and 23 per cent reporting being on a diet at the time of study. A further 6 per cent claim to be dieting all the time. The intensity and duration of dieting is also variable, with some diets lasting only a few days, but other girls reporting continuing their diets for more than 4 weeks.

Dieting practices may be variable. Some may reduce fat, snack or total energy intake, and increase fruit and vegetable intake. However, up to 15 per cent are reported to use extreme weight loss measures, such as fasting, skipping meals (usually breakfast), vomiting and using diet pills. Filling up on diet drinks to prevent hunger is also reported. Dieting can become a habit, establishing a pattern of chaotic eating. The food intake is continually restrained; if the restraint slips, a binge may occur, with large amounts of 'forbidden' foods being eaten. However, restraint is very soon re-established. Changing to a vegetarian diet may be part of a dieting strategy and be perceived as a means of weight management.

This type of dietary intake pattern can lead to inadequate energy and nutrient consumption, with subclinical deficiencies developing and implications for future health. In particular, poor nutritional status at the beginning of pregnancy may harm the fetus. Low iron status may lead to poorer cognitive abilities, and low zinc status may depress immune function and lead to higher rates of infection. Finally, poor status of antioxidant nutrients may facilitate damage at cellular level, which may in years to come result in degenerative diseases. In its most severe form, disordered eating can develop into bulimia nervosa or anorexia nervosa, both of which carry serious health risks. In the extreme, anorexia may result in death. Adolescent girls tending towards thinness should be counselled about the dangers for their future health. A body mass index of 18 or less is a useful criterion for the need to intervene.

Dieting is less of a problem among boys, although anorexia has been reported in up to 5 per cent. In some, an obsessional preoccupation with sport as a means of weight control may replace the vomiting and purging used by girls.

Usually adolescent boys are more concerned about becoming taller and stronger, and concentrate more on body building than restricting their body size.

Nutrition and IQ

In the late 1980s, research was published which suggested that supplementing the diets of schoolchildren with vitamins and minerals could improve results in non-verbal intelligence tests. However, the results of these studies have not been supported by other work. In addition, there is no information about the original nutritional status of the children who were supplemented. It is possible that children who are malnourished could benefit from supplementation and show improved mental functioning. However, there is no persuasive evidence currently available that, in children who have a normal diet, supplementation with minerals and vitamins can improve mental abilities.

Smoking and alcohol use

Both smoking and the use of alcohol are becoming more common among older children and teenagers in the UK. A quarter of 15-year olds are reported to be regular smokers and the rate is higher among girls. Alcohol interferes with the absorption and metabolism of a number of nutrients including amino acids, calcium, folate, thiamin and vitamin C. If the intake is modest, these effects are probably of little concern. However, binge drinking may have a more serious impact on nutrient levels. Among 15–16-year olds, 15 per cent of girls and 26 per cent of boys claim to be drinking more than 10 units per week, often in binges. This sort of drinking may also be accompanied by vomiting, which removes nutrients from the body. Ultimately, nutritional status may be affected. In addition, alcohol itself will have damaging effects on the organs of the body, just as in an adult.

Smoking increases the free-radical load in the body and, therefore, the requirement for vitamin C. This should be provided in greater amounts to those teenagers who smoke. A particularly vulnerable situation exists in those teenagers who are dieting and smoking, to help control their hunger and their weight. In this case, nutrient intakes may be inadequate to offer protection against the harmful free radicals in cigarette smoke.

SUMMARY

1   The transition from infant to teenager and young adult involves enormous changes in body size and composition. The constituents of the new tissues must be obtained from the diet. Thus, at all stages of this process, nutritional requirements are high.

2   Human and formula milk can provide the nutritional needs of the infant, although human milk confers some immunological and developmental advantages.

3   The process of weaning should start at 4 months. It parallels stages of development but is nutritionally important.

4   Between the years of 1 and 5, the child consolidates the early experience with food, and becomes more independent. Growth rates are slower but, because appetite can be small, the nutrient density of the diet is of great importance.

5   The diet of the school-age child is increasingly affected by external influences. It is important that well-balanced diets are provided at home. It must be recognized that children need to exercise choice in their food intake, as part of development. However, a sound foundation of education about food can make these choices healthier.

6   Teenagers are more vulnerable than the other age groups to peer pressure and may pass through phases of experimentation with food. Again, a core of well-balanced food provided at home can ensure that good nutrient intakes are maintained.

STUDY QUESTIONS

1 a Prepare a table summarizing the nutritional and non-nutritional differences between human milk and formula milk.

   b Do you have more points under the nutritional or the non-nutritional heading? Try to account for this.

2 Write a short article for a 'Parenting' magazine in answer to the question 'Why does my 18-month-old child have an erratic appetite?' Include some practical advice.

3 a What are the main nutritional principles underlying the balance of the diet suitable for children aged between 5 and 10 years?

   b What problems might be encountered?

   c Which nutrients might be most at risk?

4 At what ages are teenage boys and girls most nutritionally vulnerable and for what reasons?

5 Suggest some ways in which teenagers could be targeted for nutritional advice.

6 For the 11–16 year age group, how important nutritionally do you consider the following meals to be? Explain your viewpoint:

   a midday meal

   b breakfast

   c snacks.

REFERENCES AND FURTHER READING

Anderson, J.A., Johnstone, B.M., Remley, D.T. 1999: Breast feeding and cognitive development: a meta-analysis. *American Journal of Clinical Nutrition* **70**, 525–35.

Barker, D.J.P. 1994: *Mothers, babies and diseases in later life.* London: British Medical Journal.

Child Growth Foundation 1995: *Boys/girls growth charts.* London: Child Growth Foundation.

Decsi, T., Koletzko, B. 1994: Polyunsaturated fatty acids in infant nutrition. *Acta Paediatrica* **83**(Suppl. 395), 35–7.

DfES (UK Department for Education and Skills) 2001: *Healthy school lunches for students in secondary schools.* London: DfSE.

DoH (UK Department of Health) 1989: *The diets of British schoolchildren.* Report on Health and Social Subjects 36. London: HMSO.

DoH (UK Department of Health) 1991: *Dietary reference values for food energy and nutrients for the United Kingdom.* Report on Health and Social Subjects No. 41. Report of the Panel on Dietary Reference Values of the Committee on Medical Aspects of Food Policy. London: HMSO.

DoH (UK Department of Health) 1992: *The health of the nation: a strategy for health in England.* London: HMSO.

DoH (UK Department of Health) 1994: *Weaning and the weaning diet.* Report on Health and Social Subjects 45. Report of the Working Group on the Weaning Diet of the Committee on Medical Aspects of Food Policy. London: HMSO.

EEC 1991: Commission Directive on infant formulae and follow-on formulae. *Official Journal of the European Communities* L**175**, 35–49.

Food Standards Agency 2001: *The balance of good health. Information for educators and communicators.* London: Food Standards Agency.

Gregory, J.R., Collins, D.L., Davies, P.S.W., Hughes, J.M., Clarke P.C. 1995: *National diet and nutrition survey: children aged 1.5 to 4.5 years.* Volume 1: Report of the diet and nutrition survey. London: HMSO.

Gregory, J., Lowe, S., Bates, C.J. et al. 2000: *National Diet and Nutrition Survey: Young people aged 4–18 years.* Volume 1. Report of the Diet and Nutrition Survey. London: The Stationery Office.

Hamlyn, B., Brooker, S., Oleinikova, K., et al. 2002: *Infant feeding 2000.* London: The Stationery Office.

Hill, A.J. 2002: Developmental issues in attitudes to food and diet. *Proceedings of the Nutrition Society* **61**, 259–66.

MAFF (Ministry of Agriculture, Fisheries and Food) 1995: *The infant formula and follow-on formula regulations.* Statutory Instrument 77. London: HMSO.

Parker, L., Fox, A. 2001: The Peterborough Schools Nutrition Project: a multiple intervention programme to improve school-based eating in secondary schools. *Public Health Nutrition* **4**(6), 1221–8.

Robinson, S. 2000: Children's perceptions of who controls their food. *Journal of Human Nutrition and Dietetics* **13**, 163–71.

Ruxton, C.H.S., Kirk, T.R., Belton, N.R. 1996: The contribution of specific dietary patterns to energy and nutrient intakes of 7–8 year old Scottish schoolchildren. *Journal of Human Nutrition and Dietetics* **9**, 5–31.

Sharp, I. 1993: *Nutritional guidelines for school meals.* Report of an Expert Working Group. London: The Caroline Walker Trust.

CHAPTER 13

ADULTS AND THE ELDERLY POPULATION

The aims of this chapter are to:

- ❏ review the dietary guidelines that have been made for adults in the UK;
- ❏ identify the particular needs of men and of women;
- ❏ review the nutritional aspects of a vegetarian diet;
- ❏ consider the effects of alcohol consumption on the achievement of dietary goals;
- ❏ discuss some human situations that may influence diet and so affect the attainment of the guidelines, including belonging to an ethnic minority group, having a low income, retirement and ageing.

On completing the study of this chapter, you should be able to:

- ❏ discuss the dietary recommendations and guidelines that are in existence in the UK for adults, and explain the reasoning behind them;
- ❏ explain the background to the special dietary needs of men, and particular diet-linked diseases, which the guidelines are aiming to prevent;
- ❏ discuss why women may be considered a nutritionally vulnerable group at certain stages of their life, and whether the dietary guidelines address their problems;
- ❏ discuss the advantages and disadvantages of following a vegetarian diet;
- ❏ explain why members of some ethnic minority groups consume different diets and the implications of this for dietary guidelines;
- ❏ discuss the implications of living on a low income in meeting dietary recommendations and goals;
- ❏ show how social, psychological and emotional circumstances may affect an older person's diet and the implications of these for meeting nutritional guidelines.

Dietary reference values and nutritional guidelines have, of necessity, been devised for the population as a whole. It would be both impractical and confusing to set a great number of different recommendations for various subgroups in the population. The guidelines current in the UK are very much in line with those in other Western countries and are the result of a wide consensus.

As discussed in Chapter 3, the progress towards achieving these guidelines is slow and in some cases trends in consumption appear to be moving contrary to the desired direction. It has been suggested that the guidelines are too ambitious as they set goals that only a very small amount of the population currently meet. An intermediate set of guidelines, closer to the actual patterns of consumption in the population, may be a more realistic target.

It is also important that a 'whole-diet' approach is adopted. Many people at present mistakenly believe that, if they change just one aspect of their diet, they are already eating more healthily. For example, there has been an increase in use of low-fat spread and semi-skimmed milk. These changes are desirable, but they do not go far enough towards a healthier diet. Such changes may result in a lower energy intake from dairy fat, which is then replaced by fats

Activity 13.1

Refer back to Chapter 3 to remind yourself of the basics of a healthy diet.

What are the dietary reference values – what are they based on?

- Are they to be used for assessing the diets of individuals?
- Why are healthy eating guidelines produced?
- What is the difference between dietary reference values and healthy eating guidelines?
- What were the nutritional targets set in the 'Health of the nation' report?
- How are these converted into a practical way of planning diets?
- How does the Balance of Good Health help consumers to achieve a healthy diet?

contained in biscuits or processed convenience foods. More extensive changes to the diet, for example, becoming vegetarian may have a number of positive health effects but, at the same time, increase risks from unforeseen consequences in the diet.

In addition, it should be recognized that there are many groups within the population who, for a diverse number of reasons, cannot achieve the targets. All of these groups will be considered in this chapter, exploring the reasons why they may have different needs, and considering some of the barriers that prevent them achieving dietary guidelines.

ADULT MEN

Many dietary guidelines around the world originated from a concern about morbidity and mortality from coronary heart disease. Consequently, they were based largely on findings from studies of men, since almost all the early studies targeted groups of men. In addition, their primary focus was related to intakes of fat, which for many years has been the major dietary factor linked to coronary heart disease development. Only in more recent years have dietary guidelines widened to include other dietary components,

such as starchy carbohydrates, alcohol, salt and other micronutrients, including the antioxidant vitamins.

Do men have problems achieving these guidelines and are they appropriate?

Most men understand that they are at risk of heart disease, although many adopt the attitude that 'it won't happen to me'. Consequently, motivation to change dietary habits may not be very great. This may be sustained by social norms, which, in some cultural subgroups, expect men to have a traditional diet that contains plenty of meat and not to eat the more 'feminine' salad, fruit and vegetables. Some acceptance of a need to change spreading fat was achieved by the initial advertising of a polyunsaturated margarine in the UK as the 'margarine for men'.

Among some men there is also a general reluctance to be concerned about their health, reflected in lower attendance rates to health services by men than by women and a lower uptake of screening services. Exposure to information about healthy eating is generally less among men, as women gain this information from magazines (often in association with articles on cookery or weight loss), from information at health centres and supermarkets. In all cases, men have less access to these sources.

Further, traditional education philosophy excluded boys from learning about food and nutrition at school; the National Curriculum in the UK has introduced some teaching about health and diet to all children.

Concern about body weight is much less amongst men, although current trends in the UK show that more men than women are overweight. In addition, the distribution of body fat in men, with a greater tendency to deposit abdominal fat (apple-shape) means that overweight is a greater health risk.

Traditionally, more men have been smokers and heavy drinkers, although in both cases rates in women have increased in the last two decades. These are lifestyle factors, which may compound risk in several chronic diseases that also have nutritional risk factors. Men, therefore, are at nutritional risk and it is important

Activity 13.2

Work with a partner on this activity. Imagine you are given the brief of tackling one aspect of health promotion for a group of men (it could be reducing alcohol intake, losing weight, taking more exercise or altering the diet). Make some suggestions about:

- which group of men you would like to use as your client group;
- which aspect of health promotion you would like to tackle;
- how you might go about identifying the problem, and trying to suggest solutions.

What do you think are going to be the main barriers to success?

that attempts to change to a healthier diet are made, encompassing whole diet changes.

Studies show that, when changes are made, results are better in the younger age group than in older men. In addition, men in the higher social classes are more likely to make changes. Therefore, greatest benefits are seen here. There is a need to target men to increase their awareness of the importance of dietary change as well as exercise, and other lifestyle factors, such as drinking and smoking, in a more active approach to disease prevention. This will be easier to achieve in some groups than others; regrettably those with the greatest need for change are often the ones who are most difficult to reach. Imaginative approaches on the part of primary health care teams and health promoters are needed. These can include health promotion in the workplace or through social clubs, perhaps related to support of sporting activities.

ADULT WOMEN

There is a dilemma in trying to devise an optimal diet for women, as different stages in a woman's life may require different nutritional priorities.

A very important point to remember is that women generally have a smaller food intake than men, related to their lower energy needs. Within this smaller intake, however, they still need to obtain all of the nutrients essential for good health. Consequently, they have less margin for error in their diet – most of what they eat has to be nutrient rich. Eating too much 'empty energy' will result in an insufficient intake of micronutrients and possible health risks.

Most of the specific health issues for women have been discussed in other parts of this book; they are highlighted here to remind the reader of the vulnerability of the female to poor nutrition at various ages.

A female adolescent requires a certain amount of body fat to be present for normal reproductive activity to begin. Yet, during this time of life, many adolescent girls feel an enormous pressure from society to restrict their weight gain and achieve a slim body shape. These two goals are difficult to reconcile, with the result that some girls do not start to menstruate or, having started, stop again, as their body weight falls. This has implications for bone health in later life, in particular, because adolescence is also the time when the bone assimilates its minerals and achieves most of its final mass. Once into her early twenties, a woman is no longer able to add significant amounts of calcium to her bones, with the result that, if the bone mass is not optimal, she may develop osteoporosis in her early old age.

In early adult years, a woman may want to have children. Research dating back to the Dutch hunger winter in 1944–45 (when the population of Holland suffered severe food shortages for a period of 8 months), but replicated in many studies since then, has shown that an adequate amount of body fat is needed for normal fertility. The normal development of the fetus is threatened if the woman is underweight. More recent work shows that various vitamins and minerals must be present in sufficient amounts from the beginning of the pregnancy to avoid low birthweight and associated risks to the child, both in its early and later life.

Certain diseases are also a particular threat for women. Women experience anaemia much more commonly than men, principally because the iron lost in blood during menstruation is not replaced adequately from the diet. Both cancer of the breast and heart disease cause a large number of deaths, and are believed to have a dietary component. In addition, osteoporosis is a condition that causes disability in many more elderly women than men.

Physical activity, which is beneficial in promoting health, has for many years been more socially acceptable for men than for women. There is now an increase in women taking part in sport, but problems of time and access to sports facilities still bar many women from being more active. There may be a reluctance also to expose a less than perfect body in the gym.

Social research shows that a woman's food choices tend to be dictated more by the likes and dislikes of her partner and children than by her own preferences, even when she is the one with the major responsibility for food provision within the household. Thus, even if a woman might want to eat a healthier diet, she may experience pressure from her family to minimize change.

Finally, it must be recognized that women represent the majority (in the UK, 65 per cent) of those living in poverty, with its associated effects on nutrition. As a result of these conflicts and dilemmas, women generally have more nutritional problems than men.

VEGETARIANS

There has been a steady increase in the UK in the number of people who reject meat from their diet and follow some variant of the vegetarian diet. Surveys suggest that between 5 and 10 per cent of the population may be following some form of vegetarian diet. Numbers tend to be greatest in females and among teenagers and young adults, although people of all ages are represented. The move to vegetarianism may initially include the rejection only of red meat, but might further also exclude white meats, fish and, occasionally, other animal products such as eggs and cheese. Thus, the diet is based on cereals, pulses, nuts, vegetables and fruit. Many vegetarians, but not vegans, also include dairy products and eggs. Various categories of vegetarianism have been defined according to the foods of animal origin that are included in the diet (e.g. a lacto-ovo-vegetarian will eat cheese and eggs, a pescarian will eat fish).

The reasons for adopting a vegetarian diet vary, but may include:

■ compassion for animals and concerns about animal welfare;
■ rejection on ethical grounds of the intensive production methods used in animal husbandry and food production;
■ concern over Western overindulgence in food, and exploitation of poorer countries and world resources;
■ dislike of the taste, texture or smell of meat;
■ concern over the safety of meat and animal products in the light of 'food scares', such as *Salmonella*, bovine spongiform encephalopathy (BSE) and the use of antibiotics;
■ religious or cultural reasons.

From a nutritional perspective, an ideal diet is one that contains a wide variety of foods, providing maxiumum opportunities to meet nutritional requirements. However, it cannot be said that foods of animal origin are an essential part of such a diet, and there are many populations around the world who exist on diets that are exclusively plant based. Problems of deficiency may arise when there is overreliance on a limited number of foods, or foods of limited nutritional value, for example, cassava, yam and maize. Where the quantity of food supplied by such a diet is sufficient, and the diet contains a variety of plant foods, then nutritional adequacy is not a problem. This is generally the case in Western societies and a well-planned vegetarian diet may provide a greater diversity of foods than one based around meat, including more vegetables, pulses and nuts. As a result, many nutrients may be present in greater amounts than in an omnivorous diet. However, meat and animal products are rich in a number of minerals and vitamins that may not be sufficiently replaced in a vegetarian diet.

In general, a well-balanced vegetarian diet containing grains, vegetables and nuts is likely to provide more of the following nutrients: folate, vitamin C, carotene, thiamin, vitamin E and potassium.

Nutrients about which there may be some concern, especially if the diet lacks dairy products, include the following: protein, iron, calcium, iodine and zinc, vitamin B_{12}, vitamins A and D, and n-3 fatty acids.

It is particularly important that attention is paid to these nutrients in the diets of vegetarian infants, children and adolescents (see Chapter 12). For adults, there is little evidence for a deficiency of most of these nutrients; however, a number are discussed below.

Vegetarians are probably more prone to iron deficiency anaemia because of the poorer bioavailability of iron from plant-based diets. Attention should be paid to maximizing absorption by including enhancing factors, such as foods containing vitamin C in the diet. Vitamin B_{12} occurs only in foods of animal origin and, therefore, their strict exclusion will be a risk factor for deficiency. Many foods designed for vegetarian diets, such as meat substitutes, are fortified with the vitamin, but vigilance is needed to ensure an adequate intake.

Vitamin D status may be compromised when the vegetarian diet is also very high in phytate and low in calcium, as has been reported in some macrobiotic diets and among people of Asian origin in the UK.

Lower intakes of the long-chain n-3 fatty acids are also a feature of vegetarian diets that exclude fish. Levels of these fatty acids are lower in plasma of adult vegetarians and also in the milk during lactation. These fatty acids have a role in the development of the retina and central nervous system in the infant, and the significance of these lower levels for infant development is being studied.

More interest has been focused on the positive aspects of a vegetarian diet, in relation to some of the chronic diseases prevailing in Western societies. Studies of adult vegetarians show that they have similar energy intakes compared with omnivores. However, the body mass index of vegetarians is on average $1 \, \text{kg/m}^2$ lower than in matched omnivores. The reasons for this are unclear, but may be attributable to lower fat or alcohol intakes. One of the reported consequences of the lower body weight is a lower blood pressure, which may confer advantages in terms of stroke and coronary heart disease.

Data from five cohort studies (Key et al., 1998), including 76 000 subjects, has shown that vegetarians had a 24 per cent reduction in mortality from coronary heart disease. Mortality in semi-vegetarians, who ate fish only or meat less than once per week, was intermediate between meat eaters and vegetarians. It is proposed that these differences can be attributed to lower intakes of saturated fat in vegetarians, and related lower plasma total cholesterol concentrations. In addition, vegetarians tend to have higher intakes of polyunsaturated fatty acids, especially linoleic acid and dietary fibre. Both of these will also affect cholesterol levels, and the risk of coronary heart disease.

Higher intakes of dietary fibre are also possibly responsible for lower rates of constipation, diverticular disease, appendicitis and gallstones that have been reported among vegetarians. At present, there is no firm evidence that vegetarian diets protect against cancers.

Overall, a planned vegetarian diet can meet many of the dietary guidelines and contribute to better health. There are a number of possible shortcomings from the exclusion of meat and dairy products, and these nutrients should be replaced from other foods. A badly constructed vegetarian diet will, however, carry no health advantages and may be hazardous to long-term health. The possible advantages and disadvantages of a vegetarian diet are summarized in Figure 13.1.

MINORITY ETHNIC GROUPS

Many people around the world for a variety of political or economic reasons move to and settle in a country that is not their own. In doing so, they become immigrants to that country. If the culture of the host country is similar to that of the immigrant's own mother country, settlement is relatively easy. If there are many cultural, religious and language difficulties, the immigrant may experience alienation in the host country. If the immigrant is a refugee forced to leave the home country, the psychological challenges of adjustment may also create difficulties with the diet.

Food habits are one of the aspects of an immigrant family's culture that may undergo little adjustment, resulting potentially in some nutrition-related problems. These may be the

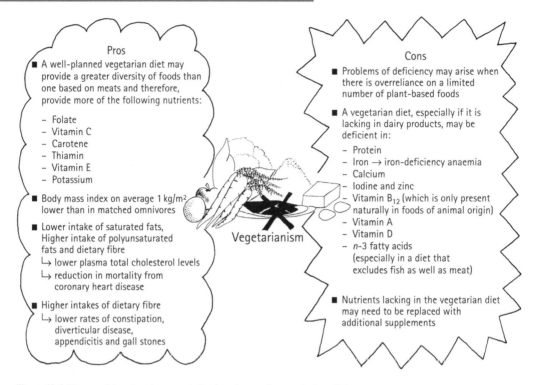

Pros

■ A well-planned vegetarian diet may provide a greater diversity of foods than one based on meats and therefore, provide more of the following nutrients:

– Folate
– Vitamin C
– Carotene
– Thiamin
– Vitamin E
– Potassium

■ Body mass index on average 1 kg/m^2 lower than in matched omnivores

■ Lower intake of saturated fats, Higher intake of polyunsaturated fats and dietary fibre
↳ lower plasma total cholesterol levels
↳ reduction in mortality from coronary heart disease

■ Higher intakes of dietary fibre
↳ lower rates of constipation, diverticular disease, appendicitis and gall stones

Vegetarianism

Cons

■ Problems of deficiency may arise when there is overreliance on a limited number of plant-based foods

■ A vegetarian diet, especially if it is lacking in dairy products, may be deficient in:

– Protein
– Iron → iron-deficiency anaemia
– Calcium
– Iodine and zinc
– Vitamin B$_{12}$ (which is only present naturally in foods of animal origin)
– Vitamin A
– Vitamin D
– n-3 fatty acids (especially in a diet that excludes fish as well as meat)

■ Nutrients lacking in the vegetarian diet may need to be replaced with additional supplements

Figure 13.1 The possible advantages and disadvantages of a vegetarian diet.

result of a number of factors that impinge on the diet.

When traditional foods are eaten, the dietary mix may seem quite different from that of the typical host country diet. Consequently, some of the guidelines that have largely been created around a 'British' diet may not be applicable. It is necessary, therefore, to explore two main issues:

■ what do some of the larger minority ethnic groups in Britain eat, and what consequences does it have for their health?

■ should the dietary guidelines be applied to the traditional diets eaten, and how can this be achieved?

The main groups of immigrants in the UK are Europeans (including people from Southern Ireland and those of Eastern European and Mediterranean origin), Asians from the Indian subcontinent (including Indians, Pakistanis and Bangladeshis), people of Afro-Caribbean origin from Africa or the West Indies, and Chinese people, from Singapore, Hong Kong and Vietnam as well as some from China. There are many other groups that have settled in the UK from every

country in the world, but numerically these are much smaller, and have not been studied as an identified group, although it is possible that nutritional issues do exist. People belonging to minority ethnic groups including those of mixed race in the UK represent about 8.8 per cent of the UK population (2001 figures).

The Europeans, together with the small groups of immigrants from various parts of the globe not mentioned above, have not as a group been reported to experience nutritional difficulties or possible deficiencies in Britain. It is possible that, like any other individual, they may experience personal dietary problems, which may be exacerbated by factors related to their ethnic origin.

Features common to many members of ethnic minority immigrant groups

Newly arrived immigrants may share the common feature of belonging to a socially disadvantaged sector of society, even if they were relatively well off in the home country. This may be reflected in various aspects of life, including low income or unemployment, poor housing, poor educational opportunity and less access to health care. All of these may have a bearing on nutrition. In those who maintain the traditional diet, the higher cost of some imported foods and the need to travel to specialist shops may limit the amount of food eaten.

The traditional diet may be modified by the substitution of some 'British' foods to replace unavailable traditional items. Unfortunately, the British foods chosen are often those of poorest nutritional quality, such as highly refined processed items like cakes, biscuits, crisps and soft drinks. These are not nutritionally comparable to the traditional items they may be displacing. In this way, a well-balanced traditional diet, by attempting to become integrated into the British diet, becomes nutritionally poorer. It is important that, where some adaptation to the British diet occurs, the foods chosen should be nutritionally adequate.

For the children of some of these families, especially those new to the UK, school meals may pose a major dilemma. If the child has been brought up from infancy eating only a traditional diet, foods presented in school may be completely unfamiliar both in content, style of presentation and expected way of being eaten. In time, peer pressure may encourage these children to sample British foods and, if they enjoy them, they may eventually request them at home. It should be pointed out, however, that many of the children in British schools who are of minority ethnic group origin are second- or even third-generation children of former migrants, who no longer consider themselves as anything other than British, and have perhaps been eating the typical British diet for the whole of their life. Traditional foods may be something that they eat only in the presence of members of the older generation or occasionally at home.

A different problem exists at the opposite end of the age spectrum, as some of the early migrants into Britain in the late 1950s and 1960s reach retirement and old age. For many of these, life has remained very traditional. This is particularly true for the women who may have never worked, or integrated much with the local population. Services such as meals on wheels or luncheon clubs may not provide appropriate meals. Because of this, the person may be excluded from receiving this provision. In some parts of Britain, special 'ethnic' meals on wheels are provided for the local population, but this service is not widespread. In most cases, the older generation of immigrants rely on their children and grandchildren to provide them with food, if they cannot cope themselves. Welfare services are gradually recognizing the need to encompass the needs of ethnic elders in their provision.

Asian immigrants

Much attention has been focused by nutritionists on the South Asian immigrants from Bangladesh, India and Pakistan. In addition, smaller numbers came to Britain from Africa, in particular Uganda and Kenya.

Religion is an important part of the culture for most of these groups, and many are followers of one of the three major religions found in Asia: Hindu, Islam and Sikh. All three have specific dietary laws, which have an impact on the foods consumed and may result in nutritional consequences. The main features of the religions and their dietary prescriptions are outlined below.

Hindu religion

This is an ancient religion, one of whose main precepts is the sanctity of life and the transmigration of the soul. As a consequence, there is a prohibition on the taking of life, including that of an animal for food. Thus, traditionally Hindus are vegetarian, eating only plant foods, or foods from animals that do not include killing – for example, dairy products. Eggs may be avoided by some Hindus, particularly women, as they are seen as a potential source of life. The cow is deemed sacred, and its products are prized in the diet. Orthodox Hindus will adhere strictly to the dietary laws, but some who are less strict may eat meat, but usually not beef or pork (the pig is considered unclean).

Fasting, which means either total abstinence from food, or alternatively the eating of 'pure' foods – fruit, yoghurt, nuts and potatoes – may be a regular occurrence.

Islam

Followers of Islam are Muslims. The religious teachings in the Koran encompass most aspects of life, including dietary laws, as well as rules on fasting. Muslims are permitted to eat the flesh of ruminant animals (which excludes pork), poultry and fish (some but not all exclude shellfish). The animal must be ritually slaughtered by a registered butcher; the meat is bled and sacrificed to Allah. It is thus made 'halal'. Meat prepared in this way is available in Britain, either fresh or frozen. Milk and dairy products are not a major part of the Muslim diet in the UK, although they are eaten increasingly, as the diet becomes more British. Even though meat is allowed in the Muslim diet, the amount actually eaten may not be very large. This is especially true for women who normally eat last, giving the larger share to the men in the household.

All Muslims over the age of responsibility (early adolescence) are required to fast from sunrise to sunset for a 4-week period each year known as Ramadan. The actual number of hours of fasting depends on the time of year in which Ramadan falls. When it occurs in the summer months, there may be up to 16 hours of fasting a day, but perhaps less than 8 hours in the winter. In the early years of the twenty-first century, the fast falls in October/November/December, and is moving back through the year into the Autumn months. Ramadan is associated with eating during the hours of darkness, with special foods being prepared, many high in fat and sugar. Families rise before dawn to eat; this alleviates the problems of hunger during the day. Ramadan finishes with special celebrations, again involving particular foods prepared only at this time of the year.

Sikhism

This religion developed comparatively recently (in the sixteenth century) and incorporates some features of both the Hindu religion and Islam. Dietary restrictions are less than in either of these religions: eggs or meat are not prohibited, but some Sikhs may believe in the transmigration of the soul and are vegetarian.

Very few eat beef, and pork may be considered unclean, as with the other religions described above. Animals for meat must be killed in a prescribed manner by a single blow to the head; meat produced in this way is known as 'khatka'.

General features

Traditional Asian meals may consist principally of the staple (a rice or wheat dish), together with one or several side dishes, which provide the garnish or flavour part of the meal. Fruit is more likely to be eaten for dessert rather than a sweet cooked dish. Sweets may be prepared for special occasions, rather than everyday. The most Westernized meal may be breakfast, which might include cereals and toast, rather than the traditional leftovers from the previous day. In the Health Survey for England 1999 (DoH, 2001), which considered the health of minority ethnic groups, consumption of red meat and fried foods was reported to be high among Bangladeshi groups, and the diet was also low in fibre. The Indian diet contained least amounts of red meat (for religious reasons), lowest fat levels and had a higher fibre content.

Asian women tend to have a more marked domestic role in the traditional household. Particularly for these women, integration with the British community may be slow. Change occurs most quickly in those communities where the women have roles outside the house: going out to work, or meeting others.

Afro-Caribbean immigrants

Immigrants to Britain from the Caribbean are predominantly of African descent, although some may be of Indian origin. The cultural outlook of these groups has been influenced by life both in the Caribbean and Britain. Several ethnic subcultures exist, linked to the island of origin. Traditional Caribbean food habits may be kept by significant numbers of this population and are likely to be diverse. Generally, they pose few nutritional problems, apart from obesity.

The diet is largely based on cereals, such as corn, rice and wheat, and starchy vegetables including potatoes. These may be served in the form of spicy stews or soups, containing many different vegetables. Many of the traditional foods, such as mangoes, breadfruit, cassava, green bananas, plantain and yams, are available in West Indian specialist shops, indicating that they have remained an important part of the diet. The diet is higher in carbohydrate (50 per cent), lower in fat (32 per cent) and alcohol (2 per cent) than the equivalent white British diet. Food patterns may be different among this population and dietary assessment requires specialist knowledge (see Sharma and Cruickshank, 2001).

One of the subgroups of the West Indian community are the Rastafarians who aspire to return to Ethiopia, which is seen as the African homeland. There is a strong adherence to the Bible, and many of the dietary laws are based on a very strict interpretation of Bible writings. In its strictest form, the diet is vegetarian, containing no meat or animal products. It is based predominantly on fruit, vegetables and cereals. However, because pulses are not a major item in the West Indian diet, the vegetables tend to be starchy roots and leafy vegetables, both of which contain little protein. There can be a lack of vitamin B_{12} in the diet. In other ways, however, the diet may be considered healthy, with a prohibition on alcohol, convenience and processed foods, and a low salt intake. As with all dietary laws, the extent to which the diet is kept will vary between individuals. However, as Rastafarianism is perceived as conferring an identity to the individual, there is a considerable motivation to keep to the dietary laws.

Chinese immigrants

The Chinese have a food culture very different from that of the indigenous British population, which has remained largely unchanged despite long periods of settlement in Britain. Although some British foods are included in the diet, usually being requested by the children, these form only a small part of the daily intake. The diet includes rice as a staple, and meat, fish, fruit and vegetables prepared in many diverse ways.

Food is perceived by older Chinese as not just providing nutrients but contributing to the overall balance of the energy in the body. This is

described in terms of hot and cold (or male and female, yin and yang) properties. Foods are ascribed such properties according to the effects they are believed to have on the body (not on the actual temperature of the food). In addition, particular stages of life, such as pregnancy, as well as illness, alter the body's balance. An appropriate selection of foods can restore the balance. For example, if children eat a school meal that is considered 'hot', they will be given a 'cooling' food to restore their balance when they return home. Thus, rather than avoiding British foods, the Chinese simply accommodate them, and adjust other foods eaten accordingly. There are no reports in the British literature of nutritional problems associated with the Chinese diet.

Potential nutritional consequences

Vitamin D deficiency began to appear among children of Asian immigrants in the early 1970s. Initially, it was believed that the cause was linked to the skin pigmentation, which reduced the synthesis of vitamin D on exposure to sunlight. However, this was not supported by results of measurements of vitamin D synthesis after ultraviolet exposure in light- and dark-skinned individuals. A further possibility was that the traditional dress of many Asian immigrants required that the body be covered, allowing little exposure of the skin and minimizing vitamin D synthesis. This may contribute to the deficiency, but is unlikely to be the sole explanation.

Investigation of the diet of affected and unaffected individuals has shown that most vitamin D deficiency occurs in those who follow the most strictly vegetarian diet. Diets that contain no meat, eggs or dairy produce appear to be the most rachitogenic (rickets causing) among the Asian population. It has been suggested that the high content of dietary fibre and phytate reduces the availability of calcium and removes vitamin D from the body in the faeces. In addition, the lack of animal products directly reduces vitamin D intake. A strict vegetarian diet has also been found to lead to rickets among Rastafarian children. Health promotion campaigns among the Asian population have largely reduced the occurrence of rickets among the children, although low plasma vitamin D levels are still recorded. The problem of osteomalacia in adults (women, in particular), however, remains and appears to be difficult to prevent by education.

Anaemia arises in these groups from inadequate intakes of iron, folic acid or vitamin B_{12}, or a combination of these. Iron deficiency arises in infants because of prolonged milk feeding, and inadequate use of iron-rich weaning foods. This has been found in both Asian and Afro-Caribbean families. Pregnant women are also at risk, in particular those who are vegetarian. Language barriers, especially among those newly arrived in the country, may prevent them seeking or accepting medical advice to treat the anaemia.

Folic acid deficiency also occurs in pregnant women, whose needs are increased to support fetal cell division. Prolonged cooking of vegetables and reheating from day to day destroys all potential folate in these foods. This is particularly a problem when the diet is vegetarian.

Vitamin B_{12} deficiency is particularly found in vegetarian immigrants, being seen most in the Hindu population in the UK. It may coexist with iron and folate deficiency, and has also been linked to a higher than average occurrence of tuberculosis.

Studies on the incidence of dental caries show that pre-school children in immigrant groups throughout Europe tend to have a higher prevalence of dental caries than the indigenous population. This is particularly true among the Asian communities and is believed to be associated with a higher intake of sugar-containing drinks, including milk, and a higher frequency of consumption of sugar products.

Obesity, diabetes and heart disease are the newer diseases among the Asian population at present. Central obesity is particularly common among the South Asian groups, especially among women (DoH, 2001). The incidence of both diabetes and heart disease is higher among members of Asian minority groups than the indigenous British population. This may seem surprising, since the traditional diet is rich in starchy carbohydrate and contains large amounts of vegetables, in line with dietary guidelines.

Recent work has shown that Asians have higher plasma levels of lipoprotein(a) than Europeans. This increases coronary heart disease risk. In addition, the Westernized diet and lifestyle contribute to increasing body mass index with central fat deposition, insulin resistance and raised blood lipids. These combine to produce an elevated risk for both heart disease and diabetes. A key factor in prevention is physical activity, which can help to reverse many of these trends. However, uptake of physical activity is low in many members of these groups.

For all of the immigrant groups, the traditional diet more closely resembles the dietary guidelines than does the current British diet. It is important that minority ethnic groups are encouraged to retain their traditional dietary practices, perhaps incorporating some of the staple foods available in Britain. They should be discouraged from including the unhealthy British dietary practices into their traditional patterns.

One of the most disadvantaged groups are refugees, who may come from many different countries. There is a high level of food insecurity in these households, particularly within the first two years of arrival in the UK. It is difficult to reach people in these groups, but child hunger is likely to be common, and significantly associated with recent arrival and receipt of fewer benefits.

LOW INCOME AND NUTRITION

People on a low income may be living in poverty. This is a relative term: it can be taken to mean an absolute lack of material possessions but, in Western society, it is more commonly used to reflect disadvantage in relation to the rest of society. In practice, the definition varies between different organizations. Two definitions that are used are:

- people receiving less than half of the average income (whether from employment or state benefits); and
- people having to spend more than 30 per cent of income on food.

Numbers of people in poverty have been increasing in Europe throughout the last decades.

It is documented that people in these situations have poorer health in almost every measure used to assess health, with excess morbidity and mortality at all ages. Various groups are particularly vulnerable to poverty. These include the following.

- Families with children, in particular, where there is a lone parent or where neither parent is in employment.
- Women, owing to the traditional dependence of women on a male breadwinner, their traditional role as carers of children and their poorer pension rights as a result of incomplete employment records. In two-adult households where the woman is the sole wage earner, the income is usually lower than in those with a male wage earner.
- People with a disability, owing to poorer employment prospects and higher than average living costs.
- Members of minority ethnic groups, owing to a higher unemployment rate and a greater representation among the low paid. In addition, there are now many refugees and asylum seekers throughout Europe who are often in severe financial hardship, which also reflects on their nutritional intakes.
- Young people who have left school but have not been able to find work. They have very low entitlements to benefits and may not be supported by their families, leading perhaps to homelessness and a life in poverty.
- Homeless people have major problems in achieving an adequate food intake. They may have additional problems that compromise nutritional status, such as alcohol or drug abuse. Alcohol may provide a substantial proportion of the energy intake. Studies on this group find that they are up to four times more likely to be underweight and have a diet that is low in a wide range of nutrients. Shelters for the homeless and soup kitchens are an important source of nutritional provision and attention to the quality of the food could make a difference to the status of this group.

Income is not the only factor contributing to poorer health experienced by people in these groups. One of the main factors is likely to be their diet, but poorer housing, low self-esteem, poorer educational opportunity and lifestyle habits detrimental to health, such as smoking, all make a contribution.

Characteristics of the diet

Expenditure on food is described as elastic, which means that when income is limited and other, fixed, expenses have to be met, the food budget can be trimmed accordingly. However, those on a limited income may spend up to three times more, proportionately, on food compared with the average UK family.

The expenditure on food is cost efficient; the annual National Food Survey consistently shows that the lowest income groups obtain more nutrients per unit of money spent. Table 13.1 shows some of the foods typically bought by the low-income and high-income groups, and in Table 13.2 the amount bought per 1 pence of expenditure is shown.

Studies such as these of the foods eaten typically show that low-income families rely more heavily on white bread, whole milk, sugar, eggs, meat products and margarine, and consume less reduced fat milk, poultry, carcass meat, fish, fresh vegetables (excluding potatoes), fruit, brown and wholemeal bread. Vegetables and potatoes are more likely to be processed rather than fresh. There is also less variety of foods eaten; for example, among pregnant women in Edinburgh and London, the poorest had only half the number of different foods in their diet compared with the richer women. The diet is, therefore, more likely to be monotonous, with few new additions.

Table 13.2 shows that, for every food group, those households with a lower income buy more (by weight) for their money. This applies to even simple products, such as confectionery or soft drinks. Overall, expenditure is also less, with a mean expenditure of £22.03 by group A and £14.07 by group D recorded by DEFRA (2001).

This cost efficiency often necessitates shopping around to find the best value for money, which may be time consuming. Some poorer residential areas may have limited shopping facilities, and the term 'food deserts' has been coined to describe this situation. Access to the wider choice of foods in larger supermarkets may be limited by

| TABLE 13.1 | Types of foods eaten by the highest (A) and lowest (D) income groups studied by the National Food Survey 2000 (consumption in g/person per week) (calculated from DEFRA, 2001) | |

Food	Income group	
	A	D
White bread	175	375
Wholemeal, brown and other bread	258	174
Breakfast cereal	155	110
Biscuits	108	143
Milk	464	833
Cheese	111	88
Meat and meat products	849	971
Fats and oils	149	200
Sugars and preserves	90	142
Potatoes (fresh)	568	776
Fresh green and other vegetables	857	581
Processed potatoes and vegetables	462	581
Fruit	895	573
Fruit juice	483	211

| TABLE 13.2 | 'Value for money' of foods bought by high-income (A) and low-income groups (D) (amount purchased in grams per 1 pence spent) (calculated from DEFRA, 2001) | |

Food	Income group	
	A	D
Milk, cream and cheese	9.3	13.8
Meat and meat products	1.9	2.8
Fish	1.3	2.0
Fats and oils	3.8	6.0
Sugar and preserves	7.0	12.9
Vegetables and potatoes	6.3	10.4
Fruit	6.8	9.0
Bread	7.8	11.5
Cereals	4.2	6.3
Soft drinks	22.1	31.3
Alcoholic drinks	2.3	3.8
Confectionery	1.6	2.0

lack of transport or insufficient resources to make the trip worthwhile. In general, about 30 per cent of the British population have no access to a car and are, therefore, dependent on public transport for their access to more distant shops. In addition, the temptation of a large variety of foods on offer makes a stark contrast with the amount of money available. Consequently, local and often smaller shops may be used, where both choice and value for money are likely to be less. There may also be a problem of a lack of storage facilities, necessitating frequent purchases of perishable items. Shopping becomes a chore, with little scope for enjoyment. It should also be noted that 'value for money' in terms of quantity of food purchased does not necessarily equate to nutritional value.

TABLE 13.3	Cost of common snack foods, in pence, to supply 420 kJ (100 Calories). Values calculated from Food Standards Agency (FSA, 2002b) and at 2002 supermarket economy prices

Food	Costs to provide 420 kJ (100 Calories) (pence)
Digestive biscuits	2
Wholemeal bread	2
Kit Kat (chocolate wafer)	6
Crisps	7
Milk	7
Banana	10
Chocolate bar	12
Peppermints	13
Coca cola	13
Sponge cake	15
Yogurt	21
Orange/satsuma	35
Apple	42

The cheaper foods bought may have poorer nutritional content; for example, cheaper meat products contain more fat and salt, cheaper vegetables may be less fresh and have lower vitamin contents.

Nevertheless, families try to maintain conventional eating patterns to lessen the impact of low income, often eating cheaper versions of 'mainstream' meals. Also, parents endeavour to protect their children against the effects on the diet of poverty, buying foods that the children prefer. As a consequence, children in low-income families may actually receive more of their favourite foods than children from better-off households. To achieve this, parents in several studies record missing meals. Protecting the children also means that the family meal is focused on what the children prefer and will eat, rather than the likes and dislikes of other family members. Eating may cease to be a pleasure and becomes simply a means to ward off hunger.

Food selection is made from a rational perspective, with a view to the meal it can produce in the most economical way. Therefore, foods that may require preparation and addition of several other ingredients to constitute a meal are less attractive. A ready-made product, such as a meat pie, needs few additional items to make it into a complete meal, in contrast to a leaner meat, which itself contains less energy and requires vegetables, pasta, potatoes, bread, etc. to make a meal. Predictability of portion size and number also helps in meal planning.

As one of the primary concerns is to feel satiated after a meal, foods that provide a large amount of energy for a small financial outlay may be preferred. Consequently, foods high in fat and sugars will be more satisfying than a low-fat, low-sugar food and will provide a cost-efficient source of energy. The cost to supply 420 kJ (100 Calories) from a variety of snack foods is shown in Table 13.3. Not all are nutritionally poor; for example, bread and milk can provide a cheap nutritious snack.

Nutritional implications

Current dietary advice (discussed in Chapter 3) is to eat more fruit, vegetables and starchy carbohydrate, and to reduce the intake of fats, particularly from whole fat dairy products and meats rich in saturated fats. In addition, the consumption of fish is encouraged. The National Food Surveys show that the trend towards a healthier pattern in the diet is more marked in the higher income groups surveyed and, in many cases, is moving in the opposite direction in the poorer groups. Thus, although there is a small downward trend in fat intake in poorer families, more of that fat is still saturated, and fruit and green vegetable consumption in one study was found to be equivalent to two apples and ten Brussels sprouts per person per week.

Evidence collected in many centres around the UK has shown that the costs of a 'healthier basket' of foods are greater than for a 'less healthy' basket. The difference in price varies between regions of the country, but may represent an excess cost of 20 per cent for the 'healthier' basket. In addition, the access to many of the healthier items may be more limited in the areas where the poorer families may shop.

The stresses of living on a low income mean that health concerns are not one of the highest priorities, even though evidence suggests that the desire to eat more healthily exists. Knowledge about what constitutes a healthier diet is also present among poorer families, although it may be fragmentary. Reports have shown that, if there was more money to spend, then this would be used to buy more fruit, vegetables and leaner meats. At present, for such families, the cost of the food takes precedence over issues of taste, cultural acceptability and healthy eating.

Members of these families run the risk of having lower intakes of many of the micronutrients. In particular, these include iron, zinc, calcium, magnesium and potassium, as well as the vitamins, especially vitamin C, folate, riboflavin, niacin, beta-carotene and vitamin E. Many of these are the 'antioxidant nutrients', which are believed to be especially important to health. At the same time, the diet may be low in non-starch polysaccharides (NSPs) and polyunsaturated fats, but contain excessive amounts of saturated fat and sugars. The consequences for health are likely at all ages. Links with nutrition have been discussed also in the relevant sections of the book; a summary is provided here.

- Infants are less likely to be breastfed, although there has been an increase in prevalence reported in the Infant Feeding 2000 Survey (Hamlyn et al., 2002). Breastfeeding

is protective against infection in early life, enhances gut development, and may protect against allergy and eczema. It is also associated with better school performance in childhood and a higher IQ for children born pre-term.

- Infants in low-income families have a higher consumption of infant formulae, potatoes, confectionery, squashes and soft drinks, and a lower consumption of milk products and fruit. Nutrient intakes are higher in saturated fats and cholesterol, and lower in carotene and vitamin C.

- Toddlers have slower growth and slower recovery from infection, but also more have a high body mass index (BMI), more dental caries and higher blood lipids. Their diets are higher in saturated fatty acids, sugars, starch and sodium (present in higher amounts in processed foods that form a larger part of the diet). There are lower intakes of NSPs, beta-carotene, vitamin C, iron, zinc, calcium and iodine.

- Older schoolchildren have lower intakes of most vitamins and minerals, lower levels of activity and poorer bone accretion. There are higher rates of anaemia among teenage girls and lower iron status, which probably impacts on cognitive ability. If the poor iron status continues into pregnancy, there are higher risks of stillbirth, low birthweight, and increased risk of hypertension and heart disease in the offspring later in their lives.

- Lone parents have a greater likelihood of falling below the lower reference nutrient intake (LRNI) for many nutrients, the greater their 'poverty index'. (This was assessed on a number of lifestyle factors associated with low income.) Pregnant women have generally lower intakes of energy and nutrients, poorer weight gain and higher occurrence of low birthweight babies. This has implications for their future health and perpetuates the intergenerational effects of deprivation.

- Older adults have lower nutrient intakes, poorer immune status and higher risk from all diet-related diseases.

- Special dietary requirements are more difficult to follow.

Keep a record of your expenditure on food for a period of 1 week. Use the Balance of Good Health (FSA, 2001) to break down this expenditure into the main food groups.

■ Which of the groups costs you the most and which the least?

■ Is it possible for you to change your expenditure on food?

■ Could you spend less during the following week?

Prepare a plan of which food groups you could buy less and which more during the next week. How easy do you find this exercise?

Make a list of the constraints that operate for you in trying to be more economical in your food expenditure. Which could you overcome, and which are beyond your control?

Practical help

Attempts have been made to devise sample diets that would be nutritionally sound and at the same time cost no more than a low-income budget could afford. One such was the 'ten pound diet' produced by Ministry of Agriculture, Fisheries and Food (MAFF; see Leather, 1992), which gave precise amounts of 26 different food groups/items, which could be used to plan meals for 1 week within this budget. Many people felt that this diet was socially unacceptable, as it expected people on a low income to eat differently from the rest of society.

More practical help is reported by the National Food Alliance, which brings together many local projects engaged in empowering people on low income and enabling them to work together in low-cost cafes, food cooperatives and other support groups. In this way, access to and education about food are improved, the feelings of isolation are reduced and self-esteem can be enhanced. In association with these more social improvements, there can be a better diet and a greater interest in food and eating healthily.

Further work was undertaken on a strategy on food and low income by the Low Income Project Team (DoH, 1996). This aimed to bring about a better understanding of the costs of healthy eating and facilitate access to healthier foods by involving policy makers and providers of the food. As part of this initiative, ways of mapping price and availability of healthy food have been developed. This can then be used to identify areas that serve their local community poorly in terms of healthy food and attempt to address this. Local projects as part of the Governments initiative on Social Exclusion in the UK are helping local groups around the country to improve their access to better quality food; this may be through, for example, local street markets, 'Get Cooking' clubs or community cafes.

OLDER ADULTS

In this discussion, the term 'elderly' is used to refer to men and women of pensionable age. In the UK, this generally means 65 years or over for men and over 60 years for women. The upper end of this age spectrum is not defined, but there are increasing numbers of people over 100 years old in the UK (the majority are women).

In 2001, 18.3 per cent of the population in the UK or 10.8 million people, was over retirement age (65 in men and 60 in women). The total numbers of the elderly are increasing in most Western countries: by 2030, it is estimated that one in four of the adult population will be aged over 65 years. In the UK, the greatest increase in the early part of the twenty-first century will be particularly in the over-85 age group, with a smaller relative increase in the over-75s. The numbers between 60/65–74 will fall slightly, reflecting the lower birth rates in the 1930s and during the Second World War. The over-85 group are the most vulnerable sector of the retired population, and the most likely to experience nutritional problems. However, it is anticipated that the increased knowledge of nutrition among younger adults, and the consumption by some of a healthier diet, will reduce the occurrence of nutritional problems as they get older. Current statistics suggest that an average of 13 years of disability for men and 16 years for women may be expected at the end of their life. The proposals of the 'Health of the nation' white paper of adding 'years to life and life to years' are particularly relevant in this group.

In making general statements about the vulnerability of the elderly population, it is important to remember that there is considerable variation between individuals, as at any age. Preparation for retirement and a healthy old age should have begun earlier in life, with the acquisition of good eating habits and a healthy lifestyle, involving both physical and mental stimulation. Several studies confirm that health and good nutrition coexist in the elderly, and when one begins to deteriorate, often so does the other.

Why are some elderly persons at risk?

Elderly people are at increasing risk of having marginal nutrition resulting from the ageing process itself and its impact on social factors, as well as an increased incidence of disease. These factors are summarized in Figure 13.2. Ageing is believed to be the result of an increase in oxidative stress and dysregulation of cellular function over time. Supplementation with several antioxidants, most notably vitamins E and C has been associated with a reduced risk of age-associated chronic diseases as well as maintenance of cognitive function.

It is helpful to consider how ageing affects some of the body's systems, which may in turn contribute to poor nutritional status.

Sensory system

Changes to the sensory system will have an impact on both the ability to obtain food as well as its enjoyment. Loss of hearing or visual acuity may restrict shopping as well as social contacts, leading to isolation. Loss of sensitivity to taste and smell, which is a normal feature of ageing, can reduce the attractiveness of food. Elderly people may actually complain that food does not taste 'as it used to'. This is more likely to be a reflection of their failing sense of taste, rather than a change in the food itself. Enhancing flavours with herbs and spices can overcome some of these problems. However, it should also be recognized that a zinc deficiency can contribute to loss of taste acuity.

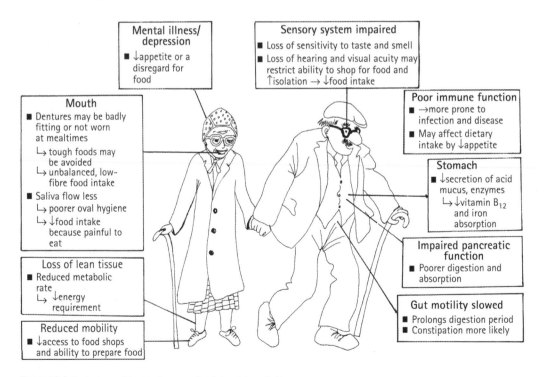

Figure 13.2 Factors resulting in increased risk in older adults.

Gastrointestinal system

The loss of teeth and wearing of dentures should not have a major impact on food intake. It is reported that 57 per cent of the 65–74 age group have none of their own teeth, with 75 per cent of those over 75 similarly affected. Although more elderly people are keeping their teeth for longer, there is still a substantial proportion of this group dependent on dentures. If the dentures are badly fitting, not checked regularly or even not worn at mealtimes because of discomfort, the dietary intake may suffer. Foods that are coarse, tough or require prolonged chewing may be avoided, possibly resulting in unbalanced intakes. Saliva flow is less in an older person, which may result in poorer oral hygiene and associated infections adding to oral discomfort.

There is a reduced secretion of acid, mucus and enzymes in the stomach in old age, and a decrease in pancreatic function. Gut motility is slowed and this may prolong the digestion period to compensate for the poorer enzyme secretions, but a more likely result is constipation. An adequate intake of dietary fibre (NSPs) as well as sufficient fluids is, therefore, desirable. The use of laxatives is to be discouraged, especially those based on mineral oils, which can deplete the body of fat-soluble vitamins. The reduced gastric secretion may produce a lower level of intrinsic factor for vitamin B_{12} absorption, as well as reduced solubilization of iron and its consequent absorption.

Kidney function

The amount of active renal mass declines with age and is on average 30 per cent less at 80 than at 30 years. Consequently, the kidneys may have a poorer ability to concentrate the urine, as well as eliminating waste products more slowly. Therefore, fluid balance will be under less precise control. In addition, thirst mechanisms are less sensitive. Thus, an elderly person runs the risk of dehydration, if fluid intake is not consciously maintained. Sometimes, the added problem of incontinence, or even a reluctance to have to get up in the night to empty the bladder, may discourage an individual from drinking enough. Consequences of dehydration include confusion, dry lips, sunken eyes, increased body temperature, dizziness and low blood pressure. An intake of eight cups (1.5–2 L) of drink per day is recommended.

Lean tissue

There is a progressive loss of lean tissue throughout life, although the actual extent depends on lifestyle factors. On average, 40 per cent of the peak tissue mass may be lost by the age of 70 years. This results in reduced basal metabolism and, consequently, a reduced energy requirement. The loss of lean tissue also results in a loss of strength and this may discourage an elderly person from engaging in even gentle physical activity. Thus, it is clearly important to minimize the loss of lean tissue by maintaining physical activity throughout life. This also maintains appetite and promotes an adequate nutritional intake. There may be little change in total body weight associated with losses of lean tissue because of an increase in the amount of body fat with age. The loss of lean tissue also represents a reduction in both total body water and potassium in the overall composition of the body.

Mobility

It is estimated that over 50 per cent of adults over the age of 65 years suffer from one form of disability and 33 per cent suffer at least one type of severe disability. Arthritis, hypertension, heart disease, hearing and visual impairments, orthopaedic impairments and diabetes are the most frequent problems that pose difficulties for this age group in carrying out daily activities. In addition to these, older adults suffer from progressive bone loss, leading to increased bone fragility and susceptibility to fractures, known as osteoporosis. This is discussed in greater detail in Chapter 10. There is an increased risk of sustaining fractures with age. After the age of 50 years, the lifetime risk of an osteoporotic fracture is 40 per cent for a woman and 14 per cent for a man. Hip fracture has the highest costs in terms of morbidity and mortality. It nearly always necessitates hospital admission, with an average length of stay of 30 days. Only about one-third of these patients regain their former mobility. Deaths within the first 6 months after a hip fracture are approximately 20 per cent.

There are many factors that interact to increase susceptibility to osteoporosis that results in a fracture. Genetic factors play a role, and these interact with environmental and dietary factors. Prevention of fracture depends on attention to long-term diet, as well as maintenance of muscle strength and balance in old age to reduce the risk of falling. Supplementation of elderly people with calcium and vitamin D has been effective in reducing fracture risk, and is a well tolerated treatment. The use of drugs that slow bone resorption may also be preventative. It is important for the nutritional well-being of this age group to maintain mobility as long as possible.

The immune system

This becomes less efficient with age, with the result that there is a higher risk of infection. In particular, there are lower levels of T-lymphocytes, as well as an increased production of autoantibodies. A poor nutritional status, in particular, with relation to protein, zinc and vitamin levels, can contribute to poor immune function. This may expose the individual to more minor infections, but also increase the risk of more serious problems, such as pneumonia or wound infections.

The brain and nervous system

Cognitive function may decline with age and this is another factor that hinders independent living. Dementia is the most common cause of cognitive impairment, and is defined as a significant memory impairment and loss of intellectual functions. Increased oxidative stress and an imbalance in antioxidant status may both contribute to the decline in cognitive function. A study in the USA found that plasma levels of vitamin C, E and A, carotenoids and selenium were correlated with memory function among people aged over 60 years (Perkins et al., 1999). The same survey found that 7 per cent of elderly Americans suffered from poor memory. Antioxidants protect the integrity of blood vessels in the brain and, therefore, maintain circulation. This may also be effective in protection against stroke, which is the most common cause of vascular dementia. Other studies have shown that oxidative injury is present in the brains of patients with Alzheimer's

disease and may play a role in its development. Various components of brain tissue appear to be affected, including lipids, proteins and DNA, and it is likely that several different antioxidants may be needed to protect the whole range of molecules. In addition, a number of B vitamins especially vitamin B_6, B_{12} and folate may play a role in the development of dementia through their involvement in the metabolism of homocysteine. Elevated levels of homocysteine have been implicated in development of cognitive impairment. Therefore, maintenance of an adequate diet before old age may be protective against some of the degenerative changes in the brain, and in turn facilitate better nutrition in old age.

Other factors

In addition, an elderly person is more vulnerable to many degenerative diseases, which often develop over a considerable number of years. These may include atherosclerosis, arthritis, lung diseases and cancers. All of these may directly affect dietary intake. Drug treatment for the disease may have an effect on appetite, digestion, absorption, excretion or metabolism of nutrients. Patients suffering from a number of chronic conditions may be taking several drugs, which can interact with one another and produce side-effects, such as nausea, diarrhoea, constipation or confusion.

Factors affecting nutritional status

In addition to ageing and its consequences, social and environmental factors may affect the nutritional status of an elderly person.

Inadequate intake

There are many contributory factors influencing a poor food intake. These are summarized in Table 13.4.

Physical/medical factors
- Reduced mobility, from rheumatism, arthritis or as a consequence of a stroke or lung disease, may be sufficiently severe to make the individual housebound or even bedfast.
- Dentition and the state of the mouth play an important part in the food intake.

TABLE 13.4	Factors contributing to poor food intake in the elderly	
Physical/medical factors	**Social factors**	**Psychological factors**
Mobility	Money available	Depression
Selection of foods bought	Food storage/preparation facilities	Bereavement
Food preparation	Education/knowledge of nutrition	Mental illness
Dentition	Social isolation	Alcoholism
Appetite		
Disease		
Drugs		

- Appetite may be reduced by coexisting disease or by its treatment, for example, disease of the gastrointestinal tract, associated with nausea and vomiting or discomfort after eating, will severely limit appetite.
- Various drugs used in the treatment of a variety of illnesses may also have a depressing effect on the appetite.
- Mental illness and depression are also likely to affect food intake; there may be a complete disregard for eating with a loss of time sense so that mealtimes are ignored.

Social factors
- Availability of money: many of the retired live on a fixed income. They may spend in excess of 30 per cent of their income on food – considerably more than the UK average of 9.5 per cent.
- Lack of education about the importance of nutrition and the existence of out of date beliefs about food may prevent the elderly individual having a healthy diet, and may render them vulnerable to cranky notions that they see in the media.
- Social isolation may be the result of retirement, re-housing, death of friends and relatives, breakdown of the nuclear family or illness. Several studies have shown that food intake was less and nutritional status poorer among those living alone and experiencing isolation. In particular, the widowed and men were more acutely affected than the long-term single and women. Conversely, where an effort was made to share food and eat in company, the food intake was better.

Psychological factors
- Depression, often the result of bereavement, is probably one of the major causes of inadequate food intake in an otherwise healthy person and may persist for many years, resulting in malnutrition.
- Altered mental function, with memory loss and unusual behaviour, may also occur and result in erratic eating. There is an increase in the numbers of people cared for in the community rather than in institutions. It is important that the nutritional needs of these individuals are addressed. Severely demented patients are cared for in nursing homes and hospitals, where food and care are provided. It is still important, however, that nutritional intakes are monitored and checked for adequacy.
- Consumption of large amounts of alcohol may be a coping mechanism for depression or bereavement. The problems associated with excessive drinking may worsen other consequences of ageing.

Less efficient digestion and absorption
Relatively little is known about the effects of ageing on the functioning of the digestive tract. Reduced secretion of stomach acid and pancreatic enzymes may result in poorer digestion and absorption. There may also be minor malabsorption syndromes, associated with a decrease in the intestinal mucosal surface and broader, shorter villi. Absorption may also be reduced as a result of chronic use of laxatives. The extent of these changes in a normal elderly person is, however, unknown.

Altered needs

Many bodily functions become less efficient with ageing.

- There is decreased nutrient uptake by cells, so that an apparently adequate intake for a younger person may not produce the same levels in the cells in an elderly person.

- Energy needs decrease with ageing because of the reduction in basal metabolic rate consequent on reduction in lean tissue mass as well as reduced activity. The latter is a cultural phenomenon and attempts are being made to change perceptions about the importance of physical activity in older people. In many societies, people remain active to a very old age, yet in Britain activity levels are generally very low in this age group. A reasonable level of activity will ensure adequate energy intake to cover the expenditure and incidentally provide sufficient other nutrients in the diet to meet requirements. Conversely, a low activity level may result in such low intakes of energy that basic nutritional requirements cannot be met. Thus, there is an important nutritional argument for maintaining activity levels. In addition, activity will help to promote cardiovascular fitness and maintain muscle mass.

- Protein needs may be higher as protein synthesis, turnover and breakdown all decrease with advancing age. Homeostatic mechanisms regulating protein levels in the body may be less efficient in elderly people. In addition, ill health, trauma and disease states may upset the equilibrium. Insufficient energy intake may also compromise protein balance, as protein will be used to meet energy needs.

- The presence of disease and its treatment by drugs may affect nutritional needs and the effects may be exacerbated by drug interactions. Further problems may arise in a confused patient who fails to take drugs at prescribed times. Up to 60 per cent of drugs taken by the elderly are obtained without prescription. One of the commonest is aspirin, which interferes with the absorption of vitamin C and may cause bleeding along the gut. It may thus cause a vitamin C deficiency or anaemia. Laxatives are also frequently obtained without prescription and can deplete the body of potassium, causing depression and affecting cardiac function.

What is the nutritional state of older adults?

A major survey of diet and nutrition in people aged over 65 was carried out in Britain between 1994–95 as part of the National Diet and Nutrition Survey programme. The results were published in 1998 (Finch et al., 1998). The study covered free-living individuals as well as a sample living in institutions. Some of the main findings are summarized.

- The foods and drinks consumed by the largest proportion of the sample were: tea (95 per cent), potatoes (87 per cent), white bread (74 per cent) and biscuits (71 per cent). Whole grain breakfast cereals were eaten by 50 per cent of the sample, and the most commonly used type of milk was full fat. Butter was the most popular fat used. The most commonly consumed meats were ham and bacon, followed by beef, veal and meat dishes. Fish was eaten by 36 per cent of the sample. Cooked vegetables were consumed by up to 66 per cent of the group. Less than half the group ate fruit. Sugar was used by 55 per cent of the sample. Alcoholic beverages were consumed by fewer than 20 per cent of the sample. In general, these findings suggest a dietary pattern that is quite traditional and shows relatively low uptake of foods such as semi-skimmed or skimmed milk, low-fat or polyunsaturated spreads, or salads. The eating pattern of the older subjects and those living in institutions was even more traditional.

- More people are retaining their teeth into old age than was the case in the past. The state of dentition has an impact on the foods chosen, and limits intakes of fruit and uncooked vegetables. The quality of the diet was strongly related to the oral health of the subjects, with higher nutrient intakes in those subjects with some natural teeth. The difference in nutrient intake with dental state was not significant in the group in institutions. However, these subjects had more dental plaque and caries, and consumed more sugar than the free-living subjects.

■ Energy intakes were generally below the estimated average requirements (EAR) and were 15 per cent less than recorded in the previous survey, 25 years ago. However, more of the subjects were overweight (65 per cent of free-living sample) than previously and it is assumed that energy intakes were adequate for needs. More people in institutions (16 per cent) than in the community (4.5 per cent) were underweight. In general, energy intakes decreased with age in men but not in women.

■ Proportions of macronutrients in the diet were in line with intakes across the adult population and did not comply with dietary guidelines. Intakes of NSP did not meet the dietary reference value (DRV), and there was a positive correlation between NSP intake and number of bowel movements.

■ Average intakes for minerals and vitamins exceeded the reference nutrient intake (RNI). However, in both groups, there were numbers of individuals in whom the intakes fell below the LRNI. In general, subjects in institutions were less likely to have such low intakes. This could be linked to the use of milk and fortified foods in the menus. The findings are summarized in Table 13.5.

■ Intakes of sodium and chloride were above the RNI in both groups of subjects. In the free-living group, systolic blood pressure levels were positively associated with urinary sodium/potassium ratio.

■ In those subjects whose intake of non-milk extrinsic sugars (NMES) was within the normal population range of 8-15 per cent of total energy, there was no evidence that micronutrient intakes were compromised. Micronutrient intakes were however marginally lower at NMES intakes outside this range. In general, micronutrient intakes reflected energy intake.

■ Biochemical assessments showed suboptimal indices for a number of nutrients. These are indicated in Table 13.6.

■ Subjects from the community who were in manual social groups had lower average intakes of nutrients per unit of energy, but higher intakes of sodium.

■ Lower intakes of energy were seen in both men and women who lived alone, compared to those who lived with others. In men living alone, this also resulted in lower intakes per unit energy of some nutrients. This was not the case in women.

Overall, these findings demonstrate that the diet of older adults in Britain is largely comparable to that of younger adults. However, dietary choice may be affected by factors such as social class, household composition and dentition, as well as state of health and age. Changes in dietary intake will lead to poorer indices of nutrients and

TABLE 13.5	Percentages of elderly subjects with nutrient intakes from food sources below the LRNI (data adapted from Finch et al., 1998)	
Nutrient	Free-living subjects (average for men and women)	Subjects in institutions (average for men and women)
Vitamin A	4.5	1
Thiamin, niacin, vitamin B_{12}	<1	<1
Folate, vitamin B_6	4	5 (folate), <2 (B_6)
Riboflavin	7	3
Vitamin C	2	<1
Iron	3.5	5.5
Calcium	7	0.75
Phosphorus	22	30
Potassium	28	65
Zinc	6.5	8.5

TABLE 13.6	Prevalence of suboptimal indices for nutrients in elderly subjects (adapted from Finch et al., 1998)	
	% in institution	% in free-living
Folate	40	15
Vitamin C	40	15
Riboflavin	40	40
Thiamin	10–15	10–15
Vitamin D	37	8
Zinc	7–15	2
Iron (low haemoglobin)		
Men	52	11
Women	39	9

may lead to poorer health. Institutional care can help to maintain nutrient intakes.

What are the nutritional requirements for the elderly?

There is still a lack of reliable data about the specific nutritional needs of elderly people and research is needed. In part, this is related to the heterogeneity of the group, which makes generalized recommendations difficult. In practice, most recommendations for nutrients are extrapolated from those for younger adults and, as such, may be inappropriate.

The principal guidelines for a healthy diet apply equally in those past retirement age. In many ways, it becomes even more important that nutrient-dense foods are eaten, since a smaller food intake increases the risk of nutrient needs not being met.

It should also be remembered that dietary reference values (DoH, 1991) and comparable figures published in other countries apply to healthy individuals. It may be that the presence of disease in certain older people may alter their nutritional needs. Therefore, it can be concluded that nutritional requirements are probably similar in the elderly to those in younger adults, but individual differences may occur, owing to particular circumstances. These may include health problems, decreased physical capacity, presence of drug–nutrient interactions, possible depression and economic constraints.

Advice about diet to people who have retired could include the following:

- enjoy food;
- follow basic healthy eating guidelines relating to fat, fibre, salt and sugar by using the Balance of Good Health (FSA, 2001);
- recognize that snacks can be an important part of the diet;
- make sure that fluid intakes are adequate;
- keep some food stocks in the house for emergencies;
- try to spend some time outdoors, especially in the spring and summer;
- if alone, try to arrange to share meals with friends/neighbours;
- ask for help with shopping when necessary;
- try to keep active;
- remember that food provides warmth.

In planning diets for an elderly person, particular attention should be paid to nutrients that have been identified as being 'at risk' in studies of this age group. These include: vitamin D, vitamin E, thiamin, pyridoxine, folate, vitamin C and vitamin B_{12}, as well as iron, zinc and calcium. Energy and protein intakes must be adequate to allow protein to be used for wound healing and tissue repair rather than for energy needs. In patients receiving diuretic therapy, potassium or magnesium levels may be at risk. A diet containing a variety of foods fitting in with the Balance of Good Health, a sufficient intake of fluids and a moderate activity level will ensure good nutritional status in an elderly person.

It should be recognized, however, that probably the most common nutritional disorder among the elderly in Western society is obesity. As at any other age, this is multifactorial in origin and is detrimental to health. If the overweight is very longstanding, the likelihood of successful, significant weight loss in an elderly person is small. Nonetheless, in cases of diabetes, hypertension and arthritis, weight loss is desirable and should be actively encouraged.

The most vulnerable elderly people are those who are ill and frail. It is necessary to identify those at risk as rapidly and efficiently as possible, before they enter a spiral of deficiency and inadequate intake, leading to further deficiency. Ten major risk factors have been identified:

- depression/loneliness;
- fewer than eight protein-containing meals/week;
- long periods without food;
- little milk drunk;
- high level of food wastage;
- disease/disability;
- low income;
- inability to shop;
- sudden weight change;
- fruit and vegetables rarely in the diet.

The presence of several of these factors points to increased nutritional vulnerability and the need for intervention.

Community services available for the elderly in the UK include the provision of luncheon clubs and day centres for those who are reasonably mobile, and 'meals on wheels' and home helps for those elderly who cannot get out, or are incapable of fully looking after themselves. They provide social contact as well as helping the nutritional status.

Approximately 5 per cent of the elderly in Britain are in institutions, including hospitals and residential or nursing homes. These are the most vulnerable subgroup, since it is largely because they are ill, infirm and incapable of caring for themselves that they live in these settings. The diet provided by the institution may be nutritionally incomplete, particularly with respect to vitamins C and D, although other nutrients have also been shown to be low. There may be problems for the individual with appetite, eating and swallowing. Many disease processes may make an adequate nutritional status difficult to achieve, or assess. However, every effort should be made to ensure that the elderly in institutions are properly fed. National Care Standards, including nutritional standards, were introduced in 2002 in the UK.

Finally, it should be remembered that, although some of the retired population do encounter nutritional problems, the great majority live a reasonably healthy life and succeed in caring adequately for themselves. A positive outlook and a continued interest in life are important prerequisities. When interest in food wanes, a decline in health will surely follow.

SUMMARY

1   The principles of the balanced diet apply to all adults; however, particular emphasis may be needed on some aspects rather than others in certain situations.

2   Men may have less access to information and be less prepared to make changes for a variety of reasons.

3   For women, nutritional needs differ at stages of the life cycle. Pressures from society, demands of pregnancy and their own health may provide conflicting messages about how to interpret the dietary guidelines.

4   Ethnic minority group members may have a traditional diet that is healthy but, by becoming Westernized, there is a reduction in nutritional quality of the diet.

5   A vegetarian diet can be a positive contributor to health but may lack some nutrients if not well planned.

6   Low income may be a major barrier to consuming a healthy diet.

7   A nutrient-dense diet is important with increasing age, as nutritional needs remain high but appetite decreases. Maintaining physical activity can help to promote appetite.

STUDY QUESTIONS

1   a The female body can experience several major biological changes during the life cycle. In what ways might these affect the dietary advice given to women?

    b Do you believe that dietary advice given to men should vary with their life stage?

2   a What are the main threats to health affecting members of the Asian community in the UK?

    b What changes to diet and/or lifestyle could be of benefit?

3   For what reasons does living on a low income pose a threat to eating healthily and/or having a healthy lifestyle?

4   Prepare a leaflet designed for those who care for the elderly, summarizing the main principles of eating healthily at this age.

5   a Discuss with a group of fellow students, or your tutor, some of the reasons why people generally appear to have difficulty achieving the dietary goals. What sources might you use to check how well goals are being achieved to help you in this discussion?

    b Identify ways in which meeting goals could be made easier.

    c Who might need to be involved in b above?

REFERENCES AND FURTHER READING

Appleby, P.N., Key, T.J., Thorogood, M. et al. 2002: Mortality in British vegetarians. *Public Health Nutrition* **5**(1), 29–36.

British Nutrition Foundation 1995: *Vegetarianism, a briefing paper.* London: British Nutrition Foundation.

Buttriss, J., Hyman, K. 1995: *Focus on women: nutrition and health. Proceedings of a conference.* London: National Dairy Council.

Davies, L., Knutson, C.K. 1991: Warning signals for malnutrition in the elderly. *Journal of the American Dietetic Association* **91**, 1413–17.

DEFRA 2001: *National Food Survey 2000 Annual report on food expenditure, consumption and nutrient intakes.* London: The Stationery Office.

DoH (UK Department of Health) 1991: *Dietary reference values for food energy and nutrients for the United Kingdom.* Report on Health and Social Subjects No. 41. Report of the Panel on Dietary Reference Values of the Committee on Medical Aspects of Food Policy. London: HMSO.

DoH (UK Department of Health) 1996: *Low income, food, nutrition and health: strategies for improvement.* A Report by the Low Income Project Team for the Nutrition Task Force. Wetherby: Department of Health.

DoH (UK Department of Health) 2001: *Health survey for England. The health of minority ethnic groups.* London: The Stationery Office.

Dowler, E., Calvert, C. 1995: *Nutrition and diet in lone-parent families in London.* London: Family Policies Study Centre.

Dowler, E.S., Turner, S., Dobson, B. 2001: *Poverty bites; food health and poor families.* London: Child Poverty Action Group.

Finch, S., Doyle, W., Lowe, C. 1998: *National Diet and Nutrition Survey: people aged 65 years and older.* Volume 1. Report of the diet and nutrition survey. London: The Stationery Office.

Food Standards Agency 2001: *The balance of good health.* London: FSA.

Food Standards Agency 2002a: *Food portion sizes*, 3rd edn. London: The Stationery Office.

Food Standards Agency 2002b: *McCance & Widdowson's The composition of foods*, 6th summary edn. Cambridge: Royal Society of Chemistry.

Gonzalez-Gross, M., Marcos, A., Pietrzik, K. 2001: Nutrition and cognitive impairment in the elderly. *British Journal of Nutrition* **86**, 313–21.

Grundman, M., Delaney, P. 2002: Antioxidant strategies for Alzheimer's disease. *Proceedings of the Nutrition Society* **61**, 191–202.

Hamlyn, B., Brooker, S. Oleinikova, K. et al. 2002: *Infant feeding 2000*. London: The Stationery Office.

Hill, S.E. 1990: *More than rice and peas. Guidelines to improve food provision for black and ethnic minorities in Britain.* London: Food Commission.

Key, T.J., Fraser, G.E., Thorogood, M. et al. 1998: Mortality in vegetarians and non-vegetarians: a collaborative analysis of 8300 deaths among 76000 men and women in 5 prospective studies. *Public Health Nutrition* **1**, 33–41.

Leather, S. 1992: Less money, less choice: poverty and diet in the UK today. In *National Consumer Council, Your food: Whose choice?* London: HMSO, 72–94.

National Food Alliance 1994: *Food and low income: a practical guide for advisers and supporters working with families and young people on low incomes.* London: National Food Alliance.

Nutrition Society 1995: Nutrition for the elderly (Symposium). *Proceedings of the Nutrition Society* **54**(3), 617–99.

Perkins, A., Hendrie, H.C., Callahan, C.M. et al. 1999: Association of antioxidants with memory in a multiethnic elderly sample using the Third National Health and Nutrition Examination Survey. *American Journal of Epidemiology* **150**, 37–44.

Ritz, P. 2001: Factors affecting energy and macronutrient requirements in elderly people. *Public Health Nutrition* **4**(2B), 563–8.

Schofield, C., Stewart, J., Wheeler, E. 1989: Dietary variety during and after pregnancy in Scotland and England. *Journal of Human Nutrition and Dietetics* **2**, 7–18.

Sellen, D.W., Tedstone, A.E., Frize, J. 2002: Food insecurity among refugee families in East London: results of a pilot assessment. *Public Health Nutrition* **5**(5), 637–44.

Sharma, S., Cruickshank, J.K. 2001: Cultural differences in assessing dietary intake and providing relevant dietary information to British African-Caribbean populations. *Journal of Human Nutrition and Dietetics* **14**, 449–56.

Van Staveren, W.A., de Groot, L.C., Burema, L. et al. 1995: Energy balance and health in SENECA participants. *Proceedings of the Nutrition Society* **54**(3), 617–29.

Williams, B. 1995: Westernised Asians and cardiovascular disease: nature or nurture? *Lancet* **345**, 401–2.

14

DIET AND CORONARY HEART DISEASE

The aims of this chapter are to:

❏   define what is meant by coronary heart disease and describe its development;
❏   describe the lipid hypothesis for heart disease aetiology;
❏   study some of the ways in which evidence about heart disease causation has been collected;
❏   identify some of the suggested risk factors;
❏   describe the suggested role of dietary factors in the development and prevention of heart disease.

On completing the study of this chapter, you should be able to:

❏   explain the physiological processes involved in the development of heart disease;
❏   discuss the origins of the lipid hypothesis of heart disease;
❏   describe some of the other dietary factors that play a part in heart disease aetiology;
❏   explain the suggested interaction of antioxidant nutrients as protective factors;
❏   propose and explain dietary advice for the prevention of coronary heart disease.

Coronary heart disease, together with other diseases of the circulatory system, is one of the major causes of death in the Western world. Worldwide mortality due to coronary heart disease and stroke accounts for approximately 20 per cent of all deaths, and numbers are increasing as the world population becomes relatively older. Throughout Europe, cardiovascular disease accounts for about 40 per cent of overall mortality, the majority of these deaths are attributable to coronary heart disease, most of the remainder to stroke. Across Europe there is an East–West gradient, with higher mortality rates in central and Eastern Europe than in Western Europe. The differential between the highest and lowest mortality approaches a factor of 5. There are also higher rates of coronary heart disease, but not stroke, in Northern Europe than in the South, and the variation between North and South is approximately 2.5.

Death rates from coronary heart disease vary between the countries of the UK. The rates are highest in northern parts of England, Scotland and Northern Ireland, and lowest in the southeast and London. Heart disease rates among women in the UK are some of the highest in the world. In Scotland, the rate amongst women aged 35–74 is ten times greater than that in Japanese women.

People born in the Indian subcontinent living in the UK have heart disease rates 36 per cent higher than those in the population as a whole. Those in people originating from the Caribbean countries are lower than in the population as a whole, by 55 per cent in males and 24 per cent in females.

In the UK, the age-standardized death rate of people under 65 from circulatory diseases was 70 per 100 000 of the population in 1995. In France, which has the lowest rate in Europe, the death rate at the same time was 36 per 100 000. In 2001, there were 120 891 deaths in the UK from coronary heart disease alone. All of the circulatory diseases taken together account for 41 per cent of mortality in England. In addition, angina and other circulatory disorders, some resulting in stroke, are leading causes of ill health and disability.

CHANGES IN RATES OF CARDIOVASCULAR DISEASE

Most Western European countries, including the UK, have experienced a downward trend in heart disease rates since the 1980s and early 1990s. The most encouraging trends have been among the younger age groups. Rates have fallen by 40 per cent in the under 65s in the last decade. However, in the countries of Eastern Europe, such as Hungary, Poland and Romania, rates increased.

In the USA, Australia, New Zealand and Japan, rates have shown a dramatic reduction in the last 15–20 years, but the causes are unclear. The White Paper, Saving Lives – Our Healthier Nation (DoH, 1999) has set the target in the UK to reduce deaths from circulatory diseases by 40 per cent by 2010. This is estimated potentially to save 200 000 lives over this period.

Traditionally, coronary heart disease has been viewed as a disease of men because, in middle age, mortality is higher in men. However, after the menopause, women become increasingly susceptible to the disease and death rates of the two sexes are similar. Since women generally live longer than men, many more suffer from heart disease in old age. As a result of this perception, much of the early research has been focused on the disease in men, and both research and treatment in women has lagged behind. More recent studies have included women among the subjects.

There are many changes that occur in diet and environmental influences that make it very difficult to pinpoint those having the major effects. Positive factors may include health education that affects, for example, the intake of fats, fruit and vegetables and increases physical activity. On the other hand, negative factors may include the societal shift in dietary intake to more 'fast food', as well as political changes (such as in Eastern Europe during the 1990s), which cause stress, and increase alcohol intake and smoking rates.

Projections for the future indicate that prevalence of cardiovascular disease will continue to rise, despite some encouraging trends. This is attributable to the better treatment and survival after heart attack, albeit with increased morbidity. A further reason is the age profile of most populations, with an increase in the proportion of older people, who are at increased risk of these diseases.

This chapter will focus on coronary heart disease, as this is the major manifestation of cardiovascular disease in Western Europe. In addition, much more of the research in this area has been on the dietary determinants of coronary heart disease, rather than stroke.

WHAT IS CORONARY HEART DISEASE?

A heart attack (myocardial infarction) can result in sudden death. It occurs when the blood and hence oxygen supply to a part of the heart fails, because of a blockage in the vessels supplying the muscular walls of the heart. This makes the heart unable to continue working normally to supply blood to all the parts of the body and, most crucially, to the brain. If a large part of the muscle is deprived of oxygen, the heart attack may be fatal. Failure of a smaller part of the heart muscle may allow the rest of the heart to continue working and maintain the circulation.

These events are, however, the culmination of a process that may have been developing gradually over a long period of time, involving a series of changes to the walls of the coronary arteries. The process may be described in terms of atherogenesis and thrombogenesis (see Figure 14.1).

Injury to the coronary arteries

The blood vessel walls are continually exposed to wear and tear by the flow of blood. The wall is not completely smooth, especially where there are divisions of the vessels into smaller channels and associated branching. Blood flow becomes turbulent here, rather like the flow of a river where streams are joining or there is some obstruction to the flow.

Prolonged raised blood pressure will also increase stress on the walls. As a result, the wall of the vessel is continually repairing itself in response to the damage, using the blood platelets

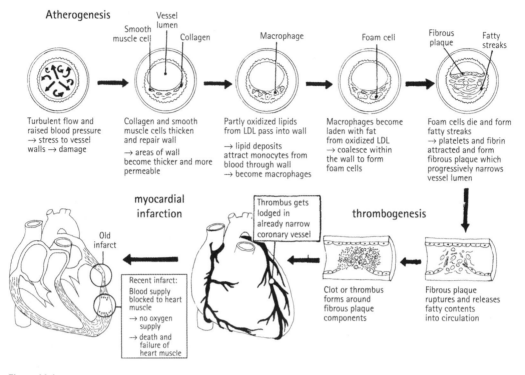

Figure 14.1 The development of coronary heart disease. LDL, low-density lipoprotein.

and forming minute blood clots. New collagen and smooth muscle cells may be laid down to strengthen the wall. Over a long period of time, these areas may become thicker and, since they are no longer perfect, become more permeable to substances and particles in the blood. Many factors contribute to the normal functioning of the endothelial surface of the blood vessel, including relaxing factors and growth factors, and these are considered to be important in maintaining functional integrity.

Fibrous plaque formation

The progression from the previous stage is not completely clear. It is normal for blood vessel walls to be permeable to substances required by the tissues, such as lipid-soluble material needed for metabolic processes. It is now believed that partly oxidized lipids present in low-density lipoprotein (LDL) entering the blood vessel wall are recognized as 'foreign' and are not allowed to pass through the endothelium of the blood vessel. Their presence attracts monocytes (a type of

white blood cell), which adhere to and then enter the blood vessel wall. Various factors are now known to influence the adhesion of the monocytes, including nitric oxide (endothelial relaxing factor) and antioxidants (particularly vitamin E).

Having penetrated the blood vessel wall, the monocytes are converted to macrophages, which are scavenger cells whose purpose is to destroy the damaged lipids. However, the macrophage itself then cannot leave the wall and so these scavenger cells accumulate, laden with fat, and gradually coalesce to produce 'foam cells'. When these die, the fat they contain remains in the wall and becomes the origin of the fatty streaks that are believed to be a contributing factor in the atherogenesis of the heart disease process.

The fatty streaks also attract blood platelets and fibrin, which attempt to 'seal off' the damaged area. In the process, these clot-forming entities actually contribute to thickening, producing a fibrous plaque and ultimately hardening the blood vessel wall. Smooth muscle cells are laid down under the influence of growth factors, derived from platelets and other blood components. The plaque area grows, protruding progressively into the lumen of the vessel and further interfering with the blood flow.

Thrombosis and heart attack

Eventually the fibrous plaque becomes unstable and ruptures, releasing fatty contents into the circulation. These attract components of the clotting mechanism and a thrombus (or clot) is likely to form. If the blood vessel is already narrow at this point, the clot may block the flow of blood. The fibrous plaque components themselves may also become lodged in the vessel. Both of these processes will cause a myocardial infarction, if the blockage is in a coronary blood vessel. When the narrowing and thrombosis occur in a blood vessel supplying the brain, a stroke (or cerebrovascular accident) will be the result.

Various physiological and dietary factors are involved in the processes described above. An understanding of these is emerging from the many studies of coronary heart disease and its associated risk factors. The developments in molecular biology have added a new dimension to these studies, so that mechanisms that were originally only suggested as a possibility are now being described in detail at the molecular level. As more information becomes available, it clarifies some aspects but it also demonstrates that the picture is highly complex.

STUDYING CORONARY HEART DISEASE

The study of coronary heart disease is hampered by the absence of a close animal model for myocardial infarction, although aspects of the disease process can be mimicked in various animals. However, to obtain the most relevant data, studies are performed on human populations and, for ethical reasons, are limited in the scope of experimental work that can be done. Much of the research is, therefore, based on epidemiological data obtained from populations with high and low rates of heart disease, and attempts to associate these with diet and lifestyle characteristics. A number of approaches have been used. Dietary lipids have been the main focus of

attention because of the lipid nature of the fibrous plaque contributing to the narrowing of the blood vessels.

Origins of the lipid hypothesis

Cross-community comparisons

The most widely known of the early studies is Keys' Seven Country Study, which compared fat intakes and serum cholesterol levels with subsequent 10-year coronary heart disease incidence in men aged 40–59 from seven countries (Keys, 1970). The strongest correlation was found between the percentage of energy derived from saturated fat in the diet and increased risk of heart disease. These results were compared more recently in a 25-year follow up of the subjects. In communities with a high incidence of heart disease, the intake of saturated fatty acids typically ranges between 15 and 25 per cent of the energy intake. At the extremes, saturated fat intakes in East Finland are 22 per cent and in Crete are 8 per cent of the energy. The corresponding rates of coronary heart disease are 1074 and 26 per 10 000 (age standardized rate), respectively. There was also a weaker, negative correlation between intake of polyunsaturated fats and heart disease.

Although these relationships could be seen across different population groups, with varying diets and cultures, they are more difficult to find in comparisons of individuals within one country. Nevertheless, it has been possible to produce an equation that predicts the change in serum cholesterol, given changes in the dietary intake of saturated and polyunsaturated fats. Two such equations have been produced by Keys and Hegsted. The Keys formula shows that saturated fatty acids (excluding stearic acid, C18) raise plasma cholesterol levels by twice as much as polyunsaturated fatty acids can lower it. This may not always be exactly so predictable for any one individual because of other behavioural or genetic factors. However, the ratio of polyunsaturated (P) fatty acids to saturated (S) fatty acids is a useful means of expressing the desirable proportion in the diet. Where the ratio is low (P/S = 0.2), the population generally has a high blood cholesterol level and a high risk of coronary heart disease. Increasing the P/S ratio to 0.5–0.8 has been considered a desirable goal, as heart disease rates are lower in populations where the normal diet approaches these proportions.

This basic premise is the first principle of the lipid hypothesis and is widely accepted. The corollary and the second principle, that both risk and mortality from heart disease can be reduced by lowering cholesterol, is still debated. Views have become polarized and the lack of consensus has been widely publicized in the media, with resulting confusion for both health professionals and the general population.

Prospective studies

These involve studying a cohort of individuals over a number of years and measuring those parameters that are believed to be related to heart disease. Over time, some individuals will develop the disease; it is assumed that they share particular characteristics, not seen in the unaffected members of the population. One of the best known of these studies is that in Framingham, Massachusetts, where a cohort of over 5000 individuals were first recruited in 1948. Data regarding their cardiovascular health and many possible causal factors have been systematically collected, using standardized methods of measurement. Data from the Framingham study have shown that raised serum cholesterol, high blood pressure and cigarette smoking are three major contributory risk factors in heart disease. The study also showed the comparative level of risk with increasing serum cholesterol levels. As newer risk factors are discovered, the data from Framingham can be reviewed to investigate other relationships. A newer data set is information from a sample of over 100 000 female nurses in the USA, from whom medical and dietary information has been collected, and who are being followed up prospectively. A review of ten within-population studies (Caggiula and Mustad, 1997), showed a positive significant relationship between intakes of saturated fat and coronary heart disease.

Intervention studies

The second principle of the lipid hypothesis suggests that, if a raised serum cholesterol level is associated with an increased risk of heart disease, then lowering it should reduce the risk. Many trials have attempted to demonstrate this by using advice, dietary manipulation, lifestyle changes or drug intervention either separately or in varying combinations.

In some studies, those with no pre-existing evidence of heart disease have been targeted (primary prevention). The main drawbacks of this approach are the size of the subject group needed to demonstrate any benefits and the difficulty of evaluation.

Some community projects have been successful, most notably the North Karelia project in Finland, where a programme of health education was targeted at the whole community, aimed at reducing the very high incidence of heart disease. Evaluation has found measurable improvements in the average values for key parameters, most notably a 13 per cent decrease in serum cholesterol. This was attributed to changes from butter to vegetable oil margarines, from whole fat to low-fat milk and from boiled to filtered coffee. In addition, blood pressure fell as a result of reduced salt intakes, and an increase in fruit and vegetable intake. Overall, coronary heart disease mortality declined by 55 per cent in men and 69 per cent in women. These results imply that some individuals have achieved substantial changes. However, such large projects can also have very disappointing results. For example, the World Health Organisation (WHO) Collaborative study, targeting factory workers in several European countries, achieved some reduction in heart disease mortality in Belgium and Italy, but not in the UK.

More specifically, focused trials recruiting those at high risk of heart disease have had mixed results. The Multiple Risk Factor Intervention Trial (MR FIT) found that both the study and control groups showed an improvement in mortality rates. This demonstrated the difficulty of human studies, where diet is not a constant variable. Figure 14.2 shows the relationship between plasma cholesterol and heart disease from this study.

A review by Truswell (1994) of 14 studies from the 1960s and 1970s, in which saturated fatty acids were exchanged with polyunsaturated fatty acids, found that the average cholesterol level was lowered by 10 per cent. This was

Figure 14.2 The increase in risk with increases in serum cholesterol levels. CHD, coronary heart disease. (From Martin et al., © 1986 The Lancet Ltd 1986. Reproduced with kind permission.)

associated with a 13 per cent reduction in coronary events and a 6 per cent reduction in mortality. Where cholesterol reduction was more than average, there was an even greater decrease in coronary events and mortality.

Trials using cholesterol-lowering drugs (e.g. Helsinki Heart Study, Lipid Research Clinic Trial) have also demonstrated that it is possible to reduce heart disease mortality. However, both of the trials mentioned also found an increase in non-cardiovascular mortality in the study group. Findings of this nature led to concern about the safety of cholesterol lowering in subjects who have not experienced heart disease. The Scandinavian Simvastatin Survival Study (1994) achieved a 25 per cent reduction in plasma cholesterol and 42 per cent fewer coronary deaths, and no excess mortality in the treated group.

Secondary prevention targets those who already possess signs or symptoms of heart disease, or who have suffered a heart attack. In recent years, interventions have introduced other dietary manipulations as the lipid hypothesis has become more sophisticated. Some of these studies have achieved excellent results. The DART study (Burr et al., 1989) showed that advice to eat fatty fish resulted in a reduction of 29 per cent in mortality within 2 years; this was not seen in a group advised about fat intakes or about cereal fibre intake. The Lyon Diet Heart Study (De Lorgeril et al., 1994) increased the levels of alpha-linolenic acid as part of the dietary intervention, and achieved a 70 per cent reduction in mortality and 73 per cent fewer non-fatal coronary events. Addition of long-chain *n*-3 fatty acids to the diet, resulted in a 20 per cent reduction in coronary heart disease mortality (GISSI Prevenzione Investigators, 1999).

It is clear that the lipid hypothesis does not fully explain all the causes of coronary heart disease. In particular:

■ the saturated/polyunsaturated fat relationship is an oversimplification of the link between diet and heart disease;

■ some of the saturated fatty acids have more potent effects than others;

■ the role of different polyunsaturated fatty acids in the atherosclerosis process is determined by the position of the first double bond in the chain and hence the fatty acid family;

■ further evidence suggests that monounsaturated fatty acids are important in determining development of coronary heart disease;

■ the *trans* fatty acids that are found in the diet may also have a role.

We shall return to these issues later in the chapter.

RISK FACTORS

Coronary heart disease is a multifactorial condition, determined by the interaction of different combinations of factors, known as risk factors. Many of these have now been identified. A risk factor does not necessarily cause the disease nor does its presence mean that an individual will definitely develop heart disease. They can, however, help to explain cross-cultural and inter-individual differences. Although the factors are modulated by individual susceptibility, the presence of several factors in any one individual does suggest that there is a greater chance of developing disease. In addition, there are synergistic effects between the risk factors. For example, the calculated risk from smoking is much greater in an individual who also has raised blood cholesterol levels than in one whose levels are in the normal range. Adding the extra risk factor of raised blood pressure further elevates the risk by an amount greater than that seen for hypertension alone. This is illustrated in Figure 14.3.

It should also be remembered that the development of heart disease is a process and that risk factors may be involved at different stages. Therefore, some may contribute to the laying down of fatty deposits in the blood vessels, and others influence the formation of a thrombosis or determine the response of the heart muscle to a lack of oxygen supply.

The main risk factors associated with heart disease are shown in Figure 14.4. Some of the factors are believed to increase risk and others to reduce risk. Therefore, any high risk factors can be ameliorated by enhancing those that reduce the risk.

Genetic predisposition

This may be associated with increased risk. Often those who develop heart disease have a strong

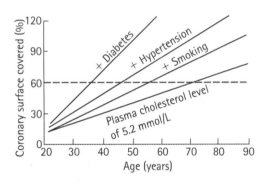

Figure 14.3 Additive effects of risk factors on damage to coronary arteries. (From Grundy, 1988. Copyright 1988, American Medical Association. All rights reserved.)

family history of the disease. It has even been suggested that any advice to reduce heart disease risk should only be targeted at those with a family history, as this will account for most of the new cases. Equally, it should be remembered that there may be a genetic predisposition to not develop heart disease.

Age

It was stated earlier in this chapter that the risk of heart disease increases with age in both men and women. Morbidity statistics show the peak age in men to be 55–64 and in women 75–84. This implies that the disease develops over a period of time, which is in line with the proposed mechanisms described earlier. In women, there is a relative protection against the disease during the reproductive years and an increase in incidence after the menopause. This also accounts for the gender differences in risk in middle age, with a higher risk seen in men than women before the ages of 50–55.

Social class

Contrary to the common perception, it is not the 'stressed businessman' who is most likely to develop heart disease. The highest incidence of the disease is in the lowest social class and shows an inverse class gradient. Standardized mortality ratios for England and Wales show this quite clearly for both genders. Furthermore,

Background
(uncontrollable)
factors

- Genetic predisposition
- Increasing age
- Men at greater risk between age 55–64
- Low social class
- Low birthweight
- More northern latitudes of geographical location
- Some particular ethnic groups
- Disease, e.g. diabetes
- Inflammation

HEART DISEASE

Behavioural
(modifiable)
factors

- Smoking
- High blood pressure
- Raised blood lipids
- Obesity (especially with central fat deposits)
- Sedentary lifestyle
- Stress and lack of social support
- Dietary factors

Figure 14.4 Main risk factors in the development of coronary heart disease.

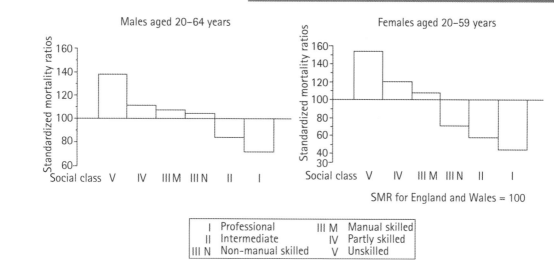

Figure 14.5 Social class and gender differences in heart disease mortality. SMR, standardized mortality ratio; it compares the true mortality of population with the experience that would have been expected if it had a standard mortality rate. An SMR in excess of 100 indicates mortality rates higher than expected in a standard population. (From DoH, 1994. Crown Copyright is reproduced with the permission of the Controller of Her Majesty's Stationery Office.)

improvements in heart disease rates have been largest in the professional classes, so that the gap between these and the unskilled groups is widening (Figure 14.5). There is also a difference in height between social classes in the UK, those in the higher social classes being taller. This results in an inverse relationship between heart disease and height.

Birthweight

Individuals who were born small for gestational age have been shown in a number of studies to have a higher risk of coronary heart disease. In addition, there is an increased risk of many of the risk factors, such as hypertension, raised cholesterol levels and higher levels of the blood clotting factors. Those individuals who were thin at birth, with less well-developed skeletal muscle are also at risk of glucose intolerance, which may result in Type 2 diabetes in adult life. This in its turn may also result in a higher risk of coronary heart disease, as it is associated with some of the other factors mentioned above. The risk seems to be greatest in those people who become overweight as adults having been small infants. Maintenance of a normal body weight helps to minimize the risk. More information about these associations is presented in Chapter 11.

Geographical location

Crude heart disease prevalence trends indicate that the disease occurs more commonly in northern latitudes and is less common nearer the equator. It has been suggested that low levels of ultraviolet light during winter months may in some way be responsible perhaps via a mechanism involving vitamin D levels. This would also link with the increased incidence of heart attacks in winter. Immigrants tend to experience the heart disease risk of their host country after a relatively short period of time. However, as has already been mentioned, it has been found that some of the immigrant groups in the UK have much higher heart disease rates than the indigenous population. Thus, although environmental factors play an important part, other mechanisms are also involved.

Disease

Of the many diseases affecting humans, diabetes is one of the most prevalent and people with Type 2 diabetes have an increased risk of heart disease, often associated with obesity and raised lipid levels. The insulin resistance syndrome that occurs in these cases is associated with central obesity and a number of metabolic abnormalities, affecting carbohydrate and fat metabolism, and resulting in raised lipid levels and poor oxidative capacity in skeletal muscle and liver (see Chapter 5). The current guidelines on dietary management of diabetes stress reduced fat intakes to minimize the risk. Previously, recommended diets controlled carbohydrate intakes strictly and allowed much higher fat intakes, which exacerbated the problem of heart disease.

There is some reported evidence that a chronic inflammatory state associated with the presence of infective organisms (e.g. *Helicobacter pylori*, found in the stomach, *Chlamydia pneumoniae*, which can cause respiratory infection, or even oral bacteria that cause gum disease) may elevate cytokine levels, which affect the endothelial function of the blood vessel, and may facilitate immune responses and trigger clotting mechanisms. Patients with periodontal disease have been shown to have higher levels of plasma clotting factors. Conversely, bacteria responsible for periodontitis have been found in atherosclerotic plaques. C-reactive protein (CRP), a marker of inflammation has now been shown to correlate with incidence of heart disease.

Smoking

Similar proportions of men and women (28 per cent) are smokers in England. Smoking is much more prevalent in manual social classes and in lower income groups. Persuading at-risk subjects to stop smoking can result in a significant reduction of their heart disease risk. It is thought that the free radicals that enter the body from cigarette smoke contribute to the disease process by causing peroxidation of lipids. The altered lipids are then taken up by macrophages in the blood vessel walls and contribute to the fatty streaks. A further potential effect of smoking is the reduction in oxygen-carrying capacity of the red blood cells owing to higher levels of carbon monoxide, which can exacerbate ischaemia in tissues fed by narrowed blood vessels. Dietary intake studies also show that smokers tend to have poorer diets and consume lower levels of antioxidants from fruit, which compounds the risks from free radicals. There appears to be a clear linear relationship between the numbers of cigarettes smoked per day and heart disease risk.

High blood pressure

The Health Survey for England (Erens and Primatesta, 1999) showed that 40.8 per cent of men and 32.9 per cent of women were hypertensive, with a higher prevalence of high blood pressure in more economically deprived groups. A higher proportion of those subjects with high blood pressure were also found to be physically inactive, have high total cholesterol and lower levels of high-density lipoprotein (HDL) cholesterol.

Raised blood pressure is one of the main contributors to heart disease, possibly because it potentiates the damage to blood vessel walls and increases the transfer of substances across the blood vessel wall. Both of these may play a part in the development of the fibrous plaque. Reduction of blood pressure by drug treatment, weight loss or dietary modification is likely to be of benefit. Better control of hypertension may account for some of the reduction in heart disease seen in Western countries in recent years.

Raised blood lipids

Above normal levels of cholesterol, especially in the low-density lipoprotein fraction, are strongly linked with increased risk of heart disease, as evidenced by many studies. Those individuals with familial hyperlipidaemias have a well-recognized high risk of developing heart disease, often at a very young age. Recent interest has focused on the possible role of lipoprotein(a), closely related to LDL, but carrying an additional apoprotein molecule. Raised levels of this molecule appear to be more strongly linked to myocardial infarction than even LDL. These may explain the high incidence of heart disease in South Asians in the UK. Chylomicrons and very low density lipoprotein (VLDL), both of which are rich in triglycerides, are elevated in some individuals, resulting in prolonged lipaemia (presence of fats in the blood) after meals. These raised levels seem to be caused by a defective rate of clearance from the circulation by the enzyme lipoprotein lipase (LPL). Both chylomicrons and VLDL are likely to be atherogenic and constitute risk factors. More attention is now being focused on dietary factors that contribute to raised levels of the VLDL fraction. Measures to reduce blood lipid levels in individuals as well as population groups could result in reduced incidence of heart disease.

Weight

Early studies, such as the Seven Countries Study by Keys, failed to find a causative effect of overweight on heart disease risk because many of the other risk factors are also aggravated by a higher body fat content. Using more sophisticated analyses, it is now clear that excess body fat is a direct contributor to coronary heart disease, as well as acting indirectly through many of the risk factors, such as diabetes, hypertension and raised blood lipids. In particular, when body fat distribution is taken into account, and people are divided into 'apples' (those with predominantly abdominal fat deposits) and 'pears' (peripheral fat deposits, mostly around the buttocks and hips), a strong relationship with heart disease is seen for 'apples'. In general, the relative risk of cardiovascular disease for individuals with a body mass index (BMI) >30 is about 2–3 times that of people with a BMI <25. The use of waist circumference as a guide to the need for weight loss is a useful quick measure to indicate increased risk. Action levels for weight loss based on waist measurements are discussed in Chapter 8. Weight loss by dietary restriction and with physical activity can improve all the modifiable risk factors and thus reduce the risk of coronary heart disease.

Physical activity

A proportion of people have been shown to have minimal levels of physical activity. The Health Survey for England (Erens and Primatesta, 1999) found that 20–25 per cent of men and women reported no physical activity in the 4 weeks prior to the survey. However, 37 per cent of men and 25 per cent of women reported activity at the recommended level. This includes activity of moderate intensity for at least 30 minutes on at least 5 days of the week. The remaining subjects had activity levels between these limits.

Many long-term studies have found lower mortality in those who have a more active lifestyle, compared with more sedentary controls and, therefore, exercise has been promoted as desirable in the reduction of heart disease risk. Changes to activity levels are followed by changes in risk of death, with an improvement of risk seen in previously sedentary subjects who begin an activity programme. Even moderate levels of activity appear to confer benefit, although the evidence is stronger for men than women. The mechanisms involved are unclear but, at a basic level, activity helps in the maintenance of energy balance and prevents development of overweight. Exercise has been shown to increase the beneficial high-density lipoprotein. Abdominal fat deposits appear to be particularly sensitive to mobilization by exercise and, in individuals with central obesity, even moderate exercise can produce improvements in the metabolic profile. Other possible beneficial effects include changes in clotting factors (linked to endurance-type exercise) or in the density of capillaries in the tissues, which provides protection against ischaemic damage, if blood vessels become narrowed. Inactivity may be as important a risk factor as hypertension, smoking or hypercholesterolaemia.

Psychosocial factors

These are less well defined than other factors. Data from the Whitehall studies show higher rates of heart disease in lower employment grades, with the gradients being steeper for women than men (see Ashwell, 1996; DoH, 1994). It is suggested that stress and lack of social support may be linked to coronary heart disease.

Dietary factors

There are several constituents of the diet for which there is evidence of a link with heart disease. Most notably this applies to the fats that have been linked with lipid levels in the blood. In addition, other components, such as total energy intake, dietary fibre (non-starch polysaccharides), sugar, salt, alcohol and antioxidant nutrients, have all been studied in

Possible promoting dietary factors

- High intake of dietary cholesterol
- High intake of saturated fatty acids
  - Myristic acid
    +
    Palmitic acid → ↑ serum cholesterol
  - Lauric acid
    +   → suppress clearing of
    Myristic acid   LDL cholesterol
  - Stearic acid
    +   → Thrombogenesis
    Myristic acid
- High intake of *trans* fatty acids
  (in processed foods and fat spreads)
  ↳ ↑ LDL cholesterol
    ↓ HDL
    (but to a lesser extent than
    lauric or palmitic acids)
- Low energy intake diets
  (because lacking in protective
  nutrients and indicative of
  sedentary lifestyle)
- High salt intake
  ↳ hypertension
- Heavy drinking of alcohol
  (>55 units for men, >35 units for
  women per week)
  ↳ ↑ triglycerides and VLDL levels
    (binge drinking → sudden death)
    from MI)

Possible protective dietary factors

- A diet high in monounsaturated fatty acids,
  low in saturated fats
  ↳ ↓ LDL cholesterol
    (half as effective as *n*-6 PUFA substitution)
  ↳ ↑ HDL cholesterol
  ↳ ↓ clotting factor activation
  ↳ resistant to free-radical damage
    which may trigger fibrous plaque
    formation
- *n*-6 PUFAs (in plant sources)
  ↳ ↑ HDL:LDL cholesterol
    (but PUFAs vulnerable to free radicals)
- *n*-3 PUFAs (in plant and marine sources)
  ↳ ↓ VLDL·············> ↓LDL
  ↳ ↓ inflammation, thrombosis and
    susceptibility to high blood pressure
  ↳ stabilizes rhythm of heart
- Potassium, calcium and magnesium
  ↳ ↓ blood pressure
- Calcium (especially in dairy products)
  ↳ binds dietary fats and stops their
    absorption
  ↳ ↓ platelet clotting activity
- Moderate alcohol (especially red wine)
  ↳ ↑HDL levels
  ↳ ↓ platelet aggregation
  ↳ antioxidants
- Soluble fibre
  ↳ ↑ sterol excretion
  ↳ ↓ serum cholesterol
- Fibre in general
- Antioxidants from dietary sources
  e.g. fruit, vegetables, seeds, nuts
  containing beta-carotene,
  vitamins C and E
- Folate (in fruit and vegetables)
  ↳ ↓ homocysteine levels
  ↳ ↓ fatty streaks and coagulation

HEART DISEASE

Figure 14.6 A summary of dietary risk factors for coronary heart disease. HDL, high-density lipoprotein; LDL, low-density lipoprotein; MI, myocardial infarction; PUFA, polyunsaturated fatty acid.

relation to stages in the development of heart disease. The dietary risk factors are summarized in Figure 14.6.

Fats

Dietary cholesterol

Meat, egg yolks and dairy products contain fairly large amounts of cholesterol and many people concerned about their blood lipids have in the past attempted to reduce their intake of these foods. However, changing the amount of cholesterol in the diet has only limited effects on blood cholesterol concentrations in most people. This is because several compensation mechanisms exist. Only about half of the cholesterol ingested is absorbed from the gut; a typical dietary intake of 400 mg/day will, therefore, only result in the absorption of 200 mg of cholesterol. The essential nature of cholesterol in the body means that the body synthesizes the remainder of its needs, about 1 g of cholesterol per day. If dietary intake increases, the amount synthesized is reduced to compensate; this is achieved by regulating one of the enzymes – hydroxymethyl-glutaryl coenzyme A (HMG-coA) reductase – in the cholesterol synthesis pathway in the liver through a negative feedback mechanism. In addition, HDL activity can also increase to scavenge excess cholesterol from the tissues for removal in bile.

However, control is not exact and an increase in cholesterol intake in the diet can raise blood cholesterol levels. It has also been shown that there are individual, genetically determined differences in response to dietary cholesterol, with hyporesponders and hyperresponders. This makes it difficult to generalize about the effect of dietary cholesterol.

Saturated fatty acids

Originally, it was postulated that all saturated fatty acids in the diet were equally harmful, causing an elevation of blood cholesterol/LDL levels. It is now recognized that myristic acid (C14) is the main fatty acid responsible for raising the serum cholesterol level. This contributes to the formation of fibrous plaques and is described as atherogenic. Both lauric acid (C12) and myristic acid also suppress the clearing mechanism at LDL receptors, which removes LDL cholesterol from the circulation, thus contributing to raised circulating levels. Palmitic acid (C16) has probably less effect on cholesterol levels in the blood than originally suggested by Keys. However, palmitic acid is the main saturated fatty acid in most diets and, therefore, has an important effect because of its prevalence. In addition, the different fatty acids appear to have varying effects on the formation of thrombi in the blood. Myristic acid and stearic acid (C18) are considered to be the most thrombogenic, together with *trans* fatty acids. A reduction in thrombogenic effects is associated with monounsaturated fatty acids, seed oils and fish oils.

Monounsaturated fatty acids

Monounsaturated fatty acids (MUFAs), particularly oleic acid (18:1), were originally believed to be neutral in their effect on blood cholesterol levels and were not included in the original equations of Keys and Hegsted. Studies of heart disease prevalence among peoples in Mediterranean countries showed a lower rate than expected. The diet in these countries (particularly Greece and southern Italy) contains more MUFAs, especially oleic acid from olive oil, than is found in northern European diets. This led to the suggestion that this type of fatty acid may be protective against heart disease. It should, however, be remembered that there are many other features of a Mediterranean diet and lifestyle, such as large intakes of fruit, vegetables and wine, which may better explain the lower prevalence of heart disease. However, a number of studies have now confirmed that substitution of some of the saturated fats in the diet by MUFAs results in a reduction of LDL cholesterol, equal to about half of that achieved by *n*-6 polyunsaturated fatty acid (PUFA) substitution. In addition, however, there is an elevation of HDL cholesterol, an effect not obtained with *n*-6 PUFAs.

The proposed mechanism is an increase in LDL clearance by the liver as a result of increased receptor activity. In addition, as MUFAs contain only one double bond, they are more resistant to the harmful effects of free radicals, which attack PUFAs and can lead to the early stages of fibrous plaque formation. Observed effects on thrombogenesis have also been reported, with reduced levels of clotting factor activation. Overall, MUFAs are considered to be a beneficial component of the diet, with no harmful effects on the known risk factors for coronary heart disease. New equations predicting the change in total serum cholesterol consequent on modifications to the dietary intake of MUFAs, in addition to saturated fatty acids (SFAs) and PUFAs, have now been developed based on metabolic ward studies (e.g. Mensink and Katan, 1992). It should, however, be remembered that, in terms of weight control, the intake of MUFAs, as of other fats in the diet may need to be regulated.

Polyunsaturated fatty acids

Polyunsaturated fatty acids in the diet originate from two main sources: *n*-6 acids from plant foods and *n*-3 acids mainly from marine foods, and it is now recognized that the two families have different effects on coronary heart disease risk factors. Other roles in the body have been discussed in Chapter 5.

n-6 PUFAs. Fatty acids from this family have a LDL cholesterol-lowering effect, independent of any change in saturated fat intake. The effect is achieved, it is believed, by increasing the removal of LDL from the circulation by enhancing the activity of the LDL receptor sites, which thus opposes the effect of the saturated fatty acids on these receptors. Although *n*-6 PUFAs are also reported to reduce HDL levels in the blood, this is to a smaller extent than the effect on LDL and, consequently, the HDL/LDL ratio increases.

The *n*-6 PUFAs in membrane lipids are, however, vulnerable to free radical attack, resulting in peroxidation. Once established, this produces a chain reaction with further peroxide formation and potential for further damage. At present, there is little evidence that high intake of n-6 PUFAs in any way contributes to enhanced peroxidation in the body, but the vulnerability of the double bonds in these molecules suggests that this could be a possibility. Accordingly, it is advisable to be cautious about excessively high intakes of PUFAs and intakes should be below 10 per cent of total energy. European recommendations (EURODIET, 2001) are that intakes of n-6 PUFAs should not exceed 5 per cent (range 4–8 per cent) of total energy.

n-3 PUFAs. The n-3 fatty acids reduce VLDL levels and hence may eventually cause a reduction in LDL. The effect is linked to a more rapid clearance of VLDL rich in n-3 PUFAs than those containing SFAs, resulting in less post-prandial lipaemia on a n-3 PUFA-rich diet. However, the main interest in these fatty acids is associated with their action on blood clotting, which arose from studies on Greenland Eskimos who, despite a diet high in fat, have very low rates of heart disease. In addition, these subjects have prolonged bleeding times. Their diet contains a large amount of marine foods providing high levels of long-chain n-3 PUFAs. Chapter 5 describes the role of the essential fatty acids in the formation of prostaglandins and related eicosanoids. The n-3 series of prostaglandins and eicosanoids has less aggregating potency than those made from the n-6 family. In addition, the vasoconstricting effects on blood vessel walls are less. The overall effect is that the n-3 series is less likely to produce inflammation, thrombosis or increases in blood pressure. All of these responses are likely to reduce the risk of heart attack. Ingestion of significant amounts of n-3 PUFAs is believed to displace the n-6 series from enzyme sites, so that n-3 series eicosanoids are produced. Research has attempted to ascertain the ratio of n-6:n-3 PUFAs in the diet that could ensure optimal outcomes in respect of coronary heart disease. Current advice for populations based on EURODIET (2001) is that n-3 PUFAs should constitute 1 per cent of total energy, providing a n-6:n-3 ratio of 5:1.

Data from the DART study (Burr et al., 1989) also suggested that the higher intake of n-3 acids

stabilizes the rhythm of the heart and allows it to continue beating normally during a heart attack, ensuring a higher chance of survival. The Lyon Heart Study (De Lorgeril et al., 1998) demonstrated a significant protective effect of additional alpha-linolenic acid together with a Mediterranean diet. Supplementation with long-chain n-3 PUFAs in the GISSI trial (GISSI Prevenzione Investigators, 1999) caused a reduction in total mortality. It is on the basis of studies such as these that an increase in n-3 PUFA intake is recommended, either by increasing fish consumption, or inclusion of more sources of alpha-linolenic acid in the diet.

Trans *fatty acids*

As discussed in Chapter 5, the naturally occurring unsaturated fatty acids have a *cis* orientation; *trans* fatty acids are produced by chemical alteration of the molecule. This occurs in the stomachs of ruminants and result in a dietary intake of naturally formed *trans* fatty acids in foods such as milk, dairy products, beef and lamb. In addition, the diet contains artificial *trans* fatty acids produced during food processing or manufacture of fat spreads by hydrogenation (approximately 65 per cent of the total intake). These fats are used in the manufacture of biscuits, pies, cakes and potato crisps. Most *trans* fatty acids have so far been monounsaturated, predominantly *trans*-oleic acid. The manufacture of high PUFA margarines, using emulsifier technology and the deodorizing of vegetable oils has resulted in increased levels of *trans* PUFAs, including both n-6 and n-3, and there could be an increased intake of *trans*-alpha-linolenic acid in the future.

Studies suggest that large amounts of *trans* fatty acids (greater than currently consumed in the UK) raise LDL cholesterol and depress HDL, albeit to a smaller extent than seen with lauric and palmitic acids. Other evidence points to an elevation of lipoprotein(a) by up to 30 per cent. Current intakes in the UK are in the range of 4–6 g per person, but the top 2.5 per cent of consumers may take in more than 12 g/day. Intakes are higher in the USA, with an average of 8.1 g/person per day.

Overall, *trans* fatty acids have an adverse effect on both LDL and HDL, and this appears to be greater than that following an equal amount of saturated fatty acids. Nevertheless, since saturated fat represents a greater proportion of fat intake, reducing these is of greater importance. Consideration should perhaps be given to including information about *trans* fatty acids in nutritional labelling. It is recommended that *trans* fatty acids should comprise no more than 1 per cent of total energy intake.

Conjugated linoleic acid (CLA) is a *trans* fatty acid formed during the conversion of linoleic acid to oleic acid by rumen bacteria. It is found in milk and dairy produce, and in beef and lamb. Animal studies have shown an anticancer and antiatherogenic activity by this acid, and current research is investigating potential health benefits.

Total fat

When total fat intake was studied by Keys (1970) in the Seven Countries Study, it was found that there was an association with serum cholesterol levels and heart disease mortality. However, this effect was dependent on the saturated fat intake. More recent data have suggested that the total fat intake may be closely linked with the activity of Factor VII, one of the clotting factors, and may thus have a role to play in the thrombosis phase of the aetiology of heart disease. The current view is that total fat intake needs to be controlled in individuals who are not within the ideal body weight range. In these cases, a reduction in fat, together with increased physical activity is a useful contribution to reducing the risk of coronary heart disease. In people who are at or near their ideal body weight, the balance of fats should be the main focus, rather than aiming to change total fat intakes.

Total energy

A low energy intake has been associated with a high incidence of heart disease. Low levels of food intake not only contain small amounts of energy, but also low nutrient levels, including many of the other protective factors that are necessary to sustain normal physiological functioning in the body. It is thought possible that this level of intake is a consequence of a low energy output and a sign of a sedentary lifestyle.

In addition, low levels of physical activity are associated with increased body weight, which in itself is considered to be a risk factor. The incorporation of physical activity into everyday life is probably the best way to escape from this cycle.

Salt

The possible links between salt intake and hypertension have been discussed in Chapter 10. Since hypertension is a recognized risk factor in coronary heart disease, it can be argued that reducing salt intake in those who are susceptible might reduce their risk of heart disease. However, it is now clear that a broader dietary approach can be more effective in reducing blood pressure. Data from the Dietary Approaches to Stop Hypertension (DASH) trial showed a dietary change that included low-fat dairy products, nuts, fruit and vegetables resulted in greater reductions in blood pressure than salt restriction alone (Appel et al., 1997). The DASH diet included increased intakes of potassium, calcium and magnesium, as well as lower sodium intakes, and it is now recognized that all of these factors are effective in changing blood pressure. These findings add further support to the importance of potassium intakes in the control of blood pressure.

Calcium

For many years it has been noted that the incidence of coronary heart disease is lower in those geographical areas that have hard water. Several mechanisms have been put forward, with supporting evidence. Dietary calcium combines with fats, especially saturated fatty acids producing soaps, which remain unabsorbed and are excreted from the body. In a study of British and French farmers, calcium intake was inversely related to blood levels of triglycerides. In addition, there was an inverse relationship with platelet clotting activity. Finally, as discussed above, calcium intakes are inversely related to blood pressure, as has been demonstrated in a number of large cohort studies. In general, calcium intakes, especially from dairy produce, appear to be associated with a lower risk of coronary heart disease and low-fat cheese may be considered a constituent of healthy diets.

Alcohol

Heavy drinking in excess of 55 units for men and 35 units for women per week is associated with raised triglyceride and VLDL levels, and thus increases heart disease risk. In addition, binge drinking has been associated with sudden death due to myocardial infarction or stroke. However, a moderate alcohol intake (within 'safe' limits) has been shown to have a protective effect against heart disease. The mechanisms appear to involve both the atherogenesis and thrombogenesis aspects of coronary heart disease. A number of studies have found an increase in HDL levels on alcohol consumption, which falls within 24 hours when alcohol intake stops. The elevation of HDL is approximately similar to that achieved by physical activity. In addition, moderate alcohol intake has been shown to reduce platelet aggregation. In large amounts, alcohol can cause platelet aggregation. In this case, alcoholic beverages that contain antioxidants, such as red wine, may be protective.

The relationship between alcohol consumption and heart disease is usually found to follow a J-shaped curve, with increased risk in non-drinkers and heavy drinkers. The lowest risk occurs in the middle range of alcohol intakes, taking 2–4 drinks per day on 3–4 days per week. Ideally, consumption should be with meals, as is seen in Mediterranean countries. There has been debate about the type of alcoholic drink that may be most beneficial, and many studies suggest that red wine has the greatest protective effects. However, in general, it appears that the consistent effects are attributable to the alcohol per se, rather than additional constituents particular to a specific beverage. However, antioxidants in red wine, most notably resveratrol, may contribute an additional protective benefit.

Some concern has been expressed by health educationists about the desirability of promoting alcohol consumption as a means of preventing heart disease because of the implications for health of alcohol in amounts greater than 'moderate'.

Fibre (non-starch polysaccharides)

Sources of soluble fibre, especially from oats, have been shown to reduce serum cholesterol levels, although the effects are not large. Insoluble fibre does not appear to have a similar effect on cholesterol. Nevertheless, a significant inverse relationship between fibre intake and myocardial infarction and coronary mortality has been demonstrated in two prospective studies, in Finland and the USA, in large cohorts of men. The relationship was strongest for cereal fibre and persisted when confounding variables were taken into account. It has been suggested that the effects occur due to the satiating effect of fibre-rich foods that results in a lowered fat intake and possibly a reduced total energy intake.

However, soluble fibre may increase sterol excretion from the body, thereby lowering cholesterol levels. High fibre intake has been associated with a decrease in the level of insulin and increased insulin sensitivity, thus improving metabolic function. Additionally, a high-fibre diet also affects the clotting factors and may be associated with a lower blood pressure. Overall, it is likely that the effects of fibre on heart disease are not mediated through a single mechanism and no adverse harmful effects have been reported from increased sources of fibre in the diet.

Antioxidants

The inability of the lipid hypothesis to explain the link between diet and heart disease fully, and the completion of studies that show inconsistent or contrary results have led over the years to a search for other influencing factors. Several studies demonstrated that levels of antioxidants in both diet and serum exhibit good correlations with heart disease incidence – often higher levels of correlation than are seen in the same studies for fat indices. In particular, the MONICA study (Gey et al., 1991) has shown inverse relationships between heart disease mortality and intakes of beta-carotene, vitamin C and vitamin E. The strongest correlations ($p < 0.001$) were seen with alpha-tocopherol, vitamin C and beta-carotene in food supplies and the rate of coronary heart disease. Correlations also existed with the dietary sources of these nutrients, most notably vegetables, vegetable oils, sunflower seed oil, seeds, nuts and fruit. In the USA, two large prospective studies (of male health professionals and female nurses) found a lower incidence of coronary heart disease in the subjects who consumed vitamin E supplements.

However, these results were not replicated in a series of intervention studies in various countries, in which supplements of the major antioxidants, mainly vitamin E and beta-carotene, were assigned to subjects. In general, these studies showed either no beneficial effect of supplementation with these antioxidants or an adverse effect of supplementation, with a higher rate of coronary heart disease or cancer than the control groups. It is suggested that antioxidant nutrients can act as pro-oxidants in certain conditions, which may include the administration of large amounts of a single antioxidant.

Thus, it is likely that antioxidants work together to produce the effects seen in whole diet studies, and that advice should be targeted towards fruit and vegetable consumption. It is possible that fruit and vegetables contain other substances that have not yet been taken into account and that have even more effect on heart disease development. There is interest in other factors found in fruit and vegetables, such as polyphenols or flavonoids. The recommendation of the WHO is to eat five servings of fruit and vegetables per day.

There are good grounds for believing that the antioxidant nutrients do play a preventive role in the formation of fibrous plaques. It is appropriate at this point to summarize all of the functions of antioxidants in protection against free radicals.

Mechanisms of action of antioxidants

Free radicals are produced by most of the oxidative reactions in the body. The most important of these radicals are:

- the hydroxyl radical. OH
- superoxide radical. O_2
- singlet oxygen. $^1O_2$
- nitric oxide. NO.

Also included are the peroxyl radical, hydrogen peroxide and hydroperoxyl. All share the common property of having an exceedingly short lifespan and, therefore, are very unstable. They can attack vital cell components, inactivate enzymes and damage genetic material. It is, therefore, reasonable to assume they play a part in degenerative diseases.

The body has a complex antioxidant defence system to counteract these radicals. This is made up of endogenous and exogenous components.

- Endogenous antioxidants are mainly enzymes that catalyse radical quenching reactions (many of these are dependent on dietary minerals for activation) or bind pro-oxidants, which might catalyse free-radical reactions.
- Exogenous antioxidants are mainly vitamins that quench free radicals.

Endogenous antioxidants

The antioxidant enzymes include:

- superoxide dismutase (SOD), which neutralizes the superoxide radical and which requires zinc and copper, or manganese for activation;
- catalase, which is specific for hydrogen peroxide and requires iron for its activity; and
- glutathione peroxidase, which removes peroxides and is a selenium-requiring enzyme.

Many minerals are clearly involved in activating these enzymes. However, copper and iron can also act as pro-oxidants when freely present. This explains why there are binding proteins present to prevent this happening, most notably caeruloplasmin and albumin to bind copper, and transferrin and ferritin to bind iron.

Exogenous antioxidants

The most important of these are vitamins C and E, and the carotenoids. Plant flavonoids are possible members of this group.

Vitamins C and E quench free radicals by providing H atoms to pair up with unpaired electrons on free radicals. This inactivates the vitamins, which then need to be regenerated. Glutathione is believed to regenerate vitamin C and vitamin C can regenerate vitamin E (Figure 14.7). In its turn, vitamin E may promote the antioxidant activity of beta-carotene against lipid peroxidation. It is suggested that vitamin C is the primary antioxidant in the plasma and is consumed first in destroying free radicals. Vitamin E is the major antioxidant in the lipid parts of membranes. Lipid peroxidation does not begin until after the vitamin C has been used. It is important that regeneration can take place, however, so that a continued supply of the vitamins is available. These interactions highlight

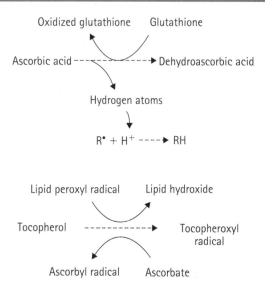

Figure 14.7 Interactions between glutathione, vitamin C and vitamin E during antioxidant activity. R• free radical.

the importance of maintaining a balance between the different exogenous antioxidants supplied to the body.

In conclusion, the theories about antioxidants allow some of the other factors discussed earlier to be linked together. It has been suggested that the desire for weight loss, which preoccupies so many women and which encourages them to eat low-calorie fruits and vegetables, helps to protect them from heart disease by adding more antioxidants to their diet. Smokers, who have a greatly increased risk of heart disease, are recorded as having very low intakes of fruit and vegetables and consequently poor vitamin C status. When linked to the increased burden of free radicals, this may explain their greater risk. Finally, alcoholic beverages, most notably wines, contain phenolic substances that also act as antioxidants. This may explain why there are lower rates of coronary heart disease among populations in wine-drinking countries.

Homocysteine

It has been known since the late 1960s that raised levels of homocysteine in the blood are associated with severe arteriosclerosis. Initially, this was considered to be a problem in individuals with inborn errors in the metabolism of homocysteine. However, in recent years, it has been found that raised homocysteine levels are an independent risk factor for vascular disease, and the effect is graded. The evidence for this comes from a range of different studies, including retrospective case-control, cross-sectional and prospective studies. The metabolism of homocysteine is linked to that of methionine and cysteine, and utilizes a number of B vitamins as cofactors. These include folate, pyridoxine, riboflavin and vitamin B_{12}. Deficiencies in the metabolism of homocysteine, with resultant elevated plasma levels, are associated with mutations in one of the enzymes (methylene tetrahydrofolate reductase; MTHFR) involved in the metabolic pathway (see Chapter 9 for more details). Lower activity levels of the enzyme have been identified in approximately 30 per cent of the population, with a smaller percentage being homozygous for the mutation. The reference range of homocysteine in the plasma is still debated, but the following are generally accepted:

5–15 μmol/L	normal range
15–30 μmol/L	moderate elevation
30–100 μmol/L	intermediate elevation
>100 μmol/L	severe elevation

It has been proposed that homocysteine may be directly toxic to endothelial cells, through a mechanism involving nitric oxide that normally causes endothelial relaxation. This would facilitate monocyte adhesion and promote the process of fatty streak formation. A further possible mechanism is through an increased coagulation tendency, by an inhibition of the normal fibrinolytic mechanisms that disperse blood clots. However, neither of these mechanisms has yet been conclusively proven and much remains to be discovered about the relationship of homocysteine to the processes of vascular disease.

Dietary interventions can lower homocysteine levels. Most importantly, folate status is inversely associated with homocysteine levels, with as little as 200 μg/day of folate causing a reduction in plasma homocysteine levels. Evidence is less conclusive for supplementation with riboflavin, pyridoxine or vitamin B_{12}, although a combination of these may be beneficial. It should also be remembered that folate is provided by fruit and vegetables in the diet, so that an increase in these foods in line with other aspects of dietary intervention will also help to increase folate status. Fortification of grain products with folic acid, at a rate of 1.4 μg/g of product has been introduced in the USA since 1999. Early indications are that, in the first year after this was introduced, there was a 3.4 per cent reduction in mortality from stroke and heart attack. Mean homocysteine levels have fallen, and mean plasma concentrations of folate have increased.

More controlled studies in this field are still required.

FUTURE DIRECTIONS

There is still a huge amount to learn about coronary heart disease. Developments in molecular biology and the human genome project may in the future allow research to identify the interaction between risk factors and particular genes. Animal models with specific genetic modifications are already being used to study mechanisms to understand existing knowledge. Improved targeting of dietary intervention and drug therapy may be a consequence.

SUMMARY

1 The role of diet in the aetiology of coronary heart disease is complex.
2 Early hypotheses about links with fat have been discovered to explain only part of the relationship.
3 New findings about the roles of other fats, such as monounsaturated fatty acids, n-3 fats and *trans* fatty acids have modified the original lipid hypothesis.
4 The importance of other dietary factors, in particular the antioxidants, provides opportunities to link some of the earlier findings together.
5 Dietary guidelines promoting lower fat, and increased fruit and vegetables intakes address many of the postulated mechanisms relating to coronary heart disease. Weight control and promotion of physical activity remain important preventive factors.

STUDY QUESTIONS

1 Distinguish between atherogenesis and thrombogenesis, and describe the mechanisms that are currently offered as explanations of these processes.
2 Which dietary factors are thought to be involved in:
   a atherogenesis
   b thrombogenesis?
3 What are the main tenets of the lipid hypothesis and what changes to it have been suggested in recent years?
4 a Explain what you understand by the antioxidant nutrients.
   b Produce a diagram to show how they might play a part in protecting against heart disease.
5 Discuss with a colleague how you believe the theories about the dietary links with heart disease are reflected in current dietary guidelines. Can you explain all of the guidelines on a scientific basis?
6 Produce a poster or leaflet to summarize the main aspects of dietary advice for the prevention of coronary heart disease. Make the information as practical as possible.

REFERENCES AND FURTHER READING

Appel, L.J., Moore, T.G., Obarzanek, R. et al. 1997: A clinical trial of effects of dietary patterns on blood pressure. *New England Journal of Medicine* 336, 1117–24.

Ashwell, M. (ed.) 1996: *Diet and heart disease: a round table of factors*, 2nd edn. London: Chapman & Hall.

Bellizzi, M.C. 1995: Wine and vegetable oils: the French paradox revisited. *British Nutrition Foundation Nutrition Bulletin* **20**, 256–65.

Brown, A.A., Hu, F.B. 2001: Dietary modulation of endothelial function: implications for cardiovascular disease. *American Journal of Clinical Nutrition* **73**, 673–86.

Burr, M.L. 1993: Fish and ischaemic heart disease. *World Review of Nutrition and Dietetics* **72**, 49–60.

Burr, M.L., Fehily, A.M., Gilbert, J.F. et al. 1989: Effects of changes in fat, fish and fibre intakes on death and myocardial infarction: Diet and Reinfarction Trial (DART). *Lancet* **ii**, 757–61.

Caggiula, A.W., Mustad, V.A. 1997: Effects of dietary fat and fatty acids on coronary artery disease risk and total and lipoprotein cholesterol concentrations: epidemiologic studies. *American Journal of Clinical Nutrition* **65**(Suppl.), 159–610S.

De Lorgeril, M., Renaud, S., Mamelle, N. et al. 1994: Mediterranean alpha-linolenic acid-rich diet in secondary prevention of coronary heart disease. *Lancet* **343**, 1454–9.

DoH (UK Department of Health) 1992: *The health of the nation: a strategy for health in England.* London: HMSO.

De Lorgeril, M., Salen, P., Martin, J.L. et al. 1998: Mediterranean dietary pattern in a randomised trial. Prolonged survival and possible reduced cancer rate. *Archives of Internal Medicine* **158**, 1181–7.

DoH (UK Department of Health) 1994: *Nutritional aspects of cardiovascular disease.* Report on Health and Social Subjects No. 46. Report of the Cardiovascular Review Group of the Committee on Medical Aspects of Food Policy. London: HMSO.

DoH (UK Department of Health) 1999: *Saving lives – our healthier nation.* London: The Stationery Office.

Erens, B., Primatesta, P. (eds) 1999: *Health survey for England: cardiovascular disease '98.* Volume 1: Findings. London: The Stationery Office.

EURODIET 2001: Report and proceedings. *Public Health Nutrition* **4**, 2(A).

Gey, K.F., Puska, P., Jordan, P. et al. 1991: Inverse correlation between plasma vitamin E and mortality from ischaemic heart disease in cross-cultural epidemiology. *American Journal of Clinical Nutrition* **53**, 3265–345.

GISSI Prevenzione Investigators, 1999: Dietary supplementation with n-3 polyunsaturated fatty acids and vitamin E after myocardial infarction, results of the GISSI Prevenzione trial. *Lancet* **354**, 447–53.

Grundy, S.M. 1988: Cholesterol and heart disease: a new era. *Journal of the American Medical Association* **256**, 2849–58.

Halliwell, B. 1994: Free radicals, antioxidants and human disease: curiosity, cause or consequence? *Lancet* **344**, 721–4.

Hardman, A.E. 1999: Physical activity and cardiovascular risk. Review in depth. *Journal of Cardiovascular Risk* **2**, 285–329.

Hegsted, D.M., Ansman, L.M., Johnson, J.A. et al. 1993: Dietary fat and serum lipids: an evaluation of the experimental data. *American Journal of Clinical Nutrition* **57**, 875–83.

Hu, H., Stampfer, M.J., Manson, J.E. et al. 1997: Dietary fat intake and the risk of coronary heart disease in women. *New England Journal of Medicine* **337**, 1491–9.

Hulshof, K.F.A.M., van Erp-Baart, M.A., Anttolainen, M. et al. 1999: Intake of fatty acids in Western Europe with emphasis on trans fatty acids. The TRANSFAIR study. *European Journal of Clinical Nutrition* **53**, 143–57.

Jacob, R.A. 1995: The integrated antioxidant system. *Nutrition Research* **15**(5), 755–66.

Keys, A. (ed.) 1970: Coronary heart disease in seven countries. *Circulation* **41**(Suppl.), 11–211.

Kinane, D.F., Lowe, G.D.O. 2000: How periodontal disease may contribute to cardiovascular disease. *Periodontology* **23**, 121–6.

Kromhout, D. 2001: Epidemiology of cardiovascular disease in Europe. *Public Health Nutrition* **4**(2B), 441–57.

Law, M.R., Wald, N.J., Thompson, S.G. 1994: By how much and how quickly does reduction in serum cholesterol concentration lower risk of ischaemic heart disease? *British Medical Journal* 308, 367–72.

Martin, M.J., Halley, S.B., Browner, W.S. et al. 1986: Serum cholesterol, blood pressure and mortality: implications from a cohort of 361 622 men. *Lancet* ii, 933–36.

McKinley, M.C. 2000: Nutritional aspects and possible pathological mechanisms of hyperhomocysteinaemia: an independent risk factor for vascular disease. *Proceedings of the Nutrition Society* 59, 221–37.

Mensink, R.P., Katan, M.B. 1992: Effect of dietary fatty acids on serum lipids and lipoproteins – a meta-analysis of 27 trials. *Atherosclerosis and Thrombosis* 12, 911–19.

Renaud, S., Lanzmann-Petithory, D. 2001: Coronary heart disease: dietary links and pathogenesis. *Public Health Nutrition* 4(2B), 459–74.

Rimm, E.B., Klatsky, A., Grobbee, D. et al. 1996: Review of moderate alcohol consumption and reduced risk of coronary heart disease: is the effect due to beer, wine or spirits? *British Medical Journal* 312, 731–6.

Scandinavian Simvastatin Study Group 1994: Randomised trial of cholesterol lowering in 4444 patients with coronary heart disease: the Scandinavian Simvastatin Survival Study (45). *Lancet* 344, 1383–9.

Schaefer, E.J. 2002: Lipoproteins, nutrition and heart disease. *American Journal of Clinical Nutrition* 75, 191–212.

Shaper, A.G., Wannamethee, G. 1991: Physical activity and ischaemic heart disease in middle-aged British men. *British Heart Journal* 66, 384–94.

Slavin, J., Martin, M.C., Jacobs, D.R. et al. 1999: Plausible mechanisms for the protectiveness of whole grains. *American Journal of Clinical Nutrition* 70, 459S–63S.

Troisi, R., Willett, W.C., Weiss, S.T. 1992: Trans fatty acid intake in relation to serum lipid concentrations in adult men. *American Journal of Clinical Nutrition* 56, 1019–24.

Truswell, A.S. 1994: Review of dietary intervention studies: effects on coronary events and on total mortality. *Australia and New Zealand Journal of Medicine* 24, 98–106.

Various authors 2000: Symposium on reducing cardiovascular disease risk: today's achievements, tomorrow's opportunities. *Proceedings of the Nutrition Society* 59, 415–40.

CHAPTER 15

DIET AND CANCER

The aims of this chapter are to:

❑   describe what is meant by cancer;
❑   discuss the ways in which the relationship between diet and cancer is studied;
❑   identify the main relationships that have been indicated;
❑   describe the guidelines on healthy eating for the reduction of cancer risk.

On completing the study of this chapter, you should be able to:

❑   discuss the links between certain specific cancers and dietary patterns and explain the suggested mechanisms, where appropriate;
❑   discuss some of the problems inherent in studies on diet and cancer;
❑   advise the practical changes needed in a Western diet to reduce the risk of cancer.

Cancer affects one in three people in the UK at some time in their life, and is responsible for approximately one-quarter of all deaths, numbering some 160 000 cases per year. Lung cancer accounts for almost one-quarter of all cancer deaths and it is the leading type of cancer in men, followed by cancer of the prostate. In women, breast cancer causes most deaths, followed by lung cancer. In both men and women, cancer of the colon and rectum is the third major type of cancer.

More people now die from cancer than was the case 100 years ago. However, this is a reflection of a longer life expectancy and larger numbers of elderly people in the population. Because risk increases with age, the majority of cancer deaths occur in people aged over 65 years. Different cancers show different trends, however. Deaths from lung cancer are clearly linked to smoking and these have followed trends in smoking throughout the century. Melanoma, a cancer of the skin, has increased in recent years, probably as a result of increased exposure to the sun as more people take holidays abroad. On the

other hand, stomach cancer rates have declined dramatically since the 1950s. Several explanations may be offered for this, including dietary changes. However, a major factor recently discovered is the role of *Helicobacter pylori* in the development of the disease. Antibodies to this bacterium are much more common among people brought up in overcrowded housing conditions, who then have a higher risk of stomach cancer. Improvements in housing provision may have had the added benefit of reducing exposure to this bacterium and, consequently, contributed to reduced rates of stomach cancer. This example illustrates the often multifactorial nature of the aetiology of cancer, and the consequent difficulties of study.

Other factors that need to be taken into account in studying statistics on cancer are the improvements in detection and diagnosis, and advances in treatment, both of which may increase figures for the apparent incidence of the disease. Thus, we are not working with a static baseline from which to explore trends. It is also important to note that changes in the environment and lifestyle factors may impact on cancer statistics, and these must be continuously studied to give more clues about the aetiology of cancer at various sites.

According to the statistics, there have been no marked changes in cancer incidence rates that could be attributed to toxic hazards, such as pesticides and pollution at average levels of exposure. However, when groups of individuals are exposed to abnormal levels, for example of radiation, as happened after the nuclear accident in Chernobyl in 1986, then higher rates of particular cancers are found. Unusual occurrences of cancer in a community are always suspicious, since they may be coincidental or linked to a particular environmental event. Finding an answer can help to further our understanding of the development of the disease.

Around the world there are also differences in the occurrence of particular cancers. In Africa, Asia and Latin America, there tends to be a higher rate of cancers of the upper respiratory and digestive systems (aerodigestive system) (mouth, pharynx, larynx and oesophagus), the stomach, liver and cervix. Conversely, cancers of the breast, endometrium, prostate, colon and rectum are more common in Europe, North America and Australia. Cancers of this latter group are now increasing in the urbanized areas of the developing countries. Lung cancer is the commonest cancer worldwide. Migration from one type of community to another is often associated with a change in the pattern of cancers seen in the migrants.

WHAT IS CANCER?

Cancer is now accepted as a genetic disorder of somatic cells, in which an accumulation of genetic changes causes a normal cell to give rise to one which is abnormal in form or function. Generally, several changes have to occur for cancer to develop, varying between different types of cancer. The fundamental change occurs within the genetic material and may be inherited or, in the great majority of cases, occurs sporadically.

The resulting abnormal cells fail to respond to some or all of the regulatory signals that control division, growth, differentiation and programmed cell death (apoptosis). In addition, the affected genes may malfunction in their role, for example, as tumour suppressors, 'proof readers' of encoded material or repair genes. There are many types of cancers. They have different characteristics, probably originate in varying ways, occur in different parts of the body, have different courses of development; and require various treatments.

The developing tumour causes damage to its host by interfering with the normal functioning of the tissue or organ where it grows. It also draws on the host for nutrients to support its growth. Some cancers produce factors, which cause increased catabolism of the body's own tissues, resulting in a state of rapid weight loss and deterioration.

Although the process of development of cancer (or carcinogenesis) is not fully understood, it is clear that there are several stages that take place over a period of time (Table 15.1). The boundaries between the stages may not be as clear as implied here, but they provide a useful framework. The exact duration of each stage is unknown, but opportunities may arise for the process to be stopped, and possibly reversed, before it reaches the later stages.

STUDYING THE RELATIONSHIP BETWEEN DIET AND CANCER

In 1997, the World Cancer Research Fund (WCRF) and the American Institute for Cancer Research (IARC) published a report in which studies relating to diet and cancer from the previous 15 years were reviewed and their scientific evidence assessed in a consistent manner. Such a systematic review is an important tool for exploring existing research findings. This evidence was used as the basis for recommendations. Various approaches to the study of cancer exist and new evidence is continually emerging. The WCRF are currently developing a systematic methodology for the identification, assessment and recording of information from the scientific literature to form the basis of a new review. Worldwide, the occurrence of cancer is greater in the industrialized than in the developing countries, with up to 30-fold differences

TABLE 15.1 Summary of stages in cancer development

Stage of development	Associated change
Initiation	Exposure to harmful agent (e.g. chemical carcinogen, virus, free radical, radiation) or error in transcription: may permanently alter the DNA material
	The cell may remain in this state for a long period
	It is also possible for the DNA damage to be repaired, or the damaged cell to be destroyed by the body's normal regulatory systems
	Molecular biology research suggests that there are genes that can both promote and suppress these changes. This may explain the increased risk of certain cancers in families
Promotion	Substances that increase the rate of cell division may cause the damaged DNA to replicate before it has been repaired or destroyed
	This may not happen for 10–30 years after the first step
	Promoters are believed to include oestrogens, dietary fat, alcohol
	There may also be inhibitory agents, including antioxidants, dietary fibre, calcium, other constituents in plant foods, additives
Progression	The cells undergo further development and begin to grow in an uncontrolled manner, producing a tumour

in rates of particular cancers. This suggests that there may be important environmental factors involved in the aetiology. Many of these have been investigated in observational studies comparing different communities, groups within communities and migrant groups moving from one community to another. However, such studies do not provide evidence of causality or information about biological mechanisms, and must be supported by experimental findings. Developments in identification and measurement of biological markers and rapid gains in information about human genetics will provide opportunities to link observational data with molecular mechanisms.

Much of the current evidence is based on many epidemiological studies, whose results allow researchers to calculate the relative risk, or odds ratio of disease, resulting from exposure to a particular factor. It is on the basis of such data that risk factors for the development of various cancers can be proposed.

Ecological or correlational studies

These aim to show an association between the incidence of cancer in a population with a high or low occurrence of a particular environmental factor. This type of evidence can only point to the need for further, more detailed studies as the existence of a correlation does not imply causality. Changes over time in either the diet or the incidence of the cancer may provide further clues.

Case-control studies

These attempt to identify individuals with cancer and closely match each one with a control individual without disease. Comparison of environmental factors, including diet, can then be made, with the objective of identifying differences that may have contributed to the development of the cancer. In addition to the difficulties of obtaining accurate measurements of dietary intake, there are a number of other drawbacks to this approach.

- Studies that rely on information about dietary intake several years ago are imprecise. This is particularly true for a person who has recently been given a diagnosis of cancer, which tends to be a devastating event. In addition, the development of symptoms associated with the disease may have already resulted in dietary changes.

- Cancer is believed to develop over a long period of time; differences in diet a short time before the diagnosis may not reflect differences when the cancer was initiated or promoted.

Prospective cohort studies

These offer the most promising approach. They involve the recruitment of a large cross-section of the population and follow up the sample over a number of years, thus monitoring development of disease. Data about diet and lifestyle factors, together with biochemical measurements are taken initially and at intervals. The use of bio-markers, for example, biological function tests, blood or urine levels of substances, carries less risk of measurement error. Thus, if and when disease does occur, data will be available that cover the period when the disease was developing. A study of this type – the European Prospective Investigation into Cancer and Nutrition (EPIC) – is currently taking place in ten countries in Europe. Recruitment started in 1992, with a target of 500 000 subjects and first results were reported in 2001. The study will continue to collect data for a further 10 years. The major disadvantage of this type of study is the need for very large numbers of subjects. Research on 'fetal programming' and evidence from studies on growth that point to relationships with later disease, may indicate that even a prospective study over 10 or 15 years may be of insufficient duration to identify factors that may trigger the cancer process.

Meta-analysis

Data from separate studies can be reanalysed by 'meta-analysis'. By cooperating with the investigators, it is possible to record all the outcomes of a number of studies in a similar way and thus increase the power of the analysis. In this way, it may become possible to quantify the relationship between exposure to a hazard and the risk of a particular disease obtained by epidemiological study, even when that risk is only moderate. It is important that only those studies that have similar methodologies are used, and that all relevant studies are included, irrespective of their results,

for the analysis to be unbiased and worthwhile. More such analyses will no doubt be carried out in the future.

ENVIRONMENTAL CAUSES OF CANCER

Various attempts have been made over the last 20 years to evaluate the environmental contribution to the development of cancer; some estimates suggest that this may be up to 80 per cent. Of these, the most important factors are:

- diet, which may account for an average of one-third of cancer deaths (although the suggested range for different cancers is between 10 and 70 per cent);
- smoking, which is causal in 30 per cent of cancer deaths (range between 25 and 40 per cent);
- physical activity, which contributes to maintenance of a normal body weight, prevention of excessive adiposity and is an important protective factor.

In comparison, other factors believed to be important causes of cancer, such as food additives, pollutants, industrial products and geophysical factors, taken together probably account for 6 per cent of all known cancer deaths (range 0–13 per cent). It should be noted that some food additives, like antioxidants and preservatives, may actually be protective against cancer.

In looking at the above data, it is not surprising that there is a growing interest and urgency in modifying diets and lifestyles in an attempt to reduce cancer risk. The World Cancer Research Fund estimated that attention to diet, smoking and physical activity could reduce cancer incidence by 30–40 per cent, preventing 3–4 million cases of cancer worldwide annually.

Role of diet

Food or nutrients may contribute to the development of cancer in a number of ways, broadly classified as follows.

- Foods may be a source of pre-formed (or precursors of) carcinogens.
- Nutrients may affect the formation, transport, deactivation or excretion of carcinogens.

■ Nutrients may affect the body's resistance to carcinogens and, therefore, be important protective factors.

Diets are extremely complex and their measurement is subject to error. This is particularly a problem in a population whose diets are relatively similar. If the error is not consistent and is greater than the variation in intakes, it can result in misclassification of individuals and a miscalculation of risk. Random errors can also reduce the power of studies to detect relationships between intake and disease, but these errors can be minimized by repeated measurements or the use of large cohorts. Other difficulties arise because of the co-variation in particular nutrients. For example, fat intakes and energy intakes may change simultaneously, meat intakes may reflect the protein content of the diet, fruit and vegetables in the diet affect the overall intake of non-starch polysaccharide (NSP). Finally, there is good evidence from many studies that subjects tend to underreport their dietary intake, and this does not happen in a systematic manner with some nutrients more likely to be underreported, in particular protein, sugars and fat missed from a diet record. Again, this can be taken into account in large prospective studies, if they are well designed. Despite these difficulties, epidemiological evidence from the last 15 years has identified a number of consistent trends in the relationship between diet and some cancers. Detailed mechanisms underlying these associations remain to be elucidated.

Possible promoting factors

Total energy intake

Restricting the food intake of mice without modifying the proportion of the individual nutrients has long been known to halve the incidence of spontaneous tumours of the mammary gland and lung and to reduce susceptibility to known carcinogens. This effect of restricted energy intake appears to be independent of any reduction in fat content of the diet. In mice, increased activity was as effective at reducing tumour development as restricted energy intake. Increased exercise may promote activity of the immune system, thereby increasing resistance.

In humans, rapid growth in childhood, and especially growth in height may also, in ways as yet unknown, contribute to a higher risk of cancer. Data from the National Health and Nutrition Examination Survey (NHANES) 1 study found a positive correlation with height and a number of cancers, including colorectal cancer. Follow-up of children under 16 years, first studied by Boyd Orr in 1937–39, has also shown a significant positive association, with a 20 per cent increased risk of all cancers not associated with smoking, for every 1 MJ greater daily energy intake (Frankel et al., 1998). Potential confounding variables, such as social class and household size, were taken into consideration in the analysis.

High energy intakes also contribute to risk by leading to greater adiposity and therefore overweight, if not accompanied by increased energy expenditure. Therefore, restriction of energy intake and avoidance of overweight are probably important at key stages of life. In women, being overweight at puberty and after the menopause appears to be linked to increased breast cancer risks, but pre-menopausal overweight may be protective. These findings are linked to pre-sensitization of breast tissue to oestrogens in the young adolescent, and unopposed production of oestrogens by adipose tissue after the menopause. Both may promote the development of oestrogen-dependent tumours. Levels of ovarian hormones appear to be influenced by nutritional status; thus, a high caloric intake may increase production and thereby risk of breast cancer. A correlation between breast cancer risks, sex hormone levels and energy intakes has been found in countries across the world. Sex hormones produced or modified by adipose tissue may also play a part in cancer of the endometrium in women and possibly the prostate in men.

A review of data on energy intake and cancers also indicates a positive relationship with large bowel cancer. This may reflect greater exposure to carcinogens with the greater food intake but more evidence is needed in this area.

Fat intakes

Fat has been described as a promoter of carcinogenesis, although the effect of dietary fat is often difficult to distinguish from that of energy intake, as fat obviously contributes to the total energy content of the diet. Associations with fat intake have been reported for cancers of the breast, colon and prostate, as well as weak relationships for cancer of the ovary, kidneys and pancreas.

In the case of breast cancer, there is still considerable controversy. Estimated fat consumption in different countries of the world shows a strong positive correlation with age-adjusted death rates from breast cancer. In the USA, the Nurses Health Study (Willett et al., 1992) found no association between total fat intake or intake of fibre and the incidence of breast cancer in both pre- and post-menopausal women. It is possible that the prevailing higher fat intakes lead to earlier menarche in girls, thereby prolonging the exposure of breast tissue to circulating oestrogens and increasing risk. This has not, however, been fully investigated. Although in animals there is evidence of a promoting effect of *n*-6 fatty acids and an inhibitory effect of *n*-3 fatty acids on mammary tumour growth, this effect has not been demonstrated in humans. It has been suggested that *n*-6 fatty acid intakes may already be above the threshold of this promoting effect, after which no further increase is seen. This may explain the absence of evidence in women. Nevertheless, it is probably prudent to limit fat intakes, even if this simply reduces total energy intake, and thereby provides some protection.

Dietary changes in Japan in the last 40 years have included a dramatic increase in fat intake, paralleled by a reduction in complex carbohydrates. Associated with these dietary changes has been an increase in colon cancer, suggesting a link. Evidence for the involvement of fat intake is stronger in the case of colon cancer, particularly in relation to fat of animal origin, cholesterol and red meat consumption. Further evidence from the US Nurses Health Study has shown a 2.5-fold increase in risk of colon cancer in women consuming beef, pork and lamb daily, compared with those eating these meats less than monthly. Association with chicken and fish was negative, and there was no association with cholesterol intakes. It has been proposed that dietary fat causes a greater secretion of bile acids; these may be fermented by anaerobic bacteria in the colon to produce mutagenic compounds, leading to abnormal cell proliferation in the colon. However, other dietary factors may modify this process, most notably NSPs and protective factors in fruit and vegetables. The lowered pH of the bowel as a result of soluble NSP fermentation may be protective.

Prostate cancer has also been weakly associated with a high fat intake, but more evidence is needed to support this. Overall, it remains problematic to separate the effects of higher fat intakes from those of a high energy intake and overweight.

Alcohol

There is an association between consumption of alcohol and cancers of the aerodigestive tract (mouth, throat and oesophagus), as well as the liver. The EPIC study has confirmed that the risk of these cancers is nine times greater in those drinking 60 g ethanol or more (7–8 units) a day compared with those drinking 30 g or less. The effects of alcohol as a causative agent are potentiated by smoking, with those smoking more than 20 cigarettes a day having a 50-fold greater risk than non-smoking, moderate alcohol drinkers. The risks of oral and pharyngeal cancers can be offset to some extent with a high intake of fruit and vegetables.

Oesophageal cancer has been increasing since the early 1970s in the UK, which parallels the increase in alcohol consumption, with a latency of 15–20 years. It is not clear if the relationship is simply with the amount of alcohol consumed; some evidence suggests that spirits are more harmful than beer and wine. Oesophageal cancer also occurs in parts of the world where alcohol consumption is low. In these cases, it is thought to be related to micronutrient deficiencies in the diet.

Alcohol consumption, above a moderate level, has also been shown in the EPIC study to be associated with a rise in breast cancer, although there was no evidence of a dose–response relationship with wine consumption.

Salt

Salt has been suggested as a causative factor in stomach cancer because it was noted that mortality from this cancer was closely related to the incidence of stroke in communities. This was found to be true between countries, between different regions of the same country and different subgroups of the population. Salt has high osmotic activity and has been reported to cause gastritis in animals, resulting in early damage to the mucosa. Other factors are also important, most notably the presence of *Helicobacter pylori*, which is now known to be a major cause of chronic atrophic gastritis and which must be taken into account in future studies on the exact role of salt as a factor in causation of stomach cancer.

In addition to sodium chloride, other forms of preservation using nitrates and nitrites as well as pickling have been associated with stomach cancers. Nitrates occur in the diet as preservatives in foods, such as ham, bacon and sausages, in beer, and are naturally present in vegetables as well as in the drinking water, particularly in agricultural areas owing to contamination from fertilizers. Dietary nitrates may not cause cancer per se, but it has been proposed that the conversion to nitrites and subsequently to carcinogenic nitrosamines is more likely in the presence of low gastric acidity. Both *H. pylori* infection and a high salt intake are thought to cause low gastric acidity and this may complete the link with nitrites.

The decline in both stroke mortality and gastric cancer over the last 20–30 years may be explained by decreases in salt intake with advances in food preservation. Refrigeration and deep freezing have reduced the use of salt as a preservative for meat, fish and vegetables. In addition, there has been much greater all year round availability of fruit and vegetables. The vitamin C content of these inhibits the formation of nitrosamines in the stomach, and may be an important protective factor. Conversely, nitrosamine formation is promoted by thiocyanates from cigarette smoke and smokers have been shown to have higher rates of gastric cancer. The decline in smoking may also have had an effect on the incidence of this disease.

Meat and fish

Nitrogenous residues from meat digestion, as well as other proteins, may be metabolized in the large bowel to produce ammonia and the amount produced increases with meat consumption. Ammonia has been shown to induce cell proliferation in human colonic cells and to produce adenocarcinomas in rats. Other products from meat ingestion that may contribute to the promotion of colon cancer are N-nitrosocompounds, which increase with red meat (but not white meat or fish) intake, and heterocyclic amines. The latter are formed during the cooking of meat, and are dependent on temperature, duration and amount and type of fat in the meat. High-temperature cooking, for example, grilling, barbecuing and frying, also produces polycyclic hydrocarbons and has been associated with higher cancer risk. Molecular biology has identified 'fast' and 'slow' acetylators among human subjects. The conversion of heterocyclic amines to carcinogenic products in 'fast acetylators' appears to increase their risk of developing adenomatous polyps, which are considered to be pre-cancerous. Subjects who are slow acetylators appear to be much less at risk.

Processed meats, including ham, sausages, bacon, have also been linked to moderately increased risk of colon cancer, which has been shown in the EPIC study to be 50 per cent greater in those subjects consuming 60 g/day of processed meat than in those consuming none. Early results from the EPIC study have not, however, shown a significant increase in colon cancer with red meat intake, but some protective effect was indicated from white meat and fish intakes, and further results are awaited. A number of other cancers have been linked in some studies with meat consumption. These include cancer of the breast, lung, prostate and pancreas, but in all cases the evidence for an association is weak. There is some evidence that stomach cancer may be linked with consumption of processed meat (see 'Salt' section above). The great variety of ways in which people preserve and cook meat across the world, makes this a particularly challenging area for study.

Other promoters of cancer

A number of other dietary factors have been linked with the promotion of cancers (Table 15.2), although the data so far are equivocal and no firm connections have been proved. In most cases, it is

TABLE 15.2 Some proposed links between dietary components and cancers

Dietary component	Suggested link with cancer site	Mechanism/interpretation
Moulds: aflatoxin	Liver	Grows on peanuts: important cause of cancer in some countries in Africa
Caffeine	Bladder, pancreas	Relationship very weak, at normal levels of consumption May be protective in colon cancer
Iron	Colon and rectum	Relates to tissue levels of iron, not dietary intakes; may represent a breakdown of iron regulatory mechanisms
High levels of maternal nutrition/adiposity	Testicular cancer	Endocrine environment of developing fetus affected, predisposes both to undescended testes and cancer
Calcium	Colon and rectum	Weak relationship; possible action through binding of intestinal fats and thus reduces bile acid secretion
Vitamin D	Colon and rectum	May control cell growth and differentiation; weak association
Folate	Colon and rectum	Inverse relationship between plasma levels and colorectal polyps; aggravated by high alcohol intake

difficult to separate the effect of the proposed factor from that of associated dietary components.

Possible protective factors

Non-starch polysaccharides (dietary fibre)

Early observations, such as those of Burkitt et al. (1972), found a low incidence of diseases of the bowel in communities that had a large consumption of plant foods. This was developed into a theory about the protective effects of dietary fibre in a number of diseases, as discussed in Chapter 6. Knowledge about this fraction, now called 'non-starch polysaccharides' in the UK, is currently much more extensive. It is believed that NSPs may protect against colon cancer by three possible mechanisms.

■ High levels of NSP in the diet lead to increased bulk, mainly due to an increase in colonic bacteria, and, therefore, faster transit time through the colon. As a result, potentially harmful carcinogenic substances are present in a more dilute form and are in contact with the colonic mucosa for a shorter time.

■ Fermentation of soluble NSP (as well as resistant starch) in the colon yields a number of short-chain fatty acids, which influence epithelial cell function. Most notable is butyric acid, which has been shown to be an antiproliferative and differentiating agent, able to induce apoptosis (programmed cell death) in the large bowel epithelium.

■ As a result of the formation of the short-chain fatty acids, NSP in the diet reduces the pH of the bowel. This allows primary bile acids to bind to calcium, preventing them from being converted to mutagenic secondary bile acids. The lower pH also increases the number of aerobic bacteria, which do not produce carcinogenic products from bile acids. More of the bile acids are excreted, bound to components such as lignin. Studies in which subjects were supplemented with wheat bran showed a reduced mutagenicity in stool samples.

Problems with interpreting studies on intakes of 'fibre' and the incidence of cancer arise because of confusion over the definition of the fractions of fibre in the diet and the lack of detailed food composition data on this. Controversy over which fractions of fibre intake are more important in prevention of colon cancer continues, with some studies supporting a role for fruit and vegetables, and others for cereal fibre. Further difficulties arise from the effects of a change of NSP content in the diet on its other constituents, which may also be involved in cancer development.

It is also possible that a high intake of vegetables and fruit, and perhaps cereals, indicates an increased intake of other substances, such as antioxidants or flavonoids, which may be protective, rather than just the NSP they contain. The EPIC study has reported a 40 per cent lower incidence of colon cancer in subjects eating a high-fibre diet (32.5 g), compared with those eating only 12 g of fibre.

In the case of breast cancer, women consuming 'high-fibre' diets have been found to excrete more inactivated conjugated oestrogen in the faeces, with resultant lower plasma levels. However, evidence that high-fibre diets are protective against breast cancer is weak. Recent evidence suggests that soya products may offer some protection against breast and prostate cancer because of the presence of phyto-oestrogens. These are believed to increase the synthesis of oestrogen-binding proteins, and thereby reduce the levels of these hormones in both men and women. Related compounds called lignans may be found in whole cereals, seeds and fruit, and may in part account for some of the findings attributed to 'dietary fibre' in protection against breast cancer.

Fruit and vegetables

One of the most consistent findings in all of the literature on diet and cancer is that incidence is lower where fruit and vegetable intakes are high. Conversely, there is no recorded increased risk of any cancer associated with fruit and vegetable consumption. The initial understanding of the mechanisms involved was that the antioxidant nutrients present in fruit and vegetables were responsible for the protective effect. The suggested mechanism links the antioxidant nutrients to the prevention of oxidative damage to the DNA by free radicals, and hence the initiation of damage. These nutrients also protect lipids in cellular membranes and may contribute to the stabilization of cells (see Chapter 14). Fruit and vegetables are also a source of NSPs and many other nutrients, which may play a role through different mechanisms. In addition, fruit

and vegetables contain a wide variety of other chemically active substances that may play an important role in the overall effect, and research in this area is still relatively new (see Chapter 17). A problem associated with studies of fruit and vegetables is the inconsistency of definition of terms used. For example, potatoes or pulses may or may not be included in the vegetables group. Tomatoes may be included as either fruit or vegetables and in some studies, fruit and vegetables are subdivided into smaller groups by colour. In reviews of evidence, therefore, the whole group of fruit and/or vegetables may be considered in general.

There is moderately strong evidence that colorectal and stomach cancers are fewer in incidence in communities where there is a high level of intake of fruit and vegetables (above 500 g/day). These findings have been confirmed by early data from the EPIC study. There is also some evidence for a protective effect against breast, lung and oesophageal cancers. Finally, although there are too few data at present to draw any firm conclusions, there is also a probable protective effect against prostate, cervical, pancreatic and bladder cancers.

Antioxidant nutrients

Fruit and vegetables provide the three most studied antioxidants, namely vitamin A (and carotenoids), C and E. Proposed mechanisms of action for a protective effect have been explored, but no firm conclusions have been possible.

Retinoids (vitamin A family) regulate epithelial cell differentiation and could, therefore, influence tumour growth in tissues. Carotenoids are powerful quenchers of singlet oxygen and, therefore, act as antioxidants to minimize damage. It has also been postulated that the role of carotenoids may be mediated through potentiation of immune system activity.

Initial epidemiological studies had suggested that vitamin A (as retinol) was protective against lung cancer. More recent data have shown a consistent inverse relationship between the incidence of lung cancer and intakes of various carotenoids (precursors of vitamin A) as well as high plasma levels of beta-carotene. Nevertheless, results of supplementation trials have not been encouraging. Supplementation of 30 000 Finnish male smokers with either beta-carotene and/or vitamin E or placebo resulted in an increased mortality from lung cancer and coronary disease in the carotene group (Alpha-tocopherol, Beta-carotene Cancer Prevention Study Group, 1994). Similar results have occurred in at least two other trials. Studies on lung cancer are often difficult to interpret because of the strong confounding effect of smoking. However, excessive amounts of any single antioxidant are undesirable, since an imbalance can promote some pro-oxidant activity. Supplementation with beta-carotene has also been associated with an increased risk of colon cancer in two studies.

The Nurses Health Study in the USA found a 20 per cent rise in breast cancer rates between the highest and lowest intakes of vitamin A and carotenoids. Among women with the lowest dietary intake of vitamin A, the use of a supplement reduced the risk of breast cancer. Results for stomach and prostate cancers, however, do not show a consistent trend.

Vitamin C may also be an important protective factor against cancers of the oesophagus, stomach and pancreas. This role may be linked to its antioxidant properties, especially in association with vitamin E. It also has a protective role for the mixed function oxidase systems in the liver, which are important for destroying foreign and harmful substances. The most researched function of vitamin C is its role in inhibiting nitrosamine formation in the stomach, thereby reducing the risks of stomach cancer. Levels of vitamin C in the stomach are reduced by *H. pylori* infection, which results in a loss of gastric acid secretion and consequent increase in stomach pH. This situation favours bacterial colonization and increased formation of nitrites and nitroso-compounds.

Results of studies into the relationship between vitamin E and cancers at various sites are inconclusive, with better results obtained in smokers than non-smokers. Results are complicated by the interaction of vitamin E with selenium status and plasma cholesterol levels. A supplementation study with various combinations of nutrients in a poorly nourished population in Linxian, China, achieved a significant reduction in mortality from stomach cancer in those subjects receiving vitamin E, beta-carotene and selenium (Blot et al., 1993). It is likely that initial intakes were low, thus contributing to the positive finding.

Most of the findings described above relate to fruit and vegetable intakes as part of the whole diet. It is perhaps unsurprising, therefore, that attempts to replicate the results with single constituents of these foods have been unsuccessful. What is more concerning is that unexpected adverse effects have occurred. This emphasizes once again the need for a balance of nutrients in the diet, to provide appropriate amounts for their metabolic role at cellular level.

Other chemically active constituents

A number of phenolic compounds are found in fruit and vegetables. These include flavonoids, such as quercetin and catechins, which act as antioxidants and may have roles in gene blocking or suppression. However, no convincing evidence exists at present of a protective role in cancer. Phyto-oestrogens are also a class of phenolic compounds, the most important examples are isoflavones, found in soya, and lignans, which occur in linseed, lentils, asparagus, broccoli and leeks. These compounds can act as oestrogen agonists (promote or mimic the action) and antagonists (oppose the action), depending on the receptors to which they bind. It is this potential to prevent a normal oestrogen response that may offer protection against hormone-dependent tumours, such as breast and prostate. However, the evidence base to support this proposal is weak at present.

Members of the brassica vegetable family (cabbage, broccoli, cauliflower, Brussels sprouts) are particularly rich in glucosinolates, which have been shown to have blocking and suppressing properties in the development of cancers. However, large amounts may also be potentially toxic, so a cautious approach and more research are needed. Garlic, onions and leeks, all of which belong to the Allium family, also have potential blocking and suppressing properties, which have been demonstrated in rats to suppress the formation of gastric cancer. Epidemiological studies suggest a possible protective role in humans.

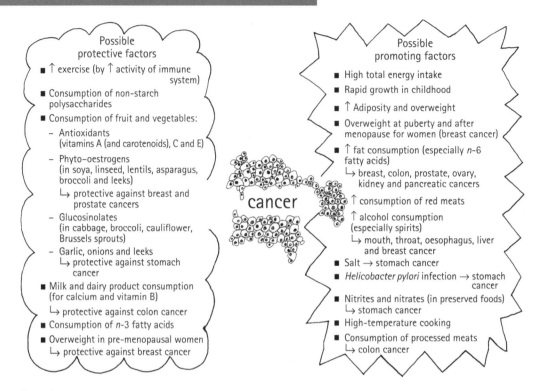

Figure 15.1 Possible promoting and protective factors in the diet in relation to cancer development.

Further research is needed, however, to demonstrate if the positive effects of fruit and vegetables in the prevention of cancer may be attributed to any of these constituents.

Calcium

In recent years, a number of studies have indicated an inverse relationship between the intake of calcium, particularly in the form of dairy products, and colon cancer. It is suggested that calcium binds fatty acids and bile acids in the colon, preventing them from causing damage to the mucosa. It is possible that calcium itself has an antiproliferative action on the colonic cells, thus preventing tumour formation. In addition, a role for vitamin D in prevention of colon cancer has also been proposed, linked to its function in control of cell proliferation. Milk may produce benefits in other ways. Whey proteins are rich in cysteine, which is a precursor of the antioxidant glutathione. In addition, milk contains lactoferrin, which can bind iron in the digestive tract, making it less available to act as a pro-oxidant.

Supplementation studies have again produced equivocal results, once more indicating that attention to foods rather than individual nutrients may be the key to prevention. Figure 15.1 summarizes possible promoting and preventive effects of nutrients.

PREVENTION OF CANCER

In the UK, healthy eating policy is embodied in the 'Eight Guidelines for a Healthy Diet', the Department of Health Dietary Reference Values (DoH, 1991) and the Balance of Good Health. All of these give advice about a diet that aims to reduce the intake of foods containing fats and sugars and to increase the intakes of starchy carbohydrates, fruit and vegetables. Ensuring a moderate intake of sources of protein, from meat, fish, dairy products and their alternatives for vegetarians, will also provide other minerals and vitamins. Maintaining a normal body weight through adequate, but not excessive energy intakes and exercise is also important.

TABLE 15.3 Summary of diet and health recommendations (WCRF, 1997)

Factor	Public health goal	Advice to individuals
Food supply and eating	Populations to consume nutritionally adequate and varied diets based primarily on foods of plant origin	Choose predominantly plant-based diets rich in a variety of vegetables and fruits, pulses and minimally processed starchy staple foods
Maintaining body weight	Population average BMI throughout adult life to be within the range 21–23, in order that individual BMI be maintained between 18.5 and 25	Avoid being underweight or overweight, and limit weight gain during adulthood to less than 5 kg
Maintaining physical activity	Populations to maintain throughout life, an active lifestyle, equivalent to a PAL of at least 1.75, with opportunities for vigorous physical activity	If occupational activity is low or moderate, take an hour's brisk walk or similar exercise daily and also exercise vigorously for a total of at least 1 hour each week
Vegetables and fruit	Promote year-round consumption of a variety of vegetables and fruit, providing 7% or more of total energy	Eat 400–800 g or five or more portions a day of a variety of vegetables and fruit, all year round
Other plant foods	A variety of starch or protein-rich foods of plant origin, preferably minimally processed, to provide 45–60% total energy. Refined sugar to provide less than 10% total energy	Eat 600–800 g or more than seven portions of a variety of cereals, pulses, roots, tubers and plantains. Prefer minimally processed foods. Limit consumption of refined sugar
Alcoholic drinks	Consumption of alcohol is not recommended and excessive consumption is to be discouraged. For those who drink alcohol, restrict it to less than 5% total energy for men and 2.5% for women	Alcohol consumption is not recommended. If consumed, limit drinks to less than two drinks per day for men and one per day for women
Meat	If eaten at all, red meat to provide less than 10% total energy	If eaten at all, limit intake of red meat to less than 80 g daily. Choose fish, poultry or meat from non-domesticated animals in place of red meat
Total fats and oils	Total fats and oils to provide 15% to no more than 30% total energy	Limit consumption of fatty foods, particularly those of animal origin. Choose modest amounts of appropriate vegetable oils
Salt and salting	Salt from all sources should amount to less than 6 g/day for adults	Limit consumption of salted foods and use of cooking and table salt. Use herbs and spices to season foods

BMI, body mass index; PAL, physical activity level.

In 1998, the Department of Health Report on Nutritional Aspects of the Development of Cancer published a number of specific recommendations in this area. In essence, they do not differ from the broader guidelines on healthy eating.

They are:

- to maintain a healthy body weight within the body mass index (BMI) range 20–25 and not to increase it during adult life;
- to increase intakes of a wide variety of fruit and vegetables;
- to increase intakes of non-starch polysaccharides (dietary fibre) from a variety of food sources;
- for adults, individuals' consumption of red and processed meat should not rise; higher consumers should consider a reduction and, as a consequence of this the population average will fall.

These recommendations should be followed in the context of the Committee on Medical Aspects of Food Policy (COMA)'s wider recommendations for a balanced diet rich in cereals, fruits and vegetables. In addition, it was recommended that:

- beta-carotene supplements as a means of avoiding cancer should not be used;
- caution should be exercised in the use of high doses of purified supplements of other micronutrients, as they cannot be assumed to be without risk.

The World Cancer Research Fund has identified the 'five-star' foods for cancer prevention:

- foods rich in beta-carotene – spinach, carrots, broccoli and tomatoes;
- foods rich in vitamin C – citrus fruits, berries, melons, green vegetables, tomatoes, cauliflowers and green peppers;
- foods rich in selenium – bran, wheat germ, tuna fish, onion, garlic and mushrooms;
- foods rich in vitamin E – wholegrain cereals, wheat germ, soya beans and leafy greens;
- foods rich in complex carbohydrates – bread, cereals, beans and peas.

These foods should be eaten in place of fattier items and can help to reduce overweight. They may also contain other important substances that may help the body's resistance to cancer.

The World Cancer Research Fund Report, published in 1997, took a global perspective on the prevention of cancer and made recommendations that were also consistent with the prevention of other diseases. They contain policy goals and advice for individuals. It was, however, intended by the report that the relative importance of the different recommendations would vary in different parts of the world, for their populations. They are summarized in Table 15.3.

In addition to the recommendations detailed above, the WCRF also identified safe storage, preservation and preparation of foods as well as the presence of additives and residues as important areas for public health policy. Recommendations were also made against the use of dietary supplements and tobacco use. Overall, the recommendations shown in Table 15.3 go further than those of the UK in recommending a move to a more plant-based diet. Many of these changes would be difficult to implement for the majority of people in the UK. However, selecting a diet from the Balance of Good Health in the proportions recommended will provide a good balance of the nutrients needed. What is also needed is the motivation and the desire to be healthy! Although much research is still required to further elucidate the role of dietary factors in certain cancers, we already have sufficient information to make recommendations that can significantly reduce the risk.

SUMMARY

1. Diet may play a major role in the development of cancer.
2. Particular aspects of the diet that may be involved as promoters and protective factors have been identified.
3. Dietary guidelines for the prevention of cancer have been proposed. These include a high intake of fruit and vegetables and avoidance of excess intakes of fat and energy. Protein intake, especially from meat sources, should also be moderated. Lifestyle changes, including regular physical activity are needed to support the dietary adjustments.

STUDY QUESTIONS

1 Why is it difficult to study the relationship between nutrition and cancer?
2 a In what ways have dietary fats been linked with the development of cancers?
   b Why is it difficult to distinguish the effects of fats from those of total energy intake in cancer causation?
3 List the reasons why an increase in non-starch polysaccharides (dietary fibre) intake might protect against some cancers.
4 How does the advice on diet for cancer prevention compare with general healthy eating guidelines?
5 a In what ways might the antioxidant nutrients be useful in the prevention of cancers?
   b Does the scientific evidence currently support this theory?

REFERENCES AND FURTHER READING

Alpha-tocophcrol, Bcta-carotene Cancer Prevention Study Group 1994: The effect of vitamin E and beta-carotene on the incidence of lung cancer and other cancers in male smokers. *New England Journal of Medicine* **330**(15), 1029–35.

Bingham, S.A. 1999: High meat diets and cancer risk. *Proceedings of the Nutrition Society* **58**, 243–8.

Blot, W.J. Li, J.-Y., Taylor, P.R. et al., 1993: Nutrition intervention trials in Linxian, China: supplementation with specific vitamin/mineral combinations, cancer incidence and disease specific mortality in general population. *Journal of the National Cancer Institute* **85**, 1483–92.

Burkitt, D.P., Walker, A.R.P., Painter, N.S. 1972: Effect of dietary fibre on stools and transit times and its role in the causation of disease. *Lancet* **ii**, 1408–12.

Burr, M.L. 1994: Antioxidants and cancer. *Journal of Human Nutrition and Dietetics* **7**, 409–16.

DoH (UK Department of Health) 1991: *Dietary reference values for food energy and nutrients for the United Kingdom*. Report on Health and Social Subjects No. 41. Report of the Panel on Dietary Reference Values of the Committee on Medical Aspects of Food Policy. London: HMSO.

DoH (UK Department of Health) 1998: *Nutritional aspects of the development of cancer*. Report on Health and Social Subjects 48. London: The Stationery Office.

Frankel, S., Gunnell, D.J., Peters, T.J. et al. 1998: Childhood energy intake and adult mortality from cancer: the Boyd Orr cohort study. *British Medical Journal* **316**, 499–504.

Key, T. 1994: Micronutrients and cancer aetiology: the epidemiological evidence. *Proceedings of the Nutrition Society* **53**, 605–14.

National Dairy Council (NDC) 1995: *Nutrition and cancer*. Fact File 12. London: NDC.

Riboli, E. 1991: Nutrition and cancer: background and rationale of the European prospective investigation into cancer and nutrition (EPIC). *Annals of Oncology* **3**, 783–91.

Riboli, E., Norat, T. 2001: Cancer prevention and diet: opportunities in Europe. *Public Health Nutrition* **4**(2B), 475–84.

Willett, W.C., Hunter, D.J., Stampfer, M.J. et al. 1992: Dietary fat and fibre in relation to role in breast cancer. *Journal of the American Medical Association* **268**, 2037–44.

Williams, C.M. 1996: Nutrition and breast cancer: facts and controversies. In Buttriss, J., Hyman, K. (eds) *Focus on women: nutrition and health*. London: National Dairy Council.

World Cancer Research Fund 1997: *Food, nutrition and the prevention of cancer: a global perspective*. Washington, DC: World Cancer Research Fund and American Institute for Cancer Research.

CHAPTER 16

CHALLENGES TO NUTRITIONAL STATUS

The aim of this chapter is to:

❏   identify situations that provide an additional challenge to the maintenance of the nutritional status. This may be as a result of obstacles to food intake, difficulties in digestion and absorption, or altered metabolic states that affect what the body can obtain from the food ingested.

On completing the study of this chapter, you should be able to:

❏   identify a number of conditions or situations that impose an additional challenge to nutritional status;
❏   use the framework of nutrient 'intake–processing–utilization' to explain how each of the situations creates a threat to nutrition;
❏   provide some practical solutions to help people in these situations.

In considering challenges to nutrition, it is useful to consider the stages through which food has to travel to achieve its purpose of providing our bodies with the necessary nutrients. A useful framework is that of 'intake–processing–utilization', which summarizes this pathway from food in the marketplace or kitchen to metabolism at the cell level. Obstacles or problems at any of the stages of this pathway will affect the ultimate achievement of satisfying nutritional requirements. This framework will be used in the following discussions.

ADVERSE REACTIONS TO FOOD

Since the 1980s there has been a considerable growth of public interest in adverse reactions to food, all of which are often (mistakenly) grouped together as 'food allergy'. The extent of these problems is difficult to ascertain precisely, as levels of self-reporting are invariably greater than can be confirmed by rigorous testing.

It is useful to start with some definitions of terms that are consistent with current practice in the UK. It should be noted, however, that there

are variations in these classifications within Europe and the USA.

Adverse reactions to food may be of three types:

■   food poisoning – includes reactions resulting from contaminants within the food;
■   food aversion – includes psychological reactions, which may not be reproduced on covert introduction of the food;
■   food intolerance – includes reproducible adverse reactions to food.

The first of these occurs as a result of triggers from outside the individual and is believed to be the most commonly occurring of the adverse reactions. The remaining two types relate to responses that are initiated within the individual in response to the food eaten and are considered to be less common.

Food poisoning

This occurs as a result of the consumption of contaminated food or water that results in disease of an infectious or toxic nature. In the UK and Europe, the causative agents are most likely to be microorganisms. However, in other parts of the world, food poisoning may occur as a result of chemical contamination, parasites or toxins naturally present in the food or acquired within the food. Bacterial food poisoning occurring in the UK includes that caused by *Campylobacter*, *Salmonella* spp. and *Escherichia coli*. Some bacteria produce toxins, which cause the symptoms; these include *Staphylococcus aureus*, *Bacillus cereus* and *Clostridium botulinum*. Foods that may be contaminated include eggs, poultry, cold meats, rice and spices. Among the viral causes of food poisoning, the most widespread are highly infectious, small round structured viruses (SRSVs), which may contaminate shellfish, but more probably are introduced into food from infected food handlers. Consumers in semi-closed communities, such as hospitals, hotels and schools are particularly vulnerable.

Contamination of food can occur, for example, from use of dirty water, sewerage overspill, and agricultural chemicals. Some plant foods may contain toxins, for example, uncooked red kidney beans or some fungi, or may be contaminated with moulds, for example, aflatoxins, which affect groundnuts (peanuts).

Most commonly, food poisoning causes rapid vomiting and diarrhoea, although a few of the agents can cause serious damage to the liver, kidneys, nervous system and may even be fatal. The young, sick and elderly are the most vulnerable to serious consequences from bacterial food poisoning.

Food aversion

Many people may be able to list foods that they avoid, generally because of a sensory preference or dislike. This may be taken to an extreme avoidance of almost all foods in the case of anorexia nervosa. In some cases, an individual believes that the food causes them unpleasant symptoms, perhaps as a result of an experience in the past where the food was temporally associated with sickness or gastrointestinal upset. In this case, the food is avoided because of an aversion to it and an associated psychological belief that the food is harmful. When tested blind, however, it is generally not possible to reproduce any alleged

symptoms, and the conclusion must be drawn that this is a psychosomatic adverse reaction rather than one that has a true physiological basis.

Aversion may also be applied to foods that are believed to affect other aspects of health, for example, tiredness, sleep problems, palpitations, bloatedness and flatulence. The individual excludes particular foods to correct these symptoms, although double-blind testing generally fails to find any scientific basis for this practice. To date, in most of these cases, there is no evidence to support a link between the food and the symptoms.

Food intolerance

This is the only group of adverse reactions to food for which reproducible responses can be produced on challenge. Precise figures for prevalence are difficult to obtain because:

- questionnaires are unreliable because of bias from respondents;
- diagnosis is time consuming (e.g. use of elimination diets followed by challenge);
- there are no simple reliable tests and these also may not be particularly sensitive;
- there is an almost limitless number of foodstuffs and additives that can provoke a response;
- reactions vary between individuals and, especially in children, may change over time;
- responses may occur immediately or after a considerable period after ingestion; these are poorly understood and difficult to diagnose.

Although many studies have attempted to quantify the extent of food intolerance, a lack of consensus over definitions and methodologies has made it difficult to arrive at reliable results on prevalence.

In 1994, a study in the UK found that, in a sample of over 18 000 people, 20 per cent complained of food intolerance, commonly citing eight different foods (Young et al., 1994). When tested with a controlled challenge, food intolerance was confirmed in only 1.4–1.8 per cent of the total. This is in line with the generally accepted figure of 1–2 per cent of the adult population exhibiting food intolerance, with a higher prevalence in children of perhaps 5–8 per cent.

Food intolerance may be further subdivided into:

- allergic reactions – immunoglobulin E (IgE)-mediated and non-IgE-mediated;
- pharmacological reactions;
- enzyme reactions.

The clinical presentation of food intolerance may be immediate or delayed onset, and is likely to affect the following tissues and systems (see Figure 16.1 for a summary).

- *Gastrointestinal system.* Symptoms include mouth tingling or swelling, abdominal pain, bloating of the abdomen, vomiting and diarrhoea or constipation. In chronic intolerance, there can be bleeding or loss of plasma protein into the gut lumen, with damage to the gut mucosa.
- *Skin.* Dermatitis, urticaria, angio-oedema and eczema are common consequences.
- *Respiratory system.* Rhinitis, laryngeal oedema and asthma (including wheezing, breathlessness) may occur.
- *Central nervous system.* Symptoms include migraine and possibly some behavioural abnormalities (including hyperactivity and depression), although the evidence for these is controversial.

Food allergy is a form of specific food intolerance that causes reproducible symptoms and includes an abnormal reaction by the immune system. Our diet contains a variety of substances that can stimulate immune responses. They are usually proteins or simple chemicals bound to proteins and are termed allergens. Usually these allergens are prevented from being absorbed by secretory immunoglobulin A (IgA) lining the gut. However, IgA is absent in the first months of life, so that allergens can be absorbed. Breast milk contains IgA, and may offer some protection. Avoidance of contact with potential allergens is important at this age, especially where there is a family history of allergy, although complete protection is unlikely. However, in general our immune system has evolved responses that allow it to be tolerant to the antigen burden represented by ingested food. This is known as oral tolerance. In some cases, these allergens induce an immune response, usually producing antibodies, which can be detected in the serum, but which are not pathogenic – known as immunological acceptance.

In a minority of individuals, however, this response is abnormal and results in pathological changes when the allergen is ingested, resulting in a food allergy. The immune system responds inappropriately against the allergen to stimulate IgE antibodies sensitized to the particular allergen. These are mainly attached to mast cells and on stimulation cause immediate degranulation of the mast cells and the release of a range of chemical mediators. These include histamine and prostaglandins, which have potent effects.

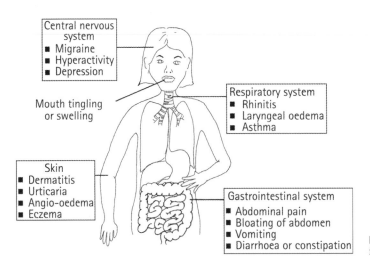

Figure 16.1 Symptoms of food intolerance.

The consequent reaction depends on the size of the dose, the speed of absorption and the distribution of the allergen in the body.

The response to the release of histamine and prostaglandins generally includes some or all of the following:

- dilation of small blood vessels (redness);
- increased permeability of blood vessels (swelling/oedema);
- contraction of smooth muscle in the airways (breathing difficulties) or intestines (causing abdominal pain); and
- stimulation of nerve endings in the skin (itching and pain).

Reactions may be seen in the following:

- the mouth, immediately following ingestion;
- the gastrointestinal tract, when the allergen reaches this area;
- one of many other sites, including the skin and respiratory system, including the nose and airways;
- several other sites, causing a widespread and possibly life-threatening reaction (see Figure 16.2).

The severity of the reaction varies between individuals and may range from mild to life threatening (anaphylactic shock), resulting from a severe fall of blood pressure and possibly

Figure 16.2 IgE-mediated food allergy.

difficulties in breathing. Immediate help in the form of an adrenaline injection is required for anyone suffering from such a major allergic reaction. Fortunately, most are not so extreme and recovery follows, resulting from the body's own homeostatic mechanisms, which cause endogenous adrenaline release.

Why do individuals develop food allergy?

Genetic predisposition is an important determinant of susceptibility to allergic disease, also called atopy. The susceptibility is more likely to be inherited from the mother than the father but, with two atopic parents, the likelihood is greatly increased. However, although the susceptibility is inherited, the actual allergens to which a child is sensitive are not necessarily the same as its parents. Babies that are born small for gestational age are more at risk of developing allergies in their first year. This suggests that growth faltering in the womb may play a role in poorer immunocompetence.

Studies suggest that the risk of atopy in a child can be reduced by avoidance of potential allergens in the mother's diet from very early pregnancy. In addition, breastfeeding for more than 4 months can reduce the development of atopic disease. Delaying the introduction of solids until after 4 months is also recommended, as well as the use of low allergen foods, such as baby rice, potatoes, fruit and vegetables.

There has been a general increase in the incidence of food and other allergies over the last 30 years. An explanation that is gaining acceptance is that modern children are exposed to fewer infectious diseases and live in a generally clean environment. This does not challenge the immune system, which is less well developed as a result, and reacts inappropriately when presented with harmless antigens, resulting in an allergic reaction.

A further explanation offered for the rising incidence of allergy is the change in balance between n-6 and n-3 fatty acids in our diets. The n-6 fatty acids are more predominant and fewer n-3 acids are consumed. The former are associated with more pro-inflammatory eicosanoids, including prostaglandins, which have an important role in allergic responses.

Foods associated with allergic reactions

Almost any food can produce an allergic reaction but some are much more likely to cause problems than others.

In children, the most common causes of food allergy are cows' milk, eggs, peanuts, fish, wheat, tree nuts, soya beans, soya products, vegetables or fruits. Milk allergy has been reported in 2–3 per cent of infants in Western countries, although in the majority (about 80 per cent), the allergy disappears by the age of 3 years. This is not surprising, as milk forms the basis of the infant's diet and cows' milk protein is often the first foreign protein to be introduced. Children with persistent milk allergy may develop hypersensitivities to other foods, especially egg, soya, peanuts, citrus, fish, tomato and cereals, as these are introduced into their diet. It is estimated that the prevalence of true food allergy in young children is about 1.4 per cent (range 0.5–3.8 per cent in the literature). Although children may grow out of some allergies, those to peanuts, tree nuts, fish and shellfish may persist into adult life.

Apart from the foods listed above for children, adults may experience cross-reactions between similar proteins in different foods. For example, tree and grass pollens can provoke reactions to fruits and vegetables. Clusters of hypersensitivities to members of the same botanical family can occur. Reports exist of allergy to apple and pear, kiwi fruit and avocado, potato and carrot, celery, cucumber, carrot and watermelon. These rarely cause anaphylactic reactions, although some have been reported.

Of great concern is the growing prevalence of peanut and tree nut allergy, both of which are associated with severe life-threatening reactions more commonly than the more traditional foods associated with allergies. In some individuals, sensitivity to peanuts is so great that as little as 100 µg of peanut protein can provoke symptoms. At present, the exact prevalence is unknown, but a prevalence of 0.5 per cent among UK children in 1996 was reported. The UK Department of Health (1997) has recommended that pregnant women with any history of atopy in the family should avoid eating peanuts during pregnancy.

The increased prevalence is reportedly linked to the increased exposure of young children to peanut proteins in peanut butter, cereals, confectionery and baked goods. Cold pressed peanut oil used in cooking may contain peanut protein. Many children appear to have become sensitized at a very young age, possibly from peanut oils in infant foods. There have been reported deaths from peanut allergy, resulting from rapid anaphylaxis affecting the larynx. Avoidance of peanuts is vital, as well as other pulses (or legumes) and other nuts. The use of adrenaline syringes in emergency is essential.

Non–IgE-mediated reactions

Adverse responses to food may not always involve IgE, and mast cells and other parts of the immune system may be involved, such as T-lymphocytes and scavenger cells. The reaction is generally delayed and may take several hours or even days to develop. In addition, the reactions to trigger foods may involve one system or several and may, therefore, imitate the reactions to IgE-mediated allergy described above. It is very difficult to identify and confirm the relationship between particular foods and an adverse reaction that occurs some time later and that also may be initiated by a number of different foods and possibly also environmental conditions.

The best defined example in this group is gluten sensitivity, whereby the immune system of genetically susceptible individuals reacts inappropriately to dietary gluten, causing a variety of problems. In coeliac disease, the target organ is the gastrointestinal tract, predominantly the region of the small intestine, in which a variety of changes are seen, resulting in malabsorption of nutrients. The skin may be affected, with an itchy blistering rash on the knees, thighs and elbows. There have also been reports of neurological manifestations of gluten sensitivity, although the evidence of this is not scientifically strong, and these disorders may be a result of nutritional deficiency consequent on malabsorption. Diagnosis of coeliac disease has classically been by small-bowel biopsy, but serological tests for antibodies found in the circulation are now also used. Exclusion of gluten from the diet resolves the changes affecting both the gut and the skin. A gluten-free diet should be maintained for life and lists of permitted foods are provided

by the UK Coeliac Society. It is estimated that the prevalence of gluten sensitivity is 1 in 300 in Europe, with a 10 per cent risk of the condition in first-degree relatives of those already diagnosed. Although often identified in young children, the condition may be 'silent' and not diagnosed until adulthood. In this case, there may already be a number of existing nutritional deficiencies, such as folate or iron deficiency leading to anaemia, or inadequate calcium absorption resulting in poor bone development.

Other conditions for which a non-IgE-mediated allergic response has been investigated, but not confirmed include:

- urticaria and dermatitis;
- infantile colic;
- irritable bowel syndrome;
- asthma;
- migraine;
- hyperactivity and attention deficit hyperactivity disorder (ADHD);
- rheumatoid arthritis.

In all of the above, where there is an apparently strong history of food intolerance in the individual, it is important to test thoroughly with appropriate scientific techniques, if specific foods are causing the symptoms of illness. It is likely that, in some of these conditions, food is one of a number of triggers for the symptoms, which makes the diagnosis very difficult. Once identified, if a food has to be eliminated, this should be done with qualified professional advice to ensure the maintenance of adequate nutritional intake.

Pharmacological reactions

Some foods contain pharmacologically active agents or may cause the production of such agents in the body. Usually these are harmless unless ingested in relatively large amounts. Even when released in the body, the amounts needed are much larger than those involved in the IgE-mediated allergic reaction discussed earlier. For example, foods such as cheese (Roquefort, Parmesan, mature Cheddar), wine (and other fermented products), bananas, yeast extract, avocados, chocolate, oranges and some fish products (e.g. pickled fish) contain biogenic amines, such as histamine, tyramine, phenylethylamine and octopamine. Other foods may directly cause the release of histamine from mast cells; this has been shown to occur with chocolate, tomatoes and strawberries. Caffeine is another agent that can produce this type of intolerance, resulting in tachycardia (increased heart rate), irritability, sleep disturbances and intestinal colic. The dose at which this occurs may be as little as two cups of coffee or three cups of tea. Prunes contain hydroxyphenylisatin, which is a stimulant of intestinal motor activity and can produce rapid transit through the gut. Sodium nitrite present in preserved meats can cause intolerance symptoms, including flushing, headaches, urticaria and abdominal symptoms.

Food additives

Many people believe themselves to be sensitive to food additives. Mentioned most often in this context are

- colouring agents, such as tartrazine;
- preservatives, such as benzoic acid and benzoates;
- antioxidants, such as butylated hydroxytoluene (BHT) and butylated hydroxyanisole (BHA).

The diagnosis of these reactions is very difficult, as no immunological effect is involved. Moreover, additives are rarely consumed singly, so individual reactions are difficult to identify. However, concern has been expressed that, for their size, children who eat a large amount of processed foods containing additives may be consuming an unacceptably high level of additive 'cocktail', which could have adverse effects. Often, where apparent sensitivity exists to food additives in children, it accompanies other allergic conditions, such as eczema, and may exacerbate their symptoms.

Sulphite used in preservation of wine, other acidic drinks or fruit and vegetables may liberate sulphur dioxide, which may aggravate asthmatic reactions. Some people believe they are sensitive to monosodium glutamate, which is used as a flavour enhancer in many foods and is present in large amounts in some Chinese dishes. Responses described include tachycardia, flushing and wheezing, but blind trials have failed to show a consistent link with a specific array of symptoms.

Food safety requires that some additives are used in food preservation but it is important that their safety for humans is reviewed regularly, and their use controlled. Without additives, foods would be hazardous, owing to bacterial contaminants and deterioration, and food-transmitted infections actually already cause more reactions in people than any effects of food additives.

Enzyme defects

The most common of these is the inability to digest lactose in milk, generally due to the disappearance of lactase after infancy (this is discussed in Chapter 6). Congenital lactase deficiency, when active lactase is absent from birth, is rare. Other disaccharidase enzyme activities in the gut may be compromised, for example, by some drug therapies and in chronic or binge alcohol consumption. In all of these cases, symptoms of intolerance occur when sugars are consumed. These result from the bacterial fermentation of lactose (or more rarely other sugars) in the colon and the resulting osmotic effects, causing bloating and diarrhoea.

Other enzyme defects that occur may be inborn and have systemic effects when metabolic pathways cannot be completed. Examples include alcohol dehydrogenase deficiency, which affects metabolism of alcohol, or fructose intolerance where fructose metabolism is incomplete and results in hypoglycaemia. In addition, there are a number of inherited disorders of amino-acid metabolism that require lifelong dietary modification to prevent serious consequences.

Diagnosis

To obtain a reliable diagnosis, strict criteria must be adhered to. An adverse reaction to a food can only be confirmed if the symptoms disappear when the food is removed from the diet and reappear when it is re-introduced. Great care must be taken if there is any risk of anaphylaxis, and patients who believe they are at risk may refuse to undergo testing. Because of the risk of a severe reaction on re-introduction, this should be carried out under supervision. A careful history of diet and symptoms needs to be taken to identify possible triggers. The testing procedure should be

| ① History of diet and symptoms taken to indentify possible triggers | ② Double-blind food testing | ③ Skin prick tests or assay of IgE levels (RAST method) | ④ Intestinal biopsy or intestinal permeability measured, if appropriate |

Figure 16.3 Diagnosis of food intolerance.

performed by a double-blind technique, so that neither the clinician nor the subject knows when the suspect food is introduced, within a range of food testing. If several foods are involved and if the reaction is delayed, the procedure may take many weeks to complete. Where there is a suspected allergy, skin prick tests or assay of IgE levels – radioallergosorbent test (RAST) method – may be used as laboratory tests. Even with these, failure to obtain a positive result may not necessarily indicate the absence of hypersensitivity. Intestinal biopsy or intestinal permeability may also be measured in the clinical setting, if this is considered appropriate (see Figure 16.3).

A large number of other tests are available directly to the public. Most of these have not been scientifically validated and, therefore, are not considered to be of value in the diagnosis of food allergy. They are potentially dangerous as they are likely to result in misdiagnosis of food allergy and potential harm from restricted diets. Even without testing, individuals may be tempted to use self-diagnosis and elimination of foods from the diet. This can readily result in omission of key foods and nutrients, which can produce deficiencies and is particularly hazardous in children. Dietary manipulation should only be undertaken under the supervision of a dietitian.

NUTRITION AND THE IMMUNE SYSTEM

There are close links between the nutritional status of the individual and the effectiveness of the immune system in providing an appropriate response in the event of challenge. It has been recognized for many centuries that infectious disease was more common in undernourished populations and that famines were associated with epidemics. The understanding of the two-way relationship between nutrition and immunity is now much greater as new challenges have emerged that demonstrate their interdependence (see Figure 16.4). The inappropriate response to food components that leads to adverse reactions has been discussed above. The appearance of human immunodeficiency virus (HIV) infections and the acquired immunodeficiency syndrome (AIDS) has provided a further example of how immune status and nutrition are related. Other nutritional challenges have an impact on immune function, for example, in chronic disease, in the very young and the elderly.

A brief outline of the role of nutrition in immunity is given here.

Effect of infection on nutritional status

The presence of infection has a potential impact on nutritional state. This can be as a consequence of:

- loss of appetite and poor dietary intake;
- failure to digest or absorb nutrients, either through loss by vomiting or diarrhoea, or loss of digesting/absorbing ability through lack of enzymes, damage to the mucosa of the gut or intestinal hurry caused by infestation with parasites;

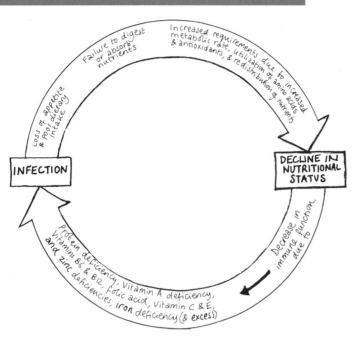

Figure 16.4 The relationship between infection and nutrition.

increased requirements owing to raised metabolic rate consequent on fever, increased utilization of certain nutrients, such as amino acids and antioxidants, or a redistribution of nutrients between different body compartments as part of the immune response.

Therefore, nutritional state may decline during an infection and compromise the body's ability to combat it and recover. This is one of the reasons for a higher mortality from infections in poorly nourished individuals, compared to those with better nutritional status.

Effect of nutritional status on immunity

The most studied aspect of this relationship is that between protein energy malnutrition and immune function. Almost all aspects of the immune system depend on adequate protein status. This includes the organs of the immune system, such as the thymus, spleen and lymph nodes, which produce phagocytic white blood cells. In addition, the biologically active proteins, such as immunoglobulins, acute-phase proteins and cytokines are dependent on adequate protein status. Cytokines are a large and diverse group of proteins secreted by cells for the purpose of altering its own function or that of adjacent cells; cytokines may have

multiple activities, and include tumour necrosis factor and interleukins. It is, therefore, not surprising that protein deficiency makes the individual vulnerable to almost all infections. Specific amino acids have also been identified as particularly important in sustaining an immune response during acute infections, and following trauma or surgery. These are the sulphur-containing amino acids (methionine and cysteine), arginine and glutamine. Some enteral feeds have been developed containing these amino acids for use in hospital patients.

The role of dietary fat in immune function has received considerable interest. In experimental studies, a reduction of total dietary fat intake, from 40 to <30 per cent of energy, resulted in improved immune activity in a variety of subjects. This has led to the suggestion that high-fat diets may have a suppressing effect on human immune function. Polyunsaturated fatty acids (PUFAs) of the *n*-6 series, when consumed in amounts typical of the Western diet, have no clear effects on immune function. However, *n*-3 PUFAs, such as those found in fish oils and linseed oil, have been reported to have a suppressing effect on immune responses. For this reason, there is interest in their role as potential antiinflammatory agents for use in conditions where the immune system is responding inappropriately to triggers and causing chronic disease states. These include rheumatoid arthritis, Crohn's disease, ulcerative colitis and psoriasis. Results of trials to date are inconclusive and further work is still needed.

Among the micronutrients, both vitamins and minerals are important in immune function.

Vitamin A deficiency is closely linked with susceptibility to infection, especially of the respiratory system in malnourished children. The role of vitamin A appears to be widespread, in maintaining the integrity of epithelial surfaces as well as in the production and function of both cellular and humoral aspects of the immune system. Other vitamins that have been proposed and studied with regard to an immune function role are vitamins B_6 and B_{12}, folic acid, and vitamins C and E.

The most important mineral in relation to immune function is zinc and subjects who are deficient have immune impairment. Supplementation with zinc of malnourished children decreases the risk of diarrhoea and increases the number of T lymphocytes. In small for gestational age infants, a supplement of zinc (5 mg/day), given for 6 months increased immune function. However, it should also be noted that excess intakes of zinc (300 mg/day) can impair immune function.

Iron deficiency has also been associated with impaired immune function. However, excess iron may inhibit immune function, although the mechanisms are unclear. Selenium is concentrated in tissues involved in the immune system, such as lymph nodes, spleen and liver, and various components of the immune system have been shown to be impaired in selenium deficiency. The bactericidal activity of phagocytes is impaired. There have been reports also of benefits of selenium supplementation in HIV-infected subjects.

Overall, it is clear that adequate nutritional status is needed for correct immune function. Supplementation with multi-nutrient mixtures can improve immune function in those individuals whose previous intakes were poor. However, there is little evidence to support enhancement of immune function by the use of supplements in those who are adequately nourished. Indeed, there is a possibility that for some nutrients an excess intake may result in suppression of immune action. More research is needed in this area.

NUTRITION IN HIV INFECTION AND AIDS

Nutritional status is an important consideration in patients with HIV infection, and improvements or maintenance of nutritional adequacy may have important implications for survival. A major advance in the management of patients with HIV infection has been the development of highly active antiretroviral drugs, which have been able to significantly improve the prognosis. Many patients with HIV, however, have no access to these drugs and, for this group, attention to nutrition can make a difference. Malnutrition can affect the length of survival by:

- reducing immune responsiveness;
- causing organ damage;
- reducing the effectiveness of therapies;
- contributing to progressive debility.

Body weight

One of the most readily available markers of nutritional status is body weight. Weight loss is reported as a major clinical sign in HIV infection, and has for some time been considered inevitable and irreversible. There is now a better understanding of the variations in weight as more of the components of the weight change have been studied. Survival appears to be increased in patients with a higher body mass index (BMI; in the range 25–30), although deliberate overeating and development of obesity is not encouraged. The composition of this body weight is probably also important, with a higher lean body mass being more advantageous than increased fat stores. An exercise programme may help to boost the amount of lean tissue.

Weight loss can occur at all stages of the HIV infection and is not constant, but rather occurs intermittently, suggesting that it is not simply caused by the underlying HIV infection. The initial loss is of fat but, in later stages, may be predominantly of lean body mass. There can be periods of weight stability and significant weight gain is also possible.

Several factors are thought to be responsible for weight loss in HIV infection:

- increased resting energy expenditure, owing to the 'hypermetabolism of the disease';
- concurrent infections;
- reduced food intake – this may arise for a number of reasons, including difficulties of obtaining and/or eating food, and loss of appetite;
- malabsorption.

Increased metabolism

Although the metabolism may be increased, by approximately 10 per cent in patients with HIV infection, and perhaps up to 30 per cent during periods of opportunistic infections, it is now thought not to be the main cause of weight loss. Careful studies have demonstrated that the increase in resting energy expenditure is more than outweighed by the reduction in physical activity. In addition, and especially during periods of infection, there is a marked reduction in food intake that contributes to the negative energy balance and weight loss. To maintain body weight, the periods of reduced food intake need to be compensated by increases following recovery from infection. It is proposed that these periods would be an ideal time for aggressive nutritional support to help re-establish body weight. This can be by enteral or even parenteral feeding, if necessary and appropriate. It is also important that other nutrients are provided at this time and that the aim is not simply to gain weight.

Patients with HIV infections appear to lose protein during weight-loss episodes. Usually, when food intake is low, the physiological response after the first 3 days is for protein to be spared and for fat stores to be predominantly used for energy. In HIV infection, however, the response is similar to that seen in trauma or physiological stress, with the breakdown of body protein and negative nitrogen balance. Reversing this loss should aim at optimizing the anabolic processes, perhaps by the use of hormones, as well as the use of appetite stimulation. Resistance exercise can help increase lean body mass in these cases.

Patients with HIV infection have also been found to have abnormal lipid metabolism, with raised plasma triglycerides, which becomes more elevated as HIV progresses to symptomatic AIDS. Conversely, cholesterol and phospholipid levels are lower in HIV-infected subjects. Treatment with antiretroviral drugs has also been found to lead to a metabolic syndrome, termed lipodystrophy, with abnormal lipid levels, reduced glucose tolerance and insulin sensitivity. In addition, there is a redistribution of body fat, with a loss of subcutaneous fat, including the legs, arms and face, and increased abdominal adiposity and deposition of fat across the back (buffalo hump) and on the breasts. The development of this condition in patients treated successfully for HIV infection is a paradox, and raised future health problems, which are similar to those seen in obese individuals, who are at risk of coronary heart disease, diabetes and pancreatitis. The causes of this metabolic syndrome are unexplained but may be due to a delay in clearance of lipids from the circulation, with resulting consequences of raised circulating lipids. Low-fat diets, exercise and drugs to reduce plasma lipids may be a way forward.

Concurrent infection

Opportunistic infections and cancer are causes of major, rapid weight loss in patients with AIDS. Treatment of the infection can reverse the weight loss. The management of these has become better as knowledge has increased.

Reduced food intake

This may arise for a number of reasons, including:

- a loss of desire to eat due to anxiety or depression;
- a deliberate desire to lose weight;
- an inability to obtain food or afford to buy food;
- problems with eating, owing to painful mouth or throat infections, or side-effects of drug therapy;
- the consequences of eating, with nausea, gastric pains, and diarrhoea.

Malabsorption

Abnormal function of the gastrointestinal tract is a fairly common aspect of AIDS, although it may only affect nutritional status in later stages of the disease. Common features include fat mal-absorption together with episodes of diarrhoea, which may be linked to malabsorption of bile salts. Where malabsorption is an important feature, there is chronic progressive weight loss. Pathogens may be present in the gut, depending on the degree of immunosuppression of the patient. They may interfere with all aspects of gut functioning, including chewing and swallowing, cause gastric pain and consequent reluctance to eat, reduce absorption, cause nausea and vomiting, general malaise and anorexia.

As with any condition where the body is faced with a reduced food intake and increased needs, maintaining good nutrition whenever possible is important. Food provides not only nutritional support, but also psychological support and social activity, and this should be recognized in any nutrition therapy.

Studies have shown that low plasma vitamin A levels are associated with accelerated progression of HIV and increased risk of mortality. Vitamin A supplementation has significantly reduced mortality and morbidity in HIV-infected children. Other studies have shown that low serum vitamin B_{12}, vitamin E, selenium and zinc levels are associated with increased risk of progression to AIDS. Multivitamin supplementation of pregnant women, improves the survival chances of their babies with fewer low birthweight and preterm deliveries.

Although as a general principle an optimal diet may well prolong a person's survival, it is possible for someone in this vulnerable state to fall prey to nutritional misinformation, and perhaps end up consuming a very unbalanced diet. Many supposedly beneficial diets have been proposed, including supplementation with very large doses of vitamin C, use of 'live' yogurt, macrobiotic diets or herbal supplements. At present, there is no evidence that any one feature of these diets will be especially beneficial in HIV infection. However, a patient's desire to help themselves through the diet is important to respect and may encourage them to take an interest in other aspects of their food intake. It is important that adequate levels of all nutrients are provided and not compromised. The development of antiretroviral drugs has brought a new approach to the management of patients with HIV infection, with better survival, but with new complications resulting from metabolic disturbances that increase risks of other diseases.

DRUG–NUTRIENT INTERACTIONS

Drugs used in medical treatment may affect nutritional status by influencing food intake or metabolism; similarly, their action and effectiveness may be altered by a person's pre-existing nutritional state.

These interactions between drugs and nutrients have been a focus of interest only in the last two decades. They can occur within the gastrointestinal tract, in the blood or at the cellular site of action of the drug. The consequence of any interaction will vary with the drug, its formulation, the timing of food intake, and the nutritional status and disease state of the individual concerned.

Effects of diet on drugs

Most drugs are taken into the body by mouth and, therefore, are processed by the gastrointestinal tract. Many drugs have to be solubilized by the digestive secretions before they can be absorbed. In a fasted subject, drugs will pass quickly through the stomach, reaching the small intestine within minutes. Drugs taken with food or after meals are likely to be more slowly absorbed than those taken following a period of fasting. The presence of food and fluid also facilitates the solubilization of solid drugs. The increased flow of blood in the splanchnic circulation associated with eating may enhance the bioavailability of some drugs, for example, some of the beta blockers.

Nevertheless, there are some drugs that are better absorbed in the fasting state, such as penicillin and tetracycline. In particular, tetracycline is less well absorbed when taken with foods containing calcium, magnesium, iron or zinc, and should, therefore, not be taken within 2 hours of food containing dairy produce or protein. The presence of protein in the meal reduces the absorption of L-dopa, but a low-fat diet enhances the effectiveness of the lipid-lowering agent lovastatin. Unpleasant flushing can occur when chlorpropamide is taken with alcohol or nifedipine (a calcium-channel blocking agent) with a high-fat meal. A high-fibre diet can bind some drugs; this may be of benefit, protecting against harmful effects, or a disadvantage, if absorption is too slow.

Dietary factors affecting drug metabolism

Adequate protein intake is required for normal drug metabolism and a low protein status may be linked with prolonged drug action. Fat-free diets may also reduce the activity of drug-metabolizing enzymes. Vitamin C is required for hepatic cytochrome P450, a key component of the microsomal oxidizing system, which metabolizes drugs. Many of the other enzymes involved in the phase I (oxidation, hydroxylation, reduction or hydrolysis) reactions, which alter the functional groups on the drug molecules, require vitamins, especially the B complex, and minerals to act as cofactors. Dietary factors are also needed to supply the groups needed to conjugate drugs in phase II reactions. These include glucuronate, glutathione, acetate and sulphate, all of which facilitate the solubilization and excretion of drugs.

This presents a potential problem for individuals with a chronic disease. If the disease affects their food intake, yet is treated by drugs, the effectiveness of the drugs and their potential side-effects may be significantly influenced by the nutritional status. In other words, those who require the drug therapy may well be in the most nutritionally vulnerable state and least able to metabolize the drugs.

Dietary factors affecting drug excretion

A low-protein diet may alter urinary pH, decrease renal blood flow and reduce the excretion of certain drugs. Some drugs are preferentially excreted in acidic conditions and reabsorbed when the pH of the urine becomes more alkaline. Lower clearance via the kidney may increase levels in the blood, resulting in side-effects. This has been reported in patients with gout, who are taking allopurinol and a low-protein diet. When several drugs are taken, there may be competition between drugs for renal excretion, with higher levels remaining in the blood.

Effects of drugs on nutrition

Food intake

One of the most important influences of many drugs is their effect on appetite. In some cases, this may be the declared aim of using the drug, when weight loss is required. However, other drugs may induce nausea or cause oral ulceration, which makes food intake painful. A notable example of this group of drugs are those used in cancer chemotherapy. Effects further along the gastrointestinal tract, such as abdominal pain, bloating or diarrhoea, may also reduce the desire to eat.

Some drugs can increase appetite as an unwanted side-effect. Major examples are the benzodiazepine tranquillizers and lithium used in manic depressive illness. Cyproheptadine is an antihistamine drug that has been used to encourage individuals with a wasting condition to increase their food intake.

Gastrointestinal function

Drugs may affect absorption from the digestive tract. Examples of such effects include:

- an alteration in pH (by antacids) and thus a change in the solubility of minerals for absorption;
- inhibition of folate deconjugating enzymes by sulphasalazine, which is used in inflammatory bowel disease, thus preventing liberation of folate from foods or competition with carrier molecules for folate transport;
- induction of catabolism of 25-OH vitamin D by anticonvulsants, reducing circulating levels and interfering with calcium absorption;
- binding of fat-soluble vitamins to mineral oil laxatives;
- destruction by long-acting antibiotics, such as neomycin, of gut flora that synthesize some vitamins;
- reduced vitamin B_{12} absorption owing to interaction with peptic ulcer drugs (H2 antagonists);
- damage to mucosal surfaces of the gut and small intestinal enzymes by excessive intakes of alcohol.

Metabolic effects of drugs on nutrients

Some drugs may be specific antagonists of the metabolic role of vitamins and may result in alterations in mineral status by specific effects on excretion. Specific vitamin antagonists include those that are intended to inhibit the vitamin or those that affect the vitamin as a side-effect. The most important of the specific antagonists are those for folic acid, which are used in cancer chemotherapy, against *Pneumocystis carnii* infection in AIDS, and as antimalarial and anti-inflammatory agents. Coumarin derivatives, used as anticlotting agents, are vitamin K antagonists.

Nitrous oxide used as an anaesthetic and the antituberculosis drug isoniazid, however, have unwanted side-effects, interfering with B_{12} and B_6, respectively.

Drugs may also lead to excessively high levels of sodium, potassium, calcium and magnesium by interfering with normal regulatory mechanisms. This may be a particular problem with drugs used in cardiac patients receiving diuretic therapies or when several drugs are used together. Diuretics can also result in mineral depletion. In both these cases, the mineral intake of the diet may need to be monitored.

The group in the population most at risk from these many interactions are the elderly. It has been reported that nursing home residents consume on average eight different medications per day. This may also be seen in elderly people living elsewhere, who may take a range of both prescribed and non-prescribed drugs. Interactions between the pharmacological effects of these substances are inevitable. If, at the same time, the physiological processes to cope with the metabolism of the drugs are beginning to be less efficient and maybe the nutritional intake is not as good as it could be, there is potential for undesirable side-effects. These may take the form of excessively large or inadequate therapeutic effects, both of which have medical implications.

NUTRITION AND THE ATHLETE

High levels of energy expenditure impose unusual physiological demands on the body. There is an increased need for energy and associated nutrients for increased metabolism as well as adequate fluids to maintain body temperature in the face of large amounts of heat production in exercising muscles. Exercise generates large amounts of free radicals because of the increase in oxidative processes. Thus, there is an increased need for antioxidant factors in the body and these should be plentiful in the diet.

To enable the body to make the most of its nutrient supplies, regular training facilitates the development of a more profuse blood supply in the muscle and shifts metabolism to more energy sparing pathways. In addition, physical activity confers a number of health advantages. A large follow-up study of 1800 British male civil servants showed that those who took vigorous exercise in their leisure time had less than a quarter of the fatal heart attacks seen in the inactive group.

In addition, exercise promotes a sense of well-being, believed to be related to altered levels of neurotransmitters in the brain. There is generally less body fat and more lean body mass than in comparable non-exercisers and a healthier blood lipid profile, with higher levels of high-density lipoproteins (HDLs). Those who exercise can consume more fat in their diet without increasing their adipose tissue levels. People who exercise regularly may also adopt other aspects of a healthier lifestyle, particularly not smoking.

The dietary needs of the athlete are, in essence, very similar to those of the average individual. Differences may arise, however, because of increased energy needs, the timing of meals to ensure an adequate intake around a busy schedule, and the importance of maintaining a high intake of carbohydrate during training and after competition. Fluid balance is also important.

Athletes can be very vulnerable to suggestions about their diet and may follow a succession of dietary fads and ideas, often spending a huge amount of money on pills and potions. When dietary advice is proposed, they may be reluctant to change what they believe to be a 'winning' diet, even if this is not nutritionally sound. If an athlete can be persuaded to adopt a sound healthy diet, it could remove a whole area of worry from the training programme and allow the focus to be concentrated on the physical training regime. In addition, careful attention to nutrition can make the difference between winning and coming second. It is the responsibility of the nutritionist to work with the athlete, to identify specific nutritional goals that are achievable and to provide strategies that match individual circumstances.

Energy needs in sport

The key consideration in any sports performance is the need for energy that is additional to that required for maintaining normal metabolism and everyday physical activity. Not all individuals undertaking sport have high energy requirements: in some sports, energy expenditure may be little more than is found in a moderately active person. Total amount of energy used is also dependent on body size, so a lightweight athlete will use less energy than one with a large body size. Exercising intensively on an energy-restricted diet can cause increased protein breakdown and may cause physiological stress. This, in turn, can result in a suppression of immune function. It is also very important to remember at this point that energy needed for

growth must also be met. In teenage athletes, high levels of activity and inadequate intakes will compromise growth. Thus, adequate levels of energy must be provided.

Provision of energy for sport (Figure 16.5)

At the cellular level, the muscles use adenosine triphosphate (ATP) in their contraction. A constant supply of this must, therefore, be maintained. In the first moments of exercise, the body will use its store of ATP, contained in the muscles, but after 3 seconds this has been exhausted. The next source is generation of ATP from creatine phosphate, also stored in the muscle, which can provide about 15 seconds' worth of ATP. This may be enough for a short burst of activity, such as a single jump, throw or lift. After this, ATP must come from other metabolic substrates, namely carbohydrates, proteins and fats. All of these can be transported to the muscle cell and broken down for energy; however, they are not used in equal amounts. Proteins do not usually contribute much to total energy expenditure in

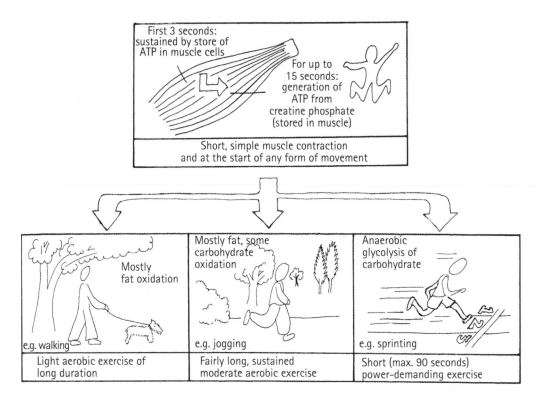

Figure 16.5 The provision of energy in sport.

exercise except in very prolonged, endurance events or in very intense exercise, when they may supply about 10 per cent of the total energy. The major supply comes from fats and carbohydrates. The choice of fuel is made on the basis of several aspects of the exercise, of which the most important is the intensity.

At rest, almost all the body's energy is supplied from fat oxidation. This is the most efficient source of energy, providing 80–200 units of ATP per molecule. Its main drawback, however, is that it is a slow producer of energy and uses more oxygen than carbohydrate metabolism does. Energy obtained from fat has been likened to a steam engine – it can use up fuel for long periods of time and maintain a steady pace. Even at low rates of exercise, the body has to use a small amount of carbohydrate to complete the oxidation of fats. Thus, stores of carbohydrate in the form of glycogen are important.

As exercise intensity increases, ATP must be produced more quickly to maintain energy supplies. This can be achieved by using increasingly more carbohydrate, which can produce 38 units of ATP per molecule of glucose as long as the oxygen supply is adequate, that is, under aerobic conditions. If the intensity of exercise becomes so great that the production of energy outstrips the supply of oxygen, glucose can still be broken down, albeit very inefficiently (no other substrate can be broken down in this way), but will only produce 2 units of ATP per molecule of glucose, by anaerobic metabolism. Such a burst of energy can be harnessed for a short and intense exercise, such as a 100-m race or a power lift. However, it is an incomplete metabolic process and lactic acid is produced. This has several consequences, particularly in the production of fatigue. A buildup of lactic acid reduces the pH in the muscle to the point where contraction can no longer occur. This terminates the exercise, so anaerobic exercise is of necessity of short duration (a maximum of about 90 seconds). The body's tolerance to lactic acid also increases with training, increasing the length of time the exercise can continue. Once the need for a rapid energy supply stops, oxygen can once again meet the needs of the metabolic pathways and the 'incomplete' oxidations can be brought to a conclusion, with the

further oxidation of lactic acid into pyruvic acid, and thence via the Krebs cycle. This has been termed 'repaying the oxygen debt'.

To maintain muscle contraction at a rapid rate, the following two conditions must be met.

- The oxygen supply must be as great as possible. This is improved by training, which allows a greater utilization per minute of oxygen, as lung capacity increases.
- There must be adequate supplies of glycogen. This is also improved by training, since the ability to use fat as fuel increases in a trained athlete and, therefore, extends the period of availability of carbohydrate.

In summary, whatever the intensity of the exercise, both fat and carbohydrate are generally used. At low levels, the balance is mostly in favour of fats, with little carbohydrate used. At high intensity, the exercise is fuelled mostly by carbohydrates, unless it is at maximal intensity and proceeds anaerobically, when carbohydrate is the sole fuel. Most exercise will predominantly occur at a level between these extremes, with perhaps only short bursts of intense action. However, the longer the duration of exercise, the greater the proportion of fat:carbohydrate used. Eventually, the supply of carbohydrate is exhausted and exercise has to stop. In addition to supplying the muscles, carbohydrate is also needed to maintain blood glucose levels, to meet the energy requirements of the vital organs, most notably the brain. These levels are maintained by the liver, which uses stored liver glycogen, but also manufactures new glucose from glycerol (from fat metabolism) and amino acid residues, in a process known as gluconeogenesis. Falling blood glucose levels contribute to fatigue. Low blood glucose levels also cause physiological stress, which results in release of hormones, such as cortisol, which in turn have a negative effect on immunity.

From the above it can be seen that maintaining a high level of stored glycogen in the muscle is important to extend duration of exercise. Many studies on exercising subjects, first carried out in the 1930s, have shown that exercise time to exhaustion can be lengthened in subjects consuming a diet containing a high proportion of carbohydrate. This increases exercise times compared with times achieved by subjects on normal

Figure 16.7 Effects of different amounts of carbohydrate in the diet on muscle glycogen levels during three consecutive periods of exercise over 72 hours. (From Wootton, 1988. Reproduced with kind permission of Simon & Schuster, London.)

Figure 16.6 Effects of different amounts of carbohydrate in the diet on the refuelling of muscle glycogen in the 24–48 hours after exercise. (From Wootton, 1988. Reproduced with kind permission of Simon & Schuster, London.)

diets, which in turn are greater than those in subjects fed a high fat/protein diet with low levels of carbohydrate. It has subsequently been shown that exercised muscle is capable of taking up carbohydrate in increased amounts in the first 1–2 hours after activity, which helps to replenish stores and permits exercise to be repeated on the following day (Figure 16.6). This increased capacity to store carbohydrate is believed to be at least partly the result of increased blood flow to muscles in the post-exercise period. Cell volume, influenced by osmotic changes is also a determinant of carbohydrate synthesis after exercise. These two findings highlight the importance of carbohydrate in the diet of the athlete.

During training

In practical terms, the diet during training should be based on carbohydrates, ideally supplying 55–60 per cent of the energy. This means that, if levels of protein are 10–15 per cent of energy, the amount of fat is 25–35 per cent. This is clearly very close to the general healthy eating guidelines. The carbohydrate should be a mixture of both simple and complex sources. In reality, an athlete who has very high energy

needs would find it very difficult to consume the volume of complex carbohydrate this would represent. This would be exacerbated by the usual lack of time for eating, which is common among amateur athletes. Nevertheless, adequate intake of carbohydrate is essential if daily exercise is taken (Figure 16.7). A daily requirement of 8–10 g carbohydrate/kg body weight is recommended during periods of hard training. For training sessions that last for more than 60 minutes, it is also important to take carbohydrate at intervals starting after the first 30 minutes. This helps to maintain circulating blood glucose levels and prevents depletion of liver glycogen stores. Once these have been depleted, they cannot be replaced until exercise has stopped.

After exercise

When exercise stops, the muscles need to be refilled as quickly as possible with glycogen. The first priority after exercise is thus to consume some carbohydrate-containing food, which will be readily absorbed and deliver its glucose content to the muscles. The food chosen should have a high glycaemic index, which will cause a quick rise in blood sugar. During this time, it is recommended that at least 50–100 g carbohydrate is consumed (1–2 g/kg) within the first hour. (Foods grouped according to glycaemic index are given in Table 16.1.)

TABLE 16.1 Grouping of some commonly eaten foods according to glycaemic index

Foods with high glycaemic index (above 85)	Foods with moderate glycaemic index (60–85)	Foods with low glycaemic index (less than 60)
Bread (white or wholemeal)	Pasta and noodles	Apples, grapefruit, peaches, plums
Rice	Porridge	Beans
Breakfast cereals (e.g. cornflakes, muesli, Weetabix)	Grapes, oranges	Milk, yogurt and ice cream
Raisins, bananas	Crisps	Fructose
Potato, sweetcorn	Biscuits	Tomato soup
Glucose, sucrose, honey		
Soft drinks		
Maltodextrin drink (20%)		

Adapted from Williams and Devlin, 1992. Reproduced with the kind permission of the publisher.

Many athletes find that they do not want to eat immediately after exercise; in this case, a carbohydrate-containing drink is useful. This helps to achieve the goal of replenishment of carbohydrate stores, as well as providing some rehydration. Small carbohydrate-containing snacks eaten at frequent intervals are also helpful. It should be remembered, however, that too many high-sugar foods may pose problems for dental hygiene and appropriate advice should also be given on this. Where possible, a meal or large snack high in carbohydrate should be consumed within 2 hours.

Later on, foods with a lower glycaemic index are acceptable, as they cause a slower but more sustained increase in blood glucose levels, which can enter the muscles over a longer period of time to maintain the refuelling process. Protein supply is also important at this time to ensure sufficient levels of amino acids in the circulation for tissue repair and protein synthesis. This does not need to come from special protein supplements, but can readily be supplied from normal foods, such as a sandwich with cheese, lean meat or fish, a baked potato with beans, or a pasta dish with a meat- or cheese-based sauce. All of these provide a combination of protein and carbohydrate.

Protein needs

Many athletes believe that, to make full use of their muscles in exercise, they require a high

Activity 16.1

An athlete requires a daily intake of approximately 21 MJ (5000 Calories). Calculate the amount of carbohydrate this would represent according to the above guidelines.

Devise a day's menu to supply this amount of carbohydrate:
- using predominantly sources of complex carbohydrate
- including some simple carbohydrate.

Repeat the calculation using a target energy intake of 10.5 MJ (2500 Calories).

Compare the practicalities of consuming the two diets.

protein intake. This stems from the idea that muscles are used up in some way in exercise and, therefore, require extra protein to restore them.

Protein makes a very small contribution to energy supply in exercise and is hardly used up at all. However, an exercising muscle does increase in mass over a period of time, so that when a person first starts to take regular exercise, more protein will initially be retained by the body. However, when equilibrium is reached, the additional food consumed to meet the energy needs should provide more than enough protein to meet the needs of the muscles for repair. Recommended levels for protein intake are in the region of 1.5 (1.2–1.7) g protein/kg body weight. There is no advantage in exceeding more than

2 g/kg, and such a high level may compromise the carbohydrate intake. Consequently, there will be insufficient glycogen for the muscles to exercise in training and any potential benefit of the extra protein will be lost anyway. The protein should always be balanced by an adequate energy intake, equal to 170 kJ (40 Calories) per gram of protein. There are many successful vegetarian athletes whose protein intakes are derived only from plant foods, and also athletes whose protein intakes do not exceed 10 per cent of the energy intake. It is the training that increases muscle size, strength and exercise capacity, and not the increased protein intake. Many athletes from developing countries do not have access to such high levels of protein, yet compete effectively on the world stage.

Dietary supplements

Athletes use a wide range of supplements, and surveys from various countries indicate that over 90 per cent of athletes studied are currently using, or have used dietary supplements in the past. Usage varies with the particular sport, level of competition and gender of the athlete.

Very few of the supplements used by athletes have been scientifically evaluated for efficacy to enhance performance, although, if the diet is inadequate, there may be a valid case for using the supplement.

Vitamin and mineral supplements

There is little evidence that vitamin supplements are of any benefit in an adequately nourished athlete. Studies that have claimed to show an improvement often give no indication of the initial nutritional status of the athlete and, therefore, their findings prove little.

The following two points are, however, important:

- Athletes who consume very little food in an attempt to maintain a low body weight appropriate to their particular sport may not meet their nutritional requirements for all micronutrients. A supplement may be indicated in this case.
- Intense physical activity produces free radicals, which may represent a health risk to the

individual, if insufficient levels of antioxidant nutrients are present. Attention should be paid particularly to vitamin E and C intakes to ensure adequate status. There is some evidence that immune status is poorer in athletes who undertake heavy training. This may be linked to low levels of certain micronutrients needed for the components of the immune response, although stress responses may also be an important factor.

Mineral status is of concern in terms of calcium and iron, especially in female athletes, who may consume diets deficient in both of these nutrients. Low calcium status in young women, together with a low body weight, which results in amenorrhoea (loss of menstrual periods), may compromise bone density and lead to fractures and early osteoporosis. This condition has been described as 'fit but fragile'. The drive to maintain a low body weight may be so intense that a type of anorexic behaviour is seen, with obsessive avoidance of food that might cause weight gain, compulsive exercise, and amenorrhoea with resulting low bone density that may lead to frequent fractures. This is sometimes described as the female athlete triad. When competitive sport participation stops, normal menstrual activity is likely to return but it is possible that bone density does not recover to that expected for age. Most at risk are young females in whom high levels of exercise delay menarche and disrupt the phase of most rapid bone mass accretion.

Iron needs are higher in women because of menstrual losses; low-weight female athletes may cease to menstruate and thereby conserve some iron. However, evidence exists of a higher turnover of iron in athletes, possibly owing to increased destruction of red blood cells. This may result in increased needs and, if these are not met, then stores will decline and anaemia can develop, which will affect performance.

Creatine

Creatine phosphate is an important energy source for muscles during intense exercise. However, the content in muscle is limited. Creatine is obtained from the diet, predominantly in meat and animal products, but is also synthesized in the body from amino acid precursors, such as glycine and arginine. Vegetarian athletes have to rely on endogenous synthesis, which can provide enough creatine. However, since the early 1990s, creatine supplements have been available, which have been shown to enhance the content in muscle by up to 50 per cent. The scientific evidence supports a positive effect of creatine supplementation in repeated short bursts of intense activity. It does not enhance duration of prolonged effort. Creatine supplementation can result in an initial gain in muscle bulk of 1–2 kg after a loading dose (4 × 5 g doses daily) for 4–5 days. This is probably due to swelling of cells, which may be accompanied by increased protein synthesis. A maintenance dose of 1–2 g daily is recommended. Subjectively, heaviness of muscles may be a reported side-effect. No clinically significant negative effects have been reported to date.

There are many other dietary supplements which are used by athletes. Some of these are mentioned in Chapter 17.

Fluid

Fluid is also an important consideration for athletes. Sweating is essential to lose heat and maintain body temperature. The sweat contains electrolytes, most notably sodium, potassium and chloride ions, derived from the plasma. However, the concentration of electrolytes in the sweat is different from that in the plasma, with the result that the remaining plasma may actually have higher concentrations of some electrolytes at the end of the exercise. Consequently, the top priority for replacement after exercise is water, to restore normal concentrations in plasma.

The issue is complicated by the observation that the best way to increase water absorption from the gut is to include some electrolytes in solution. This enhances water uptake and speeds rehydration. Many rehydrating solutions are available; most of them contain electrolytes (at less than 2.6 g/dL), together with varying amounts of carbohydrate. The carbohydrate is present in amounts that may be:

- lower than concentrations in body fluids (hypotonic solutions);

- the same as body fluids (isotonic solutions); or
- greater than body fluids (hypertonic solutions).

Absorption of these is most rapid from the hypotonic solution and slowest from the hypertonic solution. Drinking a hypertonic solution will not provide rapid rehydration and may actually aggravate matters, as fluid from the body is drawn into the digestive tract. However, hypotonic and isotonic solutions are useful in providing quick rehydration. The added benefit of the carbohydrate content when taken at the end of exercise is its contribution to refuelling the glucose stores. These solutions are also useful during prolonged exercise, when they help to maintain blood glucose levels and prevent dehydration, thus enabling performance to continue at an optimal level. Solutions that contain glucose polymers are now available; this enables more glucose to be contained in the drink without compromising the tonicity and, therefore, provide more potential energy in the drink.

Overall, many athletes do not consume a diet that is appropriate to optimize their sporting performance. This may be due to a variety of factors, including a lack of practical knowledge and time as well as a reluctance to take advice. More education about diet and nutritional needs of both athletes and those who have responsibility for their training is needed.

ALCOHOL ABUSE

Moderate amounts of alcohol (e.g. taken within the UK recommended limits of 2–3 units or 3–4 units per day for women and men, respectively) are believed to be beneficial to cardiovascular health, as described in Chapter 14. One unit of alcohol, as defined in the UK contains 8 g of alcohol, and is usually interpreted as the amount of alcohol in one standard drink (a half pint of regular beer, one glass of wine or one measure of spirits). However, amounts in excess of this taken over a period of time are likely to result in harm and to compromise health. The exact level of intake that may cause harm is difficult to define, as it is variable between individuals and depends on genetic predisposition. However, chronic intake of over 55 units per week for men and

35 units per week for women is defined as 'unlikely not to cause harm'.

It is very difficult to obtain a true assessment of the number of people whose health is damaged by alcohol. In Britain, figures quoted suggest that there are 250 000 people dependent on alcohol and a further one million at risk of dependence. The diagnosis may be difficult because so many people with an alcohol problem conceal this from those around them, often continuing to work and maintaining an external appearance of normality. It is only through alcohol-related disease, such as liver disease or encephalopathy (brain disease), that alcoholism may be diagnosed. In addition, alcohol taken in excess contributes to other diseases, such as cardiovascular disease and hypertension, ulcers, cancer and mental illness, as well as accidents and violence.

The pattern of alcohol abuse has changed in the last decade in Britain, with a rapidly increasing incidence in women. This reflects both the increased economic independence of women as well as the increased access to alcoholic drinks. Drinking among women has possible implications for the health of the fetus, if it is continued throughout pregnancy. High levels of alcohol ingestion may result in 'fetal alcohol syndrome', characterized by developmental abnormalities of the face, brain, heart and kidneys.

Young people are also drinking more, particularly in a 'binge' drinking pattern, when large amounts of alcohol are consumed in a relatively short space of time. Such high intakes may accelerate the damage caused.

The elderly, especially if affected by loneliness, are also recognized as a group at increased risk of excessive drinking. This may go unnoticed by primary health care staff until there is a crisis, such as a fall.

Nutritional implications

Food intake

Food intake can be affected by alcohol consumption in various ways, including the following.

■ There is likely to be a reduced appetite or an overall lack of interest in food as a result of a preoccupation with alcohol. Inflammation of the stomach lining (gastritis) may result in pain on eating or cause vomiting.

■ Access to food may be difficult, especially if the alcoholic has left home. Cafe or takeaway food may form a large proportion of the diet; this may not be particularly healthy or nutrient rich.

■ Money available to buy food may be scarce and be preferentially spent on drink.

Digestion and absorption

Alcohol is an irritant to living tissue, resulting in a permanent state of inflammation along the digestive tract, and leading to vomiting and diarrhoea. Gut contents tend to be moved along rapidly and enzyme production may be impaired. This is particularly the case for the enzymes produced in the wall of the small intestine, which complete carbohydrate and protein digestion. The villi may be flattened and absorptive areas reduced. There may be secondary intolerance to sugars, which remain undigested and ferment in the large intestine.

Metabolic changes

Liver damage is recognized as one of the main consequences of alcohol abuse. The liver is also the site of activation, storage and metabolism of many of the nutrients in the body. These will be adversely affected. Some nutrients are specifically needed to metabolize and detoxify the alcohol, and requirements for these will increase.

Alcohol is a diuretic agent, increasing urine production. This will cause the loss of more water-soluble nutrients from the body. The pancreas may be inflamed, resulting in pancreatitis. Although this predominantly affects the production of digestive enzymes, there may also be implications for insulin release and thereby control of blood sugar levels.

Energy balance

There is controversy about the utilization of the energy content of alcohol. The theoretical energy yield is 29 kJ (7 Calories) per gram of ethanol. However, individuals consuming large amounts of alcohol in addition to a moderate food intake do not exhibit the weight gain one might expect from the excessive energy intake. This has led to the proposal that some of the potential energy from alcohol is liberated as heat rather than being converted into usable ATP. Some alcohol is metabolized via the microsomal ethanol oxidizing system (MEOS), which becomes more active at higher levels of alcohol intake. It is possible that this oxidation does not yield usable ATP, and constitutes a 'drain' for the excess energy. Alcoholics may, in fact, be underweight or overweight, and which of these occurs appears to depend on the total intake of food, rather more than the amount of alcohol consumed.

Abnormal findings

Fat metabolism by the liver becomes abnormal. The production of NADPH by alcohol metabolism drives fat synthesis, with large amounts accumulating in the liver. Circulating lipid levels, especially the very low density lipoprotein (VLDL) fraction, are elevated, increasing the risk of heart disease.

Control of blood glucose levels becomes less precise. This is partly the result of a failing production of insulin in the pancreas, but also because of reduced gluconeogenesis by the liver. There may be periods of hypoglycaemia (low blood sugar), with feelings of dizziness and faintness, and possibly blackouts.

The liver is one of the main sites for protein synthesis and degradation. In the liver of an alcoholic, protein degradation may continue at a relatively normal rate, but protein synthesis and, therefore, tissue repair declines. Levels of essential proteins will gradually decline, for example, the plasma proteins in the blood or the proteins that function as digestive enzymes.

Among the water-soluble vitamins, it is the B complex that is most affected. Multiple deficiency states may exist, involving niacin, riboflavin and pyridoxine, and resulting in sore mouth, diarrhoea, dermatitis and psychological disturbances. Megaloblastic anaemia is likely as a result of folate malabsorption. Thiamin deficiency is likely, as it is required for the metabolism of alcohol, and may, in addition, be lost in vomiting and diarrhoea. This deficiency will result in neuropathy, affecting hands and feet, making walking difficult. In its severe form,

psychological disturbances with loss of memory and psychosis (Korsakoff's syndrome) may develop. Poor vitamin C status owing to a poor diet is also possible.

Absorption of fat-soluble vitamins may also be affected, especially if the production of bile from the liver is reduced. Particularly at risk is vitamin K, as there are generally small stores of this vitamin. Low vitamin D status has also been reported; it is believed that the breakdown of active vitamin D is induced by the alcohol.

Among the minerals, zinc is important, as it forms an essential part of the alcohol dehydrogenase enzyme. Levels may become depleted, affecting alcohol metabolism, wound healing, sense of taste and immune function. Electrolyte imbalances may arise because of vomiting and diarrhoea, and can lead to changes in muscle function. Iron status may be either high or low, depending on the beverages drunk. Spirits provide no iron (or any other nutrients), but some wines and beers may contain iron. However, blood loss due to intestinal irritation may cause iron depletion, and the alcoholic may become deficient despite an apparently adequate intake (see Figure 16.8).

INFLUENCE OF DISABILITY ON NUTRITION

The term 'disability' is used to cover a very wide range of physical or mental conditions that may influence the ability of an individual to function in the able-bodied world. The disability may be present from birth, or may have affected the person as a result of an accident or disease (such as Parkinson's disease, multiple sclerosis or stroke). The degree of disablement will be reflected in the extent to which functions are compromised. The disability may be progressive and deteriorating, or there may be gradual improvement. The perception of change may influence the person's willingness to look after themselves, and take an interest in their health and possible rehabilitation.

Some disabilities will have very little impact on nutrition; others may have profound effects. Those having the greatest effects will be those

Figure 16.8 Nutritional implications of alcohol abuse.

that affect food intake, digestion and absorption, and metabolic needs.

Impact of disability on food intake

This is probably the largest area of potential difficulties. Food intake may be influenced by:

- factors affecting appetite;
- factors affecting the ability to obtain and prepare the food; or
- factors affecting the ability to ingest, chew and swallow the food.

Appetite

Appetite will be influenced by mental state, and thus can be affected by anxiety or depression. Physiological factors will also have an influence; for example, dulled sensation of taste, nausea, constipation or pain after eating will reduce appetite. A common side-effect of drug therapy is a dry mouth, which makes food ingestion difficult and unpleasant, and depresses the appetite for eating. Physical factors, such as lack of exercise and immobility, may also mean that the individual does not feel hungry.

Environmental factors, including monotonous menu presentation, especially if the diet has to be soft or puréed, and unpleasant surroundings may be off-putting. Eating snacks or sweets between meals may also be a major factor contributing to lack of appetite at mealtimes.

In a non-verbal individual affected by any of these factors, their unwillingness to eat and the carer's desire to provide food for eating may result in conflict and frustration.

Ability to obtain and prepare food

In the situation where the individual is responsible for his/her own food supply, both the mental and physical capabilities are important. Understanding what to buy to produce a meal is essential. The process of going out and buying the food may be compromised in many ways, including mobility, ability to communicate, to see/hear and to carry the food. All of these will determine the range of foods that are actually available to eat. Cooking skills and capabilities are also important.

Where a carer is responsible for all of these functions, the autonomy of the individual must be taken into account. The question of whether the food that is being prepared is actually what is desired needs to be addressed. Food is a very personal issue and another person's choice may not be our own.

Ability to ingest, chew and swallow food

Ingestion, biting, chewing and swallowing of food may be difficult in some disabilities. There may be tongue thrusting, spitting out, choking and dribbling. These may be linked, for example, to a lack of coordination, involuntary movements, lack of lip closure or cleft lip and palate. Careful techniques are required to provide useful nutrition. Appropriate modification of texture may be needed, with the use of thickeners to improve the appearance of meals and make them easier to eat. If the individual is responsible for his/her own feeding, hand to mouth coordination is needed.

Appropriate positioning is essential to facilitate swallowing and prevent regurgitation. Special feeding utensils are available to help the process; occupational therapists can help to develop skills required for feeding and advise on modified equipment. Becoming an independent feeder can lead to marked improvements in nutritional status.

Impact on digestion and absorption

Some individuals with disabilities may tend to regurgitate or ruminate food. Food that has been swallowed may later be brought back into the mouth and spat out. If this is continuous and severe, nutritional status will be threatened.

Drugs used to manage an underlying condition, such as tranquillizers, anticonvulsants, antibiotics, analgesics and antihypertensive drugs, may all affect the digestion and absorption of food from the gut. It is important that potential drug–nutrient interactions are anticipated and avoided by suitable timing of drugs and meals, wherever possible.

Laxatives may be used to treat constipation. A form of laxative that has no impact on nutrient absorption should be chosen and, if possible, dietary fibre and fluid intakes should be increased.

Impact on metabolism

Nutritional needs may be altered by increased or reduced energy expenditure, drug-induced alterations in metabolism and specific nutritional requirements related to the underlying condition. It is, therefore, important to monitor the nutrient needs of each individual. In children, growth should be monitored regularly, including height and weight; in adults, weight can be a useful indicator of adequate energy intake. However, other assessments of nutritional status may be required, particularly micronutrient status.

Nutritional consequences

If total food intake is small, there is a risk of malnutrition, resulting in poor physical and mental well-being, increased risk of infection and, in children, delayed growth. More often, however, sufficient food is eaten, but it may be low in nutrient density, perhaps because of the foods chosen or if it is diluted during purée production. Attention should also be paid to nutrient retention during preparation. Foods that are kept hot for periods of time lose vitamin content, and modification of texture may result in significant losses of water-soluble vitamins. If specific groups of food are omitted entirely, the individual may be left vulnerable to deficiencies; for example, if few fruit and vegetables are included, they may lack trace elements and folate. Constipation may be a problem if non-starch polysaccharide (NSP) intake is low. Laxative use, on the other hand, may deplete the body of fat-soluble vitamins.

Infection and the associated physiological stress will increase nutritional needs, especially for B vitamins and vitamin C, zinc and protein.

Involuntary muscle spasms may increase energy expenditure and result in weight loss, if this is not met. This is particularly common in children with athetoid cerebral palsy and autism, and with oral defects.

Specific drug–nutrient interactions should be anticipated by adjusting food intake. If appetite is very poor, a nutritional supplement may be needed to improve well-being to a point where adequate nutrition can be obtained through the diet.

In summary, there are many threats to the nutritional status of a person experiencing some disability. If these can be identified and anticipated, they should not result in nutritional deficiency. However, the most important criterion is to judge each case in the context of the specific circumstances.

SUMMARY

1 Several situations that provide an additional threat to nutritional status have been reviewed.

2 People suffering from food intolerance may need a modified diet. However, this should be devised with appropriate consultation with a dietitian, so that nutritional content is maintained.

3 In people with HIV infection or AIDS, nutrition can contribute to health, and every effort should be made to maintain nutritional status during periods of infection and debility.

4 Drugs that are used therapeutically can influence nutritional state. However, poor status with respect to nutrition in the patient may in its turn affect the metabolism of drugs and perhaps produce unexpected reactions.

5 Athletes have additional nutritional needs. These can be met from increases in food intake. A particular emphasis should be made on the carbohydrate content of the diet.

6 Disability may have short- or long-term implications for food intake. People affected by disability should have access to various aids and modifications that can improve their nutritional intake. Monitoring of health and weight is important.

STUDY QUESTIONS

1 **a** Think about the examples of challenges to nutritional status discussed in this chapter. Construct a table to identify which part of the food path (intake–processing–utilization) is actually affected in each of the cases.

   b Suggest other challenges to nutrition that could be analysed this way.

2 **a** What are the characteristic features of a food allergy?

   b Why is allergy to peanuts currently of concern?

3 Identify the main focus of nutritional advice to be given to HIV-positive subjects.

4 **a** In what ways does nutritional status affect drug utilization?

   b What are the possible implications of this in people who are ill and are receiving drug treatments?

5 **a** What do you consider to be the main difficulties encountered by an athlete that might prevent the consumption of an adequate diet?

   b How can some of these difficulties be tackled and overcome?

6 Prepare an article to appear in a newsletter for parents of children with disability, giving practical help about diet.

REFERENCES AND FURTHER READING

British Nutrition Foundation 2001: *Nutrition and sport.* Briefing Paper. London: British Nutrition Foundation.

Buttriss, J. (ed.) 2002: *Adverse reactions to food. The report of a British Nutrition Foundation Task Force.* Oxford: Blackwell Science.

DoH (UK Department of Health) 1995: *Sensible drinking. The Report of an Interdepartmental Working Group.* Wetherby: Department of Health.

DoH (UK Department of Health) 1997: *Peanut allergy.* Committee on Toxicity of Chemicals, Consumer Products and the Environment. London: Department of Health.

Gowland, M.H. 2002: Food allergen avoidance: risk assessment for life. *Proceedings of the Nutrition Society* **61**, 39–43.

Grimble, R.F. 2001: Nutritional modulation of immune function. *Proceedings of the Nutrition Society* **60**, 389–97.

Hughes, D.A. 2000: Dietary antioxidants and human immune function. *British Nutrition Foundation Nutrition Bulletin* **25**, 35–41.

Maughan, R. 2002: The athlete's diet: nutritional goals and dietary strategies. *Proceedings of the Nutrition Society* **61**, 87–96.

Prentice, A.M., Stock, M.J. 1996: Do calories from alcohol contribute to obesity? *British Nutrition Foundation Nutrition Bulletin* **21**, 45–53.

Saarinen, U.M., Kajosaari, M. 1995: Breast feeding as prophylaxis against atopic disease: prospective follow-up study until 17 years old. *Lancet* **356**, 1065–9.

Salomon, J., De Truchis, P., Melchior, J.-C. 2001: Nutrition and HIV infection. *British Journal of Nutrition* **87**(Suppl. 1), S111–19.

Semba, R.D., Tang, A.M. 1999: Micronutrients and the pathogenesis of human immunodeficiency virus infection. *British Journal of Nutrition* **81**, 181–9.

Terho, E.O., Savolainen, J. 1996: Review: diagnosis of food hypersensitivity. *European Journal of Clinical Nutrition* **50**, 1–5.

Thomas, J.A. 1995: Drug–nutrient interactions. *Nutrition Reviews* **53**(10), 271–82.

Ware, L.J., Wootton, S.A., Morlese, J.M. et al. 2002: The paradox of improved antiretroviral therapy in HIV: potential for nutritional modulation? *Proceedings of the Nutrition Society* **61**, 131–6.

Williams, C., Devlin, J.T. (eds) 1992: *Foods, nutrition and sports performance.* London: E & F Spon.

Wootton, S. 1988: *Nutrition in sport.* London: Simon & Schuster.

Young, E., Stoneham, M.D., Petruckevitch, A. et al. 1994: A population study of food intolerance. *Lancet* **343**, 1127–30.

The aims of this chapter are to:

❏ discuss the concept of optimal nutrition;
❏ describe some of the foods that are available to the consumer that may be used to optimize health;
❏ describe the evidence to support the use of these foods.

On completing the study of this chapter you should be able to:

❏ explain what is meant by functional foods;
❏ evaluate the evidence for the role of non-nutritional factors in human health;
❏ debate the advantages and disadvantages of using designed food products to optimize health.

In the last few decades, the developed world has witnessed a shift in perception about the possible roles of food and nutrition. The fundamental role of food is to supply the basic nutrients for the maintenance of physiological function (and growth) in the body and fulfilment of social activity, while at the same time satisfying sensory needs. From this understanding come concepts, such as nutritional requirement and dietary reference values, which are discussed in Chapter 2. As our knowledge of the role of nutrients in the body and possible interactions with the prevention or development of diseases has developed, a further role for food has become apparent. This is the recognition that components of food, which may or may not have specific nutritional roles, may be beneficial to health. Thus, there has been a shift from discussing 'adequate' nutrition to considering 'optimal' nutrition.

This presents a challenge to nutritional scientists to decide, where relevant:

■ how much is enough (to minimize deficiency);
■ how much is best (to meet biochemical, physiological and other functions for normal health);
■ how much can provide other benefits in non-nutritional ways;

■ how much is too much and causes harmful effects.

Suitable indices are required in order to be able to define these limits, and this brings considerable methodological, practical and ethical challenges.

Traditional approaches have included balance studies, tissue saturation studies, measurement of body stores and functional studies. Many of these methods have been used to determine minimal requirements for nutrients.

The function of a nutrient within a specific target tissue or pathway can be used to determine its level of activity, and to explore the effects on this of changes in intake or blood level of the nutrient. Generally, it would be expected that increases in intake, or blood levels, up to a certain level would cause a dose–response change in activity of the measured function. At the point where activity ceases to increase, it can be assumed that maximal physiological (or optimal) function has been achieved.

With the current state of knowledge, the role of a nutrient is likely to be assessed in a rather general way, for example, in terms of its effect on antioxidant status, muscle strength or blood clotting. This is because, in most cases, the exact first biochemical point at which a particular nutrient is involved and at which it becomes limiting in deficiency may not be known. However, with developments in molecular biology, it may be possible in the future to explore the effects of nutrients on gene expression and determine their role precisely. A general function is also likely to be used to assess possible health benefits of a nutrient, perhaps in amounts greater than meet the functional needs.

There are many difficulties, however, in translating results obtained at the laboratory level into guidelines or targets for the intake of a particular nutrient. These can include:

- interactions between nutrients and other chemical components in food;
- uncertainties about the bioavailability of nutrients at the gut level;
- efficiency of transport to the target site;
- inter-individual variation;
- potential interaction between nutrients at different stages in the life cycle.

For all of the above reasons, research on optimal levels for the majority of nutrients is still at an early stage. The Food Standards Agency in the UK has an Optimal Nutritional Status Research programme, which has a number of objectives.

The first objective is the need to understand the links between optimal nutrition status and the maintenance of good health. This will explore the potential interactions between micronutrients at different life stages in the reduction of specific disease.

The second objective is to develop accurate measures of bioavailability of nutrients from foods. This will explore the processing of nutrients at the gut level and their transport to cellular sites. There are a number of subissues within this objective that have been identified:

- to measure the fraction of an ingested nutrient that meets functional demand at the target tissues;
- to develop functional markers of status for each micronutrient or group of micronutrients;
- to use human intervention studies to determine dose–response relationships of tissue function;

- to understand the extent of inter-individual variation in order to identify optimal nutritional intakes for the whole population and, therefore, provide advice that could reduce morbidity and mortality from chronic disease.

FOODS, FOOD COMPONENTS AND HEALTH CLAIMS

The growth of interest in the use of food to promote a state of health and well-being, and reduce the risk of disease has led to the rapid development of an industry that produces foods that claim to possess these characteristics. A health claim describes a positive relationship between a food substance in the diet and a disease or other health-related condition. This may include a lessening of the condition or a reduction in the risk of that condition.

Early research on these foods started in Japan in the 1980s, with the purpose of developing foods for specific health use (FOSHU). These were defined as 'processed foods containing ingredients that aid specific bodily functions in addition to nutrition'. Legislation allowed claims to be made about specific health effects of foods in certain categories. In the USA, the Nutrition Labelling and Education Act, enforced in 1994, allowed health claims to be made for ingredients for which there was recognized evidence of a correlation between intake and cure or prevention of certain diseases, although this does not necessarily mean that the evidence can be applied to the food itself.

The promotion of foods with health claims is much more restricted in the UK, where the law separates foods and medicines so that foods cannot be described as providing a medical health benefit. Therefore, foods cannot be labelled as 'preventing' or 'curing' a specific disease. As a result of growing concern about the unregulated market in the UK, the Food Advisory Committee produced a set of guidelines. These have been developed into a Code of Practice by the Joint Health Claims Initiative (JHCI), a panel of representatives from consumer, food industry and enforcement groups. This aims to help the food industry to make health claims that are within current legislative constraints. An expert committee is to review all claims to ensure that they are supported by scientific evidence, with the aim of producing a list of approved generic health claims for use by food manufacturers whose products meet the criteria. New submissions for products will also be considered. It is anticipated that this will allow consumers to receive information about health benefits without infringing current UK legislation.

There is a relatively high degree of public suspicion of processed foods in the UK, related to a number of food-related health scares in recent years. A meeting with consumers by the Foresight Task Force, set up by the Government in the UK in 2001, indicated that there is cynicism among consumers about the need for new products developed by the food industry, and the reasons for their development. It is evident, therefore, that products that might be valuable to optimize nutrition need to be clear in their presentation to the consumer.

This puts the onus on the food industry to follow the principles of scientific research and on regulatory authorities to ensure that systems are in place to protect the consumer.

The following points summarize stages in the process of developing such products or food components.

- Fundamental research techniques can identify possible interactions between a food component and a function relevant to health, thus generating hypotheses for study. Appropriate markers of this function need to be developed for the assessment. This is a problematic area, as few such markers exist.
- The hypothetical effect needs to be tested in appropriate models, including human studies, and safety assessments carried out. Trials should be carried out in a manner similar to drug testing, with the potential to demonstrate a dose–response relationship, and any potential risk be evaluated. The cost–benefit of the use of the food component should be analysed.
- The food component being studied should be able to be included in a variety of normal diets, in amounts sufficient to produce the desired effects, that is, they should remain 'foods'.

- Possible adverse effect of an excess intake of the component must also be examined (e.g. if the same component is included in a number of products, will this still be safe?).
- The differential effects of the component in people of different ages and states of health should be considered.
- The evidence relating to the product must be evaluated by an independent authority, which is empowered to approve the use of the product, and which can determine the nature and content of the health claim being made. This is a fundamental part of any food safety and labelling regulations that exist in a country.
- The information to the consumer about the product must be both clear and informative. It should include information about the target group or condition (if this is specific), the benefit claimed and the amount to be consumed.

Terminology

There is a confusing range of terms given to foods that have been specifically developed by the food industry to meet the demand for healthier foods.

SMART FOODS

This is a term that is being used in schools in the UK as part of the Design and Technology curriculum. The food industry uses the term 'modern' or 'novel' food materials. These are foods that have been developed through new or improved processes, generally by human intervention and, therefore, not through naturally occurring changes. This classification includes:

- foods with novel molecular structures, including fat substitutes and sweeteners;
- meat analogues, including novel proteins;
- foods produced by biotechnology;
- functional foods (also known as pharmafoods or nutraceuticals).

Foods with novel molecular structures

In relation to healthy eating initiatives, the most important components in this group are fat replacers and sweeteners. Both are useful in reducing the energy content of the diet. Fat replacers can be derived from carbohydrate or protein, or be lipid-based. In the case of carbohydrate- or protein-derived products, these can be used to substitute fat in the production of low-fat meals, and additionally act as stabilizers to prevent separation of ingredients. Lipid-based fat replacers are fatty acid esters with sugars, which are not absorbed from the digestive tract. These have the advantage of being stable at high temperatures and can, therefore, be used in fried or baked products, such as crisps and biscuits. An example of this group is Olestra, licensed for use in the USA.

Sweeteners are a well-established item in the diet of people wishing to reduce their energy intake. The main products used in the UK are saccharin, aspartame, acesulfame and cyclamate. All the intense sweeteners provide the sensation of sweetness in very small amounts because of their molecular structure and can, therefore, mimic the effect of sucrose, without supplying the associated energy. Aspartame is composed of phenylalanine and aspartic acid and, therefore, yields these amino acids when digested. However, the quantity consumed produces a negligible amount of energy. Because it contains phenylalanine, aspartame should not be used by people with phenylketonuria (PKU) who cannot metabolize it. Over 2000 products available in Europe contain aspartame.

This group of smart foods also contains modified starches, which are used in many food products that need to be stabilized or thickened,

Activity 17.1

1 Look in the supermarket for examples of 'instant' and 'ready to eat' products. Identify which of these contain modified starch that is acting as a stabilizer or thickening agent.

2 Prepare a number of drinks (e.g. cups of tea) with different sweetening agents – try to use examples of each chemical type, as well as sugar. Test these on several volunteers to study any perceived differences in taste and sweetness detected.

and has extended the range of 'instant' and 'ready to eat' products on the market.

Meat analogues

This group of smart foods includes products made from soya protein (textured vegetable protein, tofu) or fungal proteins (Quorn) that have been extruded, spun, coagulated and moulded into products that resemble meat in texture. Flavours and additional nutrients may be added as part of the processing. These products are included in the diet of people who prefer not to eat meat, but may also be considered by some to be a healthier alternative to meat. This may not necessarily be the case, as levels of fat may be comparable to those in similar meat dishes and micronutrient levels may be lower.

Foods produced by biotechnology

Plant and animal breeders have for centuries tried to breed in the best characteristics of the species, and breed out the least advantageous ones. Biotechnology is the use of biological processes to make useful products. The use of yeast to make bread and beer, and microorganisms to make yogurt and vinegar are all traditional examples. In recent years, developments in molecular biology and genetics have made it possible to manipulate the genes of plants and animals to an extent that specific characteristics have been transferable. This has made it possible to produce new varieties of certain plants having desirable characteristics. Disease resistance can be enhanced by genetic modification so that insect or virus borne diseases no longer destroy the crop. This has been achieved for a substantial proportion of maize grown in the USA. Work is under way to increase disease resistance in the sweet potato, which could enhance yields three-fold.

One of the most successful 'genetically modified' (GM) plants has been the soya bean, which carries resistance to particular herbicides, thus allowing more effective treatment of the cultivated land with less herbicide and hence more efficient crop growth and less environmental damage. Varieties of maize and rice have also been developed, which have advantages in terms of nutrient composition or yield over the more traditional varieties. For example, the protein and vitamin A content of rice has been enhanced to improve dietary balance. It is anticipated that, in the future, more beneficial amino-acid profiles or higher meat yields can be engineered into animals. Higher levels of antioxidants are being bred into tomatoes. The removal of potential allergens from foods, such as wheat, is another exciting area of research, which would help individuals who are unable to consume gluten. Similarly, research on allergens in peanuts may yield a non-allergenic product. Slower ripening allows crops to be preserved better with fewer losses.

There is concern that introducing alien genes into plants may have adverse consequences for the humans who consume these, and a considerable amount of resistance to the introduction of foods containing GM components. Careful testing for safety and long-term trials are necessary to ensure that these products are safe. Clear labelling of products that contain GM ingredients is also called for by consumers, and European legislation has been reviewed in the light of concerns and will be monitored in the future.

Functional foods

This is the largest category of smart foods and also the most diverse. The functional food market in Europe was estimated to be worth $55 billion in 2000, and is rapidly expanding. A functional food may be defined as one having health-promoting benefits, and/or disease preventing properties over and above the usual nutritional value. This definition can cause difficulties in that some common foods could be considered to be covered by this definition. For example, many vegetables provide non-nutritive phytochemicals, which are believed to have health-promoting benefits but do not contribute to the accepted nutritional value of the vegetable. It has been suggested that functional foods might be better viewed as a concept that can help to optimize nutrition rather than a means to categorize them.

Nevertheless, it is useful to consider the different types of products that could come into this group.

- foods containing added (fortified) or reduced levels of nutrients – these may be nutrients that would normally be found in the product or ones that are not typical of the food;
- foods containing phytochemicals, that is, components with no known nutritional role that are promoted as such in the diet, or have added levels of some phytochemicals;
- foods containing added components that do not occur generally in the typical diet, with the specific aim of producing a functional effect;
- foods containing bacteria that are used to promote gastrointestinal tract function.

The following sections will consider examples of foods/food components in each of these categories and some of the evidence for their use as functional foods.

Fortified foods

This group includes foods that have been fortified with macronutrients or micronutrients. On a global basis, food fortification is an important strategy for combating specific nutrient deficiency that may be prevalent in a community. Notable examples of this include fortification of salt with iodine or the use of various vehicles as a medium for increasing iron intakes. In such national schemes, it is important to choose both an appropriate food for fortification, which represents a regular item in the diet, as well as the best form of the mineral or vitamin to maintain the stability of the food product, and maximize bioavailability of the nutrient.

There is no widespread single nutrient deficiency in the UK, yet there are a great number of fortified foods available aimed at promoting health rather than preventing deficiency. These include white bread and flour, which are required legally to have thiamin, iron and calcium added to restore the content to that found in wholemeal flour. This was introduced to protect the health of the population following World War II, but has been maintained ever since, although the nutritional need for this is arguable. In the USA, folate is added to flour; but this is not the

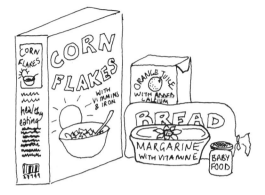

Figure 17.1 Examples of fortified foods.

Activity 17.2

1 Look at some of the foods mentioned in this section in a grocery store or supermarket. For each of the foods:

   a Note the added nutrients, how much is added and how this relates to the reference nutrient intake (RNI).

   b What fraction of the RNI does the food provide?

   c How much of the food would need to be eaten each day to meet the RNI – is this realistic and feasible?

   d Is there any indication on the label of the target consumer group for the product?

2 Try to find some examples of foods with added nutrients that would not normally be found in the food (as in the case of orange juice mentioned above). Why do you think these foods have been chosen for fortification with these particular nutrients?

3 List the advantages and disadvantages of fortifying foods with nutrients. If possible, think about the different situation in industrialized and developing countries. Discuss your findings with other members of your group.

case in the UK, following a decision taken by the Food Standards Agency in 2002, after a wide-ranging consultation. Margarine is required by law to be fortified with vitamins A and D, to provide levels of these vitamins that are comparable to those in butter. Many of the other spreading fats are also fortified with these vitamins. Breakfast cereals are voluntarily fortified with a wide range of nutrients; however, this is not a legal requirement. The range of nutrients added, and the level of fortification varies between products and from time to time in the same product (see Figure 17.1).

Infant milks and foods contain various added nutrients to enhance their nutritional value. There are guidelines on the levels of nutrients that should be provided in foods for infants. Other products that are fortified include instant mashed potato, bedtime drinks, yogurts, soft drinks, condensed milk and dried milk powder. The range of fortified foods available is not constant and it is interesting to note the information on food labels to keep up to date with products. Most of the examples mentioned above contain added nutrients that would be found in a more 'natural' form of the food. However, there are now exceptions to this, with nutrients being added that would not be found associated with the product. An example of this is the addition of calcium to orange juice. Currently, it is difficult to add some nutrients to foods because of the technological difficulties of dispersal, taint and stability of the products. However, micro-encapsulation of nutrients may expand this field further in the future. One group of nutrients being considered in this context is the *n*-3 fatty acids, which could be added to some foods in the future in this way. Similarly, calcium can be added to soya milk in an encapsulated form that avoids precipitation of the soya protein.

Reduced content of nutrients

This group contains foods mostly for the weight-reduction market, with a wide range of products that are 'low calorie' and, therefore, to be used 'as part of a calorie-controlled diet'. These include individual products, such as drinks, biscuits, yogurts and whole meals, available as 'ready meals' that have been 'calorie counted'. A further range of foods are 'low-fat' products, which represent a separate area of the market. These are not necessarily lower in energy content than a corresponding regular product, as they may contain other energy-containing constituents within the formulation, but do meet regulations of having lower percentage fat than the regular product.

Specific alterations to other constituents may include reduced sugar or salt content. A number of specific dietary products are marketed to meet the demand for foods that are free from a specific component, such as gluten-free products for people with coeliac disease. Other examples may include products that are free from lactose, sucrose, milk or egg.

Foods containing phytochemicals

Vegetables and fruit have been promoted as part of a healthy diet for many years and, since the 1990s, there has been specific advice to include five portions, or 400 g, of these in the daily diet. Both fruit and vegetables contain a number of valuable nutrients but, in addition, it has been recognized that they are rich in non-nutritive substances, known as phytochemicals. These occur in plants and products made from plants at varying concentrations. Amounts are relatively low in the storage parts of plants, higher in the fruiting parts, and highest in the seeds and parts that are dried and concentrated for use as herbs and spices. The latter, however, are generally used in small amounts and, therefore, may not represent an important dietary source. In general, the phytochemicals are produced by the plant as a defence against predators, and are bitter, acrid or astringent in an attempt to make the plant unpalatable or toxic. As a result, humans too may find these substances unpleasant, and this may be a strong disincentive to consume foods that could be good for our health but may not agree with our palate. A challenge to the food industry, both in the past and future has been to breed varieties of plants in which the bitter taste is reduced, while at the same time attempting to ensure that the beneficial effects of the phytochemicals are preserved or enhanced by selective breeding. Extracting the active agent and adding it to other products is a possible developmental step. This has already happened with the use of isoflavones from soya in some types of bread.

The interest in phytochemicals stems from the strong link between diets rich in plant foods and lower rates of cancer and coronary heart disease. The diversity of these compounds creates an enormous task to study the roles of individual phytochemicals in disease prevention or risk reduction and, at present, the evidence often relates to groups of related compounds. Several different mechanisms of action have been identified, usually by *in vitro* study. These are briefly reviewed in the following sections.

Phenolic compounds, including flavonoids

Higher concentrations of phenolic compounds are generally found in young sprouting plants or seedlings than in the mature plant, in line with their role as protection against predators. Immature fruit, such as apple or grapefruit, are very bitter because of the presence of these compounds.

There are over 5000 different flavonoids; many are responsible for the colour of flowers, leaves and fruit. They are generally bitter or astringent. The various flavonoids differ according to their molecular structure and occur in different sources. Flavones, include rutin and quercetin, and are found in apple skins, broccoli, grapes, olives, onions and parsley. Quercetin is the most important contributor to the estimated intake of flavonoids, mainly from the consumption of apples and onions. Flavanones, including hesperetin, are predominantly found in citrus fruit and their peel, and contribute to the bitterness of these fruit. The catechins occur in green and black tea, and red wine (from both the seeds and skins of grapes). They contribute substantially to the bitterness of Japanese green tea. Catechins are also thought to be responsible for the bitter taste of chocolate. Finally in this group are anthocyanins, which are darkly coloured and occur in richly coloured fruit such as berries, cherries, grapes, wine and tea.

In addition, there are high-molecular-weight polyphenols, also known as tannins, which are found in sorghum, millet, barley, peas, dry beans and legumes, fruit, tea and wine. Tannins form insoluble complexes with proteins and starches, and reduce the nutritional value of foods.

The most researched property of all of the flavonoids and phenolic compounds is their antioxidant activity. This may include limiting the production of reactive oxygen species, stabilizing white blood cells and scavenging free radicals. All of these result in less low-density lipoprotein (LDL) oxidation and potential for endothelial damage. In addition, flavonoids have been proposed as having other roles including anti-inflammatory, antitumour, antithrombogenic, and antiviral roles. However, much of the supporting evidence is based on small studies or *in vitro* research, and conclusions cannot be drawn. More research on phenolic compounds and flavonoids is required, together with more information about the bioavailability of the compounds, and more analytical techniques for measurement of intake and excretion levels.

In the meantime, it is important that the known dietary sources of these compounds are encouraged in the diet, to maximize the diversity of intake and benefit from them.

Dietary phyto-oestrogens

Phyto-oestrogens are present in plant foods; the two major subclasses are isoflavones and lignans. The majority of interest has been focused on the isoflavones, of which the major examples are genistein and daidzein, which are found in soya beans and products derived from them including textured vegetable protein, tofu and soya milk. The richest source of lignans is flaxseed (linseed); however, many fibre-rich foods contain small amounts, including lentils, sweet potato and oat bran. More accurate analytical data are needed. A more potent phyto-oestrogen has recently been discovered in hops, and more sources may yet be discovered.

Phyto-oestrogens have been shown to exert a wide range of hormonal and non-hormonal effects in animal and *in vitro* studies. In addition, epidemiological evidence indicates that, in Asian countries, where the habitual daily intake of isoflavones is between 20 and 50 mg/day, there is a lower incidence in women of many hormone-dependent diseases, such as coronary heart disease, menopausal symptoms, osteoporosis and breast cancer. Women in communities where soya beans are eaten tend to have longer menstrual cycles, by 1–2 days. This can relate to 2 fewer years of menstruating life, less ovarian activity and possibly reduced breast cancer risk. In Japanese men, the incidence of clinical prostate cancer is significantly lower than in American men and prostatic tumours develop more slowly. Benefits in terms of coronary heart disease and osteoporosis also apply in men.

Interest in the phyto-oestrogens arose because of their structural similarity to mammalian oestrogen. The compounds were shown to act both as oestrogen agonists (mimicking the effects of the hormone), as well as antagonists (blocking the action of the hormone). The varying effects are attributable to the existence of two different oestrogen receptors in specific tissues, which result in varied responses. Target tissues include breast, ovaries and uterus, brain, bone, lungs, blood vessels, kidneys, adrenals, testes and prostate. In addition to oestrogen related responses, phyto-oestrogens have also been shown to alter steroid metabolism, increase sex-hormone binding in the blood, act as antioxidants and reduce thrombogenesis. At present, these effects have not been fully tested in clinical studies, although small short-term studies have reported benefits in menopausal symptoms and bone loss. There is much to discover about the bioavailability of the phyto-oestrogens from dietary sources, the levels achieved in the blood and at active sites, and the amounts required to produce a clinical effect. Studies also indicate that there is considerable individual variation in the metabolic fate of the compounds and this may make recommendations about dosage very difficult to predict. These compounds represent a challenge to the functional food market, in trying to balance a beneficial health effect with acceptability and safety. One of the problems with soya products is their bitterness; the food industry makes attempts to reduce this, but may at the same time remove the beneficial isoflavones.

Glucosinolates

These compounds occur mostly in the cruciferous vegetables (cabbage family), including broccoli, cauliflower, turnips, Brussels sprouts, cabbage and kale. *In vitro* studies suggest that glucosinolate compounds, such as sinigrin and progoitrin, induce enzymes that inactivate carcinogens by neutralizing their toxic properties and speeding their elimination from the body. In addition, products derived from glucosinolates during digestion, including isothiocyanates, are also reported to block the effects of carcinogens. Clinical studies have so far not been able to support these findings. However, diets high in cruciferous (and other) vegetables are linked in epidemiological studies with lower cancer rates, including lung and alimentary tract. One of the major practical problems for food scientists is the bitter taste of many of the vegetables in this family. Selective breeding, genetic modification and alteration of growing conditions are all being used to decrease bitterness and increase consumer acceptability, while protecting the content of active agents.

Carotenoids

Carotenoids are fat-soluble pigments found in many fresh fruit and vegetables. Initially, they were of nutritional interest because of the role of beta carotene as a major precursor of vitamin A in the body; other carotenoids have lower levels of provitamin A activity. The total amount of carotenoids taken up from the diet is relatively small and a regular intake appears to optimize absorption. It is now known that some 600 carotenoids exist and at least 40 have been isolated in foods. The association between plasma levels of beta-carotene and cardiovascular disease has been reported in a number of epidemiological studies. However, supplementation trials using beta-carotene have not replicated the beneficial results. For example, a study in smokers resulted unexpectedly in a higher incidence of lung cancer and heart disease (Omenn et al., 1996).

Although a specific physiological role for carotenoids has not been clearly defined, they have been shown to possess antioxidant activity and, as such, are of interest in reduction of disease risk. It should be remembered that antioxidants donate an electron to stabilize a free radical. In so doing the antioxidant itself becomes unstable, with the potential to become a free radical and propagate a chain reaction. It is essential, therefore, that there are other antioxidants to repair and maintain the system. One such agent is believed to be vitamin C. This illustrates the importance of having adequate and comparable levels of various antioxidants in the body and may explain why large amounts of one of these may be more harmful than protective (see Chapter 14 for more on antioxidants). Thus, any supplement that provides additional carotenoids should also contain adequate vitamin C.

Lycopene, an acyclic form of beta-carotene, has been found to be a more potent antioxidant than beta-carotene itself. *In vitro* studies suggest that it protects LDL against oxidation. Lycopene is one of the major carotenoids in the Western diet, being found in tomato and tomato products. Intake levels are lower in developing countries. Other sources include pink grapefruit, watermelon, guava and apricot. An epidemiological association has been reported between low plasma levels of lycopene and prostate cancer in the USA. A study in Finland recently reported an excess incidence of acute coronary events and stroke in association with low levels of lycopene.

Lutein is a major pigment in chloroplasts and, as such, is one of the five most common carotenoids in the diet. Together with zeaxanthin (which is similar in structure), it is found in the macular region of the eye, which is the region of the highest visual discrimination, but also the most light-sensitive area. This area is, therefore, very vulnerable to damage by free radicals produced by light interacting with oxygen in the blood. Over time, this can result in macular generation (age-related macular degeneration; AMD) and blindness. This is the commonest cause of blindness in Western society. It is particularly common in smokers, in whom levels of lutein have been shown to be lower than the population average. Lutein absorbs blue light and, as an antioxidant, quenches free radicals. Lutein cannot be synthesized in the body and, therefore, a dietary intake is needed to maintain serum levels; active transport mechanisms concentrate lutein in the macula. There are high levels of lutein in breast milk. In addition, lutein is found in green leafy vegetables and in orange/yellow fruit and vegetables.

All of the phytochemicals discussed above have potential roles in risk reduction and health promotion. The evidence for most of them is, at present, based largely on *in vitro* or animal studies, with only a few clinical studies. However, epidemiological data support the link between intakes of fruit and vegetables in the prevention of a number of diseases. Food scientists can develop varieties in which the active agents are enhanced but, in the mean time, five servings a day of fruit and vegetables remains sound nutritional advice.

Foods with added components

Designing foods with a specific health purpose may involve adding an ingredient that is not usually present in foods, or present in only small amounts in the food.

Phytosterols are compounds that are structurally similar to cholesterol and are currently being used in a range of products as cholesterol-lowering agents. Phytosterols are thought to have been present in the diet of our ancestors in much greater amounts than occurs currently. Intakes of naturally occurring plant sterols are higher in vegetarians than in omnivores. The plant sterols currently used are extracted from soya bean oil or pine tree oil and are esterified to increase solubility. The most common are sitosterol, campesterol and stigmasterol. Products may contain plant sterol (unsaturated) or plant stanol (saturated) esters, and evidence shows that both have a similar capacity to lower circulating total and LDL cholesterol levels. The phytosterols reduce the absorption of cholesterol from the small intestine by forming insoluble particles with cholesterol, and by competing with cholesterol for bile that would facilitate absorption. Thus, a greater proportion of dietary cholesterol is excreted, although some of the phytosterol is absorbed. Absorption is estimated as no more than 5 per cent of the phytosterol. The liver does compensate for reduced cholesterol absorption by increasing synthesis of endogenous cholesterol, but the net effect is a reduction of total cholesterol in the body.

These effects are achieved with relatively small doses of the phytosterols. As little as 1 g/day may have an effective lipid-lowering effect, although a dose of 1.6 g/day of plant sterol is recommended. There appears to be a plateau effect with no further reduction of cholesterol seen at intakes above 3 g/day. The average reduction in cholesterol levels is in the region of 5–8 per cent from spread alone and, when combined with other lipid-lowering measures in the diet, or drug treatments, levels of cholesterol may be reduced by 10–15 per cent. The dispersal of the phytosterol within the food product appears to be the key determinant of its effectiveness.

There has been some concern expressed about the potential for reduced absorption of fat-soluble vitamins, as a consequence of phytosterol ingestion. Lower plasma levels of vitamin E and carotenoids have been reported, but these effects are considered to be marginal.

Although developed as an aid to the management of blood lipids levels in cardiovascular disease reduction, new evidence suggests that the plant sterols may also have a role in inhibition of tumour growth.

Plant sterols and stanols are currently marketed as a range of spreads, dairy goods, such as yogurt and cream cheese, and salad dressing.

Omega-enriched eggs

A range of eggs is on sale in the UK from chickens that have been fed on a vegetarian seed-rich diet containing *n*-3 fatty acids. This results in eggs enriched with these fatty acids. This illustrates how manipulation of the nutritional content of a product can be achieved. The eggs form a small part of the total egg sales in the UK, but can provide up to 70 per cent of the currently recommended level of *n*-3 fatty acids in one egg.

Clinical usage

In clinical nutrition, feeds are being produced that contain 'functional' components for which there is believed to be an additional need in particular circumstances. Glutamine is an important fuel source for rapidly dividing cells, for example, those lining the gastrointestinal tract and blood cells. Severely ill patients may be at risk of receiving insufficient glutamine to meet their increased demands. Supplemental glutamine may improve gut mucosal and immune functions, and reduce episodes of clinical sepsis. Trials have shown reduced mortality, lower infection rates and shorter hospital stay.

Arginine is also a conditionally essential amino acid in states of trauma and sepsis, and arginine-containing formulas may reduce complications in surgical patients.

Sports products

The sports nutrition market contains a wide range of functional foods for athletes that are promoted as supplying specific benefits over and above basic nutrition.

The development of sports drinks containing glucose polymers allowed more carbohydrate to be consumed, without undesirable effects in terms of sweetness and palatability as well as excessive osmotic effects. Products, such as high-energy bars, also provide a large amount of energy in a very small volume of food, allowing energy needs to be met. Glycerol is now included in some sports drinks as research has suggested that this can promote hyperhydration, although the evidence is equivocal.

A huge range of products that have potential use as ergogenic aids is marketed and can be considered as functional foods. Some of these are summarized in Table 17.1.

Although there is a theoretical potential for a metabolic effect for some of the functional products available for athletes, the actual ability of the substances to reach the target site and be incorporated into the cellular or subcellular metabolic machinery is usually not proven. Much more research is needed to examine possible beneficial effects of putative ergogenic agents, as well as their safety.

Foods containing bacteria

The contribution to human health of bacteria resident in the gut is increasingly recognized. More than 500 different bacterial species inhabit the human gut, amounting to about 1 kg in weight. Some of these are considered to be beneficial and health promoting, some benign and some harmful or pathogenic. The balance of these bacteria is important and a predominance of one group over another can alter the risk or progression of disease, and the health and function of the colon. Longevity had been noticed among groups of the world population who consumed fermented dairy products that were believed to reduce levels of toxin-producing bacteria, thus suggesting that the dietary intake may have an influence on the health of the bowel and the organism.

Far from being a passive excretory route, the bowel is now understood to be a metabolically active organ that provides a protective barrier for the host through effects on the immune

TABLE 17.1 Functional foods in sports nutrition		
Dietary constituent	**Suggested role**	**Strength of evidence**
Amino acids		
Arginine, lysine, ornithine	Promote growth hormone secretion and aid muscle development	Weak
Glutamine	Prevents immunodepression, reduces infections	Some experimental evidence
Caffeine	Promotes fatty acid release, sparing glycogen stores	Can be beneficial, within legal limits
Carnitine	Central role in energy production, could enhance aerobic performance	Weak
Coenzyme Q_{10}	Needed for generation of ATP	Weak
Creatine	Increases capacity for repeated bouts of high-intensity exercise	Good
Ginseng	Increase mental energy and stamina	Weak
Sodium bicarbonate	Increased alkaline reserve to buffer lactic acid produced in anaerobic exercise	May be effective in specific circumstances. Gastrointestinal effects unpleasant

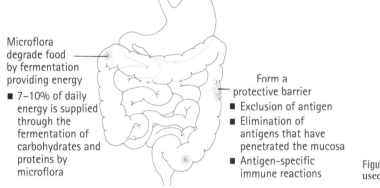

Microflora degrade food by fermentation providing energy
■ 7–10% of daily energy is supplied through the fermentation of carbohydrates and proteins by microflora

Form a protective barrier
■ Exclusion of antigen
■ Elimination of antigens that have penetrated the mucosa
■ Antigen-specific immune reactions

Figure 17.2 How microflora are used in the bowel.

system. The protection exists at various levels, in terms of physical exclusion of the antigen, elimination of antigens that have penetrated the mucosa and finally control of any antigen-specific immune reactions. In order to be able to perform these functions, the gut depends on both appropriate nutrients as well as a beneficial microbial balance.

In addition, metabolism in the bowel may provide between 7 and 10 per cent of the daily energy supply through the fermentation of carbohydrates and proteins (to a lesser extent). Some 60–80 g of the food ingested each day reaches the colon; the microflora degrade this by fermentation to lactic acid and short-chain fatty acids, as well as carbon dioxide, hydrogen, methane, phenolic compounds, amines and ammonia (see Figure 17.2).

In the past, there was a frequent challenge to the gastrointestinal tract by microorganisms present in the environment and in food, and this primed the immune system to function normally. Our increasingly clean and processed environment, with foods containing artificial sweeteners, preservatives and even antibiotic residues reduces the microbial challenge and results in an underperformance of the immune system. Modern lifestyle, with poor eating habits, stress and use of antibiotics can all contribute to alterations in the microflora. It is believed that this may be one of the mechanisms whereby there has been an increase in chronic inflammatory diseases, including eczema, asthma, allergies, Crohn's disease, inflammatory bowel disease and ulcerative colitis.

The gut of the newborn infant is sterile but becomes colonized soon after birth. The method of feeding determines the bacterial flora, with lactobacilli and coliform bacteria and bifidobacteria prevailing in the breastfed infant. Formula feeding induces a wider microflora, which additionally includes *Bacteroides*, clostridia and streptococci. After weaning the microflora becomes similar to that of the adult, with a predominance of anaerobic bacteria, which die in the presence of oxygen. Among these, the bifidobacteria and lactobacilli are considered to be beneficial to health, and some, such as certain *Eubacterium* spp., are benign but suppress the growth of harmful bacteria. Examples of the latter include proteolytic *Bacteroides* spp., many *Clostridium* spp. and pathogenic species of Enterobacteriaceae. Many other microorganisms are present in the bowel, some of which have not yet been characterized, and there is more research required.

Probiotics have been developed, therefore, as an aid to restore the immune function of the gut and to reduce the incidence or symptoms of associated clinical conditions. Thus, probiotics can be described as products that contain live microorganisms in fermented foods, which could promote good health by establishing an improved balance in intestinal microflora. The main organisms currently used are various species of lactobacilli and bifidobacteria, together with a non-pathogenic yeast, *Saccharomyces boulardii*.

A probiotic product must fulfil several criteria including safety, ease and reproducibility of production, and stability during storage.

Furthermore, the organisms should be able to survive in the digestive tract and colonize the bowel in adequate amounts to be able to provide benefit to the host. Although there is evidence from *in vitro* and animal experiments of beneficial effects of probiotics, clinical studies in humans are still at a relatively early stage. Most evidence exists for the reduction of diarrhoea and prevention of gastroenteritis, especially in infants and young children. In adults, antibiotic-induced and hospital-acquired diarrhoea has been shown to be better controlled with the use of probiotics as part of the treatment. Probiotics containing lactobacilli have also been used successfully in cases of lactose malabsorption. A study in older adults showed an improvement in several aspects of cellular immunity after 3 weeks of probiotic use, especially in those with low immune status at baseline. Some evidence of an immune system stabilising effect has also been found in inflammatory bowel conditions and atopic eczema. There is still a lack of good evidence, however, that probiotics can prevent cancer, reduce plasma cholesterol levels or reduce levels of *Helicobacter pylori* infection in the stomach. Major advances in studying the mechanisms of action of probiotics, and gut structure and function *in vivo* are needed to further clarify the potential benefits and better target specific organisms for particular health needs.

Microorganisms require a substrate on which to grow and multiply. If this is not provided in the diet, the microflora can be compromised. This is the basis of the use of prebiotics, which are non-digestible food components that reach the colon where they can selectively stimulate the growth of beneficial microorganisms. In many ways, this definition is similar to that for components of dietary fibre, although these do not support the growth of one type of microorganism alone. Candidates for prebiotics are the oligosaccharides containing fructose (fructans). A naturally occurring example of this group is inulin, although other fructans are found in wheat, onions, bananas and chicory. Oligosaccharides containing xylose, galactose and mixtures of these sugars have also been studied. The most promising results have been obtained with fructo-oligosaccharides (FOS), which were shown to stimulate growth of bifidobacteria in the colon and change the balance of microflora. Lactulose (containing galactose and fructose) has also been used in a number of clinical trials and found to promote growth of lactobacilli. Prebiotics may be useful in the management of constipation, owing to the osmotic effect associated with increased bacterial fermentation. Increased acidity in the bowel has been suggested to be beneficial in the absorption of a number of minerals, most notably calcium.

As with all of the other functional foods, however, more randomized controlled trials are needed to confirm this effect and any associated health benefits.

Prebiotics are found in a range of foods in Europe, including dairy products, infant formula and bakery products (see Figure 17.3).

ORGANIC FOOD

The concept of organic food is in many ways the opposite end of the spectrum from the functional foods discussed above. Organic foods represent more traditional food production methods, without the use of man-made chemical agents to potentiate the yield or reduce pest damage. Organic farming systems rely on traditional concepts of crop rotation, the use of animal and plant manures, and biological methods of pest control. The market in organic foods has increased rapidly in the last 5–10 years, as consumers have become concerned about the perceived safety of mass or intensively produced foods. Such concerns include the presence of pesticide, growth promoter and antibiotic residues. In addition, there may be concerns about the presence of known (such as bovine spongiform encephalopathy; BSE), or unknown disease causing factors in the foods.

Although the primary concern may be one of food safety, organic food is also perceived as having superior sensory attributes and being 'healthier'. This is taken to mean that food produced organically has a higher nutrient content. Williams (2002), in reviewing the evidence on nutritional quality of organic food, notes that there is no evidence in the scientific literature to support these claims. There are methodological shortcomings in most of the publications that

PROBIOTICS

★ Products that contain LIVE MICROORGANISMS in fermented foods

★ main organisms:
LACTOBACILLI
BIFIDOBACTERIA
SACCHAROMYCES BOULARDII

★ Organisms survive in the digestive tract & colonise the bowel to aid host defence against pathogenic organisms

★ Some evidence for reduction of diarrhoea & gastroenteritis & Lactobacilli used to treat lactose malabsorption

PREBIOTICS

★ NONDIGESTIBLE FOOD COMPONENTS that reach the colon

★ Selectively stimulate growth of beneficial microorganisms

★ Examples of prebiotic oligosaccharides:
FRUCTO-OLIGOSACCHARIDES (FOS) stimulate growth of bifidobacteria
LACTULOSE promotes growth of lactobacilli

★ may be useful in treatment of constipation

★ Increase absorption of minerals

★ Found in dairy products, infant formula & bakery products

Figure 17.3 Probiotics and prebiotics.

report on nutritional quality of organic versus conventionally produced foods. Many cover a long time period, during which there have been many changes in the production methods. Comparisons of effects of feeding experiments in animals produce inconsistent and conflicting results. No studies of effects on human health have been performed. Some data show that conventionally produced vegetables, especially green leafy vegetables may have a lower vitamin C content. This is associated with a higher water content producing a dilution effect. Conventionally grown plants grow more quickly and are harvested sooner than those grown organically, resulting in a higher water content. Nitrate levels were also higher in the conventionally grown leafy vegetables, probably associated with fertilizer use. There is no evidence of a negative impact on health from these differences. An area of potential interest that has not been studied is the level of various phytochemicals contained in plants. These are produced by plants as a protection against adverse conditions or to combat attack by potentially damaging pests or diseases. It is possible that levels may be

higher in organically grown products that are less protected by sprays. However, there has been no study of this area.

It should also be remembered that organic food may carry a higher level of microbial contamination, through the application of manure or the unchecked growth of fungi or bacterial contaminants.

Much of the organic food available for sale in the UK is imported. This has possible implications for its freshness and associated nutritional content. It is also more expensive than conventional produce. As a result, a substantial proportion of the population are unable to afford organic foods. If they choose to buy organic produce, this may be at the expense of other items in the diet that could have contributed more to a healthy balance. Where money is not an issue, individuals can buy organic produce without fear of compromising the balance of the rest of their diet.

In summary, it is more important to concentrate on consuming a diet in line with healthy eating guidelines, as there is much more good scientific evidence to support this than to worry about any risk to health of conventionally produced foods that might be avoided by eating 'organically'. At present, there is insufficient evidence to support any benefit to health of 'organic' food, and more research is needed to clarify these issues.

CONCLUSIONS

The concept of optimal nutrition opens a new era in the science of nutrition. Advances in knowledge about molecular biology and the characterization of the human genome will make it possible at some point in the future to study genetic polymorphisms that are associated with particular diseases. It is likely that these will also characterize individual responses to particular dietary components. We will also have a clearer view of the molecular mechanisms of nutrient action. An understanding of how genetic polymorphisms affect nutrient metabolism may make it possible to design specific dietary regimes to tackle nutritional problems, or disease risk. It is likely to become the responsibility of the food industry to develop products that help to fulfil these goals.

Nevertheless, although progress in recent years has been rapid, the preceding sections have indicated how little is known in some cases about mechanisms at cellular and tissue level. This is hindered by a lack of biomarkers and specific tools for identification of processes, for example, within the gut mucosa. Properly controlled large-scale clinical trials need to be performed to evaluate the potential benefits of products, and caution needs to be exercised when claims are made that have not been properly evaluated and cause confusion among consumers. Safety aspects must also be addressed, if new products are developed.

In the mean time, consuming a balanced diet following healthy eating guidelines is our best guarantee of optimizing nutrition from food. This, after all, is what has sustained the human race over thousands of years, and should not be forgotten in the rush for new designer foods that offer promises of better health and disease reduction.

SUMMARY

1 Optimal nutrition is a concept that encompasses positive benefits of food in the promotion of health.
2 Foods with altered nutritional contents have been produced to address some issues of 'healthy eating'.
3 Some of the more researched food components have been introduced into foods to produce potentially health-promoting products.
4 There are many other components of food that have no known nutritional role but may modify the risk of disease.
5 The use of bacteria to promote gut health is a novel approach to optimizing nutritional state.

STUDY QUESTIONS

1 Debate with a partner what are the arguments for and against more development of smart foods. You could consider:
   a are they useful for all people?
   b should they be targeted at specific groups? – if so, give examples
   c which foods should be promoted and which allowed to disappear?
   d are there other smart foods that you think might be useful?

2 You could imagine that you are an Expert Committee and have to decide on permission for the development of some new products. What would you need to know?
3 Survey a number of people in your community to discover how many buy organic foods.
   a Which foods are commonly bought, and what are the perceived benefits of choosing these?
   b What foods are they replacing in the diet, and does this lead to better or poorer balance of healthy items?

REFERENCES AND FURTHER READING

Buttriss, J., Hughes, J., 2000: A review of the MAFF optimal nutrition programme: aims and objectives. *British Nutrition Foundation Nutrition Bulletin* 25, 79–80.

Cassidy, A., Faughnan, M. 2000: Phyto-oestrogens through the life cycle. *Proceedings of the Nutrition Society* 59, 489–96.

Johnson, I.T. 2001: New food components and gastrointestinal health. *Proceedings of the Nutrition Society* 60, 481–8.

Kolida, S., Tuohy, K., Gibson, G.R. 2000: The human gut flora in nutrition and approaches for its dietary modification. *British Nutrition Foundation Nutrition Bulletin* 25, 219–22.

Marteau, P., Boutron-Ruault, M.C. 2002: Nutritional advantages of probiotics and prebiotics. *British Journal of Nutrition* 87(Suppl. 2), S153–7.

McConnon, A., Cade, J., Pearman, A. 2002: Stakeholder interactions and the development of functional foods. *Public Health Nutrition* 5(3), 469–77.

Omenn, G.S., Goodman, G.E., Thornquist, M.D. et al. 1996: Effects of a combination of beta carotene and vitamin A on lung cancer and cardiovascular disease. *New England Journal of Medicine* 334, 1150–5.

Rowland, I.R. 2002: Genetically modified foods, science, consumers and the media. *Proceedings of the Nutrition Society* 61, 25–9.

Schrooyen, P.M.M., van der Meer, R., De Kruif, C.G. 2001: Microencapsulation: its application in nutrition. *Proceedings of the Nutrition Society* 60, 475–9.

Various authors 1999: Symposium on optimal nutrition. *Proceedings of the Nutrition Society* 58, 395–512.

Williams, C.M. 2002: Nutritional quality of organic food: shades of grey or shades of green? *Proceedings of the Nutrition Society* 61, 19–24.

CHAPTER 18

PUBLIC HEALTH NUTRITION AND HEALTH PROMOTION

The aims of this chapter are to:

❏ review and link some of the issues discussed in earlier parts of the book in relation to increasing health through improved nutrition;
❏ consider some of the obstacles to improving nutrition that may exist;
❏ describe strategies for health promotion and nutrition education that have been developed in recent years;
❏ consider future directions.

On completing the study of this chapter, you should be able to:

❏ discuss the importance of nutrition in prevention of chronic disease;
❏ recognize the stages involved in undergoing change and the barriers that may exist;
❏ describe and evaluate some of the strategies that exist to promote better nutrition.

To develop and implement policies for the prevention of a disease, it is important at the outset to make a realistic assessment of its prevalence and the extent to which it impacts on morbidity and mortality statistics in the population. Further, if these policies are to relate to dietary intake and nutritional goals, it is also important to make an assessment of the role of the diet in the aetiology of these diseases and how much gain can be expected from changes in the diet.

These are areas of controversy, generating quite polarized opinions. At one extreme, it is suggested that, because we cannot be certain that diet plays a role in a particular disease, we should do nothing, with the implication that to change could do more harm than good. On the other hand, others suggest changes based on very weak evidence, coming from a small database. However, between these extremes there is a broad consensus on desirable dietary change, based on evidence from large numbers of studies. Many of these have been re-evaluated using the technique of 'meta-analysis', which allows a number of studies with similar research criteria

to be combined to increase the statistical power of the results.

The World Health Organisation (WHO), since its formation in 1948, has been working to improve the health of all the peoples of the world. In the last two decades, it has become clear that there have been changes in patterns of morbidity and mortality in many countries. These have arisen from:

■ reductions in maternal and infant mortality;
■ better control of infectious diseases through immunization and environmental improvements, although the spread of HIV infection has run counter to this trend;
■ increased population life expectancies owing to advances in medical technology and lifestyle changes;
■ improvements in diets in some areas.

However, in parallel with these, there has been a persistent rise in chronic non-communicable diseases, such as cardiovascular disease, cancers, diabetes, chronic respiratory diseases and osteoporosis. In the Western industrialized countries, these diseases have been well established for over

40 years and, in many of these countries, there have been decreases, especially in coronary heart disease incidence. However, there has been an upward trend in the countries of Eastern Europe and, most notably, in the developing countries.

Many countries whose traditional diet and lifestyle had been associated with a low incidence of non-communicable disease have been experiencing a period of food transition. This is typified by an increased consumption of animal protein and reduction in vegetable protein sources, generally associated with a higher fat intake. In addition, the intake of carbohydrate from the starchy staple, and minerals and vitamins from vegetables may begin to decrease. This has been noted in Japan, where the prevalence of obesity and coronary heart disease, both previously relatively rare conditions, has begun to increase. Countries such as China and those in South America are also experiencing this trend. In some of the poorer countries in the world, the gradual transition to a more Western diet, accompanied by rapid increasing urbanization and lower levels of physical activity (as well as smoking), is causing a rapid rise in chronic diseases. Because of the greater numbers of people in these countries than in the developed countries, mortality from chronic diseases has now outstripped on a numerical basis that in the developed world. There is also concern about the spread of overweight and obesity in these countries, and the potential for associated health problems, as has already happened in the industrialized world. These trends have been monitored by the INTERHEALTH programme of WHO, which studies the risk of the major non-communicable diseases in a number of populations around the world, as well as trends in diet and nutrition, and aims to promote and monitor community-based strategies for intervention.

In Europe, the WHO has been working to develop a Food and Nutrition Policy by 2005. This aims to increase awareness of the links between food growing, buying and eating, and the effects on health and environmental sustainability. This reflects a new approach inherent in many nutrition policies that incorporates concepts of social justice and the importance of fair access to food for all.

The European Community has also enshrined human health protection as a part of all its policies. This has led to the formulation of a public health framework, including an action programme, public health policies and legislation. The EURODIET project has been one aspect of this and aims to contribute towards a coordinated European Union (EU) and member-state health promotion programme on nutrition, diet and healthy lifestyles. Progress has been made on European dietary guidelines. Other objectives of this project include:

- translating these into food-based dietary guidelines within member states;
- promoting these to the population;
- identifying and overcoming barriers;
- a European Food Safety Authority to oversee the food supply from its production to consumption.

Despite some improvements in the incidence of coronary heart disease, it is estimated that, across Europe, the demand for treatment related to chronic diseases will continue to increase, because of the increases in the elderly population. It is, therefore, essential that changes in lifestyle and diet are introduced to reduce the incidence of these diseases, as clearly health services will not be able to cope with such huge increases in demand. There is, therefore, an economic benefit to be gained as well as the social gain for individuals.

Measures to prevent chronic diseases are needed and these are the goals of many strategies around the world. It is recognized that such strategies must take into account all aspects of the food chain:

- production policies;
- social policies determining access to the foods;
- education policies to increase awareness;
- dietary guidelines to inform choice.

They must, therefore, involve the governments as well as all those concerned with food. Policy makers also need to examine health impact effectiveness and cost effectiveness in their decision-making. In addition, there needs to be a commitment to the strategy, which is translated into action. Much has been learned in the last decade about public health approaches that are likely to result in changes in attitudes, behaviour, risk factors, morbidity and mortality. Attention is needed to public health nutrition, which is the promotion of good health though nutrition and physical activity, and the primary prevention of related illness in the population.

WHAT IS THE BASIS OF HEALTH-PROMOTING POLICIES AND WHAT IS PROPOSED?

There exists public concern in Europe about potential hazards associated with recent developments in a complex food chain. This concern focuses on new infections, such as bovine spongiform encephalopathy (BSE), *E. coli* 0157, novel viruses, and perceived environmental hazards from the use of genetically modified plants and food. Yet this concern is out of proportion to the effects on health from these sources, compared to the impact of dietary imbalances, which account for at least 100-fold more premature deaths and considerably more ill health. About one-third of all premature deaths in Europe are diet related and many are preventable. The cost of this burden of ill health is in excess of that caused by tobacco use. Despite this, the budget in most European countries for health promotion is on average, less than 1 per cent of the total health budget.

Dietary links

Over 100 expert reports, produced throughout the world over the previous 20 years, have been in broad agreement about both the major chronic diseases threatening health and the dietary changes that are needed to reduce their incidence. The change in disease incidence over the last 40 years has made it increasingly clear that changing environmental factors, including diet, are involved in their aetiology. Although we are now discovering more about the role of genes in the susceptibility to disease, these are rarely the sole factor in its development and, at present, are believed to play a much less important role than other environmental factors, such as activity and diet. It is also unlikely that genetic changes or mutations would have produced such

major changes in a relatively short time span. The dietary trends seen around the world point to alterations in the balance of nutrients in the diet, which parallel, in most countries, the changes in disease incidence. Inevitably, there are exceptions that need explanation. In some cases, a satisfactory explanation can be proposed; in others it awaits further research. Additional dietary concerns are also emerging, as our understanding of disease increases. Table 18.1 shows some of the proposed linkages between chronic disease and dietary factors.

Specific nutritional problems are also important. Anaemia is increasingly recognized as a problem among the female population, affecting adolescent girls in particular. Consumption of foods with low bioavailability of iron contributes to this problem, and can result in reduced physical performance and lowered cognitive function. In addition, where it exists in pregnant women, poor iron transfer to the fetus will impact on its early development.

The increasing number of older adults results in a higher prevalence of low vitamin D status. This appears to be associated with low sunshine exposure, even in Southern European countries. Bone pain, difficulty in walking and accelerated bone demineralization may all occur.

In Europe, there is still a problem with iodine deficiency, affecting populations in the central parts of the landmass and in mountainous regions. The use of iodized salt is an important public health measure but education about its need is required. The consequences for maternal health and, in particular, the normal development of the fetus are profound, if deficiency exists.

Lifestyle and social factors

In addition, other aspects of lifestyle are important. There is convincing evidence that physical activity is an essential component of health and interacts with dietary aspects in a number of ways including:
- activity increases energy expenditure and is, therefore, crucial for the maintenance of energy balance and normal weight;
- activity increases physical fitness and the sense of well-being, and may be important

TABLE 18.1	Summary of chronic diseases and other health problems with possible dietary links	
Disease	**Dietary excess**	**Dietary lack**
Heart disease	Saturated fats	Antioxidant nutrients
	Total fats	*n*-3 fatty acids
	Trans fatty acids	Dietary fibre
		Folate
Hypertension	Salt	Calcium
	?Total fat	Potassium
	Alcohol	
Diabetes (Type 2)	Energy intake (via obesity)	
Cancers	Total fat/energy	Antioxidant nutrients
	?Meat	Fruit and vegetables
	?Salt	Dietary fibre
		?Dairy products
Gallstones	Energy intake (link via obesity)	Dietary fibre
Osteoporosis	?Salt	Calcium
	?Animal protein	?Vitamin D
		Fruit and vegetables
Dental disease	Sugar	Fluoride
		Dietary fibre
Arthritis	Total energy (linked to obesity)	
Liver cirrhosis	Alcohol	?General dietary deficiency
Dementia		?Folate
		?Vitamin C

in the control of blood pressure, prevention of colon cancer, regulation of blood glucose levels and lowering of blood lipid level;

■ weight-bearing activity maintains bone health and limits demineralization of bone in later life;

■ activity helps to maintain muscle mass and sense of balance, which is important with increasing age to preserve independence and prevent falls.

The most prevailing social factor that impacts on diet and health is that of poverty. This has increased substantially throughout Europe in the last two decades, as a result of rising unemployment, more insecure and low-paid work, and pressures experienced by governments in providing social security. All the evidence shows that the health experience of these groups is worse than in the better off, with an average of 5 years lower life expectancy. This is attributable to many factors, including dietary choices, lack of physical activity, access to shops and leisure facilities, stressful life experiences and an increased burden of illness. Many dietary goals have now recognized the need to address such social inequalities.

On the basis of existing evidence, the EURODIET team has put forward population goals for nutrients, some foods and lifestyle features, consistent with the prevention of major public health problems. These are based on a review of the scientific literature and represent the consensus view. These population goals are intended to form the basis for food-based dietary guidelines to be developed, or that have already been developed within individual countries, which reflect the national diet. The population goals for Europe are shown in Table 18.2.

There has been debate about who should be the target population for dietary goals. Those

TABLE 18.2 Population goals for nutrients, foods and lifestyle factors, consistent with the prevention of major public health problems in Europe (Eurodiet Core Report, 2001)

Component	Population goal	Background information
Physical activity level (PAL)	PAL >1.75	Maintenance of energy balance and cardiovascular health
Adult body weight	Body mass index (BMI) 21–22	An optimal individual BMI may be 20, and Asians may be susceptible to weight-related diseases above BMI 23–24
Dietary fat (% energy)	<30%	The goal is for the prevention of overweight. Higher fat intakes up to 35% may be consumed with high levels of physical activity
Fatty acids (% energy)		These intakes are recommended in relation to blood lipid levels. Stearic acid has little effect on these. A lower ratio of *n*-6:*n*-3 acids than at present is recommended
Saturated	<10%	
Trans	<2%	
MUFAs	10–15%	
n-6 PUFAs	4–8%	
n-3 PUFAs	2 g linolenic 200 mg very long chain	
Alcohol (where consumed) g/day	24–36 (men) 12–24 (women)	The lower values are optimum
Carbohydrates (% energy)	>55%	Rich in non-starch polysaccharides and of low glycaemic index
Dietary fibre (g/day)	>25 (or 3 g/MJ)	Based on Southgate method of analysis
Sugary foods (occasions/day)	<4	To reduce the risk of dental decay; frequency of consumption is a major factor. Important for lifelong oral health
Fruit and vegetables (g/day)	>400	These have many health-promoting properties, including non-nutritional components
Folate from food (μg/day)	>400	Bioavailability from food is only 50% of that of folic acid; needed for pregnancy and for normal homocysteine levels
Sodium (as sodium chloride; g/day)	<6	Population benefits are greater than those obtained if only hypertensive subjects adopt the guideline
Iodine (μg/day)	150	Essential for normal development
Exclusive breastfeeding	About 6 months	Promotes immunological responses, lower risk of infection and atopic disease, reduced risk of breast cancer in mother

MUFAs, monounsaturated fatty acids; PUFA, polyunsaturated fatty acids.

individuals with most risk factors and the most severe risk factors will be in greatest need of intervention. However, they represent only a small proportion of the total population and, therefore, reducing their risk will make little impact on overall population morbidity and mortality. On the other hand, the majority of the population will have moderate levels of risk. Improvement in these risk factors will have less success on an individual basis (because the

Activity 18.1

What common themes are apparent in Table 18.1 that could form the basis for coordinated dietary advice?

If you were presented with this group of suggested links between diet and disease, what specific dietary changes might you recommend?

Check these with the targets suggested in Table 18.2.

original risk is less) but, taken for the population as a whole, will amount to a greater reduction in the population's risk of morbidity and mortality.

Hence, many strategies, such as the European goals shown here, are now targeted at the whole population, because this will bring the greatest reduction in risk. It also provides more social support for changes in dietary patterns. This does not, however, exclude an additional policy directed at those most at risk, with more intensive and specific targeting at this group. Of course, before this can happen, the problem of identifying those with greatest risk must be overcome!

From goals to guidelines

In order to achieve the population goals, practical advice must be developed. It is recognized that across Europe there are different dietary patterns, so national guidelines must take into account the existing culturally determined diet. Of course, there are many differences between intakes of individuals within any one country and these can provide an opportunity to study which existing dietary pattern comes closer to the desirable goals. In recent years, dietary guidelines have moved from being nutrient based to being food based (see Chapter 3). In other words, instead of recommending that consumers 'eat more fibre' and 'eat less fat', foods that contain these nutrients are used in the recommendations. Clearly, this is easier for the consumer to understand, as it coincides with how we buy and select our daily food.

Many countries are now publishing food-based guidelines, with the emphasis on foods and the numbers of servings to be eaten; these can

also be used to develop advice for populations at higher risk, such as those produced by the American Heart Association in 2000. These recommend the inclusion of fruits and vegetables, whole grains, low-fat dairy products, legumes, fish and low-fat meats. Achieving and maintaining a healthy body weight through physical activity is included as a guideline.

Several stages have been identified in compiling food-based dietary guidelines. These include identification of:

- the major food sources of the nutrients recommended (e.g. from tables of food composition);
- the foods contributing substantially to the intake of the population (e.g. from national food surveys);
- existing food patterns that show differing levels of intake of key nutrients (e.g. from individual dietary intakes studies);
- key foods that explain the major variation in intakes of specific nutrients in the diets of high and low consumers.

With this information, it should be possible to identify the most important foods or eating patterns that could be targeted for change in order to move all dietary intakes towards achievement of a dietary goal. If this can be done for several key nutrients or foods, then many goals can be achieved. Guidelines can be formulated to include choice of products, menu planning, portions and frequencies of eating that have a sound basis within the target population. A further strategy may be to change the supply of food, by modifications to existing products (e.g. lowering the fat content, fortifying with a nutrient) or introducing new products.

Consideration of the population goals suggests some common themes. Reduction of fat intake and attention to the balance of fats with a reduction of saturated fat, and attention to polyunsaturated fats, especially those of the n-3 family addresses a number of health issues. The reduction in energy intake that will ensue may be beneficial for weight loss but, in many people, it will have to be counterbalanced by an increase in other energy sources. Most appropriate is an increase in complex carbohydrates from cereals, grains, pulses, roots, vegetables and fruits. These will provide not only starch, but also intrinsic sugars, dietary fibre and a wide range of micronutrients. Among these will be folate, the antioxidant nutrients and other non-nutritional factors, such as the phytonutrients, which are considered to be important as protective factors (see Chapter 17). A shift in the diet to fewer, or at least lower-fat animal products may also occur as fat intakes are reduced.

Thus, a series of nutrient goals may be achieved by the same changes in the diet. In theory, this should make the giving of dietary advice more straightforward, as the basis of a 'healthy diet' will apply whatever the client's needs. Clearly, there will be differences in emphasis, for example, if weight needs to be lost, or if the appetite is small, as in older sedentary people or in young children.

In Britain, the Nutrition Task Force devised the National Food Guide (the Balance of Good Health), which has been adopted throughout many areas of nutrition education as the basic framework for achieving the nutrient goals (see Chapter 3).

The role of the Nutrition Task Force cannot, however, be viewed in isolation. It was part of an overall strategy, emanating from the 'Health of the nation' paper, which has involved many in the move towards actually 'adding years to life' and 'life to years'. Since its publication, public health initiatives related to nutrition have remained on the political agenda. The Department of Health has recognized the importance of nutrition in a series of National Service Framework documents, published since 2000. These indicate the standards of service and care in relation to coronary heart disease, mental health, older people and diabetes, and, in each case, include a role for nutrition. Most recently, the Food Standards Agency (FSA), created in 2000, has become responsible for the public's health and consumer interests in relation to food. One of the key aims is to secure long-term improvements in the health of the population by working to reduce diet-related ill health, within the UK Strategic Framework for Nutrition. The main elements of this are:

- securing a sound evidence base for action to promote a healthy diet;

- developing appropriate means of informing the general population;
- identifying and addressing barriers to changing dietary behaviour;
- evaluating and monitoring the effectiveness of action taken.

This framework is intended to form the basis for developing realistic and effective programmes for the future.

It is possible to illustrate how this might work by considering the Nutrition Strategy developed by the Food Standards Agency Wales. The strategy aims to improve the diet of all the people in Wales, but certain groups have been prioritised, owing to their poor diet and health, and, therefore, have the greatest potential gain from improved nutrition.

The top priority groups were identified as infants, children and young people, and socially disadvantaged and vulnerable groups. The second priority groups were women of child-bearing age, especially pregnant women, and men, especially middle aged men.

The main recommendations include:

- increase the uptake of a healthy balanced diet to meet recommended levels for nutrients and micronutrients;
- increase fruit and vegetable intake;
- develop and manage initiatives to prevent and manage obesity and overweight;
- ensure that schemes and policies are in place to assist improvement in healthy eating;
- provide information and training to key players;
- ensure that the public is well informed about the need for dietary improvement;
- ensure that local initiatives are in place to tackle the main barriers to improving nutrition;
- develop and promote initiatives with the food industry to improve healthy eating, especially relating to access to specific foods;
- evaluate the impact of activities resulting from the strategy.

Key players in delivering the strategy will include policy and decision-makers, health, nutrition and catering professionals, practitioners and educators at national and local levels, and the food production and the retail industry.

Recruiting and training volunteers to become involved with local projects is important. The approach is, therefore, multi-dimensional and flexible, and able to focus on specific targets and develop local initiatives suited to the needs of particular communities. Settings for the interventions can be very diverse. They may include schools, workplaces, health care locations, the commercial sector (e.g. supermarkets), local clubs or day centres, or even street markets.

A systematic review of interventions to promote healthy eating in the general population has shown that the most effective appear to:
- adopt an integrated, multidisciplinary comprehensive approach;
- involve a complementary range of actions;
- work at individual, community, environmental and policy levels.

Information provided by itself is insufficient to produce change. Thus, any attempt to implement food-based dietary guidelines needs to learn from previous work and adopt the lessons from other interventions. In so doing the difficult challenge of changing diets to improve health will make progress.

WHAT IS HEALTH PROMOTION?

The above discussion illustrates some of the principles of health promotion, these will now be considered in their own right.

The Ottawa Charter for health promotion, developed by the WHO (1986) outlines an approach to health promotion that includes:
- building healthy public policies;
- creating supportive environments;
- developing the personal skills of the public and practitioners;
- re-orienting health services;
- strengthening community action.

It, therefore, demonstrates that health promotion involves more than just providing people with knowledge about the functions of the body and ways of preventing illness, and thus helps them to maintain well-being. This part of the process can be better described as health education, or if it is carried out in the nutritional context, then it is nutrition education.

Nutrition education, in turn, has been described as the process that assists the public in applying knowledge from nutrition science, and the relationship between diet and health to their food practices. Having the knowledge, however, is insufficient in itself to effect change. This can be witnessed all around us most vividly in the context of smoking. Almost everyone knows that smoking is injurious to health, yet a substantial proportion of the population continues to smoke. For knowledge to be translated into action, the environment must be supportive of the change and thereby enable it to happen. This includes the political context, the social environment and the individual's personal environment. In addition, the person making the change must have the desire and the belief that this is achievable, by the means available to them.

Thus, health promotion must be seen in a wide context. It includes:
- having in existence the political and community structures that can make health-promoting changes possible;
- providing the information about health-promoting measures to all interested and involved parties;
- developing in the individual the desire to want to change towards a healthier set of practices;
- showing the individual that they have the ability to do this.

Briefly, health promotion has been described as 'making healthier choices the easier choices'.

In the context of nutritional improvements, the introduction of nutritional goals is accepted as the responsibility of governments in most countries of the world. This was not always so. The first advice formulated about reducing fat intakes for the prevention of coronary heart disease was developed by the American Heart Association. This government-led approach had been perceived by some as unwarranted interference by the State in food intake, which is a purely personal matter. Nevertheless, without appropriate support from the government in establishing food production policies and legislation, for example, for clear nutritional labelling, the consumer is left without adequate information to make a choice.

Activity 18.2

Applying this in the nutrition context, the nutritionist or dietitian wants people to adopt healthier eating practices. Ways must be found to make these 'the easier choices'.

- Who will need to be involved? Think of all the parties concerned in the food production chain.
- What does the consumer need to know about the healthier choice?
- How will the consumer be convinced to try this out?
- What might the obstacles be and how can they be tackled?

In working through this activity, you should find yourself referring back to the key points made above about health promotion.

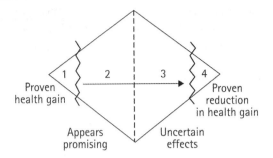

Figure 18.1 The health gain rhomboid.

Health promotion incorporates a number of related phases:

- planning;
- intervention;
- evaluation.

Planning

This is arguably the most important stage and can determine the success or failure of the programme. Most importantly, the issue that is to be addressed must be identified. In coming to this decision, the planners balance the perceived needs with the possible benefits. This may be illustrated in the form of the 'health gain rhomboid' (shown in Figure 18.1). At the two extremes, there are very few interventions that have been assessed and shown definitely to provide health gain, or to diminish it (i.e. at 1 or 4, respectively). Interventions classified as 2 would generally be considered worthwhile, but there may be an equal number at 3 that have not been fully evaluated and whose benefits to health promotion are uncertain. Where decisions have to be taken about the use of a finite amount of resources, most planners will chose interventions in the area 2, rather than 3.

A further element of the planning process is to identify the target group, since particular interventions may be more appropriate and relevant to certain groups. This type of planning and consultation was undertaken in the preparation of the 'Health of the nation' paper. During this period, a very large number of possible goals and targets were discussed, with supporters of each putting forward strong arguments. Eventually, only a small number of goals were identified, although these were chosen because they were believed to be the most appropriate to achieve the maximum health gain. This has also been described in the case of the Food Standards Agency Wales Nutrition Strategy.

A further aspect of planning includes taking account of the nature of the problem, for example, by collecting data about morbidity and mortality statistics. Perhaps also at this stage it is important to consider the lifestyle aspects of the target community. When this is being done at national level, the variation among communities within the country makes this more difficult.

Finally, general aims and specific objectives are formulated, taking into account the nature of the existing problem and the potential change expected. This, in turn, depends on existing knowledge, attitudes and behaviours of the target group. A very important consideration is the readiness to change on the part of the target. This has been studied extensively and a model developed that shows change as a process comprising several stages (Table 18.3). It will be necessary to consider what aspects of the programme will facilitate people moving from one stage to the next in the change process.

In the UK, the information about food intakes is available from National Food Survey data and from National Dietary and Nutrition Survey data.

TABLE 18.3	Model for stages of change
Stage of change	**Associated behaviour**
Pre-contemplation	Not considering any change or need for change
Contemplation	Thinking about changing, but not yet prepared to start the process
Preparation	When the change seems possible and benefits are perceived, ready to change
Action	Actually doing things differently. May need much support and reassurance; may slip back to earlier stages
Maintenance	New behaviour becomes part of the healthier lifestyle

Adapted from Prochaska et al., 1992.

Intervention

An obvious but important element of this stage of the process is the decision on the methodology to be used. This should take into account information about previous uses of this methodology and their level of success. Constraints that might exist must be taken into account. For example, if the promotional material is presented in a written form, this necessitates that the target group can, and wants to, read. Computer-based images may be more appealing to young people than the written word. Thus, the methodology must be flexible and adaptable to meet the objectives with all of the targets.

The FSA Wales is employing a variety of interventions. Breakfast clubs have been set up in some schools, which can provide a healthy start to the day and encourage children to interact. Nutrition and health education activities in the workplace are increasing awareness of the links between diet and cancer in middle-aged men. Midwives working with vulnerable groups are teaching about meal planning and budgeting to reduce the numbers of low birthweight babies. Local grocers are involved in delivering fruit to schools as part of a school tuck shop scheme. Fitness training in a local club for young people is being linked with some nutrition education as well as smoking, drugs and alcohol education.

Evaluation

The process of health promotion may be seen as cyclic. The evaluation of one programme may generate questions and proposals for an improved programme, which can start with another planning stage. No programme can be brought to a conclusion without evaluating what it has achieved. In the case of health promotion, changes in some of the measures that were used at the planning stages may be indicative of success. These may include morbidity data, measures of quality of life or, in the case of nutrition programmes, changes in patterns of food purchasing. On the other hand, outcomes may be programmes and policies that need to be taken up in subsequent interventions. In its 'Eat well II' report, the Department of Health (1996) published an evaluation of the first 2 years of operation of the Nutrition Task Force initiatives. Follow-on initiatives have since been introduced, so the original outcomes have been superseded by new interventions.

The FSA Wales Nutrition Strategy is aiming for some quantitative outcomes, for example, in terms of knowledge about portions and increased consumption of fruit and vegetables in priority groups, as well as a balance of the diet closer to recommendations by 2010.

The national progress towards a healthier diet in the UK is more difficult to follow. However, there are indications that intakes of fat are falling, although rates of obesity are increasing. Intake of fruit has increased, although vegetable intakes are static. There is increased knowledge about recommendations to increase fruit and vegetable intake and reduce intakes of fat. Yet, generally food intake patterns remain resistant to change. Many studies demonstrate that people are not making changes for a number of reasons. These include:

- confusion over the message (e.g. what is a portion);
- perception that the messages are frequently changing and the professionals cannot agree;

- belief that the subject's diet is already healthy, so the messages do not apply to them;
- inadequate/incorrect knowledge about which foods contain particular nutrients;
- concern that healthy food is unappealing;
- perceptions about the cost of healthy food;
- beliefs about the availability of healthy foods, both in local shops and in catering venues;
- lack of interest.

For all of these reasons, progress is inevitably slower than nutritionists and other health professionals would like it to be. However, if goals are made specific, measurable, achievable and realistic, then after a set time some progress is generally found to have occurred. It is important to recognize that such small steps will eventually add up to more substantial change. Trends in the incidence of chronic disease will take longer to become apparent. Evaluation is, therefore, essential to ensure that all changes are recorded and lessons learned from them.

HEALTH-PROMOTION INITIATIVES AND THE INDIVIDUAL

Most individual consumers may know little about national initiatives and are dependent on changes in their own immediate environment to provide them with opportunities to improve their nutrition. This section will consider what difference health-promotion initiatives might make to the individual.

Information and education

The National Food Guide continues to be published as *The balance of good health* (FSA, 2001). It is an example of food-based dietary guidelines and, as such, should be readily understood by consumers. It is used widely by retailers and health professionals, and has been adapted for use with groups, such as ethnic minority groups and diabetics.

Past advice had tended to focus on single nutrients. Thus, consumers heard the message that they should 'eat more fibre', for example. They follow this advice by buying wholemeal bread and eating a wholegrain breakfast cereal, but continue as before with their previous diet.

This may still be high in fat, low in fruit and vegetables, high in salt, or even all of these, but the consumer may believe that he/she is now eating 'a healthy diet'.

This focus on single nutrients has also led to an enormous increase in consumption of supplements, with up to 30 per cent of some groups in the population taking supplements regularly. This again reflects the message about 'antioxidant nutrients', which are being consumed in tablet form rather than by amending the diet. It is possible that it is the chemical substances found alongside these antioxidants that may actually be the biologically important agents.

The balance of good health moves away from this approach and provides a whole diet picture. It can be used in many ways, both as an educational tool in settings ranging from schools to antenatal clinics, a meal-planning guide or even a shopping list; and provides a non-verbal illustration of the balanced diet, which can be very useful in allowing each person to understand the guide in their own way.

Although we are exposed to many messages about nutrition and health throughout the week, some are more likely to persuade us than others. The effectiveness of a message is determined by the wording. Messages need to be:
- reasonable (we should understand the message, and the reason for it);
- practical (we should find the change possible); and
- compelling (we should want to do it).

We are more likely to be influenced by messages that fit in with existing belief systems, rather than those which seem alien to us. In devising messages, the health promoter must be sure that he or she understands the belief systems of the target group, so the messages will be understood and acted on. A common failing is that health promoters make assumptions about their target group's level of understanding; this can lead to misunderstanding of the message.

Schools

A network of 'School Nutrition Action Groups' has been set up as school-based healthy alliances between schoolchildren, staff and caterers, together with a community dietitian. These groups aim to develop a health-promoting environment in the school, establishing, monitoring and evaluating a consistent food policy with health as the main objective, and providing healthy options on the school menu, at lunchtime and for snacks. It allows pupils, caterers and teachers to have involvement and ownership of school meals provision. The existence of good examples of healthy food aims to serve as an educational model. There is now more teaching of food and nutrition in schools, and computer-based packages to facilitate this have been produced by the British Nutrition Foundation. The introduction of new guidelines on school meals in 2001 should help to integrate the educational and food-based messages.

The NHS and health professionals

It is recognized that the majority of people will turn to members of the primary health care team if they want specific nutritional advice. However, many studies have indicated that doctors may be uncertain about nutritional advice and, although they appreciate that it is important, often have not included nutrition in a consultation. This may be influenced by a number of factors, including lack of time, inadequate teaching materials, low confidence and patient non-compliance. The practice nurse in the primary health care setting is more likely to provide nutritional advice and may have more time to do so. The importance of training in nutrition for many groups of health professionals is now widely recognized and included in the curriculum. A recent report by the Royal College of Physicians (2002) confirmed that nutrition of patients was a doctor's responsibility and should be supported by appropriate training in nutrition. A study of nutrition intervention in primary care (Moore and Adamson, 2002) found that there were good levels of nutritional knowledge among members of the primary care team. Diet was discussed with a proportion of patients, although practical aspects of food were not well covered. There is thus evidence of progress in widening the availability of nutritional information to patients. Multi-disciplinary nutrition teams have been established in many hospitals to ensure adequate feeding of at-risk patients in this setting.

Media/advertising

A major source of information for the lay person is the media and advertising. Because the most eye-catching news items are the ones that aim to surprise or shock, it is the sensational aspects of nutrition that tend to reach prominence in the media. An expert opinion, which apparently disagrees with the accepted viewpoint, becomes newsworthy and is published in the press. Where a number of experts have agreed, however, this is often not considered important and so receives no publicity. Thus, the overall impression given is that 'experts' always contradict one another, and there is no point in following any advice, as it is inevitably contradicted within the next few months. Regrettably, this is believed by many and frequently cited as the reason for not following any dietary advice. Information from professionally accredited nutritionists and state registered dietitians is sound and based on scientific evidence. Unfortunately, a proportion of the information provided by the media is not.

The food chain

The food industry is in a very powerful position to determine the nutritional quality of the diet consumed. It is, therefore, essential that health promoters work with the industry. The potential for the development of modified products or new products with a healthier nutritional profile is there, and whether they appear on the supermarket shelves depends on the manufacturers.

In the UK in recent years, there has been a huge growth in the consumption of ready-made and convenience food products, and, therefore, a great responsibility rests with the food industry with respect to these. The provision of comprehensive nutritional labelling can help the consumer decide whether products are healthy or not. Eating a diet containing many pre-prepared meals makes it difficult to achieve the holistic view of the diet, as many complete dishes span various segments of the Balance of Good Health, and make it impossible to gauge exactly how much of each component has been eaten. It is probably easier to achieve the balanced diet using more basic foods than predominantly composite dishes. Unfortunately, many people have little time and/or perhaps ability to do this, and may resort to eating a largely pre-prepared diet. There is evidence that cooking skills are gradually declining in parallel with the more hectic lifestyle and the use of ready meals. This highlights the importance of the food industry in making sure that this type of diet is balanced and healthy. A further challenge for the food industry is to respond to the drive for an increase in fruit and vegetable intake. Traditionally, there has been very little profit margin for the sale of fruit and vegetables, as minimal processing is required. However, if public health is to be improved and the food industry is to be involved, new and more creative ways of promoting plant-based foods will need to be developed.

Catering outlets also have a great responsibility, as over one-third of the meals now consumed in the UK are eaten away from home. Guidelines on healthy catering practice for hospitals, restaurants, fast-food outlets and in the workplace are available, with awards for good practice. Recommendations for the training of caterers have been drawn up. These initiatives should make it easier for consumers to be able to choose healthy eating in all outside venues, although, in practice, this is not always the case.

Constraints

Change is difficult for most people. Even if the health promotion is well designed and appropriately targeted, there may be some for whom it is not appropriate or for whom it is not possible to change. Some groups that are more difficult to reach by health-promotion programmes are:

- those on a low income;
- the elderly;
- people in minority ethnic groups;
- single men;
- children – who need specifically focused programmes.

A targeted policy

It is useful to consider a more targeted policy as an illustration of how the process described above can be applied within a more specific health promotion context. The Folic Acid Campaign in the UK, initially commissioned by the Department of Health in 1995, is an example of a policy that was specifically targeted (see Figure 18.2).

The planning stage reviewed the evidence in the literature that the estimated risk of neural tube defects (NTDs) was progressively reduced with an increasing dose of folic acid intake, and that supplementation with folic acid would significantly impact on the risk of NTD in the population. A daily dose of 400 μg folic acid was indicated as appropriate to achieve a reduction in NTD incidence of at least 50 per cent. The primary target group for the campaign were women intending to become pregnant and the aim was to reduce the incidence of NTDs, such as spina bifida, in their offspring. However, since almost half of the conceptions in the UK are reported to be unplanned, the target audience was initially expanded to all women of child-bearing age, and later to young people, as future parents. It was thus intended that, as an outcome, all women would gain an awareness of the importance of folic acid supplementation.

The intervention stage of the campaign was designed to increase the baseline intake of folate from foods, as well as promote the use of folic acid supplements at the appropriate time before conception and during early pregnancy. This entailed developing cooperative partnerships with food producers and the commercial sector to increase the availability of fortified products, as well as an increased range of appropriate supplements in order to increase access to the vitamin in shops. The increased demand was to come as a result of dissemination of the message about the importance of folate, by health professionals, teachers and journalists. Manufacturers of pregnancy testing kits were also involved at this stage. Many diverse strategies were used to disseminate the message about folate. These included leaflets and posters, a new labelling symbol for foods fortified with folic acid, promotion of fortified products by advertising, and development of teaching packs for use in schools.

The campaign finished in 1998, although many elements of the promotion of folic acid remain in place as part of health promotion. Initial evaluation results indicated an increase in

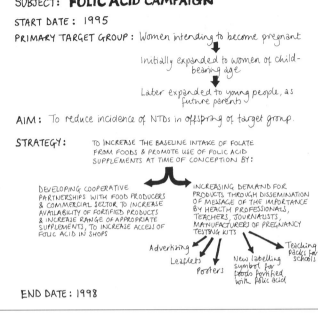

CASE STUDY REPORT

SUBJECT: **FOLIC ACID CAMPAIGN**

START DATE: 1995

PRIMARY TARGET GROUP: Women intending to become pregnant

↓

Initially expanded to women of child-bearing age

↓

Later expanded to young people, as future parents

AIM: To reduce incidence of NTDs in offspring of target group.

STRATEGY: TO INCREASE THE BASELINE INTAKE OF FOLATE FROM FOODS & PROMOTE USE OF FOLIC ACID SUPPLEMENTS AT TIME OF CONCEPTION BY:

DEVELOPING COOPERATIVE PARTNERSHIPS WITH FOOD PRODUCERS & COMMERCIAL SECTOR TO INCREASE AVAILABILITY OF FORTIFIED PRODUCTS & INCREASE RANGE OF APPROPRIATE SUPPLEMENTS, TO INCREASE ACCESS OF FOLIC ACID IN SHOPS

INCREASING DEMAND FOR PRODUCTS THROUGH DISSEMINATION OF MESSAGE OF THE IMPORTANCE BY HEALTH PROFESSIONALS, TEACHERS, JOURNALISTS, MANUFACTURERS OF PREGNANCY TESTING KITS

Advertising
Leaflets
Posters
New labelling symbol for foods fortified with folic acid
Teaching packs for schools

END DATE: 1998

Figure 18.2 The folic acid campaign. NTDs, neural tube defects.

awareness about the issue among women, wider availability of folic acid supplements and fortified products, and an increased usage of folic acid supplements. However, women whose pregnancies are unplanned remain at risk as a result of low uptake of folic acid at the critical time around conception. The campaign can thus be viewed as only partly successful and demonstrates that the challenge of achieving change, with a simple supplement and at a highly vulnerable time of life, is enormous.

ECONOMICS OF HEALTH PROMOTION

It is generally assumed that health promotion is inexpensive and will reduce health care costs. Thus, many see health promotion as a way of saving money. However, although it is possible that money may be saved through health promotion, this cannot be the primary objective. Health promotion involves various cost inputs, most obviously in the form of resources, such as health professionals, their time and materials. There generally needs to be an input in the form

of government action whether through legislation or financial 'pump priming'. In addition, better health is also achieved by efforts on the part of individuals, which are more difficult to evaluate economically.

To evaluate the cost–benefit of health promotion, it is necessary to identify what is gained as a result of the programme and what has been forgone by diverting these resources from elsewhere (see Figure 18.3).

Because the outcomes of nutritional health promotion are often difficult to measure, decisions of this nature are rarely straightforward. Various measures of health gain may need to be used that show incremental advantages, rather than simply the ultimate goal of reducing chronic disease incidence. Balanced against this are the costs of treating these diseases and the loss of earnings that chronic disease can cause. Each case may need to be evaluated separately and on its merits. However, the more information is provided about nutrition and health and the more that people can be empowered to make their own choices in an informed way, the greater will be the potential benefit for health.

A health economist might wish to compare the costs (C) of a programme to reduce obesity, against the potential saving in the treatment of diabetes (D) associated with obesity. If C is greater than D, then clearly the programme would appear not to be cost effective as it stands. However, if one also could show that reducing obesity would cause a potential saving in treatment for arthritis and hypertension (A + H), it is now possible that the combined savings (D + A + H) could be greater than the cost C. In this way, a multiple benefit can make the programme cost effective.

Figure 18.3 Economics of health promotion.

SUMMARY

1 Nutrition plays an important part in the causation of chronic disease. It is, therefore, essential that dietary change is introduced to reverse the high prevalence of some diseases.
2 Guidelines have been established by various national and international bodies that propose change.
3 The consensus on change recommends reductions in fat, increases in starchy carbohydrates, fruits and vegetables.
4 Health promotion can facilitate change.
5 Health promotion involves partnerships between the various players in the food system and the citizen, in a process of education and empowerment.

STUDY QUESTIONS

1 Improving health involves more than just an awareness of dietary guidelines. What other aspects of life must be considered and changed to make dietary improvements possible?
2 List the major participants in the food chain and indicate how you think each could be involved in promoting healthier eating.
3 Discuss with colleagues:
  a Where they have obtained information about healthy eating (if at all)?
  b Have they understood the information?
  c Have they acted on the information? If not, why?
4 Do you believe that nutrition information available generally to the public is adequate and/or an appropriate way of producing changes in the diet?
5 Survey newspaper articles describing nutritional issues over a period of 3–4 weeks. Try to look at a 'popular' newspaper and one which is considered to be of higher 'quality'.
  a Are issues handled differently and, if so, in what way?
  b Do you find either of the article types more credible?
  c As a result of reading the articles are you encouraged to change your diet?
  d What can you conclude from this investigation?

REFERENCES AND FURTHER READING

DoH (UK Department of Health) 1994: *Eat well!* An action plan from the Nutrition Task Force to achieve the Health of the Nation targets on diet and nutrition. Wetherby: Department of Health.

DoH (Department of Health) 1996: *Eat well II.* A progress report from the Nutrition Task Force on the action plan to achieve the Health of the Nation targets on diet and nutrition. Wetherby: Department of Health.

DoH (Department of Health) 2000: *Folic acid and the prevention of disease.* Report on Health and Social Subjects 50. London: The Stationery Office.

Eurodiet core report 2001: Nutrition and diet for healthy lifestyles in Europe: science and policy implications. *Public Health Nutrition* **4**(2A), 265–73.

Eurodiet Working Party 2. 2001: A framework for food-based dietary guidelines in the European Union. *Public Health Nutrition* **4**(2A), 293–305.

Food and Agriculture Organisation/World Health Organisation (FAO/WHO) 1998: *Preparation and use of food-based dietary guidelines.* Geneva: WHO.

Food Standards Agency 2001: *The balance of good health.* London: FSA.

Food Standards Agency Wales 2002: *Nutrition Strategy for Wales*, Consultation Document. London: FSA.

Gillespie, A.H., Shafer, L. 1990: American Dietetic Association position paper on nutrition education for the public. *Journal of the American Dietetic Association* **90**, 107–10.

Gregory, J., Foster, K., Tyler, H., Wiseman, M. 1990: *The dietary and nutritional survey of British adults.* London: HMSO.

HEA (Health Education Authortiy) 1994: *Introducing the National Food Guide: The balance of good health.* Information for educators and communicators. London: HEA.

Jackson, A.A. 2001: Human nutrition in medical practice: the training of doctors. *Proceedings of the Nutrition Society* **60**(2), 257–63.

James, W.P.T. 1988: *Healthy nutrition: preventing nutrition-related diseases in Europe.* WHO Regional Publications, European Series, No. 24. Copenhagen: WHO Regional Office for Europe.

Margetts, B.M., Thompson, R.L., Speller, V. et al. 1998: Factors which influence 'healthy' eating patterns: results from the 1993 HEA health and lifestyle survey in England. *Public Health Nutrition* **1**(3), 193–8.

Moore, H., Adamson, A.J. 2002: Nutrition interventions by primary care staff: a survey of involvement, knowledge and attitude. *Public Health Nutrition* **5**(4), 531–6.

Posner, B.M., Franz, M., Quatromoni, P. and the INTERHEALTH Steering Committee 1994: Nutrition and the global risk for chronic diseases: the INTERHEALTH Nutrition Initiative. *Nutrition Reviews* **52**(6), 201–7.

Prochaska, J.O., DiClemente, C.C., Norcross, J.C. 1992: In search of how people change. *American Psychologist* **47**, 1102–14.

Roe, L., Hunt, P., Bradshaw, H. et al. 1997: *Health promotion interventions to promote healthy eating in the general population – a review.* London: Health Education Authority.

Royal College of Physicians 2002: *Nutrition and patients: a doctor's responsibility.* London: Royal College of Physicians.

World Health Organization 1986: *The Ottawa Charter: principles for health promotion.* Copenhagen: WHO Regional Office for Europe.

World Health Organization 1990: *Diet nutrition and the prevention of chronic diseases.* WHO Technical Report No. 797. Geneva: WHO.

INDEX